AF812383

Minimally Invasive Surgery Trauma

Marcus Cezillo • Bruno Monteiro Pereira
Editors

Minimally Invasive Surgery Trauma

Laparoscopic and Robotic Approach

Springer

Editors
Marcus Cezillo, MD, MSc
Trauma Surgery Department
Hospital de Base do Distrito Federal
Brasília, DF, Brazil

Bruno Monteiro Pereira, MD, MSc, PhD
University of Vassouras, Surgical Group®
President, Campinas Brazil. World Society of
the Abdominal Compartment Past-President,
Campinas, Brazil

ISBN 978-3-032-28970-4 ISBN 978-3-032-28971-1 (eBook)
https://doi.org/10.1007/978-3-032-28971-1

© The Editor(s) (if applicable) and The Author(s), under exclusive license to Springer Nature Switzerland AG 2026, corrected publication 2026

This work is subject to copyright. All rights are solely and exclusively licensed by the Publisher, whether the whole or part of the material is concerned, specifically the rights of translation, reprinting, reuse of illustrations, recitation, broadcasting, reproduction on microfilms or in any other physical way, and transmission or information storage and retrieval, electronic adaptation, computer software, or by similar or dissimilar methodology now known or hereafter developed.
The use of general descriptive names, registered names, trademarks, service marks, etc. in this publication does not imply, even in the absence of a specific statement, that such names are exempt from the relevant protective laws and regulations and therefore free for general use.
The publisher, the authors and the editors are safe to assume that the advice and information in this book are believed to be true and accurate at the date of publication. Neither the publisher nor the authors or the editors give a warranty, expressed or implied, with respect to the material contained herein or for any errors or omissions that may have been made. The publisher remains neutral with regard to jurisdictional claims in published maps and institutional affiliations.

This Springer imprint is published by the registered company Springer Nature Switzerland AG
The registered company address is: Gewerbestrasse 11, 6330 Cham, Switzerland

If disposing of this product, please recycle the paper.

Foreword

Laparoscopy and robotic-assisted surgery have emerged as powerful tools, transforming both diagnostic and therapeutic approaches in emergency general surgery. The approach in this text is to present practical information for the application of these minimally invasive techniques in trauma surgery. At first glance, this book may seem like another academic treatise on trauma laparoscopy. In fact, its purpose is different. The objective is to provide practical, step-by-step guidance; a collection of tips and detailed insights on how to effectively apply minimally invasive techniques in trauma surgery. The book is comprehensive, covering every conceivable scenario in trauma. The content is also extended to special populations and settings, including combat situations. This is an invaluable resource for all those providing operative care of the injured patient. Minimally invasive approaches are the future of trauma surgery.

Ernest E. Moore Shock Trauma Center
University of Colorado Denver,
Denver, CO, USA

Ernest E. Moore

Preface

The evolution of trauma care has long been a story of relentless innovation, fueled by the unwavering pursuit of better outcomes for critically injured patients. In elective surgery, the rise of minimally invasive techniques (MIT) has transformed clinical practice, largely due to their reproducibility, precision, and the controlled environment in which they are performed. However, trauma surgery presents an entirely different challenge—a broad spectrum of clinical scenarios marked by urgency, unpredictability, and a fragile physiological balance. For many trauma surgeons, these variables were seen as limitations that hindered the application of MIT in the acute setting. For others, they represented a powerful opportunity—an invitation to bring innovation and technology into one of the most demanding fields in surgery.

The integration of laparoscopy, thoracoscopy, and robotic surgery into the high-stakes environment of trauma has been a cautious but increasingly promising journey. Today, there is a growing recognition of the value that minimally invasive approaches can bring—not only in the acute phase of trauma, but also in the post-injury period, where patients benefit from less invasive re-interventions, reduced morbidity, and faster recovery. In stable trauma patients, robotic surgery represents a new frontier, with expanding indications and a strong potential for future growth, as highlighted throughout this book.

Despite growing interest, the literature in this field often lacks the practical, technical guidance that trauma surgeons truly need—a step-by-step approach that bridges the gap between theoretical knowledge and operative execution. This is the purpose of the *Minimally Invasive Surgery Trauma: Laparoscopic and Robotic Approach,* to standardize and adapt MIT across a wide range of trauma scenarios, breaking the barrier of the so-called irreproducible surgery. Our goal extends beyond basic reproducibility. We aim to empower trauma surgeons—from residents to seasoned practitioners—with the knowledge, tools, and confidence to incorporate advanced techniques into their daily practice.

In this book, we emphasize not just the *why*, but critically, the *how*. Each chapter takes the reader through a specific trauma condition, detailing patient selection, required equipment, procedural steps, technical nuances, and potential pitfalls. We address both the acute trauma setting and the post-traumatic period, providing comprehensive perspectives on when and how to safely introduce minimally invasive interventions. We also explore the essential role of teamwork, from preoperative planning to intraoperative coordination, recognizing that successful trauma care is always a team effort.

Robotic surgery, in particular, holds enormous promise for the future of trauma care in stable patients. Its precision, enhanced visualization, and ergonomic advantages make it a valuable tool for select cases, and its role is expected to grow significantly as technology becomes more accessible and surgeon experience increases.

This is more than a textbook—it is a practical manual and a must-read for anyone passionate about trauma surgery and committed to staying at the forefront of its evolution. Whether you're beginning your journey or refining your expertise. This collection of experiences offers a clear roadmap for integrating innovation into trauma care, one careful and evidence-based step at a time. We are proud to present the collective experience of an esteemed group of authors who share a vision for safer, smarter, and more effective trauma surgery.

Marcus Cezillo, MD, MSc
Bruno Monteiro Pereira, MD, MSc, PhD

Contents

Contributors

Sameh Abogabal Hull University Teaching Hospitals, Hull, UK

Syed Fouzaan Albeez Batterjee Medical College, Jeddah, Saudi Arabia

Natalia Karolina Alvarez Emergencies, Trauma and Critical Care Surgeon, Hospital Municipal de Urgencias, Córdoba, Argentina

Andres Aponte Department of General Surgery, Central Military Hospital, Bogotá, Colombia

Gabriel Lunardi Aranha InCor—Instituto do Coração do Hospital das Clínicas da FMUSP, São Paulo, SP, Brazil

Rodrigo Caselli Belém Hospital de Base do Distrito Federal (HBDF), Brasilia, DF, Brazil

Carlos Yánez Benítez Mediclinic Parkview Hospital, Dubai, UAE

Juan García Cardo Servicio de cirugia general, Unidad cirugia HBP y trasplantes, Hospital universitario Marques de valdecilla, Santander España, Spain

Jorge Roberto Marcante Carlotto Hospital de Clínicas de Passo Fundo, Passo Fundo, Brazil

Marcus Cezillo, MD Trauma Surgery Department, Hospital de Base do Distrito Federal (HBDF), Brasília, DF, Brazil

José Ciongoli Department of Anatomy and Operative Technique, School of medicine of the ENIAC University, Guarulhos, Brazil

Federico Coccolini Department of General, Emergency and Trauma Surgery, Pisa University Hospital, Pisa, Italy

Camilla Cremonini Department of General, Emergency and Trauma Surgery, Pisa University Hospital, Pisa, Italy

Rafael L. Curado, MD, MSc Grupo Surgical, Campinas, Brazil

Paula Duarte D'ambrosio InCor—Instituto do Coração do Hospital das Clínicas da FMUSP, São Paulo, SP, Brazil

Rafael Izar Domingues da Costa Department of Medicine, Federal University of São Carlos (UFSCar), São Carlos, SP, Brazil

Bruna Amaral da Cruz Grupo de Pesquisa e Extensão em Cirurgia (GPEC), São Paulo, Brazil

Federico Davrieux School of Medicine, University of Buenos Aires, Buenos Aires, Argentina

Karine Matos de Albuquerque Faculty of Medicine, University of Porto, Porto, Portugal

Simone de Campos Vieira Department of Pediatric Surgery, Federal University of São Paulo, São Paulo, SP, Brazil

Evan DeCan Division of Trauma and Acute Care Surgery, Inova Healthcare System, Fairfax, VA, USA

Dirceu de Castro Rezende Júnior Hospital de Base do Distrito Federal (HBDF), Faculty of Medicine Unieuro DF, Brasília/DF, Brasília, Brazil

Nicolas de Cesaro Schpchacki Pontifícia Universidade Católica do Rio Grande do Sul (PUCRS), Porto Alegre, Brazil

Ricardo de Deus Honorato Grupo de Pesquisa e Extensão em Cirurgia (GPEC), Hospital Municipal Antônio Giglio (HMAG), Osasco, Brazil

Anna Gabriela Santana de Lacerda FAM (Centro Universitário das Américas) Department of Medicine, São Paulo, Brazil

Hugo Gregoris de Lima Hospital Municipal Antônio Giglio (HMAG), Osasco, Brazil

Renato de Mesquita Tauil Brazilian College of Surgeons (TCBC) and Brazilian College of Digestive Surgery (TCBCD), Rio de Janeiro, Brazil

Andrii Dinets Taras Shevchenko National University of Kyiv, Kyiv, Ukraine

Christopher Dyke Department of Surgery, Walter Reed National Military Medical Center, Bethesda, MD, USA

David T. Efron Department of Surgery – R Adams Cowley Shock Trauma. Center, University of Maryland School of Medicine, Baltimore, MD, USA

Faaleha Heba Fakruddin Batterjee Medical College, Jeddah, Saudi Arabia

Paula Ferrada Division of Trauma and Acute Care Surgery, Inova Healthcare System, Fairfax, VA, USA

Marcos Arcoverde Fortes Filho Centro Universitário UniFacid | IDOMED, Teresina, Brazil

Jaqueline Schaparini Fonini Instituto do Cancer do estado de São Paulo, São Paulo, SP, Brazil

Vinicius Cordeiro Fonseca Faculty of Medicine of USP (University of São Paulo), São Paulo, Brazil

Viktor Frieders-Justin Department of Surgery, Section for Surgical Research, Medical University of Graz, Graz, Austria

Department of Surgery, Klinik Donaustadt, Vienna Healthcare Group, Vienna, Austria

Marcelo L. Furtado Fellow of the Brazilian College of Surgeons, General, Bariatric and Digestive Surgery, Brazilian Society of Minimally Invasive and Robotic Surgery—SOBRACIL-SP, São Paulo, Brazil

Agata Grochowska Faculty of Medicine, Medical University of Lodz, Lodz, Poland

Kostiantyn Gumeniuk National Military Medical Clinical Center—Head Military Clinical Hospital, Kiev, Ukraine

Shailvi Gupta Department of Surgery – R Adams Cowley Shock Trauma. Center, University of Maryland School of Medicine, Baltimore, MD, USA

Jennifer Gurney Brooke Army Medical Center San Antonio, San Antonio, TX, USA

Nafeesa Hashim General Medicine Practice Program, Batterjee Medical College for Science and Technology, Jeddah, Saudi Arabia

John Holcomb University of Alabama at Birmingham, Birmingham, AL, USA

Steven B. Holsten Department of Surgery – R Adams Cowley Shock Trauma. Center, University of Maryland School of Medicine, Baltimore, MD, USA

Donald Jenkins University of Texas Health Sciences Center San Antonio, San Antonio, TX, USA

Mansoor Ali Khan Iqarus Gulf FZ LLC, Dubai, UAE

Sariya Khan General Medicine Practice Program, Batterjee Medical College, Jeddah, Saudi Arabia

Zain Ali Khan Nottingham University Medical School, Lincoln and Nottingham University Campus, Nottingham, UK

Igor Kryvoruchko Kharkiv National Medical University, Kharkiv, Ukraine

Diana Delgado Lindeman Department of Pediatric Surgery, Antonio Giglio Municipal Hospital, Osasco, SP, Brazil

Renato Diniz Lins Hospital de Base do Distrito Federal (HBDF), Brasilia, DF, Brazil

Antonella Lopes Department of General, Emergency and Trauma Surgery, Pisa University Hospital, Pisa, Italy

Igor Lurin National Academy of Medical Sciences of Ukraine, Kiev, Ukraine

Germano Andrade Maranduba Hospital de Base (HBDF) Brasília / DF, Brasília, Brazil

Corrado P. Marini Department of Surgery, Albert Einstein College of Medicine, Jacobi Medical Center, Bronx, NY, USA

John McNelis Department of Surgery, Albert Einstein College of Medicine, Jacobi Medical Center, Bronx, NY, USA

Jody Miller Department of Trauma and Acute Care Surgeon and General Surgery, Mediclinic Parkview Hospital, Dubai, UAE

Rodrigo Moreira e Lima Department of Anesthesia, Perioperative, and Pain Medicine, University of Manitoba, Winnipeg, MB, Canada

Ricardo Kalaf Mussi State University of Campinas (UNICAMP-SP), Campinas, São Paulo, Brazil

José Roberto Ramírez Nava Adscrito a la división de cirugía general y endoscopica, Hospital General Dr. Manuel Gea González, Mexico City, Distrito Federal, Mexico

Lais Helena Navarro e Lima Department of Anesthesia, Perioperative, and Pain Medicine, University of Manitoba, Winnipeg, MB, Canada

Marcos Dal Vesco Neto Hospital de Clínicas de Passo Fundo, Passo Fundo, Brazil

Juliana Ordoñez Department of General Surgery, Central Military Hospital, Bogotá, Colombia

Trauma and Critical Care Surgeon, Head of the Vascular Surgery Service – Central Military Hospital, Bogotá, Colombia

Pablo R. Ottolino Lavarte, MD Trauma and Emergency Unit, Dr. Sótero del Río Hospital, Pontifical Catholic University of Chile, Santiago, Chile

Andrea Pakula, MD, MPH Robotic Surgery, Simi Valley, CA, USA

Mariano Palermo Department of Bariatric Surgery, School of Medicine, Diagnomed Affiliated Institution to the University of Buenos Aires, Buenos Aires, Argentina

Olivia Parry Brooke Army Medical Center San Antonio, San Antonio, TX, USA

Bruno Monteiro Pereira, MD, MSc, PhD, FACS, FCCM University of Vassouras, Surgical Group® President, Campinas Brazil. World Society of the Abdominal Compartment Past-President, Campinas, Brazil

Mable Pereira Lincoln American University, School of Medicine, Georgetown, Guyana

Patrizio Petrone NYU Grossman Long Island School of Medicine, Mineola, NY, USA

Chairman, Research Committee, Panamerican Trauma Society, Mineola, NY, USA

José A. Pezati Tenani Unidade de Emergencia, Hospital das Clinicas of Ribeirão Preto, Faculdade de Medicina de Ribeirão Preto, University of São Paulo, Ribeirão Preto, Brazil

Rafael Dib Possiedi R Adams Cowley Shock Trauma Center, University of Maryland, Baltimore, MD, USA

Seth Rabinowitz School of Medicine, University of Maryland, Baltimore, MD, USA

Atika Rauf General Medicine Practice Program, Batterjee Medical College for Science and Technology, Jeddah, Saudi Arabia

Leonardo de Andrade Reis Board of Directors of the Latin American Society of Regional Anesthesia, São Paulo, Brazil

Marcelo Augusto Fontenelle Ribeiro Jr., MD, MSc, PhD R Adams Cowley Shock Trauma Center, University of Maryland, Baltimore, MD, USA

Rodrigo Chaves Ribeiro Department of Pediatric Surgery, Children's Cancer Hospital, Barretos Cancer Hospital, Barretos School of Health Sciences Dr. Paulo Prata, São Paulo, SP, Brazil

Luis Gustavo Capochin Romagnolo Colorectal Department of Barretos Cancer Hospital, Barretos, SP, Brazil

William Sanchez Head of the Medical-Surgical Unit, Central Military Hospital, Bogotá, Colombia

Department of General Surgery, Central Military Hospital, Bogotá, Colombia

Roberto Fernández Santiago Servicio de cirugia general, Unidad cirugia HBP y trasplantes, Hospital universitario Marques de valdecilla, Santander España, Spain

Thomas M. Scalea Department of Surgery, R Adams Cowley Shock Trauma Center, University of Maryland School of Medicine, Baltimore, MD, USA

Saniyah Shaikh College of Medicine, Alfaisal University, Riyadh, Saudi Arabia

Patrick Sheahan Division of Trauma and Acute Care Surgery, Inova Healthcare System, Fairfax, VA, USA

Justin Sleeter Brooke Army Medical Center San Antonio, San Antonio, TX, USA

Jorge Luiz Carnesecca Sobrinho Department of Surgery, Ribeirão Preto Medical School, University of São Paulo (USP), Ribeirão Preto, SP, Brazil

Philipp Stiegler Department of Surgery, Section for Surgical Research, Medical University of Graz, Graz, Austria

Kenneth Stransky Department of Surgery, Walter Reed National Military Medical Center, Bethesda, MD, USA

Federico Castillo Suescun Servicio de cirugia general, Unidad cirugia HBP y trasplantes, Hospital universitario Marques de valdecilla, Santander España, Spain

Bruno Tabajuihanski Hospital Municipal do Campo Limpo, São Paulo, Brazil

Husna Irfan Thalib General Medicine Practice Program, Batterjee Medical College, Jeddah, Saudi Arabia

Sophie Tran School of Medicine, University of Maryland, Baltimore, MD, USA

Selman Uranues Department of Surgery, Section for Surgical Research, Medical University of Graz, Graz, Austria

Oleksandr Usenko Bogomolets National Medical University, Shalimov National Institute of Surgery and Transplantology, Kiev, Ukraine

Robson Uwagoya FAM (Centro Universitário das Américas), Department of Medicine Departament of Pediatric Surgery at Antônio Giglio Municipal Hospital, São Paulo, Brazil

Adolfo Cuendis Velázquez Adscrito a la divisiõn de cirugía general y endoscopica, Hospital General Dr. Manuel Gea González, Mexico City, Distrito Federal, Mexico

Sebastian Eduardo Velez Córdoba National University, Hospital Municipal de Urgencias, Córdoba, Argentina

Luiz von Lohrmann Cruz Arraes State University of Campinas (UNICAMP-SP), Campinas, São Paulo, Brazil

Hospital Ophir Loyola (HOL-Belem/PA), Belém, Brazil

Gordon G. Wisbach Department of Surgery, Navy Medicine Readiness & Training Command, San Diego, CA, USA

Tamara J. Worlton Department of Surgery, Uniformed Services University of the Health Sciences, Bethesda, MD, USA

Anaida Xacur-Trabulce Hospital Angeles Lomas, General Surgery Department, Mexico City, Mexico

Part I

Introduction

Minimally Invasive Surgery History in Trauma and Its Advances Through Time

1

Bruno Monteiro Pereira and Marcus Cezillo

Introduction

Trauma remains one of the leading causes of death and disability worldwide, particularly among young and economically productive populations. Traditionally, the surgical management of traumatic injuries was synonymous with exploratory laparotomy, an approach that prioritized rapid access and direct intervention. However, over the past three decades, a transformative shift has occurred with the gradual incorporation of minimally invasive surgery (MIS) into trauma care. Once considered incompatible with the urgency and complexity of trauma, MIS has now carved a niche within the trauma surgeon's armamentarium.

This chapter explores the historical evolution of MIS in trauma, its resistance and acceptance within the surgical community, the pivotal milestones that shaped its growth, and the most significant technological and procedural advances that continue to redefine its role.

The Beginnings: Laparoscopy in Elective Surgery

The origins of MIS trace back to the early twentieth century with the use of diagnostic laparoscopy by gynecologists and general surgeons. However, it was not until the late 1980s and early 1990s, with the advent of laparoscopic cholecystectomy, that

B. M. Pereira (✉)
University of Vassouras, Surgical Group® President, Campinas Brazil. World Society of the Abdominal Compartment Past-President, Campinas, Brazil
e-mail: adm@gruposurgical.com.br

M. Cezillo
Trauma Surgery Department, Hospital de Base do Distrito Federal (HBDF), Brasília, DF, Brazil

© The Author(s), under exclusive license to Springer Nature Switzerland AG 2026

M. Cezillo, B. M. Pereira (eds.), *Minimally Invasive Surgery Trauma*,
https://doi.org/10.1007/978-3-032-28971-1_1

MIS gained widespread adoption in elective general surgery. The advantages—less postoperative pain, faster recovery, shorter hospital stays, and improved cosmetic results—were undeniable.

Despite its success in elective procedures, trauma surgery remained a stronghold of open techniques. The unpredictability of injuries, need for rapid intervention, and limited visualization initially rendered laparoscopy unsuitable in trauma settings.

The First Steps: Diagnostic Laparoscopy in Trauma

By the mid-1990s, pioneers in trauma surgery began to explore laparoscopy's diagnostic utility in selected patients, particularly those with penetrating abdominal trauma. The goal was to reduce the incidence of non-therapeutic laparotomies—operations that carried significant morbidity despite the absence of injuries requiring surgical repair.

Early studies showed that laparoscopy could reliably detect peritoneal violations, diaphragmatic injuries, and intra-abdominal bleeding. As a result, it began to be cautiously incorporated into the diagnostic algorithm for hemodynamically stable patients.

Key early milestones included:

- 1991: First published case reports of diagnostic laparoscopy in trauma.
- Late 1990s: Laparoscopy used to evaluate diaphragmatic injuries and peritoneal penetration.

The Early History of Laparoscopy in Trauma: From Case Reports to Clinical Strategy

The incorporation of laparoscopy into trauma care began modestly in the early 1990s, evolving from isolated diagnostic case reports into structured clinical strategies by the end of the decade. This progression laid the foundation for modern minimally invasive trauma surgery.

1991: First Published Case Reports of Laparoscopy in Trauma

The earliest published case reports describing the use of laparoscopy in trauma emerged in 1991, marking a paradigm shift in how surgeons approached hemodynamically stable patients with abdominal trauma.

One of the pivotal milestones in the history of minimally invasive surgery in trauma care was the publication by Ivatury et al. [1]. This concise yet impactful study is among the earliest to formally evaluate the feasibility, safety, and clinical utility of laparoscopy for penetrating anterior abdominal injuries, specifically stab wounds. The authors reported that laparoscopy avoided unnecessary laparotomies in a subset of patients, thus reducing non-therapeutic laparotomy rates, which had been historically high in penetrating trauma.

Study Summary and Observations

- *Patient selection*: The study included hemodynamically stable patients with penetrating abdominal trauma where the extent of peritoneal violation was unclear.
- *Methodology*: Diagnostic laparoscopy was employed to assess for peritoneal penetration and determine the need for further operative intervention.
- *Key Findings*:
  - Laparoscopy successfully identified peritoneal penetration in several cases, guiding the decision for therapeutic laparotomy.
  - Importantly, it also prevented unnecessary laparotomies in a subset of patients where no penetration or intra-abdominal injury was detected.
  - The study highlighted shorter hospital stays, lower morbidity, and better patient outcomes when laparoscopy was used appropriately.
  - Demonstrated laparoscopy could reliably assess for peritoneal violation.
  - Supported the safety of laparoscopy in hemodynamically stable patients. Raised early discussions about the learning curve and limitations of minimally invasive trauma care.
- *Impact*: At the time, non-therapeutic laparotomy rates in penetrating trauma were as high as 30–40%. This paper laid the foundation for using laparoscopy as a selective tool to reduce unnecessary surgery, thereby ushering in a new era of damage control with minimally invasive precision.

Historical Importance of Dr. Rao R. Ivatury; A Tribute

Dr. Rao R. Ivatury is widely recognized as a pioneer in modern trauma surgery, particularly in the advancement of selective non-operative management (SNOM) and the integration of laparoscopy in trauma care.

Key Contributions:

- Innovation in trauma techniques: Dr. Ivatury was among the first to challenge the dogma of mandatory laparotomy for all penetrating injuries. His work supported selective approaches based on physiology and imaging, which is now a standard principle in modern trauma algorithms.
- Champion of minimally invasive trauma care: This 1991 publication marked one of the first applications of minimally invasive techniques in trauma patients. Dr. Ivatury's foresight contributed to the progressive inclusion of laparoscopy in trauma guidelines, especially for diaphragmatic injuries and anterior abdominal stab wounds.
- Educator and global influence: As a professor and researcher at institutions such as Virginia Commonwealth University and Elmhurst Hospital / Mount Sinai

School of Medicine, Dr. Ivatury trained multiple generations of trauma surgeons. His lectures, consensus papers, and leadership in the American Association for the Surgery of Trauma (AAST) shaped contemporary trauma systems.
- Publications and leadership:
  - Over 400 peer-reviewed articles and textbook chapters.
  - Co-editor of major trauma surgery textbooks.
    Leader in advocating for damage control surgery, resuscitative thoracotomy, and urban trauma systems.

Late 1990s: Expansion to Diaphragmatic Injuries and Peritoneal Violation

By the late 1990s, laparoscopy had expanded its role in trauma diagnostics, especially in thoracoabdominal injuries and the evaluation of diaphragmatic integrity, a historically challenging diagnostic area [2].

In this landmark review, the authors provided a comprehensive synthesis of over a decade of laparoscopic applications in trauma. They emphasized laparoscopy's diagnostic value in:

- Left thoracoabdominal stab wounds, where occult diaphragmatic injuries could be easily missed.
- Blunt trauma, in selected cases, to assess internal injury without large incisions.

Another important contributor during this period was [3].

This large retrospective review provided strong evidence that laparoscopy was associated with:

- A reduction in non-therapeutic laparotomy rates.
- Improved length of stay and postoperative pain control.
- The emergence of therapeutic laparoscopy, not just diagnostic, especially for diaphragmatic repair.

Synthesis: From Innovation to Integration

By the end of the 1990s, laparoscopy in trauma had evolved from a bold innovation into a reliable adjunct in the management of trauma patients. It was no longer a theoretical possibility but a practical diagnostic and therapeutic tool—albeit still confined to select patient profiles (primarily hemodynamically stable, with penetrating injuries).

Key milestones from this era include:

Year	Milestone	Authors / Impact
1991	First case reports of laparoscopy in trauma	Ivatury et al.—Penetrating abdominal trauma
1993–1996	Increasing use for diaphragm and peritoneal evaluation	Nathens et al., Brandt et al.
1999	Comprehensive reviews and large patient series	Gazzaniga et al., Miles et al.

Legacy and Foundation for the 2000s

The experiences of the 1990s laid the essential groundwork for more aggressive laparoscopic interventions in the 2000s—including laparoscopic repair of hollow viscus injuries, control of bleeding, and trauma-specific minimally invasive protocols. They also established patient selection criteria, technical feasibility, and surgeon training requirements that are still referenced today.

Despite these advances, therapeutic laparoscopy remained rare due to concerns about missing injuries and the need for advanced skills and equipment.

The 2000s: Expansion of Indications and Technological Maturity

The early 2000s saw critical changes that allowed MIS to gain momentum in trauma surgery:

- Improved imaging (CT angiography) helped better select patients for MIS.
- Instrumentation became more refined, with high-definition optics and advanced energy devices.
- Surgeon training in laparoscopy became more widespread due to its acceptance in elective surgery.

With these improvements, surgeons began to expand indications beyond diagnosis:

- Repair of diaphragmatic lacerations
- Control of splenic bleeding or resection of devascularized segments
- Lavage of hemoperitoneum
- Identification and control of bile leaks
- Treatment of contained hollow viscus injuries

This period marked the beginning of therapeutic laparoscopy in trauma. However, success depended heavily on patient selection, institutional resources, and surgeon expertise.

Consolidation from the 2000s Onward

Advancements in the Twenty-first Century: From Diagnostics to Therapeutic Applications

Since the early 2000s, laparoscopy has gained increasing recognition not just as a diagnostic tool but also as a therapeutic strategy in abdominal trauma—especially in hemodynamically stable patients and with experienced surgical teams.

Key Highlights:

- *Laparoscopic repair* of diaphragmatic, gastric, and colonic injuries.
- Growing use in *civilian and military trauma systems.*
- Protocol development for *thoracoabdominal trauma* using minimally invasive techniques.
- *Cautious adoption* in selected blunt trauma cases [4].

One of the most significant contributions to the international body of evidence on laparoscopy in trauma comes from the landmark study by Kawahara et al., published in 2009 in the *Journal of Trauma and Acute Care Surgery*. This article presents the results of 20 years of experience in using laparoscopy for abdominal trauma at the Hospital Municipal Souza Aguiar in Rio de Janeiro, a major Latin American trauma referral center.

This retrospective observational study encompassed 1016 trauma patients who underwent laparoscopy between 1985 and 2007. The patient population included both penetrating and blunt abdominal trauma cases, and the authors evaluated the diagnostic accuracy, therapeutic potential, conversion rates, and complication profiles associated with the laparoscopic approach.

Key Findings

1. Patient Demographics and Trauma Mechanism
   - Total patients: 1016
   - Mechanism of trauma:
     - 87% penetrating (mostly stab wounds)
       13% blunt abdominal trauma
   - Most common injury site: Anterior abdominal wall
2. Laparoscopy as a Diagnostic Tool
   - Diagnostic laparoscopy was used to:
     - Determine peritoneal violation
     - Evaluate diaphragmatic integrity
       Assess for solid organ and hollow viscus injuries
   - Diagnostic accuracy: Laparoscopy demonstrated high sensitivity and specificity for peritoneal and diaphragmatic injuries.

- The study emphasized the use of laparoscopy to rule out injuries, thereby reducing unnecessary exploratory laparotomies.

3. Reduction in Non-therapeutic Laparotomy

   - Laparoscopy avoided laparotomy in 583 patients (57.4%), demonstrating its value in reducing non-therapeutic procedures.
   - This translated into:
     - Shorter hospital stays
     - Reduced morbidity
       Lower overall healthcare burden

4. Therapeutic Laparoscopy

   - In selected cases, laparoscopy was used to:
     - Control minor bleeding
     - Repair small diaphragmatic or bowel injuries
       Perform peritoneal lavage and drainage
   - *Therapeutic interventions* were possible in 83 patients (8.1%), reinforcing the concept that laparoscopy is not merely diagnostic but also potentially therapeutic in the right context.

5. Conversion to Laparotomy

   - *Conversion rate*: 10.6% (108 patients).
   - Most common reasons:
     - Intraoperative findings necessitating open surgery
       Poor visualization due to hemoperitoneum or adhesions

Complications and Mortality

- Low rate of complications attributed to laparoscopy itself.
- No deaths directly linked to the laparoscopic procedure.
- The overall mortality rate (2.4%) was attributed to associated injuries and not to the surgical approach.

Discussion and Significance

This study represents one of the largest single-institution series on laparoscopy in trauma worldwide and is the most comprehensive Latin American report on the subject to date. Its significance lies in several domains:

1. *Validation of laparoscopy in a resource-constrained environment*
   - Despite occurring in a public trauma hospital in a middle-income country, the findings demonstrate that laparoscopy can be applied safely and effectively outside of high-income, high-tech settings.

2. *Strategic patient selection and protocol development*
    - The authors describe a clear algorithm for patient triage, with emphasis on hemodynamic stability and anatomical site of injury.
3. *Expansion of minimally invasive trauma surgery in penetrating trauma*
    - The predominance of penetrating trauma in this cohort (primarily knife injuries) makes the findings especially relevant to regions with high urban violence.
4. *Legacy and leadership in Latin American trauma care*
    - This work placed Brazil at the forefront of trauma laparoscopy and demonstrated that surgical innovation can and should arise from high-volume trauma centers globally, regardless of geography.

Implications for Practice

Kawahara et al. advocate for wider integration of laparoscopy into trauma algorithms, emphasizing its benefits in:

- Reducing unnecessary exploratory laparotomy
- Improving recovery and patient satisfaction
- Facilitating direct visualization of difficult-to-assess injuries (e.g., diaphragm)
- Performing therapeutic procedures in well-selected cases

Their findings also underscore the importance of training trauma surgeons in advanced laparoscopy, especially in regions with high rates of penetrating trauma.

This Brazilian study revealed that even in high-volume trauma centers, laparoscopy can be safe and effective for both diagnostic and therapeutic purposes. The authors highlighted cases where laparoscopy helped avoid non-therapeutic laparotomies, control minor bleeding, and identify injuries not visualized on CT scans.

International Experience: How Other Countries Evaluated in the 2000s?

Israel (IDF and Civilian Hospitals)

- Integrated laparoscopy into algorithms for blast and projectile injuries.
- Military experience accelerated the adoption of minimally invasive techniques in penetrating trauma.

South Africa

- Extensive experience with penetrating trauma (urban violence).
- Studies from Durban and Cape Town report that laparoscopy reduced non-therapeutic laparotomies by up to 60%.

Table 1.1 Current indications for laparoscopy in trauma

Clinical scenario	Indication	Level of evidence
Stable penetrating abdominal injury	Assessment of peritoneal and diaphragm penetration	High
Left thoracoabdominal stab wound	Rule out diaphragmatic injury	High
Unexplained abdominal bleeding	Exploratory evaluation	Moderate
Blunt trauma with inconclusive imaging	Diagnosis of perforation or hematoma	Moderate
Small lesion management (gastric, hepatic)	Selective laparoscopic treatment	Moderate

Europe (France, Germany, Spain)

- More restricted use, focused in high-complexity trauma centers.
- Primarily used for complementary evaluation and treatment of diaphragmatic and minor hepatic injuries.

Initial Criticism and Barriers: Important Lessons

Despite its benefits, laparoscopy in trauma was not universally adopted in the early stages, due to:

- Fear of missed injuries, particularly in blunt trauma.
- Requirement for 24/7 skilled surgical teams.
- Concerns that pneumoperitoneum could worsen concealed hemorrhage.
- Lack of clear patient selection protocols.

Nevertheless, further studies confirmed that with proper criteria and surgical expertise, laparoscopy is both safe and effective in trauma care [5] (Table 1.1).

Timeline: Key Milestones in Trauma Laparoscopy

Year	Milestone	Contribution
1991	Ivatury et al. publish first trauma laparoscopy cases	Demonstrated feasibility in penetrating trauma
1995–1999	Expanded to diaphragmatic evaluation	Key studies by Gazzaniga et al., Miles et al.
2003	Leppäniemi & Haapiainen (Finland) report safe use in selected blunt trauma	Broadened indications
2009	Brazilian 20-year experience (Kawahara et al.)	Validated safety in high-volume centers
2015+	Laparoscopic treatment of liver, gastric, and splenic injuries (select cases)	Expanded therapeutic role
2020s	Integration with robotic surgery and “FAST-lap” protocols	Precision trauma surgery consolidation

The 2010s: Global Dissemination and Evidence Accumulation

In the 2010s, the global surgical community began to recognize MIS in trauma as a viable option in selected cases. Several international trauma centers began publishing their experiences, case series, and comparative studies.

Key developments:

- *Meta-analyses* began to show favorable outcomes for MIS in terms of reduced infection rates, length of stay, and postoperative pain.
- *MIS in pediatric trauma* gained traction due to the desire to avoid large incisions in young patients.
- *Use in blunt trauma* increased, particularly for liver and splenic injuries after failed NOM (non-operative management).

The American Association for the Surgery of Trauma (AAST) and the World Society of Emergency Surgery (WSES) started incorporating MIS into trauma guidelines for specific indications, further validating its role.

The Present: State-of-the-Art Minimally Invasive Trauma Surgery

Today, MIS is a recognized component of trauma care in modern surgical centers. Its current applications include:

- *Diagnostic laparoscopy* for stable patients with penetrating trauma
- *Therapeutic laparoscopy* for solid organ bleeding, bile leaks, and hollow viscus injuries
- *Thoracoscopy (VATS)* for retained hemothorax and diaphragm injuries
- *Laparoscopy-assisted procedures*, combining open and MIS techniques

Moreover, the integration of damage control strategies into MIS—such as laparoscopic packing or limited bleeding control—merged as a novel frontier. MIS has also become integral to enhanced recovery protocols, with patients experiencing less pain, faster mobilization, and reduced ICU needs.

The Role of Laparoscopy in Modern Trauma Surgery

Laparoscopy in trauma is no longer experimental or marginal. In many trauma centers worldwide, it is now an essential component of abdominal trauma evaluation and, in selected cases, minimally invasive treatment.

Its use—while context-dependent—has been shown to:

- Reduce morbidity

- Avoid non-therapeutic laparotomies
- Enhance diagnostic accuracy
- Shorten hospital stays
- Improve patient comfort and recovery

Laparoscopy does not replace clinical judgment. Rather, it enhances the trauma surgeon's toolkit, requiring precision, protocol-driven selection, and a high level of technical expertise.

The Role of Robotics and Future Directions

The last 5 years have witnessed a rapid expansion of robotic-assisted surgery in trauma. Though cost and availability remain barriers, early adopters have demonstrated that robotic platforms offer:

- Superior dexterity and precision
- Enhanced visualization
- Greater ergonomics for complex reconstructions

Future directions in MIS for trauma may include:

- Artificial intelligence for intraoperative decision-making
- Augmented reality to visualize vascular structures or organ planes
- Remote telesurgery in military or rural trauma settings
- Hybrid trauma operating rooms that combine fluoroscopy, laparoscopy, and angiography in the same suite

These advances are likely to expand MIS into more complex and unstable trauma scenarios in the future [6].

Challenges and Limitations

Despite its success, MIS in trauma faces several limitations:

- Requires surgical expertise and a learning curve
- Dependent on resource availability and institutional commitment
- Limited in cases of massive hemorrhage or unstable physiology
- Risk of missed injuries in polytrauma patients

Therefore, the surgeon must be skilled in both MIS and open techniques and capable of rapid conversion when necessary.

Conclusion

Minimally invasive surgery in trauma has evolved from skepticism to acceptance and innovation. What began as a diagnostic adjunct is now a therapeutic tool in selected patients, offering lower morbidity and faster recovery without compromising outcomes. As technology continues to advance and training becomes more widespread, MIS will likely play an increasingly central role in trauma care, complementing—but never replacing—the essential principles of damage control and surgical judgment.

The future is not about replacing open surgery, but rather integrating all available tools—open, laparoscopic, robotic, and interventional—into a tailored, patient-centered trauma strategy.

References

1. Ivatury RR, Simon RJ, Stahl WM, et al. Laparoscopy in the evaluation of penetrating abdominal trauma. Am Surg. 1991;57(9):540–2.
2. Gazzaniga AB, Bammer T, Alessandrini R, et al. Laparoscopy in trauma. Surg Clin N Am. 1999;79(6):1377–90.
3. Miles EJ, Carrillo EH, Spain DA, et al. Is laparoscopy for trauma a better approach? Evidence from 1,300 patients. Surg Endosc. 1999;13(6):500–5.
4. Kawahara NT, Alster C, Fujisaki LT, et al. Laparoscopy in abdominal trauma: a two-decade experience at a reference trauma hospital in Brazil. J Trauma Acute Care Surg. 2009;67(4):689–95.
5. Ermolov AS, Tlibekova MA, Yartsev PA, Guliaev AA, Rogal MM, Samsonov VT, Levitsky VD. Laparoscopic splenectomy in patients with spleen injuries. Surg Laparosc Endosc Percutan Tech. 2015;25(6):483–6. https://doi.org/10.1097/SLE.0000000000000207.
6. de' Angelis N, Khan J, Marchegiani F, Puglisi A, Belli F, Di Saverio S, et al. Robotic surgery in emergency setting: 2021 WSES position paper. World J Emerg Surg. 2022;17:4. https://doi.org/10.1186/s13017-021-00415-2.

The Role of Laparoscopy in Modern Trauma Care

2

Evan DeCan, Patrick Sheahan, and Paula Ferrada

Introduction: Brief History and Evolution of Trauma Laparoscopy

Laparoscopy in Elective and Emergency Surgery

Over the past decades, advances in technology, training, and accessibility have made laparoscopic surgery the standard of care for many elective procedures [1–3]. Compared to open surgery, laparoscopy offers numerous benefits in elective settings, including reduced patient discomfort, faster recovery times, and improved cosmetic results. These advantages have driven the widespread adoption of minimally invasive techniques across surgical specialties. Emerging evidence indicates that laparoscopic techniques have demonstrated improved clinical outcomes for patients undergoing acute care surgery, compared to traditional open procedures. Specifically, laparoscopic repair of perforated peptic ulcer disease has been associated with reduced postoperative pain, fewer complications such as surgical site infections and incisional hernias, as well as shorter hospital stays and earlier return to work times, when patients are carefully selected [4, 5].

Laparoscopy in Trauma

Building on these findings, the consideration of the use of laparoscopic techniques in trauma patients has gained ground over recent years, as both a diagnostic and therapeutic tool. And while historically there has been concern over potential missed injury [6] and limited visualization, its use as a diagnostic modality for injury identification in stable blunt or penetrating abdominal injury has been established

E. DeCan · P. Sheahan · P. Ferrada (✉)
Division of Trauma and Acute Care Surgery, Inova Healthcare System, Fairfax, VA, USA
e-mail: paula.ferrada@inova.org

© The Author(s), under exclusive license to Springer Nature Switzerland AG 2026

M. Cezillo, B. M. Pereira (eds.), *Minimally Invasive Surgery Trauma*,
https://doi.org/10.1007/978-3-032-28971-1_2

[7–12]. And its use as a therapeutic modality in trauma patients is quickly becoming more widespread and accepted as evidence for its use grows [13, 14]. Given this growth in popularity, several recent studies have highlighted the most appropriate clinical scenarios and patient populations that could potentially benefit most from a laparoscopic approach [10, 13–19].

The purpose of this chapter is to equip the reader with a comprehensive understanding of the clinical indications and contraindications for utilizing this modality as a first-line approach. It will explore specific clinical scenarios where its application proves beneficial, provide therapeutic recommendations and techniques tailored to those scenarios, and conclude with a discussion on its advantages and disadvantages relative to open surgery, as well as its potential future implications.

Contraindications to Trauma Laparoscopy

Absolute Contraindications

Laparoscopic surgery is well documented to exert significant physiologic effects on the cardiorespiratory system, primarily through the introduction of pneumoperitoneum with CO2 insufflation. These effects include increased intra-abdominal pressure, reduced venous return, elevated systemic vascular resistance, and compromised cardiac output, even in otherwise healthy elective surgical populations [20–23]. These physiologic changes can be particularly pronounced in trauma patients, who may already be experiencing reduced physiologic reserves due to hemorrhage, shock, or other injuries. Consequently, careful patient selection based on baseline hemodynamic stability is essential when considering laparoscopy in trauma settings to mitigate the risk of further physiologic deterioration.

In trauma care, hemodynamic instability has historically been regarded as an absolute contraindication for laparoscopy, as the physiological perturbations introduced by the procedure could exacerbate a patient's critical state [13, 15, 24, 25]. For patients presenting in extremis, immediate laparotomy remains the standard of care when operative intervention is indicated, given its ability to provide rapid access and definitive management. Laparoscopy, with its increased demand on the cardiovascular system, is not appropriate in these cases, as even brief periods of elevated intra-abdominal pressure can lead to catastrophic outcomes in patients with compromised hemodynamics. Limited research exists regarding the feasibility or safety of laparoscopy in unstable trauma patients, [26] and the lack of robust data reinforces the need for adherence to current recommendations against its use in this subgroup.

Furthermore, elevated intracranial pressure (ICP) is another critical contraindication for laparoscopy, given the well-established effects of CO_2 insufflation on increasing ICP [27]. In patients with suspected or known traumatic brain injury, the physiologic response to pneumoperitoneum could exacerbate cerebral edema and impair cerebral perfusion, leading to worsened neurologic outcomes. As such, the interplay between the physiologic demands of laparoscopy and the preexisting vulnerabilities of trauma patients underscores the importance of precise patient selection and careful consideration of the procedure's risks and benefits. While laparoscopy offers numerous advantages, its use must be judicious, especially in patients with limited physiologic reserve or conditions predisposing them to adverse responses.

Relative Contraindications

Known cardiac or pulmonary diseases, while not absolute contraindications to laparoscopy, require careful consideration due to the physiological effects of pneumoperitoneum that can exacerbate underlying dysfunction. In patients with preexisting cardiac conditions, such as heart failure or coronary artery disease, the increased intra-abdominal pressure and elevated systemic vascular resistance induced by CO2 insufflation can place an additional burden on cardiac output and myocardial oxygen demand. These effects heighten the risk of perioperative ischemia or heart failure, necessitating rigorous hemodynamic monitoring and individualized risk assessment. Similarly, arrhythmias or valvular disorders may worsen due to the hemodynamic shifts caused by pneumoperitoneum, making it crucial to evaluate the stability of these conditions prior to considering a laparoscopic approach.

For patients with baseline pulmonary diseases such as chronic obstructive pulmonary disease (COPD) or asthma, the effects of pneumoperitoneum on ventilatory mechanics are of particular concern. Elevated intra-abdominal pressure can decrease diaphragmatic excursion and functional residual capacity, leading to ventilation-perfusion mismatches and potential hypercapnia. Additionally, the CO2 used in insufflation can exacerbate respiratory acidosis, placing additional strain on compromised pulmonary function. These risks demand enhanced intraoperative ventilatory support and continuous monitoring to mitigate potential complications. The decision to proceed with laparoscopy in this patient population should be based on a thorough assessment of pulmonary reserve and the anticipated benefits of the procedure relative to its risks.

Pregnancy represents another important consideration, as the physiological changes associated with pregnancy and the potential risks to both the mother and fetus require a tailored approach. While laparoscopy is not an absolute contraindication during pregnancy, the effects of pneumoperitoneum on maternal hemodynamics, ventilation, and uteroplacental perfusion warrant careful evaluation. Increased intra-abdominal pressure can reduce venous return and cardiac output, posing a risk to maternal circulation. Moreover, the positioning required for laparoscopy and the potential for CO2 absorption into the maternal bloodstream must be managed to minimize adverse effects. Fetal monitoring and coordination with obstetric specialists are essential when laparoscopy is deemed necessary, ensuring the safety of both mother and fetus. Thus, while pregnancy is not strictly contraindicated, conditions like cardiac and pulmonary disease necessitates an individualized and multidisciplinary approach to the decision-making process for laparoscopic surgery.

Indications/Uses for Trauma Laparoscopy

The use of laparoscopy as a diagnostic utility for hemodynamically stable patients has been well established in both penetrating and blunt traumatic injuries [9, 28–31]. Several key scenarios where laparoscopy has proven beneficial include:

Equivocal CT Findings and Concerning Mechanism

The use of multidetector CT scan in the assessment of hemodynamically stable trauma patients has become the gold standard for detection of both parenchymal and hollow viscus injuries [32, 33]. However, there is still a significantly high false-negative rate, as high as 20% in some studies, leading to delay in diagnosis and increased morbidity [34, 35]. In patients where CT findings are unclear or concerning for possible solid organ, hollow viscus, or diaphragmatic injury, laparoscopy may be utilized as a complementary diagnostic tool to better risk stratify these patients and guide appropriate management.

Suspected Bowel/Mesenteric Injury (Blunt Abdominal Trauma)

Diagnosis of bowel and mesenteric injuries can be particularly challenging in the context of blunt abdominal trauma, where the subtlety of clinical presentations often complicates timely and accurate identification. Physical examination findings, imaging results, and laboratory markers may fail to consistently indicate the presence or severity of these injuries. This diagnostic uncertainty arises, in part, from the underlying ischemic mechanism of injury, which frequently leads to delayed systemic manifestations. In such scenarios, early CT imaging findings may appear equivocal or nonspecific, contributing to the difficulty in forming a clear clinical picture and necessitating additional measures to avoid missed or delayed diagnoses.

Given these challenges, laparoscopy has emerged as a definitive diagnostic modality with an impressive reported accuracy of 95% for detecting bowel and mesenteric injuries. Unlike prolonged observation, serial examinations, or repeated imaging, laparoscopy allows for direct visualization of intra-abdominal structures, enabling prompt identification and intervention for injuries that might otherwise go undetected. Its ability to facilitate timely surgical management offers a significant advantage in cases where other diagnostic approaches fall short. Incorporating laparoscopy into the diagnostic algorithm for blunt abdominal trauma cases not only enhances diagnostic precision but also helps mitigate the risks associated with delayed or missed injuries, ultimately improving patient outcomes.

Assessment of Diaphragmatic Injury (Penetrating/Blunt)

Traumatic diaphragmatic injuries, though relatively uncommon, pose a serious risk if undiagnosed, with potential for delayed and life-threatening complications. These injuries are often challenging to identify due to their subtle or absent early clinical signs, particularly in patients with concurrent traumatic injuries. Missed diaphragmatic injuries can lead to significant morbidity, including progressive herniation of abdominal contents into the thoracic cavity, which may result in respiratory compromise, strangulation of herniated viscera, and severe infections such as empycma. Mortality rates increase dramatically when these complications develop, underscoring the critical importance of timely diagnosis and management.

While CT scans are commonly used in the initial evaluation of thoracic and abdominal trauma, their sensitivity for detecting diaphragmatic injuries is limited, particularly for small or occult tears. In contrast, laparoscopy has demonstrated superior diagnostic sensitivity, offering direct and reliable visualization of the diaphragm to assess its integrity more accurately than CT imaging [9, 36]. This enhanced visualization minimizes the risk of missed injuries, providing a significant diagnostic advantage in complex trauma cases where subtle diaphragmatic tears might otherwise go unnoticed. By enabling precise assessment, laparoscopy serves as a critical tool in the trauma surgeon's diagnostic arsenal.

Beyond its diagnostic capabilities, laparoscopy also allows for simultaneous therapeutic intervention. Small to moderate diaphragmatic defects can often be repaired during the same procedure without requiring conversion to an open approach, reducing operative morbidity [37–39]. This dual diagnostic and therapeutic capability not only facilitates prompt and effective management but also spares patients the risks and delays associated with separate procedures. Given the potentially severe consequences of a missed diaphragmatic injury, the integration of laparoscopy into the diagnostic pathway for trauma patients provides a compelling approach to enhancing patient outcomes and preventing long-term complications.

Penetrating Trauma and Uncertain Peritoneal Violation

Patients with penetrating injury to the abdomen and unclear peritoneal penetration should be evaluated with diagnostic laparoscopy for evaluation of intra-abdominal injury. While prior concern for potential missed injury [6] and limited visualization are valid, a recent meta-analysis [17] examining a total of 3362 patients, 1604 who underwent laparoscopy for penetrating abdominal trauma and 1758 who received laparotomy, showed a low rate of missed injury in the laparoscopic group, $n = 2$, and $n = 1$ in the laparotomy group. The sensitivity of laparoscopy was 100% in all but one of the studies—92% [40]. Importantly, the known rates of nontherapeutic surgical exploration in the setting of penetrating trauma remain high, with a wide range of reported values from 30% to as high as 61% in some studies [41]. This meta-analysis by [17] showed that patients who underwent laparoscopy: 45.6% avoided unnecessary laparotomy, which is consistent with prior reported values of 51.8% & 63% [42, 43].

Diagnostic Laparoscopy Case Basics: Equipment and Setup

Patient Positioning

Patients' positioning should be supine to allow for immediate operative conversion to laparotomy or thoracotomy depending on the injury. Multiple patient securement straps should be used to allow for patient tilting and optimal visualization during exploration. Examination of the right abdomen (right colon, small bowel, and liver) is generally performed on the patients' left side, whereas assessment of the right abdomen is generally performed from the patients' left (diaphragm, stomach/spleen, transverse and left colon, sigmoid, rectum and bladder).

Technique

Intra-abdominal access should be obtained via open Hasson technique at the umbilicus with either a 10-mm or 12-mm trocar. Veress technique in trauma patients is ill advised given the potential for iatrogenic bowel and/or vascular injury. Insufflation pressure of a maximum of 15 mmHg is sufficient for the majority of cases. Optically, we recommend a 0-degree scope for diagnostic entry and a 30-degree scope for its use in therapeutic laparoscopy. Additional trocars (either 5-mm or 10-mm) should be inserted under direct vision as needed in appropriate locations for suspected injury/potential intervention. The abdominal cavity should then be systematically examined. Reverse Trendelenburg position should be used for assessment of the liver, gallbladder, spleen, diaphragm, lesser sac, stomach, duodenum, and pancreas. The lesser sac should be opened and the posterior stomach examined. The transverse and descending colon should be inspected, and patient positioning adjusted to reverse Trendelenburg while inspecting inferiorly from the descending colon to the sigmoid, rectum, and bladder. At this point, the transverse colon should be elevated, the ligament of Treitz identified, and the small intestine run in an anterograde fashion to the ileocecal valve in a hand over hand atraumatic fashion taking care to examine both sides of the bowel. Mesenteric injury should also be assessed at this stage. Suspicion of duodenal injury should indicate conversion to an open procedure.

Proper execution of a diagnostic laparoscopic exam, including appropriate patient positioning, access technique, scope selection, and systematic cavity exploration, requires significant training and experience in advanced laparoscopic surgery. Equally important is the clinical judgment of when it is necessary to convert to an open procedure.

Conversion to Open

The development of sustained hemodynamic instability during the procedure clearly warrants conversion to an open approach. Likewise, the identification of injuries that cannot be adequately managed through laparoscopic repair necessitates conversion. Additionally, incomplete or uncertain exploration of injuries serves as an indication for transitioning to an open procedure.

Therapeutic Applications

Hemorrhage Control and Coagulation

While laparoscopy is not generally thought of as a first-line tool for hemorrhage control, there are certain situations where it can be utilized quite effectively. The visualization provided through the laparoscope is sometimes extremely helpful in examining the upper abdomen, specifically the surface of the liver, the diaphragm, proximal stomach, and spleen. Given the magnification of the scope, small areas of bleeding can be more easily identified and controlled [38, 44]. Multiple hemostatic tools can be utilized such as regular monopolar electrocautery as well as more modern technologies such as argon beam coagulation or bipolar radiofrequency ablation (aquamantys). It is important to note, however, that conversion to an open procedure should be made quickly and without delay in the setting of significant or diffuse hemorrhage [13, 14].

Repairing Organ Injuries

In terms of repairing organ injuries, again, there is some utility in the use of laparoscopy. Much like with hemorrhage control, the best injuries that can be repaired under laparoscopic visualization are smaller, isolated injuries. Diagnostic laparoscopy truly shines in its use of identifying injuries traditionally difficult to see on cross-sectional imaging, such as diaphragmatic injury and hollow viscus injury. Diaphragm injuries are especially amenable to laparoscopic sutured repair, and it is recommended that all left-sided diaphragmatic injuries be repaired. Smaller right-sided injuries can generally be left alone if they are located superior to the dome of the liver. Additionally, small primary suture repairs can also be performed on structures such as the stomach, small bowel, or bladder. Traditionally, larger bowel injuries requiring resection have been managed with conversion to open. However, newer data supports similar complication rates following total laparoscopic management of these injuries [14]. It should also be noted that success in undertaking these more advanced laparoscopic procedures is highly dependent upon each individual surgeon's skill set, and any reservation in successful laparoscopic management should prompt a conversion to open.

Advantages and Disadvantages of Laparoscopy

Comparison with Open Surgery

The morbidity associated with unnecessary laparotomy is high, with prior studies showing a significant complication rate of approximately 40%, including surgical site infections (SSIs), hernias, dehiscence, intestinal obstruction, and even mortality [42, 45]. The selective use of laparoscopy in trauma has been demonstrated to significantly reduce the rate of nontherapeutic laparotomy without increasing patient morbidity or mortality, when compared to open exploration [17, 26, 46]. Furthermore, laparoscopic management has been shown to shorten length of stay and improve postoperative pain while decreasing rates of postoperative wound infection, pneumonia, and ileus [17, 47–49].

Limitations

Despite these demonstrated advantages, laparoscopy also has some inherent limitations. Adequate exposure of the entire abdominal cavity and retroperitoneum can be challenging, and complete visualization of all potential injury sites may not be achievable, increasing the likelihood of missed injury and necessitating open conversion. However, this risk can be mitigated with the implementation of a standardized protocol for traumatic laparoscopic exploration [24, 50–52]. The therapeutic applications of laparoscopy in trauma are further limited by the need for advanced laparoscopic skills and the availability of specialized equipment.

Future Directions

Robotic surgery has emerged as a transformative approach in modern surgical practice, offering enhanced precision, dexterity, and visualization. While traditionally associated with elective procedures, its applications have expanded to include emergency general surgery and, increasingly, trauma care in carefully selected, hemodynamically stable patients. The integration of robotic systems into emergency and trauma settings marks a significant step forward in surgical innovation, leveraging the technology's unique advantages to address complex clinical challenges.

In emergency general surgery, robotic systems are already being employed to manage acute conditions such as perforated ulcers, bowel obstructions, and appendicitis. These procedures benefit from the robot's ability to facilitate minimally invasive approaches, even in anatomically challenging cases, thereby reducing postoperative pain, hospital stays, and recovery times. The success of robotic platforms in these emergency scenarios demonstrates their versatility and the growing confidence of surgeons in utilizing this technology under time-sensitive and high-pressure conditions.

For trauma care, robotic surgery represents the next frontier, particularly for stable patients requiring definitive management of injuries. The enhanced visualization provided by robotic systems is particularly valuable in assessing and addressing injuries to complex anatomical regions, such as the diaphragm or retroperitoneum. Additionally, the improved precision and range of motion offered by robotic instruments allow for meticulous repairs that might be challenging with traditional laparoscopic techniques. Early adoption in select trauma cases has shown promising results, with the potential to combine diagnostic and therapeutic interventions in a single procedure.

As the technology continues to evolve, robotic surgery in trauma care is poised to revolutionize the field, enabling minimally invasive management of injuries that traditionally required open surgery. This approach not only aligns with the principles of damage control surgery by minimizing physiologic stress but also opens the door to expanded applications in the acute care setting. As training programs incorporate robotics into trauma education and evidence continues to build, the role of robotic surgery is expected to grow, paving the way for a new standard of care in emergency and trauma surgery.

References

1. Alkatout I, Mechler U, Mettler L, Pape J, Maass N, Biebl M, et al. The development of laparoscopy—a historical overview. Front Surg. 2021;8:799442.
2. Qayumi K. Surgical techniques: past, present and future. Surg Tech Dev. 2011;2:9.
3. Rosenberg AG. Surgical evolution: development of minimally invasive surgery. Oper Tech Orthop. 2006;16:84–6.
4. Mandrioli M, Inaba K, Piccinini A, Biscardi A, Sartelli M, Agresta F, et al. Advances in laparoscopy for acute care surgery and trauma. World J Gastroenterol. 2016;22:668–80.
5. Nakamura T, Yoshida M, Otani Y, Kameyama K, Ishikawa H, Kumai K, et al. Twelve years' progress in surgery for perforated gastric and duodenal ulcers: a retrospective study of indications for laparoscopic surgery, post-operative course and the influence of candida infection. Aliment Pharmacol Ther. 2006;24:297–302.
6. Ivatury RR, Simon RJ, Stahl WM. A critical evaluation of laparoscopy in penetrating abdominal trauma. J Trauma Inj Infect Crit Care. 1993;34:822–8.
7. Fabian TC, Croce MA, Stewart RM, Pritchard FE, Minard G, Kudsk KA. A prospective analysis of diagnostic laparoscopy in trauma. Ann Surg. 1993;217:557–65. Available from:. https://doi.org/10.1097/00000658-199305010-00017.
8. Friese RS, Coln CE, Gentilello LM. Laparoscopy is sufficient to exclude occult diaphragm injury after penetrating abdominal trauma. J Trauma. 2005;58:789–92. Available from:. https://doi.org/10.1097/01.ta.0000158243.78299.b5.
9. Madiba MDM, Oosthuizen G, Clarke D, Madiba T. Laparoscopy in the diagnosis and repair of diaphragmatic injuries in left-sided penetrating thoracoabdominal trauma: laparoscopy in trauma. Surg Endosc. 2014;29:747–52. Available from:. https://doi.org/10.1007/s00464-014-3710-8.
10. Misra PP, Kumar S, Gupta A, Bansal VK, Sagar S, Mishra B, et al. Role of laparoscopy in patients with abdominal trauma at level-I trauma center. Surg Laparosc Endosc Percutan Tech. 2017;28:20–5. Available from:. https://doi.org/10.1097/sle.0000000000000379.
11. Mohamed AMM, Kabbash MM, Al-Bokhary AAEA, Rayan YMS. Laparoscopy versus laparotomy in the management of abdominal trauma. Surg Pract. 2024;28:122–8.
12. Stefanidis D, Richardson WS, Chang L, Earle DB, Fanelli RD. The role of diagnostic laparoscopy for acute abdominal conditions: an evidence-based review. Surg Endosc. 2008;23:16.
13. Chestovich PJ, Browder TD, Morrissey SL, Fraser DR, Ingalls NK, Fildes JJ. Minimally invasive is maximally effective. J Trauma Acute Care Surg. 2015;78:1076–85.
14. Cho DK, Kim M, Lee D-S, Hong TH, Park H, Joo H. Role of laparoscopic surgery in managing hemodynamically stable abdominal trauma patients: a single level I trauma center, propensity score matching study. Eur J Trauma Emerg Surg. 2024;50(5):2517–25. Available from:. https://doi.org/10.1007/s00068-024-02642-4.
15. Sermonesi G, Tian BWCA, Vallicelli C, Abu-Zidan FM, Damaskos D, Kelly MD, et al. Cesena guidelines: WSES consensus statement on laparoscopic-first approach to general surgery emergencies and abdominal trauma. World J Emerg Surg. 2023;18(1):57. [cited 2024 Dec 19]. Available from:. https://doi.org/10.1186/s13017-023-00520-9.
16. Cirocchi R, Birindelli A, Inaba K, Mandrioli M, Piccinini A, Tabola R, et al. Laparoscopy for trauma and the changes in its use from 1990 to 2016. Surg Laparosc Endosc Percutan Tech. 2018;28:1–12.

17. Hajibandeh S, Hajibandeh S, Gumber AO, Wong CS. Laparoscopy versus laparotomy for the management of penetrating abdominal trauma: a systematic review and meta-analysis. Int J Surg. 2016;34:127–36.
18. Chakravartty S, Sarma DR, Noor MA, Panagiotopoulos S, Patel AG. Laparoscopy has a therapeutic role in the management of abdominal trauma: a matched-pair analysis. Int J Surg. 2017;44:21–5. Available from:. https://doi.org/10.1016/j.ijsu.2017.05.035.
19. Tugnoli SDS, Birindelli A, Podda M, Segalini E, Piccinini A, Coniglio C, et al. Trauma laparoscopy and the six w's: why, where, who, when, what, and how? J Trauma Acute Care Surg. 2018;86:344–67. Available from:. https://doi.org/10.1097/ta.0000000000002130.
20. Atkinson TM, Giraud GD, Togioka BM, Jones DB, Cigarroa JE. Cardiovascular and ventilatory consequences of laparoscopic surgery. Circulation. 2017;135:700–10.
21. Bajwa SJS, Kulshrestha A. Anaesthesia for laparoscopic surgery: general vs regional anaesthesia. J Minimal Access Surg. 2016;12:4–9.
22. Böttger TC, Hermeneit S, Müller M, Terzic A, Rodehorst A, Elad L, et al. Modifiable surgical and anesthesiologic risk factors for the development of cardiac and pulmonary complications after laparoscopic colorectal surgery. Surg Endosc. 2009;23:2016–25.
23. Gutt CN, Oniu T, Mehrabi A, Schemmer P, Kashfi A, Kraus T, et al. Circulatory and respiratory complications of carbon dioxide insufflation. Dig Surg. 2004;21:95–105.
24. Koto MZ, Matsevych OY, Aldous C. Diagnostic laparoscopy for trauma: how not to miss injuries. J Laparoendosc Adv Surg Tech A. 2018;28:506–13. Available from:. https://doi.org/10.1089/lap.2017.0562.
25. Li Y, Xiang Y, Wu N, Wu L, Yu Z, Zhang M, et al. A comparison of laparoscopy and laparotomy for the management of abdominal trauma: a systematic review and meta-analysis. World J Surg. 2015;39:2862–71.
26. Yakuba A, Sitnikov V, Sarkisyan B, Degtirev O, Turbin M, Cherkasov M. Laparoscopy versus laparotomy in management of abdominal trauma. Surg Endosc. 2007;22:228–31. Available from:. https://doi.org/10.1007/s00464-007-9550-z.
27. Josephs LG, Este-McDonald JR, Birkett DH, Hirsch EF. Diagnostic laparoscopy increases intracranial pressure. J Trauma. 1994;36:815–9. Available from:. https://doi.org/10.1097/00005373-199406000-00011.
28. Johnson JJ, Garwe T, Raines A, Thurman JB, Carter S, Bender JS, et al. The use of laparoscopy in the diagnosis and treatment of blunt and penetrating abdominal injuries: 10-year experience at a level 1 trauma center. Am J Surg. 2013;205:317–21. Available from:. https://doi.org/10.1016/j.amjsurg.2012.10.021.
29. Biffl WL, Leppaniemi A. Management guidelines for penetrating abdominal trauma. World J Surg. 2015;39:1373–80.
30. Khubutiya MS, Yartsev PA, Гуляев AA, Levitsky VD, Tlibekova MA. Laparoscopy in blunt and penetrating abdominal trauma. Surg Laparosc Endosc Percutan Tech. 2013;23:507–12. Available from:. https://doi.org/10.1097/sle.0b013e3182937c37.
31. Uranues S, Popa DE, Diaconescu B, Schrittwieser R. Laparoscopy in penetrating abdominal trauma. World J Surg. 2015;39:1381–8.
32. Castrillon GA, Soto JA. Multidetector computed tomography of penetrating abdominal trauma. Semin Roentgenol. 2012;47:371–6.
33. Cinquantini F, Tugnoli G, Piccinini A, Coniglio C, Mannone S, Biscardi A, et al. Educational review of predictive value and findings of computed tomography scan in diagnosing bowel and mesenteric injuries after blunt trauma: correlation with trauma surgery findings in 163 patients. Can Assoc Radiol J. 2017;68:276–85.
34. Cline MR, Cherry-Bukoweiz J, Machado-Aranda D, Chong ST. Diagnostic limits, blind spots, and pitfalls in CT imaging of blunt abdominal trauma. Contemp Diagn Radiol. 2016;39:1–6.
35. Matsushima K, Mangel PS, Schaefer É, Frankel HL. Blunt hollow viscus and mesenteric injury: still underrecognized. World J Surg. 2012;37:759–65. Available from:. https://doi.org/10.1007/s00268-012-1896-2.
36. McDonald AA, Robinson BRH, Alarcon LH, Bosarge PL, Dorion H, Haut ER, et al. Evaluation and management of traumatic diaphragmatic injuries: a practice management guideline from

the eastern association for the surgery of trauma. J Trauma Acute Care Surg. 2018;85:198–207. Available from:. https://doi.org/10.1097/ta.0000000000001924.
37. Berg RJ, Karamanos E, Inaba K, Okoye O, Teixeira PG, Demetriades D. The persistent diagnostic challenge of thoracoabdominal stab wounds. J Trauma Acute Care Surg. 2014;76:418–23. Available from:. https://doi.org/10.1097/ta.0000000000000120.
38. Matthews BD, Bui H, Harold KL, Kercher KW, Adrales G, Park A, et al. Laparoscopic repair of traumatic diaphragmatic injuries. Surg Endosc. 2003;17:254–8. Available from:. https://doi.org/10.1007/s00464-002-8831-9.
39. Koganti D, Hazen BJ, Dente CJ, Nguyen J, Gelbard RB. The role of diagnostic laparoscopy for trauma at a high-volume level one center. Surg Endosc. 2021;35:2667–70.
40. Karateke F, Ozdogan M, Ozyazici S, Das K, Menekse E, Gulnerman YC, et al. The management of penetrating abdominal trauma by diagnostic laparoscopy: a prospective non-randomized study. Ulus Travma Acil Cerrahi Derg. 2013;19:53–7.
41. Taner AS, Topgul K, Kucukel F, Demir A, Sari S. Diagnostic laparoscopy decreases the rate of unnecessary laparotomies and reduces hospital costs in trauma patients. J Laparoendosc Adv Surg Tech. 2001;11:207–11.
42. Ross SE, Dragon GM, O'Malley KF, Rehm CG. Morbidity of negative coeliotomy in trauma. Injury. 1995;26:393–4.
43. Villavicencio RT, Aucar JA. Analysis of laparoscopy in trauma. J Am Coll Surg. 1999;189:11–20.
44. Berg RJ, Inaba K, Okoye O, Pasley J, Teixeira PG, Esparza M, et al. The contemporary management of penetrating splenic injury. Injury. 2014;45:1394–400.
45. Renz BM, Feliciano DV. Unnecessary laparotomies for trauma. J Trauma Inj Infect Crit Care. 1995;38:350–6.
46. Stawicki SP, Kindel TL, Latchana N, Swaroop M, Chaudhry U, Noria S, et al. Laparoscopy in trauma: an overview of complications and related topics. Int J Crit Illn Inj Sci. 2015;5:196. Available from:. https://doi.org/10.4103/2229-5151.165004.
47. Berk JMM, Youngelman D, Berk T. Cost analysis of diagnostic laparoscopy vs laparotomy in the evaluation of penetrating abdominal trauma. Surg Endosc. 1997;11:272–6. Available from:. https://doi.org/10.1007/s004649900342.
48. Lin H-F, Chen Y-D, Lin K-L, Wu MC, Wu CY, Chen S-C. Laparoscopy decreases the laparotomy rate for hemodynamically stable patients with blunt hollow viscus and mesenteric injuries. Am J Surg. 2015;210:326–33.
49. Wang J, Cheng L, Liu J, Zhang B, Wang W, Zhu W, et al. Laparoscopy vs. laparotomy for the management of abdominal trauma: a systematic review and meta-analysis. Front Surg. 2022;9:817134.
50. Kawahara NT, Alster C, Fujimura I, Poggetti RS, Birolini D. Standard examination system for laparoscopy in penetrating abdominal trauma. J Trauma. 2009;67:589–95. Available from:. https://doi.org/10.1097/ta.0b013e3181a60593.
51. Hori Y, Committee SG. Diagnostic laparoscopy guidelines. Surg Endosc. 2008;22:1353–83.
52. Matsevych OY, Koto MZ, Aldous C. Trauma laparoscopy: a prospect of skills training (cohort study). Int J Surg. 2018;55:117–23. Available from:. https://doi.org/10.1016/j.ijsu.2018.05.033.

Minimally Invasive Surgery in Trauma Education from Basics to High Performance

3

Luis Gustavo Capochin Romagnolo, Renato de Mesquita Tauil, and Vinicius Cordeiro Fonseca

Minimally invasive surgery (MIS), notably laparoscopy, is currently the universal route of choice for elective abdominal surgery. Surgeons' exposure to laparoscopy in elective surgeries and increased experience have led to an increase in the adoption of MIS in the emergency setting [1]. The practice of emergency and trauma surgery generally requires dedicated teams with specific skills and competencies, but these may not include training in MIS techniques in their education and training [2]. On the other hand, MIS training in emergency surgery has rarely been investigated. This is probably due to the lack of well-defined benchmarks, standards, and objectives in this field [3].

When first used in trauma, laparoscopy resulted in high rates of undetected injuries (41–77%), generating considerable criticism [4]. However, as the first publications involved studies where the procedures were not standardized, the data is difficult to interpret. In addition, the learning curve of laparoscopic surgery was ignored in the initial evaluations, and surgeons' subjective preferences seem to have determined decisions during laparoscopy [5]. As the use of laparoscopy in stable trauma patients has gained acceptance, the number of scientific publications on this topic has also increased rapidly [6]. This technique is useful in blunt and penetrating trauma. Patients can benefit from shorter hospital stays, less pain, faster recovery, and lower morbidity and mortality rates [1, 7, 8]. Another benefit of using laparoscopy in this scenario is that it can lead to significant savings for the healthcare system [9, 10]. It can be a diagnostic tool to rule out intra-abdominal injuries that may

L. G. C. Romagnolo (✉)
Medical Assistant of Colorectal Department of Barretos Cancer Hospital, Barretos, SP, Brazil

R. de Mesquita Tauil
Full Member of the Brazilian College of Surgeons (TCBC) and Brazilian College of Digestive Surgery (TCBCD), Rio de Janeiro, Brazil

V. C. Fonseca
PhD in Surgery in the Faculty of Medicine of USP (University of São Paulo), São Paulo, Brazil

© The Author(s), under exclusive license to Springer Nature Switzerland AG 2026

M. Cezillo, B. M. Pereira (eds.), *Minimally Invasive Surgery Trauma*,
https://doi.org/10.1007/978-3-032-28971-1_3

be missed by CT scans, such as diaphragmatic injuries; moreover, it can be used to avoid unnecessary laparotomies in patients with penetrating injuries, where a breach of the peritoneum cannot be ruled out clinically or radiologically. Furthermore, in the presence of adequate surgical skills, laparoscopy can play an important therapeutic role [8, 11]. As surgeons gain skill, experience, and confidence, a recent retrospective study carried out at level 1 trauma center showed a progressive increase in the use of laparoscopy at the institution, as well as a progressive expansion of the indications and appreciation of the technique, thanks to its advantages, feasibility, and safety [12]. Although the feasibility and benefits of diagnostic and eventually therapeutic laparoscopy in selected hemodynamically stable trauma patients have already been demonstrated, the role of laparoscopy in this scenario is still under strong debate in the trauma community and the evidence on this topic is poor [7, 8].

Certainly, a laparoscopic approach to trauma should not be carried out unless it is performed by an experienced trauma surgeon who is able to correctly select suitable patients and deal with the immediate need to convert to open procedures, but who also has advanced laparoscopic skills and is confident in his or her ability to properly inspect the abdominal cavity, fully rule out possible injuries, and eventually decide whether to convert to an open procedure after diagnosis, for appropriate treatment, or administer a minimally invasive therapeutic procedure when it is feasible and safe to do so. Furthermore, unlike an elective surgery, the trauma surgeon needs to have the experience to frequently deal with, in addition to the anatomical problem, possible alterations to the patient's physiology, for example, due to blood loss; the existence of other associated injuries, such as pulmonary contusions or head trauma; and also the repercussions of the pneumoperitoneum on the different organs and functions, which can compromise or make the minimally invasive procedure unfeasible.

The indications for the laparoscopic approach to trauma patients are wide-ranging, as is the skill required to perform it in different scenarios, ranging from diagnostic to therapeutic procedures. Emergency laparoscopy generally requires even more proficient camera navigation, as the presence of blood or extravasation of hollow organ contents can often obscure the image on the monitor. It also requires critical skills, such as the ability to mobilize intra-abdominal organs or perform inspection by traversing the intestinal loops quickly and safely to allow proper identification of lesions and their management. Furthermore, in addition to managing intraoperative complications, laparoscopic suturing is an essential technique required in many advanced laparoscopic procedures [13]. In this way, simpler diagnostic procedures such as the assessment of peritoneum violation in penetrating wounds to the anterior abdominal wall are feasible to perform safely by surgeons who have at least the ability to traverse and assess bowel loops, and still bring the benefit of reducing non-therapeutic laparotomies by up to 73%, and their complications [8, 14]. On the other hand, in therapeutic laparoscopies, in addition to basic skills, the surgeon must have expertise in suturing and in performing the different advanced laparoscopy techniques for treating lesions in specific organs, for example, suturing to control bleeding and contamination of the cavity, enterectomies, colectomies, and splenectomies.

Retrospective studies have shown that many surgeons are able to perform minimally invasive surgery in emergency cases, but few patients use this technique [1, 3]. However, surgeons prepared to perform these cases must have reached an adequate and high level of training and proficiency in order to be successful in their procedures. When we mention these emergency cases, we are referring to cases of acute cholecystitis, diverticulitis, appendicitis, cases of perforation of hollow viscera, and some cases of trauma in which the patient is hemodynamically stable [15].

Training surgeons in the minimally invasive technique comes in various forms and models and has been investigated in various ways in studies with impressive results [16]. However, when it comes to trauma training in laparoscopy or even robotics, little has been studied or standardized. Turning specifically to the subject of this chapter, which is training in minimally invasive surgery in trauma, we should basically specify how this training should be carried out, since trauma care in an approach such as this depends on various factors, both for the patient and the surgeon, and, in this case, we are referring to their learning curve in minimally invasive surgery (laparoscopic or robotic).

Several articles have already referred to the ways and difficulties of working with this training in various specialties and have always concluded that more studies are needed to identify the difficulties and remedy them [16].

In a study carried out by the World Society of Emergency Surgery, the learning curve of beginners and senior residents in performing appendectomies using the minimally invasive technique was compared, and it clearly showed a great improvement over the years in medical residency [1]. Therefore, in order to carry out training from beginner to advanced, we have to evaluate how to do it step by step, so that the student can constantly evolve and reach advanced cases safely.

For basic methods, we must follow the initial training rules for everyone, as the concepts are the same. Before starting practical training, it's best to have an initial analysis of the student. This can include an initial assessment or even providing content in classes, whether face-to-face or virtual, with learning assessments in tests afterward. With the results of this theoretical assessment, we can set up the practical activities, which range from cognitive exercises to advanced suturing on synthetic models, and finally live models with simulations of emergency exercises.

1. Cognition exercises (Fig. 3.1)
2. Suturing exercises (Fig. 3.2)
3. Tissue manipulation exercises (Figs. 3.3 and 3.4)

Training should always be carried out with supervision and coordinated activities, respecting the gradual evolution of the surgeon, starting with the handling and manipulation of surgical optics with their various possibilities, moving on to the handling of materials with one hand, and later with the coordination of movements between the two hands. From there, training in suturing with the handling and positioning of the needle should follow, and finally, training in knots and sutures in the various possible positions and techniques.

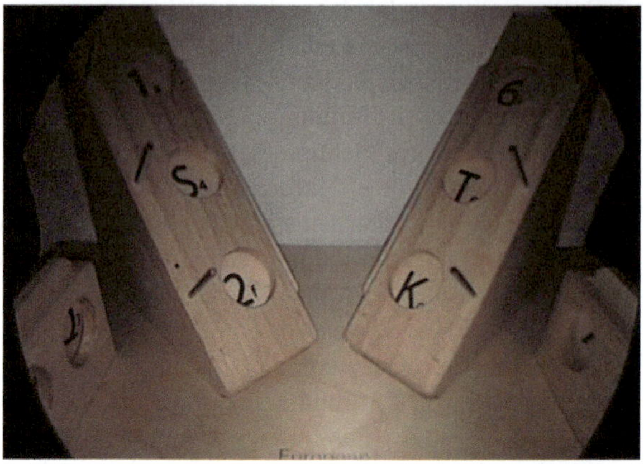

Fig. 3.1 Control training model

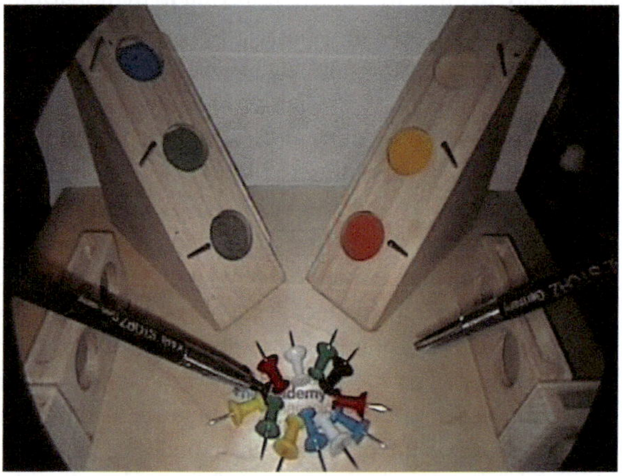

Fig. 3.2 Training model involving needle manipulation techniques at different points, as well as suture training on synthetic material simulating living tissue

All of these dry-lab exercises have one main foundation, which is to create visual and manual skills in surgeons' minds—visual, in other words—because there is a transition from the real image of open surgery to laparoscopic surgery. The notion of depth that we have directly in our eyes is lost when using the image, so this training enables surgeons to use these new platforms. Manual skills would be training with laparoscopic forceps, as we move away from direct hand contact to contact with instruments, and this must be trained through suturing exercises, instrument manipulation, camera positioning, etc.

This is followed by training on live tissue, in order to improve in situations that are increasingly close to reality (traversing intestinal loops, identifying lesions, controlling bleeding and gastrointestinal leaks, etc.), and finally, practice on the patient. At the beginning of the learning curve, this must be accompanied by a proctor (a surgeon with expertise in laparoscopy and trauma), making the training journey possible, accessible and safe.

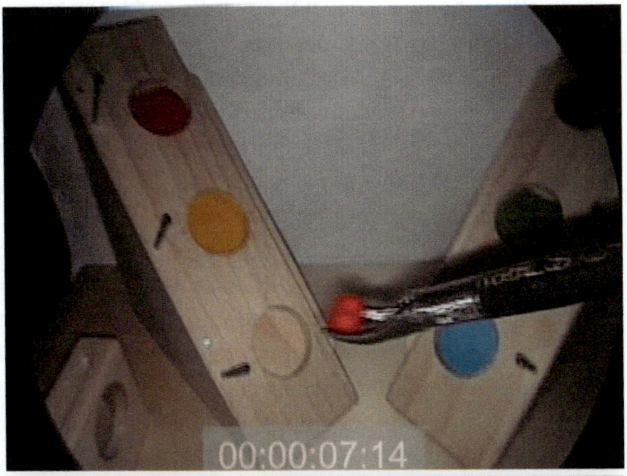

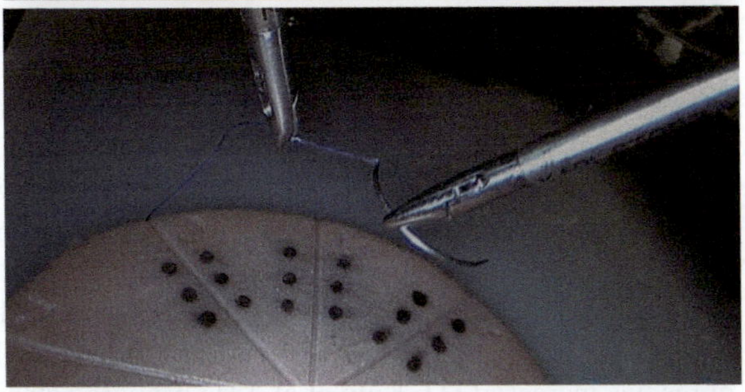

Figs. 3.3 and 3.4 Training model involving manipulation of objects with both hands, as well as control and finesse of movements

Below are some photos of standardized exercises in training courses, which are of great value in training and qualification in minimally invasive surgery.

In addition to training skills in the laboratory, proficiency in performing more complex procedures in a minimally invasive way is not usually acquired only from trauma patients but also from elective surgeries and non-traumatic emergencies. Due to the increasingly established and frequent role of non-operative treatments and interventional radiology, fewer trauma patients are operated on every day. This makes it more difficult for surgeons who work exclusively in trauma to develop, maintain, and improve their surgical skills. In addition, this surgeon will have fewer opportunities to come into contact with new technologies and equipment developed for minimally invasive, laparoscopic and robotic surgery, further distancing him or her from this experience, especially when there are no trauma centers dedicated to providing care and that have specific material and financial resources to invest in new technologies, which have a higher cost, for treating this population. A good emergency general surgeon cannot be fully trained to perform emergency procedures if they are not continually exposed to elective visceral surgical interventions. The need to know the surgical interventions and their possible variations in order to deal with emergency situations requires experience in elective general surgery. In this sense, it seems ideal for surgeons to work with trauma and non-traumatic emergencies, so that they have more opportunities to maintain a volume of surgical cases, which allow them to perfect their skills and learn how to properly use new technologies that can also bring benefits to trauma patients [17]. This type of work also brings greater personal and financial satisfaction to their career [18]. To balance the safety of today's patients with the need to promote procedural competence in future surgeons, a progressive and appropriate training plan based on simulation, proctoring, and surgical fellowships is necessary [1, 3]. All these competencies are encouraged to be taught with multiple sequential, structured and repetitive training modules and sub-modules to allow for a rapid gain in proficiency in laparoscopic skills [19, 20]. Surgical proficiency should be maintained with a minimum caseload [13], and results should be evaluated by adopting an accreditation system to guarantee quality standards. Quality laparoscopic equipment, a well-coordinated trauma team with experience in laparoscopic surgery and strict adherence to the steps previously determined for the procedure play an essential role in ensuring successful laparoscopic procedures.

There is a lack of standardization of the laparoscopic technique in trauma, part of which can be explained by the wide possibility of different scenarios due to multiple injuries or the clinical condition of the patients. In some studies, laparoscopy was used only as a screening tool before laparotomy, without completing a full laparoscopic evaluation. Recent literature, however, has shown that with the selected use of preoperative imaging, advances in technology, improvements in surgical technique and experience, along with the development of a systematic protocol of standardized laparoscopic evaluation with adherence to the predetermined steps of a procedure, the rates of missed lesions have fallen and the rate of therapeutic procedures has increased [1]. Koto et al. [21] proposed standardizing the position of the trocars and a sequence of steps for the complete laparoscopic evaluation of the cavity in order to avoid unnoticed injuries, starting with the right diaphragm and liver, moving on to the left diaphragm and spleen and then going through the entire digestive tract from the stomach to the rectum. In their study, 2 iatrogenic lesions were recorded (1.8%, both treated by laparoscopy); the conversion rate was 1.7% and there were no unnoticed lesions.

References

1. Sermonesi G, Tian B, Vallicelli C, Abu-Zidan FM, Damaskos D, Kelly MD, et al. Cesena guidelines: WSES consensus statement on laparoscopic-first approach to general surgery emergencies and abdominal trauma. World J Emerg Surg. 2023;18(1):57.
2. Ceresoli M, Pisano M, Abu-Zidan F, Allievi N, Gurusamy K, Biffl WL, et al. Minimally invasive surgery in emergency surgery: a WSES survey. World J Emerg Surg. 2022;17(1):18.
3. de'Angelis N, Marchegiani F, Schena CA, Khan J, Agnoletti V, Ansaloni L, et al. Training curriculum in minimally invasive emergency digestive surgery: 2022 WSES position paper. World J Emerg Surg. 2023;18(1):11.
4. Villavicencio RT, Aucar JA. Analysis of laparoscopy in trauma. J Am Coll Surg. 1999;189(1):11–20.
5. Lim KH, Chung BS, Kim JY, Kim SS. Laparoscopic surgery in abdominal trauma: a single center review of a 7-year experience. World J Emerg Surg. 2015;10:16.

6. Coleman L, Gilna G, Portenier D, Auyang E, Khan U, Grabo D, et al. Trauma laparoscopy from 1925 to 2017: publication history and study demographics of an evolving modality. J Trauma Acute Care Surg. 2018;84(4):664–9.
7. Ribeiro Jr MAFAF, Tebar GKTK, Rodrigues Salgueiro JL, Galindo GFC, Hughes JD, Al Sayari A, et al. Role and limitations of laparoscopy in abdominal trauma. Med Res Arch. 2023;11(8)
8. Di Saverio S, Birindelli A, Podda M, Segalini E, Piccinini A, Coniglio C, et al. Trauma laparoscopy and the six w's: why, where, who, when, what, and how? J Trauma Acute Care Surg. 2019;86(2):344–67.
9. Marks JM, Youngelman DF, Berk T. Cost analysis of diagnostic laparoscopy vs laparotomy in the evaluation of penetrating abdominal trauma. Surg Endosc. 1997;11(3):272–6.
10. Taner AS, Topgul K, Kucukel F, Demir A, Sari S. Diagnostic laparoscopy decreases the rate of unnecessary laparotomies and reduces hospital costs in trauma patients. J Laparoendosc Adv Surg Tech A. 2001;11(4):207–11.
11. Zafar SN, Onwugbufor MT, Hughes K, Greene WR, Cornwell EE 3rd, Fullum TM, et al. Laparoscopic surgery for trauma: the realm of therapeutic management. Am J Surg. 2015;209(4):627–32.
12. Birindelli A, Podda M, Segalini E, Cripps M, Tonini V, Tugnoli G, et al. Is the minimally invasive trauma surgeon the next (r)evolution of trauma surgery? Indications and outcomes of diagnostic and therapeutic trauma laparoscopy in a level 1 trauma center. Updat Surg. 2020;72(2):503–12.
13. Bilgic E, Watanabe Y, Nepomnayshy D, Gardner A, Fitzgibbons S, Ghaderi I, et al. Multicenter proficiency benchmarks for advanced laparoscopic suturing tasks. Am J Surg. 2017;213(2):217–21.
14. Kawahara NT, Alster C, Fujimura I, Poggetti RS, Birolini D. Standard examination system for laparoscopy in penetrating abdominal trauma. J Trauma. 2009;67(3):589–95.
15. Menegozzo CAM, Damous SHB, Sabioni GR, Alves PHF, Rasslan R, de Salles Collet ESF, et al. Could trauma laparoscopy be the standard of care for hemodynamically stable patients? A retrospective analysis of 165 cases. Surg Endosc. 2023;37(9):6727–35.
16. Soomro NA, Hashimoto DA, Porteous AJ, Ridley CJA, Marsh WJ, Ditto R, et al. Systematic review of learning curves in robot-assisted surgery. BJS Open. 2020;4(1):27–44.
17. Coccolini F, Sartelli M, Kluger Y, Osipov A, Cui Y, Beka SG, et al. The LIFE TRIAD of emergency general surgery. World J Emerg Surg. 2022;17(1):41.
18. Coleman JJ, Esposito TJ, Rozycki GS, Feliciano DV. Acute care surgery: now that we have built it, will they come? J Trauma Acute Care Surg. 2013;74(2):463–8. discussion 8–9.
19. Jenkins JT, Currie A, Sala S, Kennedy RH. A multi-modal approach to training in laparoscopic colorectal surgery accelerates proficiency gain. Surg Endosc. 2016;30(7):3007–13.
20. Yamada S, Shimada M, Imura S, Morine Y, Ikemoto T, Saito Y, et al. Effective stepwise training and procedure standardization for young surgeons to perform laparoscopic left hepatectomy. Surg Endosc. 2017;31(6):2623–9.
21. Koto MZ, Matsevych OY, Aldous C. Diagnostic laparoscopy for trauma: how not to miss injuries. J Laparoendosc Adv Surg Tech A. 2018;28(5):506–13.

Anesthesiology Care in Laparoscopic Trauma Surgery

4

Leonardo de Andrade Reis, Lais Helena Navarro e Lima, and Rodrigo Moreira e Lima

Background

Trauma is the leading cause of death during the first half of the human lifespan and the fifth leading cause of death across all age groups, significantly impacting global public health [1]. Approximately 25% of all abdominal trauma cases necessitate surgical abdominal exploration or treatment [2] due to the failure of non-operative management or overlooked abdominal injuries, leading to substantial morbidity and mortality. The population requiring emergency general surgery is often elderly, associated with prolonged lengths of stay, poorer outcomes, and a bimodal distribution of death. These factors considerably influence healthcare utilization rates [3]. In the absence of hemorrhagic or septic shock and indications of severe physiological derangement, the appropriate surgical approach in emergency abdominal surgery remains ambiguous. Emergency laparotomy is essential for unstable patients; however, studies have indicated that patients undergoing emergency laparotomy experience the highest rates of morbidity and mortality [4–6]. In recent years, an increasing body of evidence has demonstrated favorable outcomes with the adoption of a laparoscopic approach, when feasible, in emergency general surgery and abdominal trauma patients [7].

Laparoscopy was first introduced as a diagnostic method, primarily used to rule out peritoneal injury or hidden diaphragmatic damage in hemodynamically stable patients suffering from penetrating abdominal trauma. This is particularly relevant in cases of anterior or flank stab wounds and tangential gunshot wounds [8, 9]. By utilizing diagnostic laparoscopy, the rate of unnecessary laparotomies has significantly decreased [10–13]. For patients with penetrating injuries in the upper

L. d. A. Reis (✉)
Latin American Society of Regional Anesthesia, São Paulo, Brazil

L. H. N. e. Lima · R. M. e. Lima
Department of Anesthesia, Perioperative, and Pain Medicine, University of Manitoba, Winnipeg, MB, Canada

© The Author(s), under exclusive license to Springer Nature Switzerland AG 2026

M. Cezillo, B. M. Pereira (eds.), *Minimally Invasive Surgery Trauma*,
https://doi.org/10.1007/978-3-032-28971-1_4

abdomen and lower precordium, the laparoscopic transdiaphragmatic pericardial window has proven to be a safe and effective technique for assessing hemodynamically stable individuals who may have cardiac or abdominal injuries [14, 15]. Based on a 2016 systematic review and meta-analysis of 3362 patients [16], Hajibandeh et al. found that laparoscopy was linked to a significantly lower risk of wound infections and pneumonia, shorter hospital stays, and reduced procedure times, while maintaining a comparable risk of missing injuries in laparotomy cases.

On the other hand, the role of laparoscopy in blunt abdominal trauma has received limited focus [17], leaving its therapeutic potential uncertain due to insufficient research and prevailing views. Nevertheless, some studies suggest that since laparoscopy's introduction for blunt trauma, the rate of unnecessary laparotomies has declined further, and this approach is deemed safe and effective for hemodynamically stable patients with blunt hollow viscus and mesenteric injuries, particularly when executed by skilled surgeons [18, 19]. A meta-analysis from 2022 that compared outcomes of laparoscopy to laparotomy in 5517 hemodynamically stable patients with both penetrating and blunt abdominal trauma [20] revealed no significant differences in missed injuries or mortality rates between the two procedures, with similar risks for intra-abdominal abscesses, thromboembolism, and ileus. However, the laparoscopic group showed a lower frequency of wound infections and pneumonia, alongside shorter procedure and hospitalization durations.

Accordingly, in recent years, the use of therapeutic laparoscopy has grown among trauma patients. A systematic review and meta-analysis of 9817 laparoscopies conducted for abdominal trauma revealed that only 26.2% were converted to laparotomy. The rate of therapeutic laparotomies dropped from 69% to 47.5%, whereas therapeutic laparoscopies increased from 7.2% to 22.7% [21]. This shift has been driven by major improvements in laparoscopic skills and equipment over recent decades. According to the 2022 WSES guidelines on blunt or penetrating bowel injury [22], laparoscopy can be employed in hemodynamically stable patients and identified bowel injuries may be treated laparoscopically depending on the surgeon's expertise and the resources of the trauma center. Recent research has also confirmed the feasibility of laparoscopic interventions, including bowel resection, bowel repair, bladder repair, splenectomy, distal pancreatectomy, diaphragm repair, and hemostasis. These procedures indicate a wide range of scenarios for utilizing laparoscopy in stable patients [23–28]. An international panel of WSES experts, based on the available data, has come to a shared conclusion: for stable patients needing emergency abdominal surgery due to general surgery issues or abdominal trauma, laparoscopy is the preferred initial approach (Grade of recommendation: Strong recommendation, based on moderate-quality evidence, 1B) [7].

However, the use of laparoscopy is restricted by conditions like injuries that necessitate packing, any abdominal wall tissue loss in trauma cases, or situations where the abdomen is overly distended and cannot be expanded further [29]. The repercussions of heightened intra-abdominal pressure and hypercarbia due to carbon dioxide insufflation during laparoscopy are well recognized. Additionally, the essential use of pneumoperitoneum along with extreme patient positioning (for instance, Trendelenburg) can result in metabolic, respiratory, cardiovascular, and neurological changes, which might pose risks to hemodynamically unstable patients awaiting surgery who cannot currently undergo laparoscopic procedures [30–34]. Furthermore, the experience and confidence of surgeons in performing laparoscopy during emergencies, particularly concerning abdominal trauma, continue to be significant hurdles for the technical dissemination and standardization of the procedure. Emergency laparoscopy requires expert camera navigation skills, especially in environments where blood or the contents of hollow organs can frequently obscure visibility. It also necessitates critical skills, such as quickly and safely mobilizing intra-abdominal organs or performing bowel loop inspection ("running loops") to identify and manage injuries effectively [7].

Anesthesia Considerations in Laparoscopic Surgery

Cardiovascular System

In today's era of minimally invasive surgery, the criteria for surgical procedures have become more relaxed, leading to a notable rise in the annual number of laparoscopic surgeries. In the USA alone, laparoscopic surgery accounts for over two million procedures yearly [35]. The overall mortality rate for laparoscopic surgery remains low, estimated between 0.3% and 1.8% [36, 37]. This technique is often employed for higher risk patients, including the elderly, those who are obese, and individuals with preexisting health issues such as cardiovascular and pulmonary diseases. The advantages of laparoscopic surgery over traditional open surgery include reduced trauma, faster recovery, less intraoperative bleeding, improved aesthetic outcomes, and lower postoperative pain levels [38, 39]. As a result, over the past two decades, the application of laparoscopy in emergencies has grown significantly, thanks to improved surgical skills and ongoing technological advancements. Notably, frequently used risk assessment tools, like the Revised Cardiac Risk Index, lack validation for patients undergoing laparoscopic surgery [40]. Furthermore, recognized cardiovascular risk calculators and the American Heart Association/American College of Cardiology perioperative guidelines do not consider a laparoscopic approach when evaluating operative risk [36].

Anesthesia management for trauma patients presents significant challenges due to limited information about existing health conditions, medications, allergies, possible hemodynamic instability, hidden injuries, airway complications, and the short time frame for addressing comorbidities. Nevertheless, collecting all pertinent history alongside a thorough airway evaluation and a brief physical exam is crucial. The pre-anesthetic assessment should begin with checks on the airway, breathing, and circulation. Evaluation and documentation of mental status, focal neurological signs, heart sounds, breath sounds, arterial pressure, pulse rate, airway condition, and skin color (including pallor, icterus, and cyanosis) are essential. Collaboration with the surgeon is necessary to understand the nature and severity of the injuries. Trauma scoring systems like the Injury Severity Score (ISS), Abbreviated Injury

Scale, Revised Trauma Score, and Acute Physiology and Chronic Health Evaluation Score (APACHE) can aid this evaluation.

The trauma management team, composed of the trauma surgeon, anesthesiologists, and emergency physician, must decide which urgent procedures can wait until the patient stabilizes [41]. If feasible, preoperative assessments should be performed, including complete blood count, chest X-ray, lateral cervical spine X-ray, ECG, focused abdominal ultrasound, coagulation profile, and electrolyte levels. Blood grouping and cross-matching must also be conducted, ensuring that sufficient blood supply is available.

The OR needs to be ready for trauma victims. Besides standard OR preparations, specific arrangements for the perioperative management of trauma patients undergoing surgery are essential. Prior to moving the patient, the OR should be heated to 26–28 °C, ensuring sufficient fluids (both colloids and crystalloids), fluid warmers, rapid infusion sets, medications including vasopressors and inotropes, blood and blood products, a cell saver, a forced air warmer, and a difficult airway cart. Emergency medications and airway carts should be easily accessible. The patient should always be transported with supplemental oxygen and proper monitoring, ensuring that the cervical spine is cleared or the neck is stabilized before transportation [42].

While laparoscopic surgery is associated with a lower risk of cardiovascular mortality than open surgery, it is crucial to recognize the specific physiological effects that may increase the likelihood of cardiovascular and respiratory complications in high-risk groups. This includes individuals with congestive heart failure, ischemic heart disease, valvular heart disease, congenital heart disease, and pulmonary hypertension [43]. Understanding the impact of abdominal insufflation at different stages of laparoscopic surgery allows for the identification of patients who may be at higher risk. Strategies to reduce this risk can also be discussed. For example, heart disease is not an outright contraindication for laparoscopic procedures; however, in cases of cardiac dysfunction, maintaining low-pressure insufflation is essential [44, 45]. The most pronounced cardiovascular effects occur when pneumoperitoneum begins, with hemodynamic changes generally negligible in ASA I–II patients at insufflation pressures of 12–14 mmHg. In contrast, these changes can be significant in ASA III-IV patients, who require at least invasive arterial pressure monitoring [46].

Two main factors of CO_2 insufflation significantly impact the cardiovascular, respiratory, and renal systems: increased intra-abdominal pressure (IAP) and hypercarbia [47, 48]. Studies in humans and animals demonstrate that the hemodynamic effects of raised IAP stem from both mechanical and neurohormonal responses [49]. Elevated IAP can result in (1) inferior vena cava compression, (2) aorta compression, (3) reduced blood flow to the splanchnic region, (4) decreased renal blood flow, and (5) diaphragm displacement [34, 50]. The compression of the inferior vena cava due to increased IAP leads to complicated changes in venous return and resistance. In a swine model, inferior vena cava pressure rises alongside IAP, causing an initial elevation in right atrial pressure (RAP), which stabilizes at an IAP of 15 mm Hg [51]. Initially, an increase in venous return leads to an early increase in cardiac output (CO) at an IAP of 5 mm Hg in normovolemic animals; however, as IAP continues to climb, both venous return and CO decrease. This initial rise in venous return is attributed to the compression of the splanchnic vasculature, which shifts blood volume toward the central venous system [51]. As IAP continues to escalate, venous return to the heart reduces because of inferior vena cava compression and venous blood pooling in the lower extremities. Furthermore, hepatic arterial and portal venous blood flow decline, which further reduces splanchnic blood flow and reallocates blood volume to the central venous system, contributing to the sustained increase in RAP [34].

Pneumoperitoneum raises mean arterial pressure (MAP) and systemic vascular resistance (SVR) while potentially reducing cardiac output (CO). Research conducted on healthy subjects has demonstrated a sudden surge in SVR and MAP within the first 5 min of abdominal insufflation, attributed to compression of the abdominal aorta and neuroendocrine responses [34, 50]. Studies have revealed increases in levels of plasma norepinephrine, epinephrine, cortisol, vasopressin, atrial natriuretic peptide, renin, and aldosterone [52]. Reduced renal blood flow occurs due to mechanical compression of the renal arteries from elevated intra-abdominal pressure (IAP) and decreased cardiac output, which triggers renin release [50, 52]. The rise in renin and aldosterone parallels an increase in MAP. Cardiac output fluctuates as IAP increases during abdominal insufflation. While there is an overall trend of decreased CO when IAP exceeds 15 to 20 mm Hg, a biphasic pattern can be observed: an initial increase in CO due to heightened preload is followed by a decrease in CO due to reduced venous return and increased afterload [34]. At IAP levels of 7.5 mm Hg, right atrial pressure (RAP), left atrial pressure (LAP), and CO all rise. As IAP increases to 15 mm Hg and 30 mm Hg, RAP remains elevated, whereas LAP declines but stays above baseline, and CO drops below baseline [51]. This finding defines the critical IAP threshold of 15 mm Hg, where further increases in IAP decrease CO.

TEE has offered additional insights into the cardiac effects of elevated IAP during laparoscopic procedures. It revealed a notable increase in left ventricular preload (measured by left ventricular end-diastolic diameter) and afterload (indicated by left ventricular end-systolic wall stress) within 3 min following abdominal insufflation, along with a reduction in cardiac performance (assessed through fractional area shortening) [53, 54]. However, in healthy subjects, these alterations reverted to baseline after 30 min of insufflation [55].

Identifying patients prone to adverse hemodynamic and ventilatory shifts is crucial for formulating a comprehensive operative plan in coordination with the preoperative consultant, anesthesiologist, and surgeon. Intraoperative patient positioning, intravascular fluid volume, and preexisting cardiovascular conditions—like congestive heart failure, ischemic heart disease, valvular heart disease, congenital heart disease, pulmonary disease, and obesity—can either exacerbate or reduce cardiovascular changes [56]. For individuals with cardiovascular issues, laparoscopic surgery may result in notably increased elevations in RAP and PCWP, along with a reduction in CO [57]. Preoperative strategies to reduce these changes must be established, including sufficient hydration, appropriate positioning, use of the lowest possible IAP, and continuous hemodynamic monitoring.

Patient positioning is vital for the hemodynamic and ventilatory changes experienced during laparoscopy. When patients are placed in the Trendelenburg position, both the diaphragm and abdominal contents shift upward, leading to decreased pulmonary compliance and increased peak airway pressures. Although pulmonary compliance is compromised, the Trendelenburg position boosts venous return and pulmonary capillary wedge pressure (PCWP), aiding in the prevention of cardiac output reduction after abdominal insufflation. The neuroendocrine response associated with the Trendelenburg position features elevated noradrenaline levels and a rise in plasma NT-proANP (N-terminal proatrial natriuretic peptide), which suggests increased atrial stretch caused by increased venous return [52].

Conversely, the reverse Trendelenburg position creates beneficial changes in ventilation but negative effects on the cardiovascular system. This head-up position, combined with increased intra-abdominal pressure for insufflation, reduces venous return, subsequently lowering right atrial pressure (RAP), pulmonary capillary wedge pressure (PCWP), and cardiac output (CO). Additionally, the reverse Trendelenburg position leads to elevated plasma noradrenaline levels, causing increased systemic vascular resistance (SVR) and further diminishing CO [52].

Trauma victims may experience hemodynamic compromise, with its severity influenced by factors such as the nature of the injury, degree of systemic impact, affected organs, and the patient's response to initial resuscitation (whether they are a responder, non-responder, or transient responder). It is crucial to continuously monitor the patient's volume status and adjust fluid therapy accordingly. Securing vascular access is one of the most vital initial steps for trauma patients, particularly those who may need surgical interventions. At least two large-bore peripheral venous catheters (minimum size 18 gauge) should be placed, preferably in the forearm or antecubital region [58]. In cases where obtaining vascular access is difficult or when there is a need for high-risk medications such as vasopressors or inotropes, it is essential to establish central venous or intraosseous access. The key sites for central venous catheter (CVC) insertion include the internal jugular vein, subclavian vein, and femoral vein. Choosing the insertion site involves considering factors like accessibility, the patient's anatomy, and trauma location. The subclavian approach is typically favored as it remains patent during episodes of hypotension, can be done without ultrasound guidance, and has a lower risk of infection. A strong tunica supports the vessel walls and anchors them to adjacent ligaments, fascia, and periosteum, helping to maintain lumen patency [42].

The choice of anesthetic technique for surgery depends on the procedure and duration of the procedure, the patient's hemodynamic status, and whether the stomach is full. Rapid sequence intubation (RSI) is the preferred approach for general anesthesia. The induction agent should be administered in small, titrated doses based on the patient's response. Caution is necessary when giving propofol and thiopentone, as they can cause severe hypotension; thus, they should be used in limited amounts. Etomidate is a suitable option for hemodynamically unstable patients, although it may lead to adrenocortical suppression and myoclonus. It has minimal effects on cardiovascular and respiratory function, positively influencing cerebral perfusion and the oxygen supply-demand ratio when doses remain below 0.25 mg/kg. Ketamine is appropriate as an induction agent for trauma patients; however, in those experiencing severe shock, its cardiac depressant effects can be significant, posing a risk of cardiovascular collapse [59]. Rocuronium is the preferred neuromuscular blocker during RSI, and fentanyl is the favored opioid for these patients. Anesthesia maintenance can be managed with low-concentration volatile anesthetics, total intravenous anesthesia, opioids, and neuromuscular blocking agents [60]. Continuous volume resuscitation is essential to prevent vascular collapse. When hemodynamic changes or ventilation problems occur, the surgeon and anesthetist must assess and correct the surgical laparoscopic settings as a team, if possible, or decide whether to continue a surgical procedure or to discontinue it and convert. Devices for intermittent pneumatic compression of the lower limbs can be used to reduce venous stasis; the reverse Trendelenburg position reduces operation time; finally, stabilizing intravascular volume is beneficial.

Whenever possible, regional anesthetic techniques should be incorporated into managing patients during the perioperative phase, taking into account factors such as the type of surgery, the patient's hemodynamic condition, and whether or not there is coagulopathy or sepsis present [60]. These regional techniques offer several advantages: they mitigate the stress response and protect bowel function while ensuring neurological status remains unaffected. They also improve patient positioning, make painful procedures manageable, enhance patient transport, boost blood circulation, ensure greater patient comfort, diminish the risk of developing opioid tolerance and addiction, positively affect chronic pain conditions, reduce postoperative delirium and stress responses, and lead to shorter stays in the ICU and hospital, ultimately contributing to lower healthcare costs [61].

A hypercoagulable state can develop in severely injured patients, known as "Acute Coagulopathy of Trauma Shock." Several factors may play a role in the development of this coagulopathy. Following trauma, hypoperfusion leads to increased anticoagulation and hyperfibrinolysis due to elevated levels of protein C and tissue plasminogen activator, combined with a reduction in plasminogen activator inhibitor and thrombin-activatable fibrinolysis inhibitor [62]. Patients exhibiting an Injury Severity Score (ISS) over 25, a pH lower than 7.10, a temperature below 34 °C, and systolic blood pressure below 70 mmHg have a 98% chance of experiencing life-threatening coagulopathy [63]. Whether to extubate the trachea or transfer the patient to a critical care unit while keeping the tracheal tube depends on various factors, including the length of surgery, hemodynamic and metabolic stability, arterial lactate levels, preoperative cardiac and pulmonary health, intraoperative blood loss, and transfusion requirements [60].

Finally, desufflation, which involves the removal of CO_2 from the abdominal cavity, along with recovery, marks the concluding steps of anesthesia. Even after desufflation, minute ventilation requirements remain elevated since the body may retain up to 120 L of CO_2. The elimination of CO_2 is managed by the lungs and renal proton excretion [64]. In cases of significant hypercarbia, the anesthesiologist must decide the optimal timing for extubation to ensure effective CO_2 removal. Insufficient

CO_2 elimination can lead to considerable postoperative pain that may radiate to the left shoulder, simulating cardiac chest pain [65]. For healthy individuals, hemodynamic parameters usually return to baseline immediately following desufflation. However, patients with cardiovascular issues may experience prolonged elevations lasting 65 min or more [65]. Among elderly patients with cardiovascular disease, desufflation has been linked to increases in heart rate (HR), cardiac index, left ventricular stroke work index, and ejection fraction, along with a decrease in systemic vascular resistance. In patients with cardiovascular disease undergoing laparoscopic surgery, 20% experienced heart failure within 3 h after the procedure [57]. Those patients who developed heart failure showed a significant reduction in cardiac index (to 65% of baseline), left ventricular stroke work, and stroke volume [34]. Therefore, it is crucial to monitor for signs of myocardial ischemia and heart failure in the period immediately following surgery.

Pulmonary Effects of Pneumoperitoneum on Respiratory Function

Although minimally invasive surgeries, such as laparoscopic procedures, have become more common in trauma patients, the effects of pneumoperitoneum in this group remain under-explored. Current understanding largely stems from studies focused on non-traumatic cases. Investigating how shock and respiratory function interact during laparoscopy can illuminate this surgical method's potential limitations and risks. Generally, laparoscopic surgery minimizes postoperative impacts on respiratory function, facilitating a smoother recovery. Therefore, it can be assumed that these outcomes apply to trauma patients, as only those in stable condition qualify for laparoscopic procedures. Even for patients with COPD, laparoscopic surgeries are considered safe due to improved lung function in the recovery phase [66].

The pneumoperitoneum affects the respiratory system in several ways. The increase in intra-abdominal pressure leads to heightened intrathoracic and intratracheal pressures. This change in intrathoracic pressure can result in air leaks from the endotracheal tube cuff. In a prospective study of 70 patients undergoing elective laparoscopic surgery, Wu et al. observed an increase of 10–15 cmH_2O in endotracheal tube cuff pressures, indicating similar rises in intrathoracic pressures [67]. The diaphragm's cephalic displacement shifts the carina and causes selective positioning of the tracheal tube, complicating lung ventilation. Thus, verifying the endotracheal tube position, checking for leaks, and ensuring bilateral lung ventilation are essential.

Cephalic diaphragm displacement increases intrathoracic pressure, resulting in lung collapse. This leads to atelectasis even with normal blood flow, a condition called shunt. Conversely, some lung areas maintain normal ventilation, and pulmonary hypoxic vasoconstriction causes low blood flow in these regions, known as pulmonary dead space. The interplay of pulmonary shunt and dead space significantly disrupts the ventilation-perfusion (V/Q) relationship, resulting in hypercarbia. The end result is restrictive lung disease, which is marked by reduced residual capacity and vital capacity alongside increased dead space and atelectasis. Hypoxia is rare, as anesthetists generally use high levels of inspired O_2, often around 50%. Monitoring hypercarbia can be difficult; while gasometric evaluation is the ideal parameter, expired CO_2 levels are used to adjust ventilation during anesthesia. Capnography may yield errors, especially in obese patients and those with lung conditions [68].

Ventilation is a challenge as well. Despite current recommendations for protective lung ventilation, the effects of pneumoperitoneum imply enhancements in peak and plateau pressures [69], hypercarbia, and the need for PEEP titration. High PEEP levels reduce venous return, compromising hemodynamics, so the recommendation is to adjust PEEP levels. Low ventilation volume and pressure worsen atelectasis. Adjusting PEEP levels is crucial to prevent pulmonary complications and improve oxygenation [70]. Protective lung ventilation enhances oxygenation and compliance with no incidence of atelectasis [71]. Chen et al., in a review of a randomized controlled trial involving 708 participants, found lower pulmonary complications in the PEEP group compared to the no PEEP group (risk ratio = 0.27, 95% CI: 0.05–1.60; $p = 0.15$) and increased oxygenation and respiratory compliance [72]. Shono et al. found more homogeneous ventilation but no improvement in postoperative lung function using high PEEP levels [73]. Profound neuromuscular block is essential for surgery and allows for lower respiratory pressures, improving respiratory mechanics and lowering interleukin levels [74]. The ultimate effect is protection against inflammation and lung damage. However, setting ventilators is challenging, and any increase in volume or pressure releases more lung energy, potentially causing damage. The concept of drive pressure, which is the pressure that effectively distends the lung (drive pressure is the difference between plateau pressure and PEEP), can provide some insights. Jo et al., in a prospective study with 50 patients scheduled for laparoscopic cholecystectomy, found no difference between volume-guaranteed and volume-controlled ventilation with the same drive pressure [75]. Mechanical power (MP) represents the energy delivered to the lungs during ventilation, and limiting this energy could reduce inflammation. MP can be calculated using ventilator parameters and can be affected by body mass index, surgical position, high PEEP, high lung pressures, and volumes [76].

Electrical impedance tomography effectively optimizes ventilation [77, 78]; however, sensor presence restricts its applicability in laparoscopic surgeries, making it most suitable for the ICU. The best strategy involves adjusting and personalizing PEEP levels [79, 80], as protective lung ventilation helps minimize postoperative pulmonary complications (PPC) [81]. Comparatively, lung recruitment maneuvers do not prevent PPC as effectively as protective ventilation and may negatively impact hemodynamics by diminishing venous return [82]. Griva et al. demonstrate that recruitment maneuvers fail to restore lung compliance to baseline levels during surgery [83], although they might be necessary in certain instances to enhance oxygenation [84].

The head-up position has minimal effect on respiratory function, but the Trendelenburg position exacerbates the effects of pneumoperitoneum. In a prospective study involving 25 patients undergoing robotic surgery compared to 25 patients who underwent laparoscopic surgery, Popescu et al. found significantly elevated plateau pressure and lower compliance in the robotic surgery group, with these differences persisting into the postoperative period [85]. Arterial and expired CO_2 levels were significantly more compromised in the robotic group during and after surgery. The cumulative effect of the head-down position and pneumoperitoneum results in increased peak inspiratory pressure, plateau pressure, driving pressure, and airway resistance, while reducing pulmonary compliance [86].

Carbon dioxide (CO_2) is the main gas employed for creating pneumoperitoneum. While it is absorbed rapidly, the rise in intra-abdominal pressure compresses small vessels, hindering absorption. When pneumoperitoneum is released, the reduction in intracavitary pressure allows for the swift absorption of any remaining gas, which may cause the capnograph to indicate short-term hypercarbia. This occurrence can be risky for patients with traumatic brain injuries, as high CO_2 levels can elevate intracranial pressure. For these individuals, laparoscopic surgery can be detrimental; both Trendelenburg positioning and hypercarbia can worsen intracranial pressure, leading to increased cerebral edema. Also, CO_2 is dry and cold, leading to hypothermia and peritoneum irritation during insufflation. This irritation may necessitate analgesics, resulting in minor side effects. Hypothermia is particularly dangerous in trauma patients as it increases O_2 consumption and can lead to coagulopathies. Coagulopathies can be worsened by hypercarbia and acidosis, with possible bleeding risks, and acidosis is more likely to occur with pneumoperitoneum.

Pneumoperitoneum and Organ Perfusion and Other Physiopathologic Changes

Pneumoperitoneum, a method used in laparoscopic surgery, can impact the renal system, potentially resulting in acute kidney injury (AKI) or postoperative renal dysfunction [87]. Notably, when intraperitoneal pressure surpasses 10 mmHg, it may reduce renal blood flow and cause renal impairment along with transient oliguria. The occurrence of AKI varies widely, with rates from 0.8% to 22.4% [88–91] after abdominal surgeries and from 3.4% to 8.8% following laparoscopic procedures [92–97]. There is an inverse relationship between abdominal blood flow and intra-abdominal pressure (IAP). When IAP exceeds the arterial pressure in abdominal arteries, the perfusion of abdominal organs, including the kidneys and liver, can suffer, leading to diminished venous drainage. This decrease in renal blood flow contributes to lower glomerular filtration, which results in reduced urine output and creatinine retention. Improving intravascular volume may alleviate this issue [98].

Physiological changes in the kidneys, both direct and indirect, are associated with CO_2 insufflation, which activates important mechanical and neurohumoral responses. The kidneys receive regional perfusion through four anatomically distinct vascular zones: the cortex, the outer stripe of the medulla, the inner stripe of the outer medulla, and the inner medulla. A pressure of 20 mmHg during insufflation can lead to a 60% decrease in renal blood flow, which prompts blood to shift from the outer cortex to the juxtamedullary zone. This alteration adversely affects filtration, as most glomeruli are located in the cortex [99].

The pathophysiological hypothesis for kidney damage in surgical patients, particularly those undergoing laparoscopic procedures, involves several mechanisms. These mechanisms include renal hypoperfusion, cellular hypoxia, inflammation, and direct toxicity. The main cause of injury to tubular epithelial cells during kidney hypoperfusion stems from an imbalance between oxygen and nutrient supply and the metabolic demands of renal cells. A critical factor in the reduction of renal perfusion pressure is the drop in mean arterial pressure (MAP), which mirrors the effects of pneumoperitoneum. Specifically, pneumoperitoneum exerts pressure on the renal parenchyma, leading to a significant decline in renal blood flow and increasing the risk of kidney damage during surgery [87].

Pneumoperitoneum is associated with both local and systemic inflammation, acidosis, oxidative stress, changes in the mesothelium lining, and adhesion formation [100].

- Inflammation: The insufflation of CO_2 triggers local and systemic inflammatory responses involving cytokines such as IL-6, IL-1, and TNF-α. The severity of this response is linked to the insufflated gas's pressure, duration, temperature, and humidity. Notably, lower pressure and higher humidity appear to diminish the inflammatory response.
- Acidosis: Insufflation with CO_2 may lead to peritoneal and systemic acidosis, particularly at higher pressures. Employing heated and humidified gas might reduce acidosis effects.
- Oxidative stress: Pneumoperitoneum can trigger ischemia-reperfusion injury, resulting in heightened production of reactive oxygen species (ROS) and oxidative stress. Ensuring sufficient tissue oxygenation—possibly by supplementing oxygen in the insufflated gas—may mitigate oxidative stress.
- Mesothelial injury: The mesothelium, which covers the abdominal cavity, is prone to damage from pneumoperitoneum. This injury, evident through cellular changes such as bulging and clefts, correlates with the gas's pressure, duration, and temperature. Utilizing heated and humidified gas might help protect the mesothelium.
- Adhesion formation: Pneumoperitoneum contributes to the formation of postoperative adhesions. Employing lower pressure insufflations, using heated and humidified gas, and considering ischemic preconditioning may help lessen adhesion development.

Finally, another key change associated with pneumoperitoneum is that elevated intra-abdominal pressure (IAP) can cause gastric contents to be regurgitated, posing a risk of pulmonary aspiration. This issue is particularly critical for obese patients. Furthermore, an increase in IAP also raises intracranial pressure (ICP), which may lead to a reduction in cerebral perfusion pressure (CPP), especially if there is a drop in cardiac output [101].

Final Remarks

Laparoscopic surgery has emerged as a vital technique in contemporary operating rooms, especially for trauma patients, and provides numerous patient benefits. The primary advantage lies in the smaller incisions that result in less tissue damage due to minimally invasive methods. Nevertheless, particular prerequisites, such as extreme positioning and pneumoperitoneum, are necessary, which can pose considerable risks to the patient's physiological state. This can lead to complications not typically encountered in open surgeries and may be challenging to address. It is crucial for the anesthetist to meticulously determine which patients are eligible for these procedures and to be ready for potential intraoperative challenges, although absolute contraindications are infrequent. Additionally, smaller incisions do not automatically equate to reduced pain. Thus, the well-known sayings, "Small incisions do not equal minimal anesthesia" and "There may be minor surgery, but, typically, this is not associated with minor anesthesia," are completely accurate [100], especially in trauma surgery settings.

References

1. Rhee P, Joseph B, Pandit V, Aziz H, Vercruysse G, Kulvatunyou N, et al. Increasing trauma deaths in the United States. Ann Surg. 2014;260:13–21. https://doi.org/10.1097/SLA.0000000000000600.
2. Townsend CM Jr, Beauchamp RD, Evers BM, Mattox KL. Sabiston text book of surgery, the biological basis of modern surgical practice. 18th ed. Philadelphia: Elsevier-Saunders; 2008. p. 512.
3. Knowlton LM, Minei J, Tennakoon L, et al. The economic footprint of acute care surgery in the United States: implications for systems development. J Trauma Acute Care Surg. 2019;86(4):609–16.
4. Donohue SJ, Reinke CE, Evans SL, Jordan MM, Warren YE, Hetherington T, et al. Laparoscopy is associated with decreased all-cause mortality in patients undergoing emergency general surgery procedures in a regional health system. Surg Endosc. 2021;36(6):3822–32. https://doi.org/10.1007/s00464-021-08699-1.
5. NELA Project Team. Fifth patient report of the national emergency laparotomy audit. London: RcoA; 2019.
6. Scott JW, Olufajo OA, Brat GA, Rose JA, Zogg CK, Haider AH, et al. Use of national burden to define operative emergency general surgery. JAMA Surg. 2016;151:e160480. https://doi.org/10.1001/jamasurg.2016.0480.
7. Sermonesi G, Tian BWCA, Vallicelli C, Abu-Zidan FM, Damaskos D, Kelly MD, et al. Cesena guidelines: WSES consensus statement on laparoscopic-first approach to general surgery emergencies and abdominal trauma. World J Emerg Surg. 2023;18:57. https://doi.org/10.1186/s13017-023-00520-9.
8. Fabian TC, Croce MA, Stewart RM, Pritchard FE, Minard G, Kudsk KA. A prospective analysis of diagnostic laparoscopy in trauma. Ann Surg. 1993;217:557–64. Discussion 564–5.
9. Ivatury RR, Simon RJ, Stahl WM. A critical evaluation of laparoscopy in penetrating abdominal trauma. J Trauma. 1993;34:822–7. Discussion 827–8.
10. Simon RJ, Rabin J, Kuhls D. Impact of increased use of laparoscopy on negative laparotomy rates after penetrating trauma. J Trauma. 2002;53:297–302.
11. Chol YB, Lim KS. Therapeutic laparoscopy for abdominal trauma. Surg Endosc. 2003;17:421–7.

12. Kawahara NT, Alster C, Fujimura I, Poggetti RS, Birolini D. Standard examination system for laparoscopy in penetrating abdominal trauma. J Trauma. 2009;67:589–95.
13. Leppäniemi A, Haapiainen R. Occult diaphragmatic injuries caused by stab wounds. J Trauma. 2003;55(4):646–50. https://doi.org/10.1097/01.TA.0000092592.63261.7E.
14. Smith CA, Galante JM, Pierce JL, Scherer LA. Laparoscopic transdiaphragmatic pericardial window: getting to the heart of the matter. J Am Coll Surg. 2011;213:736–42. https://doi.org/10.1016/j.jamcollsurg.2011.09.005.
15. Anderson JE, Salcedo ES, Rounds KM, Galante JM. Getting a better look: outcomes of laparoscopic versus transdiaphragmatic pericardial window for penetrating thoracoabdominal trauma at a level I trauma center. J Trauma Acute Care Surg. 2016;81(6):1035–8. https://doi.org/10.1097/TA.0000000000001173.
16. Hajibandeh S, Gumber AO, Wong CS. Laparoscopy versus laparotomy for the management of penetrating abdominal trauma: a systematic review and meta-analysis. Int J Surg. 2016;34:127–36. https://doi.org/10.1016/j.ijsu.2016.08.524(PEN).
17. Kaban GK, Novitsky YW, Perugini RA, Haveran L, Czerniach D, Kelly JJ, et al. Use of laparoscopy in evaluation and treatment of penetrating and blunt abdominal injuries. Surg Innov. 2008;15:26–31.
18. Lin HF, Chen YD, Chen SC. Value of diagnostic and therapeutic laparoscopy for patients with blunt abdominal trauma: a 10-year medical center experience. PLoS One. 2018;13:e0193379. https://doi.org/10.1371/journal.pone.0193379.
19. Lin HF, Chen YD, Lin KL, Wu MC, Wu CY, Chen SC. Laparoscopy decreases the laparotomy rate for hemodynamically stable patients with blunt hollow viscus and mesenteric injuries. Am J Surg. 2015;210:326–33.
20. Wang J, Cheng L, Liu J, Zhang B, Wang W, Zhu W, et al. Laparoscopy versus laparotomy for the management of abdominal trauma: a systematic review and meta-analysis. Front Surg. 2022;9:817134. https://doi.org/10.3389/fsurg.2022.817134.
21. Cirocchi R, Birindelli A, Inaba K, Mandrioli M, Piccinini A, Tabola R, et al. Laparoscopy for trauma and the changes in its use from 1990 to 2016: a current systematic review and meta-analysis. Surg Laparosc Endosc Percutan Tech. 2018;28:1–12.
22. Smyth L, Bendinelli C, Lee N, et al. WSES guidelines on blunt and penetrating bowel injury: diagnosis, investigations, and treatment. World J Emerg Surg. 2022;17:13. https://doi.org/10.1186/s13017-022-00418-y.
23. Obaid O, Hammad A, Bible L, et al. Open versus laparoscopic repair of traumatic diaphragmatic injury: a nationwide propensity-matched analysis. J Surg Res. 2021;268:452–8. https://doi.org/10.1016/j.jss.2021.07.022.
24. Birindelli A, Martin M, Khan M, et al. Laparoscopic splenectomy as a definitive management option for high-grade traumatic splenic injury when non-operative management is not feasible or failed: a 5-year experience from a level one trauma center with minimally invasive surgery expertise. Updat Surg. 2021;73:1515–31. https://doi.org/10.1007/s13304-021-01045-z.
25. Trejo-Ávila ME, Valenzuela-Salazar C, Betancourt-Ferreyra J, FernándezEnríquez E, Romero-Loera S, Moreno-Portillo M. Laparoscopic versus open surgery for abdominal trauma: a case-matched study. J Laparoendosc Adv Surg Tech A. 2017;27:383–7. https://doi.org/10.1089/lap.2016.0535.
26. Huang GS, Chance EA, Hileman BM, Emerick ES, Gianetti EA. Laparoscopic splenectomy in hemodynamically stable blunt trauma. JSLS. 2017;21:e2017.00013. https://doi.org/10.4293/JSLS.2017.00013.
27. Litwin A, Coulter AP, Romanelli J, Tirabassi M. Use of minimally invasive surgery for the management of hollow viscus traumatic injuries. Surg Endosc. 2022;36(11):8421–9. https://doi.org/10.1007/s00464-022-09102-3.
28. Segalini E, Khan M, Podda M, Gallo G, Morello A, Marziali I, et al. The role of laparoscopic splenectomy in traumatic splenic injury: a narrative review. Minerva Surg. 2023;78(1):76–80. https://doi.org/10.23736/S2724-5691.22.09799-4.
29. Coccolini F, Roberts D, Ansaloni L, et al. The open abdomen in trauma and non-trauma patients: WSES guidelines. World J Emerg Surg. 2018;13:7. https://doi.org/10.1186/s13017-018-0167-4.

30. Sharma KC, Brandstetter RD, Brensilver JM, Jung LD. Cardiopulmonary physiology and pathophysiology as a consequence of laparoscopic surgery. Chest. 1996;110:810–5.
31. Gutt C, Oniu T, Mehrabi A, Schemmer P, Kashfi A, Kraus T, et al. Circulatory and respiratory complications of carbon dioxide insufflation. Dig Surg. 2004;21:95–105. https://doi.org/10.1159/000077038.
32. Böttger TC, Hermeneit S, Muller M, Terzic A, Rodehorst A, Elad L, et al. Modifiable surgical and anesthesiologic risk factors for the development of cardiac and pulmonary complications after laparoscopic colorectal surgery. Surg Endosc. 2009;23:2016–25. https://doi.org/10.1007/s00464-008-9916-x.
33. Bajwa SJS, Kulshrestha A. Anaesthesia for laparoscopic surgery: general versus regional anaesthesia. J Minimal Access Surg. 2016;12:4–9. https://doi.org/10.4103/0972-9941.169952.
34. Atkinson TM, Giraud GD, Togioka BM, Jones DB, Cigarroa JE. Cardiovascular and ventilatory consequences of laparoscopic surgery. Circulation. 2017;135(7):700–10. https://doi.org/10.1161/CIRCULATIONAHA.116.023262.
35. Tsui C, Klein R, Garabrant M. Minimally invasive surgery: national trends in adoption and future directions for hospital strategy. Surg Endosc. 2013;27:2253–7. https://doi.org/10.1007/s00464-013-2973-9.
36. Fleisher LA, Fleischmann KE, Auerbach AD, Barnason SA, Beckman JA, Bozkurt B, et al. 2014 ACC/AHA guideline on perioperative cardiovascular evaluation and management of patients undergoing noncardiac surgery: a report of the American College of Cardiology/American Heart Association Task Force on practice guidelines. Circulation. 2014;130:e278–333. https://doi.org/10.1161/CIR.0000000000000106.
37. Aminian A, Brethauer SA, Kirwan JP, Kashyap SR, Burguera B, Schauer PR. How safe is metabolic/diabetes surgery? Diabetes Obes Metab. 2015;17:198–201. https://doi.org/10.1111/dom.12405.
38. Antoniou SA, Antoniou GA, Koch OO, Pointner R, Granderath FA. Meta-analysis of laparoscopic vs open cholecystectomy in elderly patients. World J Gastroenterol. 2014;20:17626–34.
39. Kuhry E, Jeekel J, Bonjer HJ. Effect of laparoscopy on the immune system. Semin Laparosc Surg. 2004;11:37–44.
40. Lee TH, Marcantonio ER, Mangione CM, Thomas EJ, Polanczyk CA, Cook EF, et al. Derivation and prospective validation of a simple index for prediction of cardiac risk of major noncardiac surgery. Circulation. 1999;100:1043–9.
41. Dutton RP, Scalea TM, Aarabi B. Prioritizing surgical needs in patients with multiple injuries. Probl Anesth. 2001;13:311.
42. Fort AC, Zack-Guasp RA. Anesthesia for patients with extensive trauma. Anesthesiol Clin. 2020;38:135–48. https://doi.org/10.1016/j.anclin.2019.10.012.
43. Boersma E, Kertai MD, Schouten O, Bax JJ, Noordzij P, Steyerberg EW, et al. Perioperative cardiovascular mortality in noncardiac surgery: validation of the Lee cardiac risk index. Am J Med. 2005;118:1134–41. https://doi.org/10.1016/j.amjmed.2005.01.064.
44. Agresta F, Ansaloni L, Baiocchi GL, et al. Laparoscopic approach to acute abdomen from the consensus development conference of the Società Italiana di Chirurgia Endoscopica e nuove tecnologie (SICE), Associazione Chirurghi Ospedalieri Italiani (ACOI), Società Italiana diChirurgia (SIC), Società Italiana di Chirurgia d'Urgenza e del Trauma (SICUT), Società Italiana di Chirurgia nell'Ospedalità Privata (SICOP), and the European Association for Endoscopic Surgery (EAES). Surg Endosc. 2012;26:2134–64.
45. Naitoh T, et al. Emergency laparoscopic cholecystectomy for a patient with an implantable left ventricular assist device: report of a case. Surg Today. 2013;43:313–6.
46. Neudecker J, et al. The European Association for Endoscopic Surgery clinical practice guideline on the pneumoperitoneum for the laparoscopic surgery. Surg Endosc. 2002;16:1121–43.
47. Kashtan J, Green JF, Parsons EQ, Holcroft JW. Hemodynamic effect of increased abdominal pressure. J Surg Res. 1981;30:249–55.

48. Cullen DJ, Coyle JP, Teplick R, Long MC. Cardiovascular, pulmonary, and renal effects of massively increased intra-abdominal pressure in critically ill patients. Crit Care Med. 1989;17:118–21.
49. Odeberg-Wernerman S. Laparoscopic surgery: effects on circulatory and respiratory physiology: an overview. Eur J Surg Suppl. 2000;166:4–11.
50. O'Malley C, Cunningham AJ. Physiologic changes during laparoscopy. Anesthesiol Clin North Am. 2001;19:1–19.
51. Kitano Y, Takata M, Sasaki N, Zhang Q, Yamamoto S, Miyasaka K. Influence of increased abdominal pressure on steady-state cardiac performance. J Appl Physiol. 1999;86:1651–6.
52. Hirvonen EA, Nuutinen LS, Vuolteenaho O. Hormonal responses and cardiac filling pressures in head-up or head-down position and pneumoperitoneum in patients undergoing operative laparoscopy. Br J Anaesth. 1997;78:128–33.
53. Branche PE, Duperret SL, Sagnard PE, Boulez JL, Petit PL, Viale JP. Left ventricular loading modifications induced by pneumoperitoneum: a time course echocardiographic study. Anesth Analg. 1998;86:482–7.
54. Larsen JF, Svendsen FM, Pedersen V. Randomized clinical trial of the effect of pneumoperitoneum on cardiac function and haemodynamics during laparoscopic cholecystectomy. Br J Surg. 2004;91:848–54. https://doi.org/10.1002/bjs.4573.
55. Joris JL, Noirot DP, Legrand MJ, Jacquet NJ, Lamy ML. Hemodynamic changes during laparoscopic cholecystectomy. Anesth Analg. 1993;76:1067–71.
56. Hein HA, Joshi GP, Ramsay MA, Fox LG, Gawey BJ, Hellman CL, et al. Hemodynamic changes during laparoscopic cholecystectomy in patients with severe cardiac disease. J Clin Anesth. 1997;9:261–5.
57. Portera CA, Compton RP, Walters DN, Browder IW. Benefits of pulmonary artery catheter and transesophageal echocardiographic monitoring in laparoscopic cholecystectomy patients with cardiac disease. Am J Surg. 1995;169:202–6.
58. American College of Surgeons' Committee on Trauma. Advanced trauma life support. 10th ed. Chicago: American College of Surgeons; 2018.
59. Dutton RP, McCunn M, Grissom TE. Anaesthesia for trauma. In: Miller RD, editor. Miller: Miller's anaesthesia. 10th ed. New York: Churchill Livingstone; 2024.
60. Dattari R, Jain VK, Iyengar KP, Vaishya R, Garg R. Anaesthetic considerations in polytrauma patients. J Clin Orthop Traum. 2021;12:50–7.
61. Malchow RJ, Black IH. The evolution of pain management in the critically ill trauma patient: emerging concepts from the global war on terrorism. Crit Care Med. 2008;36:S346–57.
62. Sorensen B, Fries D. Emerging treatment strategies for trauma-induced coagulopathy. Br J Surg. 2012;99(Suppl 1):40–50.
63. Savioli G, Ceresa IF, Macedonio S, et al. Trauma coagulopathy and its outcomes. Medicina. 2020;56:205.
64. Henny CP, Hofland J. Laparoscopic surgery: pitfalls due to anesthesia, positioning, and pneumoperitoneum. Surg Endosc. 2005;19:1163–71. https://doi.org/10.1007/s00464-004-2250-z.
65. Beaver J, Safran D. Pneumopericardium mimicking acute myocardial ischemia after laparoscopic cholecystectomy. South Med J. 1999;92:1002–4.
66. Gautam N, Harjai M, Rai P, Tripathi M, Malviya M, Singh AK. Anaesthetic management and physiologic effects of pneumoperitoneum in patients with chronic obstructive pulmonary disease. Cureus. 2023;15:e46458. https://doi.org/10.7759/cureus.46458.
67. Wu CY, Yeh YC, Wang MC, Lai CH, Fan SZ. Changes in endotracheal tube cuff pressure during laparoscopic surgery in head-up or head-down position. BMC Anesthesiol. 2014;14:75. https://doi.org/10.1186/1471-2253-14-75.
68. Kwak HJ, Park SK, Lee KC, Lee DC, Kim JY. High positive end-expiratory pressure preserves cerebral oxygen saturation during laparoscopic cholecystectomy under propofol anesthesia. Surg Endosc. 2013;27:415–20.
69. Suh MK, Seong KW, Jung SH, Kim SS. The effect of pneumoperitoneum and Trendelenburg position on respiratory mechanics during pelviscopic surgery. Korean J Anesthesiol. 2010;59:329–34.

70. Yessenbayeva GA, Yukhnevich YA, Khamitova ZK, Kim SI, Zhumabayev MB, Berdiyarova GS, et al. Impact of a positive end-expiratory pressure strategy on oxygenation, respiratory compliance, and hemodynamics during laparoscopic surgery in non-obese patients: a systematic review and meta-analysis of randomized controlled trials. BMC Anesthesiol. 2023;23:371.
71. Nguyen TK, Nguyen VL, Nguyen TG, Mai DH, Nguyen NQ, Vu TA, et al. Lung-protective mechanical ventilation for patients undergoing abdominal laparoscopic surgeries: a randomized controlled trial. BMC Anesthesiol. 2021;21:95. https://doi.org/10.1186/s12871-021-01318-5.
72. Chen C, Shang P, Yao Y, et al. Positive end-expiratory pressure and postoperative pulmonary complications in laparoscopic bariatric surgery: systematic review and meta-analysis. BMC Anesthesiol. 2024;24:282. https://doi.org/10.1186/s12871-024-02658-8.
73. Shono A, Katayama N, Fujihara T, Böhm S, Waldmann A, Ugata K, et al. Positive end-expiratory pressure and distribution of ventilation in pneumoperitoneum combined with steep. Anesthesiology. 2020;132:476–90.
74. Kim JE, Min SK, Ha E, Lee D, Kim JY, Kwak HJ. Effects of deep neuromuscular block with low-pressure pneumoperitoneum on respiratory mechanics and biotrauma in a steep Trendelenburg position. Sci Rep. 2021;11:1935.
75. Jo YY, Chang YJ, Lee D, Kim YB, Jung J, Kwak HJ. Comparisons of mechanical power and respiratory mechanics in pressure-controlled ventilation and volume-controlled ventilation during laparoscopic cholecystectomy in elderly patients. J Pers Med. 2023;13:201.
76. Tharp WG, Neilson MR, Breidenstein MW, Harned RG, Chatfield SE, Friend AF, et al. Effects of obesity, pneumoperitoneum, and body position on mechanical power of intraoperative ventilation: an observational study. J Appl Physiol. 2023;34:1390–402.
77. Borges JB, Suarez-Sipmann F, Bohm SH, Tusman G, Melo A, Maripuu E, et al. Regional lung perfusion estimated by electrical impedance tomography in a piglet model of lung collapse. J Appl Physiol. 2012;112:225–36.
78. Rauseo M, Spadaro S, Mirabella L, Cotoia A, Laforgia D, Gaudino G, et al. Electrical impedance tomography during abdominal laparoscopic surgery: a physiological pilot study. J Clin Med. 2023;12:7467.
79. Mazzinari G, Dias-cambronero O, Alonso-Iñigo JM, Garcia Gregorio N, Ayas Montero B, Ibañez JL, et al. Intraabdominal pressure targeted positive end-expiratory pressure during laparoscopic surgery. Anesthesiology. 2020;132:667–77.
80. Li X, Liu H, Wang J, Ni ZL, Liu ZX, Jiao JL, et al. Individualized positive end-expiratory pressure on postoperative atelectasis in patients with obesity: a randomized controlled clinical trial. Anesthesiology. 2023;139:262–73.
81. Sun M, Jia R, Wang L, Sun D, Wei M, Wang T, et al. Effect of protective lung ventilation on pulmonary complications after laparoscopic surgery: a meta-analysis of randomized controlled trials. Front Med. 2023;10:1171760.
82. Jo YY, Lee KC, Chang YJ, Jung WS, Park J, Kwak HJ. Effects of an alveolar recruitment maneuver during lung protective ventilation on postoperative pulmonary complications in elderly patients undergoing laparoscopy. Clin Interv Aging. 2020;15:1461–9.
83. Griva P, Talliou C, Rougeris L, Samara D, Panagouli K, Varvarousi G, et al. Restoration of pulmonary compliance after laparoscopic gynecologic surgery using a recruitment maneuver. J Pers Med. 2024;14:451.
84. Parmeswaran P, Gupta P, Ittoop AL, Kaushal A, Kumar A, Singla D, et al. Effect of intraoperative alveolar recruitment maneuver on intraoperative oxygenation and postoperative pulmonary function tests in patients undergoing robotic-assisted hysterectomy: a single-blind randomized study. Braz J Anesthesiol. 2023;73:418–25.
85. Popescu M, Olita MR, Stefan MO, Mihaila M, Sima RM, Tomescu D. Lung mechanics during video-assisted abdominal surgery in Trendelenburg position: a cross-sectional propensity-matched comparison between classic laparoscopy and robotic-assisted surgery. BMC Anesthesiol. 2022;22:356. https://doi.org/10.1186/s12871-022-01900-5.

86. Cheng M, Ni L, Huang L, Zhou Y, Wang K. Effect of positive end-expiratory pressure on pulmonary compliance and pulmonary complications in patients undergoing robot-assisted laparoscopic radical prostatectomy: a randomized control trial. BMC Anesthesiol. 2022;22:347. https://doi.org/10.1186/s12871-022-01869-1.
87. Villa G, Fiorentino M, Cappellini LS, De Rosa S. Renal implications of pneumoperitoneum in laparoscopic surgery: mechanisms, risk factors, and preventive strategies. Korean J Anesthesiol. 2024;77:575–86. https://doi.org/10.4097/kja.24011.
88. Kim M, Brady JE, Li G. Variations in the risk of acute kidney injury across intraabdominal surgery procedures. Anesth Analg. 2014;119:1121–32.
89. Kheterpal S, Tremper KK, Englesbe MJ, O'Reilly M, Shanks AM, Fetterman DM, et al. Predictors of postoperative acute renal failure after noncardiac surgery in patients with previously normal renal function. Anesthesiology. 2007;107:892–902.
90. Teixeira C, Rosa R, Rodrigues N, Mendes I, Peixoto L, Dias S, et al. Acute kidney injury after major abdominal surgery: a retrospective cohort analysis. Crit Care Res Pract. 2014;2014:132175.
91. Long TE, Helgason D, Helgadottir S, Palsson R, Gudbjartsson T, Sigurdsson GH, et al. Acute kidney injury after abdominal surgery: incidence, risk factors, and outcome. Anesth Analg. 2016;122:1912–20.
92. Sim JH, Kang SJ, Bang JY, Song JG. Comparison of the effects of laparoscopic and open surgery on postoperative acute kidney injury in patients with colorectal cancer: propensity score analysis. J Clin Med. 2021;10:1438.
93. Abdullah HR, Tan TP, Vaez M, Deb C, Farag N, Jackson TD, et al. Predictors of perioperative acute kidney injury in obese patients undergoing laparoscopic bariatric surgery: a single-centre retrospective cohort study. Obes Surg. 2016;26:1493–9.
94. Srisawat N, Kongwibulwut M, Laoveeravat P, Lumplertgul N, Chatkaew P, Saeyub P, et al. The role of intraoperative parameters on predicting laparoscopic abdominal surgery associated acute kidney injury. BMC Nephrol. 2018;19:289.
95. Tang Y, Li B, Ouyang W, Jiang G, Tang H, Liu X. Intraoperative hypertension is associated with postoperative acute kidney injury after laparoscopic surgery. J Pers Med. 2023;13:541.
96. Paek JH, Kang SI, Ryu J, Lim SY, Ryu JY, Son HE, et al. Renal outcomes of laparoscopic versus open surgery in patients with rectal cancer: a propensity score analysis. Kidney Res Clin Pract. 2021;40:634–44.
97. Park YS, Jun IG, Go Y, Song JG, Hwang GS. Comparison of acute kidney injury between open and laparoscopic pylorus-preserving pancreaticoduodenectomy: propensity score analysis. PLoS One. 2018;13:e0202980.
98. Moon YJ, Jun IG, Kim KH, Kim SO, Song JG, Hwang GS. Comparison of acute kidney injury between open and laparoscopic liver resection: propensity score analysis. PLoS One. 2017;12:e0186336.
99. Hottenrott S, Schlesinger T, Helmer P, Meybohm AI, Kranke P. Do small incisions need only minimal anesthesia?—anesthetic management in laparoscopic and robotic surgery. J Clin Med. 2020;9:4058. https://doi.org/10.3390/jcm9124058.
100. Umano GR, Delehaye G, Noviello C, Papparella A. The "Dark Side" of pneumoperitoneum and laparoscopy. Minim Invasive Surg. 2021;2021:5564745. https://doi.org/10.1155/2021/5564745.
101. Perrin M, Fletcher A. Laparoscopic abdominal surgery. Contin Educ Anaesth Crit Care Pain. 2004;4:107–10.

Equipment and Materials: From Hardware to High Technology Materials on Laparoscopy

5

Marcus Cezillo, Robson Uwagoya, Anna Gabriela Santana de Lacerda, and José Ciongoli

Introduction

In trauma videolaparoscopic surgery, surgical instruments have been designed, developed, and structured to enable feasible procedures while respecting the clinical stability of the traumatized patient and the organization of the surgical team. The goal is to perform the procedure in the most minimally invasive manner possible, with precision and efficiency. The evolution of surgery has shown us an objective focus on precision and efficiency in surgical instrumentation, which plays a crucial role in the effectiveness and resolution of traumatic injuries. Advances in cutting-edge technology have led to safer and more cost-effective solutions. In this way, technology has created surgical environments that are less dependent on a master trauma surgeon, allowing general surgeons working in remote locations far from major trauma centers, and with less exposure to large traumatic events, to safely manage traumatic situations in their operating rooms. This is made possible through digital instrumentation with actions transmitted by electronic components capable of tissue analysis [1].

When we think about the proposal to use minimally invasive videolaparoscopic surgery in controlled trauma scenarios, there is a growing need for a properly trained

M. Cezillo (✉)
Trauma Surgery Department, Hospital de Base do Distrito Federal (HBDF), Brasília, DF, Brazil

R. Uwagoya
Department of Pediatric Surgery at GPEC, FAM (Centro Universitário das Américas) Department of Medicine, São Paulo, Brazil

A. G. S. de Lacerda
General Practitioner, FAM (Centro Universitário das Américas) Department of Medicine, São Paulo, Brazil

J. Ciongoli
Professor of the Department of Anatomy and Operative Technique, School of medicine of the ENIAC University, Guarulhos, Brazil

© The Author(s), under exclusive license to Springer Nature Switzerland AG 2026

M. Cezillo, B. M. Pereira (eds.), *Minimally Invasive Surgery Trauma*,
https://doi.org/10.1007/978-3-032-28971-1_5

team. The effectiveness of trauma management must include a surgical team, anesthetic support, a skilled surgical technologist, and qualified nursing staff responsible for monitoring and controlling the equipment hardware external to the surgical field. This multidisciplinary team is essential for ensuring greater patient and procedural safety, conducting a checklist of all devices and instruments while adhering to safe surgery protocol principles [2].

Since bioengineering has become integrated into surgery, hardware evolution has shown no signs of technological stagnation, particularly in imaging dynamics and digitalization. Initially, purely diagnostic imaging, with poorly defined vision limited by the telescope through natural orifices, was introduced in urology, gynecology, and proctology, followed by laparoscopy and thoracoscopy—practically without proper internal lighting. Today, we have striking high-definition images in 3D, 4 K, and 8 K, with increasingly impressive brightness, providing embryological tissue approximations that allow for anatomopathological diagnoses and even the visualization of perfusion and lymphatic networks in traumatized tissues or during visceral sutures and anastomoses through Firefly® filter technology [3],[4].

Videolaparoscopic Surgery Hardwares

Cameras

High-definition cameras, especially 4 K and beyond, have transformed the way surgeons visualize procedures. 4 K resolution (3840 × 2160 pixels) offers stunning clarity, making it easier to see fine details compared to Full HD. This means sharper, more precise images, enhancing safety and efficiency in minimally invasive surgeries.

For situations that demand ultra-high definition, such as large screens at medical conferences, 8 K resolution (7680 × 4320 pixels) allows for incredible magnification without losing image quality—a game-changer for teaching and live demonstrations. These cameras are usually attached to telescopes, also known as endoscopes, but newer models integrate a distal illumination chip and a 90-degree viewing angle that automatically adapts to movement. This makes them almost a flexible endoscopic optic, giving surgeons even more control. The traditional rigid telescopes are still widely used, available in 0, 30, and 45-degree angles, with thinner and more durable designs that keep up with the demands of modern surgery [5].

3D Imaging Systems

Three-dimensional equipment provides an image that allows a superior depth perception compared to previous two-dimensional (2D) imaging systems, which is essential for visual assessments of tissue trauma intensity, resulting in an important tool for therapeutic decision-making. The types of imaging systems include stereoscopic cameras, which use two lenses to capture images from different angles, creating a three-dimensional effect, as well as depth cameras that use sensors to measure the distance between structures, a device used in augmented reality situations [6].

Image Processors

Used in minimally invasive surgery, image processors play a crucial role in visualization and analysis during procedures. The most common types are video processors used to capture images from endoscopic cameras and process them in real time. Three-dimensional image processors create images from two-dimensional data, allowing visualization with greater depth perception and definition of structures, even down to the point of "embryological" macroscopic differentiation in high-definition devices [7].

Real-time image processors analyze and instantly enhance image quality by applying filters and corrections, digitizing the image, and enabling the assessment of tissue perfusion, bile flow, and even pathological characteristics of structures under investigation [8].

Image processors can also benefit from Artificial Intelligence (AI), utilizing algorithms to assist in identifying anatomical structures and detecting anomalies through scanning and surgical navigation systems. This system integrates images from different sources, such as CT scans and MRI devices, to guide surgical instruments like robotic arm forceps and laparoscopic forceps with greater precision and efficiency [9, 10].

High-Resolution Monitors

Supporting 4 K or higher resolutions and even 3D, with high refresh rates, these monitors offer clear and precise visualization, ensuring compatibility with the other equipment configurations [11].

Data Integration Platform

Systems that connect different devices to each other and enable real-time data sharing enhance performance and problem-solving capabilities in collaboration between medical and surgical teams. These platforms are designed to collect, process, and analyze data from various sources, including clinical data management systems that integrate patient information such as medical history, exams, and results, medical imaging systems transmitting information from digitized sensors, guiding the surgeon toward the goal of their procedure while preventing damage to adjacent tissues, and real-time monitoring systems that allow for faster and safer decision-making by providing access to critical patient data, particularly in trauma cases [12].

Advanced Endoscopes

Equipped with led lighting and increasingly smaller high-definition miniature cameras, these provide clear images and a wide field of view with depth of field at the examined site. Some feature automatic zoom mechanisms without the need for manual entry and exit adjustments via the trocar. As described above, there is also a high-tech camera integrated with the telescope as a single piece, featuring a distal illumination chip via led and a 90-degree digitally maneuvered viewing angle, effectively creating a flexible endoscopic optic. Traditional endoscopes remain rigid with 0, 30, and 45-degree angles. The latest endoscopes are built with three-dimensional high-definition camera technology, which, as mentioned earlier, provides a three-dimensional view of the surgical field, enhancing depth perception and precision during surgery, similar to those currently used in robotic surgery. Others are composed of spectral imaging technology, utilizing different wavelengths to identify abnormal tissues, offering a highly compatible method with histopathological diagnosis [13].

Augmented Reality Tools

Augmented Reality (AR) is a technology that overlays digital information onto the real visual field, assisting in surgical navigation. It has proven to be a valuable tool in minimally invasive surgeries, offering various functionalities that enhance precision and efficacy [14]. Despite the actual advancements in digital technology, these tools are rapidly evolving due to the continuous process.

These tools include:

- AR displays: Devices such as smart glasses that overlay digital images onto the surgeon's view, allowing real-time visualization of the structures being operated on [14, 15].
- Surgical navigation systems: Platforms that utilize AR to guide surgical instruments with precision, integrating preoperative imaging data [14, 15].
- Mobile applications: Tools that provide surgeons with real-time access to information relevant to the procedure [15].
- Interactive 3D models: Three-dimensional representations of organs or structures that can be manipulated for a better understanding of the patient's anatomy [14, 15].

Robotic Surgery

Robotic systems offer greater precision and control over surgical movements, including wrist rotations and tremor elimination. Proper training is essential to fully utilize these systems, making procedures safer and more dynamic. These technological advancements significantly improve the efficacy and reproducibility of minimally invasive interventions, reducing learning curves and financial investment, despite high institutional implementation costs [16].

In Brazil, the use of these advanced technologies in trauma surgeries is still limited, primarily present in institutions that prioritize patient safety and invest in technology to mitigate the consequences of functional incapacity and preventable deaths [16, 17].

Main benefits of robotic surgery:

- Precision in complex surgeries: Robotic technology allows for more stable and precise movements, reducing the risk of adverse events in critical situations. It is especially useful in emergency procedures involving anatomically difficult-to-access areas [16, 17].
- Reduction of surgical trauma: Minimizes the metabolic stress caused by traumatic events, reducing blood loss and, consequently, the need for transfusions, leading to faster recovery [16].
- Access to hard-to-reach anatomical sites: Robotic arms can reach areas that would be difficult or risky using conventional techniques [16].
- Agility in diagnosis and resolution in trauma surgeries: Enhances speed and precision in decision-making in cases of acute abdominal pain [16].
- Reduced surgeon fatigue: Improved ergonomics and comfort at the console allow for prolonged and efficient surgical performance in complex trauma cases [16, 17].
- Integration with imaging technology: AR-based software integrates with CT scans, MRIs, and ultrasounds to improve surgical planning and execution in emergency contexts [17].
- Remote surgery capability: When a specialist cannot be physically present, robotic surgery allows an experienced surgeon to perform procedures remotely. There have been reported cases where the surgeon operated from up to 3000 km away [17].

For these advancements to be successful, high-cost investments are necessary. Equipment quickly becomes obsolete due to constant technological development, requiring a multidisciplinary team with specialized training and impeccable infrastructure to ensure the rapid and efficient deployment of robotic systems in emergency operating rooms [16, 17].

Despite these challenges, the continuous evolution of technology motivates the expansion of robotic surgery in emergency, urgent, and trauma care [16].

Accessories Equipment

Robotic and laparoscopic surgeries rely on a variety of accessory equipment to ensure optimal outcomes. Some of the essential components include:

Gas insufflators: Devices used to create pneumoperitoneum by insufflating carbon dioxide (CO_2) into the abdominal cavity, providing adequate workspace for visualization and manipulation. These devices can be manual insufflators, which are simple and portable for emergencies, or automated insufflators, which precisely regulate intra-abdominal pressure and integrate real-time monitoring, alarms, and gas filtration to prevent biological contamination [18, 19].

We can work with three types of energy sources such as monopolar, bipolar, and advanced energy systems such as Ligasure® and Ultracision®, which analyze tissue properties and adjust energy delivery for optimal cutting and coagulation. These tools are becoming more ergonomic, safer, and increasingly digitized, requiring less human intervention. They function as robotic instruments, analyzing the tissue between their jaws, adjusting energy intensity, and performing precise cuts and coagulations with minimal tissue damage [19].

Additionally, surgical instruments such as trocars, graspers, energy devices, needle holders, and staplers have been continuously evolving through bioengineering to enhance ergonomics and precision. Selecting the appropriate instrument for each stage of a procedure is crucial, both in laparoscopic and robotic surgery [19].

Veress Needle

The Veress needle remains a critical instrument for the creation of pneumoperitoneum in minimally invasive surgery, particularly when employing the closed technique or Palmer's technique. Pneumoperitoneum should be established gradually, with meticulous monitoring of clinical parameters and in close coordination with anesthetic management. This is especially crucial in cases with a potential risk for hemodynamic instability, such as polytrauma patients or those with comorbid cardiovascular conditions [20].

During these procedures, it is advisable to work with the minimum intra-abdominal pressure necessary to ensure both safe visualization and effective manipulation of tissues and organs. This approach reduces the risks associated with elevated insufflation pressures, such as decreased venous return and compromised cardiac output, while preserving optimal operating conditions [20].

Trocars

Trocars are indispensable instruments that enable access to the peritoneal or thoracic cavities, allowing for the introduction of the laparoscopic telescope, camera, and working instruments. They vary in size, shape, and mechanisms depending on the nature of the procedure and the patient's anatomical characteristics. The internal diameters of trocars also differ based on the instruments required during surgery [20, 21].

For minimally invasive trauma procedures, it is recommended to utilize 12-mm disposable trocars with reducers accommodating instruments as small as 5 mm. This configuration facilitates greater operational versatility, enabling aspiration, the insertion and retrieval of surgical gauze, needle-handling, and the removal of foreign bodies or tissue specimens [20, 21].

Modern technology has introduced several enhancements to these essential devices:

- Bladeless trocars, reducing the risk of vascular and visceral injuries.
- Optical trocars, allowing direct visualization of tissue layers during cavity entry.
- Non-slip trocars, designed with ergonomic features to prevent displacement during manipulation.
- Accessory port trocars, enabling the passage of sutures for closing fascial puncture wounds at the end of the procedure.

Disposable trocars provide a secure access route into body cavities with real-time visualization, minimizing inadvertent injury to organs and blood vessels. This is particularly valuable in patients with altered anatomy due to adhesions, prior surgeries, or abdominoplasty. In trauma scenarios, they offer rapid diagnostic capability via direct visual inspection, often allowing for a minimally invasive approach to replace exploratory laparotomy, thereby reducing patient morbidity and length of hospital stay [21].

Limitations to their use include availability in emergency settings and cost considerations. Not every trauma operating room is equipped with these devices at all times, and adequate surgical team training is paramount. Improper trocar use can result in adverse events, complicating the management of traumatic injuries [21].

Suction and Irrigation Devices

Suction and irrigation devices are essential tools for maintaining a clear and unobstructed surgical field by aspirating fluids and debris. In trauma surgery, they are indispensable not only for suction but also for the active irrigation of the operative area, which aids in clearing blood and contaminants, thereby improving visualization and facilitating hemostasis [20, 21].

In our clinical practice, we commonly refer to multifunctional aspirator forceps as the "suction finger" due to their versatility in intracorporeal manipulation, dissection, retraction, and suction. Typically, this instrument is the first to be introduced through a 12-mm trocar by the surgeon's dominant hand, while a non-traumatic grasper is managed with the non-dominant hand. This configuration establishes the classic triangular laparoscopic working setup, with the telescope centrally placed and the surgeon positioned between the patient's legs in the French position for abdominal procedures, or on the contralateral side for thoracic interventions [21].

This technique allows for optimal ergonomics, direct instrument alignment, and effective three-dimensional manipulation within the confines of the abdominal or thoracic cavity, which is particularly advantageous in trauma scenarios requiring rapid assessment and intervention [21].

Graspers, Scissors, and Other Surgical Instruments

In both thoracic and abdominal minimally invasive trauma surgery—as well as in elective procedures—a diverse array of precision-designed instruments is employed to achieve accurate, efficient surgical outcomes. These tools typically feature fine, elongated tips with variable diameters, with 5-mm instruments being regarded as the safest standard for general use [22].

Graspers can be either directly acting or articulating, providing secure tissue manipulation. Scissors are available with different blade types for precise cutting, while needle holders are essential for hemostasis through intracorporeal suturing. For this purpose, we advocate the exclusive use of 3-mm diameter needle holders—part of mini-laparoscopy or mini-videolaparoscopy instrument sets—due to their superior ergonomics. These allow for knot tying, suturing, and anastomosis within a reduced pneumoperitoneum volume, maximizing working space and maneuverability. Only robotic graspers surpass this capability, although randomized studies validating systematic robotic use in trauma remain unavailable at present [21, 22].

Monopolar, Bipolar, and Advanced Bipolar Devices

Energy-based devices are indispensable in trauma surgery. While knots and sutures remain the gold standard for hemostasis, monopolar and bipolar energy remain essential, especially in settings where advanced technologies may not be immediately accessible. Among bipolar devices, the Ligasure Maryland® is widely favored for its reliable vessel sealing, dissection, cutting, and grasping capabilities within a single instrument [23].

Bipolar instruments deliver current only between their jaws, limiting tissue damage and eliminating the need for dispersive electrodes, unlike monopolar instruments. In robotic systems, the evolution of bipolar devices is exemplified by the Strattner Intuitive Force Bipolar Grasper, which features finer, longer jaws for deeper access, 70° articulation in all directions, and DualGrip® technology for selecting between standard and high-force grasping modes. This allows surgeons to dissect, grasp, retract, and coagulate without instrument changes, further enhanced by robotic tremor reduction and the EndoWrist® system, offering seven degrees of wrist-like freedom [23].

Ultrasonic Energy Devices

Ultrasonic energy instruments convert high-frequency vibrations into mechanical energy for simultaneous vessel sealing and tissue cutting. These tools are effective for hemostasis and dissection of vessels up to 5 mm and fibrofatty or muscular structures. Notable examples include the Ultracision® (Johnson & Johnson) and Sonicision® (Medtronic). The latter, a cordless battery-powered device, offers enhanced ergonomics without requiring external energy cables [24].

While highly multifunctional, ultrasonic instruments produce significant lateral thermal spread, posing risks during trauma surgery, especially near vital structures. Therefore, when available, advanced bipolar sealers such as Ligasure Maryland® are preferred for their superior multifunctionality and minimal thermal dispersion [24].

Intraoperative Ultrasound

Intraoperative ultrasound with laparoscopic probes transmits high-frequency sound waves to generate real-time images of internal organs, critical for identifying lesions and assessing vascular integrity in trauma patients. The probe is introduced through a trocar or a minor incision adjacent to the area of interest. Advanced systems integrate Doppler ultrasound, displaying both color and spectral images of blood flow, offering crucial information for trauma surgeons during minimally invasive interventions [25].

Endoscopic Linear Staplers

Endoscopic staplers are essential tools in minimally invasive trauma surgery, facilitating rapid, secure closure and division of tissues and vascular structures when suture control may be technically difficult or time consuming. Their utility in emergent trauma scenarios has progressively increased with the growing acceptance of minimally invasive approaches for both diagnostic and therapeutic purposes [26].

Modern endoscopic staplers typically employ either linear cutting staplers or non-cutting staplers, most commonly available in lengths of 45 and 60 mm. They deploy parallel rows of staples while simultaneously transecting tissue between the staple lines (in the case of cutting staplers). These devices accommodate variable tissue thicknesses through different reload cartridges and staple heights [27].

Contemporary staplers incorporate:

- Tri-staple or multi-row staple formation to distribute pressure gradients more evenly across the staple line, improving perfusion and reducing the risk of ischemia or staple line failure.
- Integrated cutting mechanisms within either the reload cartridge (disposable blade per reload) or the stapler body itself (blade reactivated with each firing), depending on the system architecture.
- Tissue-sensing technologies in digital systems, which adjust firing speed or compressive force according to tissue characteristics, optimizing staple formation consistency and safety.

In trauma settings, endoscopic staplers are particularly valuable for pulmonary tract injuries requiring wedge resections, control of bleeding from solid organ injuries such as spleen, liver, or kidney when repair or partial resection is indicated and bowel injury management, enabling rapid segmental resection and anastomosis in damage-control surgery [26].

The availability of stapler reloads of varying staple heights allows surgeons to tailor tissue compression according to tissue thickness and quality—a key consideration in trauma cases, where tissue edema or friability is frequent [26, 27].

Limitations and Operational Challenges

A notable limitation is the availability of appropriately sized reloads during off-hours emergency procedures. Furthermore, not all trauma centers possess comprehensive laparoscopic stapler inventories, necessitating surgeon proficiency in intracorporeal suturing techniques for situations where staplers are unavailable or contraindicated. Additionally, staple line leaks and bleeding remain potential complications, emphasizing the importance of device familiarity and staple line reinforcement in select scenarios [27].

Surgical Needles and Sutures

Advancements in suture needle manufacturing have produced biocompatible, high-performance alloys and polymer-based needles that minimize tissue reaction and improve healing outcomes. Innovations in needle geometry—including ultra-sharp tips and optimized cutting profiles—facilitate easier penetration of delicate tissues, crucial in minimally invasive trauma procedures. Low-friction coatings enhance insertion smoothness and precision [27].

Emerging technologies include controlled-release suture systems combining needle and suture, streamlining rapid hemostatic suturing in parenchymal organ injuries. 3D-printed custom needles, produced via additive manufacturing, are being explored for patient-specific, complex trauma interventions [27].

Surgical sutures remain fundamental in trauma surgery, and recent technological innovations have significantly enhanced their performance, biocompatibility, and clinical utility. Modern sutures are manufactured using advanced materials, including high-performance alloys and biocompatible polymers, which minimize tissue reaction and promote optimal healing. Improvements in needle design, such as refined geometries with sharper, atraumatic tips and specialized cutting profiles, facilitate safer and more efficient penetration of delicate or friable tissues frequently encountered in trauma procedures. Additionally, low-friction coatings on both needles and suture threads reduce tissue drag and improve handling characteristics during minimally invasive interventions [28].

Beyond their mechanical properties, sutures have evolved to incorporate bioactive functions. Antibiotic-coated sutures have demonstrated efficacy in reducing surgical site infection rates, a particularly valuable feature in contaminated wounds or emergency trauma cases where the risk of infection is heightened. Bioabsorbable sutures, which degrade naturally within the body, eliminate the need for removal, reducing patient discomfort and follow-up procedures—an advantage in anatomically challenging or damage-control scenarios [28].

Technological advancements have also led to the development of barbed sutures, which maintain tissue approximation without the need for knots. This reduces operative time, minimizes suture line tension, and improves distribution of mechanical stress, particularly beneficial in minimally invasive settings where intracorporeal knot tying can be time-consuming and technically demanding. Furthermore, the introduction of hemostatic sutures, incorporating agents that actively aid coagulation, offers trauma surgeons additional options for rapid hemorrhage control in solid organ or vascular injuries [28].

Emerging research has introduced intelligent or "smart" sutures embedded with biosensors capable of monitoring parameters such as pH, temperature, or local biochemical markers at the wound site. These devices offer real-time assessment of wound healing and early detection of complications, potentially improving outcomes through earlier therapeutic interventions. Moreover, the advent of 3D-printed, procedure-specific needles and suture delivery systems has created new opportunities for trauma surgeons requiring customized or rapid solutions in complex or emergent situations, especially in resource-limited or battlefield environments [28].

Collectively, these innovations reflect a shift in surgical suture technology from passive mechanical devices to dynamic, multifunctional tools that enhance tissue approximation reliability, reduce postoperative complications, and expedite recovery in patients undergoing minimally invasive trauma surgery [28].

References

1. Kourambas J, Preminger GM. Advances in camera, video, and imaging technologies in laparoscopy. Urol Clin N Am. 2001;28(1):5–14.
2. Huber T, Paschold M, Hansen C, Wunderling T, Lang H, Kneist W. New dimensions in surgical training: immersive virtual reality laparoscopic simulation exhilarates surgical staff. Surg Endosc. 2017;31(11):4472–7.
3. Nakayama DK. How technology shaped modern surgery. Am Surg. 2018;84(6):753–60. PMID: 29981596
4. Sagawa H, Saito M, Ito S, et al. Near infrared ray-guided surgery using firefly technology of the daVinci Xi system and intraoperative upper gastrointestinal endoscopy for subtotal gastrectomy and surgery for cancer of the gastroesophageal junction. BMC Surg. 2022;22:174. https://doi.org/10.1186/s12893-022-01633-9.
5. Ayala L, et al. Spectral imaging enables contrast agent-free real-time ischemia monitoring in laparoscopic surgery. Sci Adv. 2023;9(10):eadd6778. https://doi.org/10.1126/sciadv.add6778. Epub 2023 Mar 10. PMID: 36897951; PMCID: PMC10005169.
6. Yim C, Lo CH, Lau MH, Fan R, Lai HM, Foo DCC. Three-dimensional laparoscopy: is it as good as it looks?—a review of the literature. Ann Laparosc Endosc Surg. 2017;2:131.
7. Sinha RY, Raje SR, Rao GA. Three-dimensional laparoscopy: principles and practice. J Minim Access Surg. 2017;13(3):165–9.
8. Benavides D, Cisnal A, Fontúrbel C, de la Fuente E, Fraile JC. Real-time tool localization for laparoscopic surgery using convolutional neural network. Sensors. 2024;24:4191.
9. Knudsen JE, Ghaffar U, Ma R, Hung AJ. Clinical applications of artificial intelligence in robotic surgery. J Robot Surg. 2024;18(1):102.

10. Reza T, Bokhari SFH. Partnering with technology: advancing laparoscopy with artificial intelligence and machine learning. Cureus. 2024;16(3):e56076.
11. Damasceno NA, de França Damasceno E. Refraction and visual fatigue syndrome on watching the ULTRA HD 4k television curved screen system. Rev Bras Oftalmol. 2016;75:1–10. https://doi.org/10.5935/0034-7280.20160062.
12. Feng Z, et al. Intelligent perioperative system: towards real-time big data analytics in surgery risk assessment. DASC PiCom DataCom CyberSciTech., IEEE 15th Intl Conf on dependable, autonomic and secure computing, 15th Intl Conf on pervasive intelligence and computing, 3rd Intl Conf on big data intelligence and computing and cyber science and technology congress, Orlando, FL, USA. 2017;2017:1254–9. https://doi.org/10.1109/DASC-PICom-DataCom-CyberSciTec.2017.201.
13. Lin J, et al. Endoscopic depth measurement and super-spectral-resolution imaging. In: Descoteaux M, Maier-Hein L, Franz A, Jannin P, Collins D, Duchesne S, editors. Medical image computing and computer-assisted intervention—MICCAI 2017, Lecture notes in computer science, vol. 10434. Cham: Springer; 2017. https://doi.org/10.1007/978-3-319-66185-8_5.
14. Huang X, Liu X, Zhu B, Hou X, Hai B, Yu D, Zheng W, Li R, Pan J, Yao Y, Dai Z, Zeng H. Augmented reality surgical navigation in minimally invasive spine surgery: a preclinical study. Bioengineering. 2023;10(9):1094. https://doi.org/10.3390/bioengineering10091094.
15. Azad TD, Warman A, Tracz JA, Hughes LP, Judy BF, Witham TF. Augmented reality in spine surgery—past, present, and future. Spine J. 2024;24(1):1–13. Elsevier BV. https://doi.org/10.1016/j.spinee.2023.08.015.
16. Robinson ML, Rogers BA, et al. The role of robotics in trauma and orthopaedics. Orthop Trauma. 2023;37(4):239–45, Elsevier BV. https://doi.org/10.1016/j.mporth.2023.05.001.
17. Biswas P, et al. Recent advances in robot-assisted surgical systems. Biomed Eng Adv. 2023;6:100109, Elsevier BV. https://doi.org/10.1016/j.bea.2023.100109.
18. Tianwu Y, et al. Gases for establishing pneumoperitoneum during laparoscopic abdominal surgery. Cochrane Database Syst Rev. 2017;6(6):CD009569. Wiley. https://doi.org/10.1002/14651858.cd009569.pub3.
19. Antoun MA, et al. Outcomes of conventional and advanced energy devices in laparoscopic surgery: a systematic review. Minim Invasive Ther Allied Technol. 2024;33(1):1–12. Informa UK Limited. https://doi.org/10.1080/13645706.2023.2274396.
20. de Azevedo OC, et al. Veress needle insertion in the left hypochondrium in creation of the pneumoperitoneum. Acta Cir Bras. 2006;21(5):296–303. FapUNIFESP (SciELO). https://doi.org/10.1590/s0102-86502006000500005.
21. Sermonesi G, et al. Guidelines: WSES consensus statement on laparoscopic-first approach to general surgery emergencies and abdominal trauma. World J Emerg Surg. 2023;18(1):57. https://doi.org/10.1186/s13017-023-00520-9. PMID: 38066631; PMCID: PMC10704840
22. Palanivelu C. Art of laparoscopic surgery: textbook and atlas. Jaypee Brothers Medical Publishers; 2014.
23. Newcomb WL, et al. Comparison of blood vessel sealing among new electrosurgical and ultrasonic devices. Surg Endosc. 2009;23(1):90–6. https://doi.org/10.1007/s00464-008-9932-x. Epub 2008 May 16. PMID: 18483824.
24. Casey VJ, McNamara LM. Instrumental in surgery: a narrative review on energy-based surgical cutting devices and surgical smoke. Ann Surg. 2023;278(3):e457–65. https://doi.org/10.1097/SLA.0000000000005816.
25. van der Steen K, et al. The value of laparoscopic intraoperative ultrasound of the liver by the surgeon. Ann Laparosc Endosc Surg. 2021;6:17. AME Publishing Company. https://doi.org/10.21037/ales-20-106.
26. Cirocchi R, et al. Laparoscopy for trauma and the changes in its use from 1990 to 2016: a current systematic review and meta-analysis. Surg Laparosc Endosc Percutan Tech. 2018;28(1):1–12. https://doi.org/10.1097/SLE.0000000000000466. PMID: 28915204

27. Goto O, et al. Advancements in endoscopic treatment for gastric subepithelial tumors. Gut Liver. 2025;19(2):151–60. https://doi.org/10.5009/gnl240358. Epub 2025 Jan 8. PMID: 39774123; PMCID: PMC11907253.
28. Li Y, Meng Q, et al. Advances, challenges, and prospects for surgical suture materials. Acta Biomater. 2023;15(168):78–112. https://doi.org/10.1016/j.actbio.2023.07.041. Epub 2023 Jul 28. PMID: 37516417.

Implementing the Pneumoperitoneum and Its Physiologic Consequences

6

Mariano Palermo and Federico Davrieux

Introduction

The trauma patient, whether polytraumatized or multiple traumatized, is, in itself, a serious patient. Controlling cardiovascular, respiratory, and neurological involvement is vital for the expectations of the patient and the treating medical team [1].

Intra-abdominal hemorrhage due to abdominal trauma (either closed or open) is an emergency that is usually addressed by laparotomy. However, since the implementation of laparoscopy, its continuous development and technical improvement have allowed some reference groups from high-volume centers to operate on this group of patients in a minimally invasive approach. In this way, the benefits of this technique can be taken advantage of [2].

However, the necessary use of pneumoperitoneum for these procedures can bring physiological alterations in the organism of a traumatized individual that, in some cases, can become serious [3].

In this chapter, we will analyze the physiological consequences of pneumoperitoneum during the care of the trauma patient.

M. Palermo
Department of Bariatric Surgery, Diagnomed Affiliated Institution to the University of Buenos Aires, Buenos Aires, Argentina

School of Medicine, University of Buenos Aires, Buenos Aires, Argentina

F. Davrieux (✉)
School of Medicine, University of Buenos Aires, Buenos Aires, Argentina

© The Author(s), under exclusive license to Springer Nature Switzerland AG 2026

M. Cezillo, B. M. Pereira (eds.), *Minimally Invasive Surgery Trauma*,
https://doi.org/10.1007/978-3-032-28971-1_6

Specific Aspects of Pneumoperitoneum

Device Aspects

A pneumoperitoneum system consists of an electrically powered console that controls the flow and pressure of the gas supply to establish the pneumoperitoneum. The gas used is carbon dioxide, which is characterized by low tissue diffusion, good patient tolerance, low gas embolism capacity, and rapid postoperative reabsorption, and is nonflammable, allowing the use of energy devices during surgery. The carbon dioxide supply to the console is carried out through a central tower in the operating room. In turn, the carbon dioxide offered by the console is connected to an abdominal port through a hose. In this way, it is possible to carry out the abdominal pneumoperitoneum.

Technical Aspects

Carbon dioxide supplied by the console has 2 variables to control, flow and pressure.

Regarding flow, it is measured in liters per minute (l/m). Generally, most equipment offers a flow of 0–40 l/m. This equipment allows for a quick recovery of the pneumoperitoneum, and therefore of the operating view when for some reason, there is an abdominal gas leak (change of instruments, removal of surgical piece, introduction of sutures, etc.). It is suggested to use a flow of between 20 and 40 l/m.

About pressure, it is measured in millimeters of mercury (mmHg). The equipment offers a pressure of 0–15 mmHg. This allows for greater or lesser abdominal distension, which results in a better operating visual field. It is suggested to use a pressure of between 10 and 12 mmHg, depending on the patient's body mass.

An optional variable that some pneumoperitoneum equipment presents is temperature. Carbon dioxide gas is cold; therefore, pneumoperitoneum can generate a decrease in the patient's body temperature. Some consoles can provide warm carbon dioxide, which avoids hypothermia during surgery, and its respective physiological implications (postoperative pain and shivering, coagulation deficiencies) [4].

Patient Aspects

Pneumoperitoneum can cause cardiovascular changes in the patient. When too high, a flow is used at the start of surgery, this can cause rapid abdominal distension with vasovagal physiological changes, such as tachy or bradycardia, a drop in blood pressure (BP), and increased postoperative pain. It should also be noted that a pressure greater than 15 mmHg can compromise venous return due to collapse of the intra-abdominal veins (cava vein, iliac veins), similar to abdominal compartment syndrome.

Pneumoperitoneum causes elevation of the diaphragm, which results in a decrease in respiratory volume. This can be relevant in patients with respiratory compromise (chronic obstructive pulmonary disease (COPD) and pulmonary fibrosis) or trigger reactive bronchospasm in asthmatic patients. It is essential for the anesthesiologist to monitor oxygen saturation and capnography in these cases. Excessive pneumoperitoneum, which causes rapid abdominal distension and high pressure, can cause postoperative pain, especially at the ports. In addition, poor deflation can cause right shoulder pain due to irritation of the phrenic nerve. Postoperative pain can also be increased by cold carbon dioxide due to low body temperature [5–8].

Physiological Aspects of Traumatized Patients

Polytrauma or multiple trauma in a patient can cause several problems, but ultimately the most serious consequences are cardiovascular (including hemorrhages), respiratory, and neurological.

Any trauma can alter vital parameters, so maintaining stable BP, heart rate, airway, and body temperature, among others, is essential for the patient's survival.

Severe trauma can cause hypotension and extreme bradycardia without the need for hemorrhage. They are often due to spinal or vasovagal shock and recover quickly. One must be sure of the stability when deciding to transfer the patient to the operating room (OR) in order to avoid problems inside, because pneumoperitoneum could modify these variables. Moderate or severe hemorrhage causes hypotension and compensatory tachycardia, among other processes. If this patient is a candidate for surgery, fluid management or the need for pre- or intraoperative transfusions must be taken into consideration, since pneumoperitoneum could aggravate them.

Respiratory compromise during trauma can occur due to airway injury, direct injury to the chest, or both. Airway patency is essential, so once it is secured (either with orotracheal intubation or tracheostomy), the chest must be examined. Both severe blunt injuries and sharp-point wounds can lead to compromising situations, such as pneumothorax, hemothorax, or pulmonary bleeding. These scenarios must be taken into account before implementing pneumoperitoneum, overall elevation of the diaphragm would seriously compromise respiratory function.

Neurological injuries are very common in trauma patients. These can be peripheral or central; the latter being the ones that could compromise the patient's life. Depending on the level of injury, they may or may not affect consciousness, as well as cardiovascular and respiratory functions. It must be kept in mind because a rapidly forming or high-pressure pneumoperitoneum could exacerbate the symptoms caused by the underlying trauma.

A special section covers intra-abdominal hemorrhage secondary to trauma and the application of laparoscopy (and the pneumoperitoneum that it entails). Solid organs (liver, kidney, spleen) are the most frequently injured by closed abdominal trauma. Severe vascular injuries (aorta artery, cava vein, splenic or iliac vessels, among others) are more often due to open wounds (stab or gunshot wounds). Depending on their severity, they may or may not cause hemodynamic decompensation in the patient. Although the current trend in the main centers is to use laparoscopic approach in this kind of patient, it must be ensured that hemodynamic stability is correct, or at least controlled. This is because pneumoperitoneum could generate vasovagal syndrome that accentuates the hemodynamic compromise, already affected by abdominal hemorrhage. It should also be considered that rapid or excessive pneumoperitoneum could unblock a hematoma that has formed physiologically to counteract an eventual hemorrhage (hepatic or renal hematoma, splenic rupture). In case of any vascular injury open to the peritoneum cavity, the possibility of carbon dioxide gas embolism should be seriously considered. It is necessary to keep in mind that laparoscopic view could be diminished by the amount of abdominal blood.

Finally, an important detail is the postoperative pain experienced by the traumatized patient operated by laparoscopy. The stress inherent to the trauma, vasoplegia due to bleeding or neurological compromise, together with the consequent hypothermia, poor oxygenation due to thoracic trauma, among other factors interact to increase postoperative pain. For this reason, it is advisable to optimize the use of pneumoperitoneum in this type of patient by setting the console to low pressure, low flow, and if possible, warm carbon dioxide gas [9, 10].

Conclusion

The use of laparoscopy and therefore of pneumoperitoneum is becoming more common. The benefits of minimally invasive surgery (correct visualization of the quadrants, fewer incisions, less pain, fewer infections) are notable. However, in a polytraumatized patient or with multiple trauma, the use of pneumoperitoneum can compromise the hemodynamic stability of the patient. Nevertheless, the optimization of the resource can allow a minimally invasive approach to the patient while preserving his safety.

Disclosure Statement No competing financial interests exist.
Funding InformationNo funding was received for this article.

References

1. Mejaddam AY, Velmahos GC. Randomized controlled trials affecting polytrauma care. Eur J Trauma Emerg Surg. 2012;38(3):211–21.
2. Buunen M, Gholghesaei M, Veldkamp R, et al. Stress response to laparoscopic surgery: a review. Surg Endosc. 2004;18(7):1022–8.
3. Jones SB, Jones DB. Surgical aspects and future developments of laparoscopy. Anesthesiol Clin North Am. 2001;19(1):107–24.
4. Wildey B, Berman D, Borahay MA. Cardiovascular collapse during laparoscopy: a brief overview. Arch Gynecol Obstet. 2024;309(5):2253–6.
5. Mynbaev OA, Corona R. Possible mechanisms of peritoneal tissue-oxygen tension changes during CO2-pneumoperitoneum: the role of design, methodology and animal models. Hum Reprod. 2009;24(6):1242–6.

6. Radkowski P, Oniszczuk H, Opolska J, et al. Optimizing Anesthetic Management for Laparoscopic Surgery: a comprehensive review. Med Sci Monit. 2024;30:e945951.
7. Barazanchi AWH, MacFater WS, Rahiri JL, et al. Evidence-based management of pain after laparoscopic cholecystectomy: a PROSPECT review update. PROSPECT collaboration. Br J Anaesth. 2018;121(4):787–803.
8. Gunusen I, Akdemir A, Sargın A, et al. The effects of CO(2) pneumoperitoneum at different temperature and humidity on hemodynamic and respiratory parameters and postoperative pain in gynecological laparoscopic surgery: a prospective randomized controlled study. Asian J Surg. 2022;45(1):154–61.
9. Sermonesi G, Tian BWCA, Vallicelli C, et al. Cesena guidelines: WSES consensus statement on laparoscopic-first approach to general surgery emergencies and abdominal trauma. World J Emerg Surg. 2023;18(1):57.
10. Uranues S, Popa DE, Diaconescu B, et al. Laparoscopy in penetrating abdominal trauma. World J Surg. 2015;39(6):1381–8.

Preparation for Trauma Laparoscopy: Patients and Trocar Positions

7

Anaida Xacur-Trabulce, Atika Rauf, Nafeesa Hashim, Saniyah Shaikh, and Marcelo A. F. Ribeiro Jr

Introduction

Historically, laparotomy has been considered the conventional approach to trauma surgery, with a reported morbidity of 20–41%. However, advancements in imaging technology, improvements in surgical technique and experience, and the development of nonoperative management strategies and laparoscopic evaluation protocols have established laparoscopy as a safe and effective tool in the management of hemodynamically stable patients requiring abdominal trauma surgery [1].

One of the key breakthroughs in the surgical field is laparoscopic surgery, because of its association with less postoperative pain, a reduction of wound infections, reduced hospital stay, significant decrease in morbidity and mortality, prompt reintegration into the workforce, and enhanced quality of life [1–3]. For most procedures, minimally invasive surgery has become a standard technical approach; however, in the trauma field, its application remains evolving, even though its use is expanding in emergency surgery with hemodynamically stable patients. In this chapter, we review the key aspects of the preparation for trauma laparoscopy, emphasizing patient selection and trocar positions to optimize procedural safety [2].

A. Xacur-Trabulce
Hospital Angeles Lomas, General Surgery Department, Mexico City, Mexico

A. Rauf · N. Hashim
General Medicine Practice Program, Batterjee Medical College for Science and Technology, Jeddah, Saudi Arabia

S. Shaikh
College of Medicine, Alfaisal University, Riyadh, Saudi Arabia

M. A. F. Ribeiro Jr (✉)
University of Maryland, R Adams Cowley Shock Trauma Center, Baltimore, MA, USA

© The Author(s), under exclusive license to Springer Nature Switzerland AG 2026

M. Cezillo, B. M. Pereira (eds.), *Minimally Invasive Surgery Trauma*,
https://doi.org/10.1007/978-3-032-28971-1_7

Surgical Pearls [2]

Preoperatively: Take into consideration the use of antithrombotic prophylaxis and antibiotic prophylaxis.

Intraoperatively: Adequate patient positioning, correct distribution of the surgical team and equipment, continuous monitorization. Precise use of pneumoperitoneum, enhancing the use of technological staplers and advanced energy devices, maintaining the lowest intra-abdominal pressure possible, elude 10–15 mm ports for placing drains, ensure that the time-out is always done before starting the surgical procedure.

Postoperatively: Appropriate pain management, prompt ambulation, systematic monitoring of early warning indicators.

Importance of Patient Selection, Procedure Selection, and Patient Positioning to Ensure Safety

Patient Selection

Laparoscopic surgery is associated with increased risks due to elevated intra-abdominal pressure and extreme patient positioning. Therefore, considering a careful patient selection, optimizing positioning strategies, and monitoring intraoperative continuous are crucial to ensure safety and reduce complications. Sometimes patient comorbidities might make them unsuitable for a laparoscopic approach like severe cardiovascular and pulmonary diseases, history of multiple previous abdominal surgeries or open midline laparotomy due to an increased risk of finding adhesions, and cirrhotic liver disease with hepatic enlargement or pregnancy. In these challenging situations, the surgeon will have to face difficult decisions and must choose the most appropriate course of action, whether to step back and postpone the procedure, or to adapt and proceed with a different approach than the originally planned [1, 2].

Procedure Selection

In patients with blunt abdominal trauma, laparoscopy has been proven to be a safe and useful procedure, reducing the risks of performing a non-beneficial laparotomy and reducing mortality rates. However, its utility in penetrating abdominal trauma is still ambiguous, but it can be a valuable assessment tool to determine which patients may benefit from laparotomy [1, 2].

Patient Positioning

To perform a safe laparoscopy, proper precautions should be considered, including positioning major joints neutrally and cushioning pressure points [1, 2].

Principles of Patient Positioning in Trauma Laparoscopy

Goals and Considerations

Basic Principles of Positioning

To ensure intraoperative stability and avoid slippage, straps should be used to secure the patient's chest and thighs. Footrests should be used if the reverse Trendelenburg position is expected. In pelvic surgery, a Trendelenburg position is anticipated, maintaining a neutral position of knees and hips, with a correct paddling of pressure points and applying shoulder supports to prevent cephalad migration is essential. When using a stationary retractor, it must be firmly secured to the operating table to reduce the risk of intraoperative adverse events. The insertion and removal of these retractors should be carried out carefully to avoid complications. Transferring the patient on and off the operating table or bed should be done carefully to prevent injuries to both the patient and the surgical team. The use of air mattresses in patients with obesity can facilitate safe mobilization [2].

Trocar Positioning

Proper port placement following the triangulation principle is essential to optimize ergonomics (Fig. 7.1). Inspecting the peritoneal cavity after port placement, beginning with the structures beneath the Veress needle or trocar, is crucial for the early detection of unintentional injuries [2].

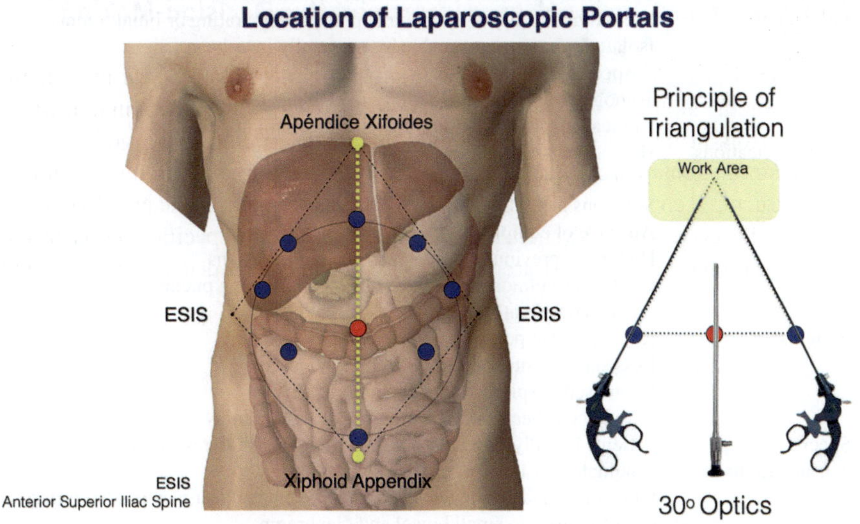

Fig. 7.1 Location of laparoscopic portals according to the principle of triangulation. (Illustration provided by Dr. Pablo Otolino)

Hemodynamic Implications of Pneumoperitoneum

The misuse of pneumoperitoneum can have negative effects on the cardiovascular system. To achieve optimal visualization while preventing adverse effects, the following factors should be considered: Informing the anesthetist when the insufflation starts. Avoid an abrupt rise of intra-abdominal pressure to avoid cardiac arrhythmias such as bradycardia resulting in hemodynamic instability. To avoid the cardiopulmonary consequences of intra-abdominal hypertension, because of diaphragmatic splinting and carbon dioxide-induced hypercarbia, it is recommended to maintain intra-abdominal pressure below 12 mmHg. Before increasing pneumoperitoneum, it is essential to ensure adequate relaxation of the abdominal wall. The adverse effects of pneumoperitoneum could be aggravated by patients' positioning, for instance, the Trendelenburg position elevates intrathoracic pressure, which can reduce functional residual capacity [2].

Most studies concluded that in hemodynamically stable patients, laparoscopy can be helpful in blunt and penetrating trauma, enabling an accurate and complete abdominal exploration (Table 7.1), decreasing the incidence of negative laparotomies in trauma patients [1–3].

Table 7.1 Diagnostic minimally invasive surgery in trauma

Category	Characteristics
General considerations	Correct patient selection is crucial Consider hemodynamic stability, injury pattern, and surgeon laparoscopic experience Successful operation: Isolated injury in a hemodynamically stable patient
Indications	Hemodynamically stable trauma patient (penetrating or blunt trauma) Isolated injuries manageable by minimally invasive repair Suspected diaphragmatic or deep pelvic injury Tomographic evidence of injury in stable patients Clinical suspicion of injury despite uncertain imaging results
Contraindications	Hemodynamic instability or shock Traumatic brain injury Surgeons lack of experience Absence of equipment History of previous surgeries suggesting adhesions Cardiac or pulmonary comorbidities conditioning pneumoperitoneum-related complications
Benefits	Reduced postoperative pain Less surgical site infections and incisional hernias Decreased hospital stay, cost, and mortality Avoids non-therapeutic laparotomy or thoracotomy
Special considerations	Patients initially unstable, who were responsive to resuscitation may be candidates for laparoscopy in selected cases Ultrasound and computed tomography: Limited accuracy in identifying occult injuries to small bowel and diaphragm Laparoscopy limits the tactile sensitivity and ability to directly visualize injuries

Common Positions

Correct patient positioning is a key factor in avoiding unintended patient movement, preventing patient injuries, ensuring clear access to the port entry site, facilitating efficient instrument handling, and allowing unobstructed movement of the surgical team around the patient. Other factors that increase the risk of positional injuries include body mass index, either over or underweight, longer operative times, procedures lasting >5 h, which are associated with the development of rhabdomyolysis, and an American Society of Anesthesiologists classification score of III–V [4].

Essential aspects to evaluate include pressure redistribution with adequate use of padding material in bony prominences, deep venous thrombosis prevention with compression devices or anti-thromboembolic stockings, correct upper extremities positioning by placing arms at the patient's sides, or, if abducted, ensure leveling them with the bed and not more than 90°, and lower extremities positioning, taking into account the next key aspects: angle of hip flexion 60–170°, angle of knee flexion 90–120°, angle of hip abduction ≤90°, and minimal degree of external hip rotation [4] (Table 7.2).

Table 7.2 Standard surgical positions and main characteristics including key aspects, body distribution, and organ access

Surgical position	Characteristics
Supine (dorsal recumbent)	Key aspects: Most common, straps above the knees Body distribution: Align head and spine horizontally, hips parallel to each other, extended legs straight and uncrossed, arms alongside the body or abducted Access: Neck, anterior access to the abdomen, inguinal region
Trendelenburg	Key aspects: Hemodynamic changes return to normal in 10 min, increases airway pressures and intracranial pressure Body distribution: Placing the body on a head-down plane with a 15–30° inclination Access: Moves the organs away from the pelvis
Reverse Trendelenburg	Key aspects: Decreases venous return, can cause hypotension and reduce cerebral perfusion Body distribution: Placing the body on a head-up plane with a 15–30° inclination Access: Move the organs away from the upper quadrants
Lateral decubitus	Key aspects: Favors ventilation of the upper lung Body distribution: Patient lies down on the side opposite to the area of intervention Access: Thorax, kidneys, and retroperitoneal space
Modified lithotomy	Key aspects: Increases risk of lower extremity compartment syndrome Body distribution: Hips flexed and legs abducted, bent knees, and buttocks at the table's edge, with arms either at the sides or abducted Access: Multiple abdominopelvic cavity quadrants and perineal area

Special Considerations in Trauma

Hemodynamic Instability

In hemodynamically unstable patients, the induction of pneumoperitoneum and extreme patient positioning can lead to metabolic, respiratory, cardiovascular, and neurological adverse effects that may result in significant clinical deterioration [1–3] (Table 7.3).

Table 7.3 Complications, intraoperative management, and preventive strategies in minimally invasive surgery

Condition	Characteristics
Cardiac dysfunction	Maintain the lowest pressure insufflation possible Carboperitoneum between 12 and 14 mmHg ASA I - II: Not significant ASA III - IV: Significant, place an arterial pressure invasive measurement
Pre-existing pulmonary disease or severe obesity (BMI > 40)	Protective ventilation: Increase minute-volume Avoid high insufflation volumes and pressures
Pre-existing cardiopulmonary disease or chest trauma	Optimization of mechanical ventilation with operative intervention Place invasive hemodynamic monitorization Radial arterial catheter Arterial blood gas Monitorization of blood pressure
Baseline elevated ICP (intracranial pressure) of severe head trauma	Maintain the lowest intra-abdominal pressure possible Evaluate the need of intracranial pressure monitorization
Gas embolism	Direct insufflation of CO_2 into a vein or abdominal organ Incidence: 0.15% Prevention: Trocars should be inserted under direct visualization through the laparoscopic camera. The periumbilical port should be placed using the open (Hasson) technique or with a trocar designed for visual entry Proper insertion of the Veress needle must be ensured using standardized safety tests to confirm correct intraperitoneal placement Management: Interruption of CO_2 insufflation Adoption of a left-side Trendelenburg position Start hyperventilation with 100% FiO_2 Central venous catheter in the pulmonary artery for gas aspiration Cardiac massage Massive embolism: Cardiopulmonary bypass Consider hyperbaric therapy After stabilizing the patient slowly restore pneumoperitoneum, if hemodynamic instability persists, convert to laparotomy
Abdominal compartment syndrome	Decompressive laparotomy

Missed Injuries

Missed injuries in trauma remain to be a significant concern in the surgical field, leading to increased morbidity and mortality. Minimally invasive surgery can be associated with a higher perceived risk of missed injuries due to a lack of tactile feedback, a limited field of view, or difficult access to certain anatomical regions. However, recent studies and multiple meta-analyses show a low missed injury rate (<1%) and no significant difference in missed injuries with open surgery when the patient is carefully selected for laparoscopy in trauma [3].

Port Placement

A proper placement of the laparoscopic ports can enhance exposure, facilitating exploration and ergonomic efficiency. The principles of triangulation should always be followed, and if the location of the injury is unclear, a 5-sided dice port configuration with a periumbilical camera is recommended [1–3].

Role of Advanced Instruments

The therapeutic capabilities of minimally invasive surgery can be easily expanded with adequate knowledge and use of laparoscopic staplers, advanced energy vessel sealing devices, and tools designed to facilitate laparoscopic suturing [3].

Minimally Invasive Surgery as a Safe First Approach

Morbidity associated with open incisions can be prevented with laparoscopy, while providing a safe approach in hemodynamically stable trauma patients. However, when exposure is limited or missed injuries are suspected, conversion to laparotomy remains an option (Figs. 7.2 and 7.3). The presence of hemoperitoneum, peritoneal disruption, or retroperitoneal organ injury is associated with a higher conversion rate [3].

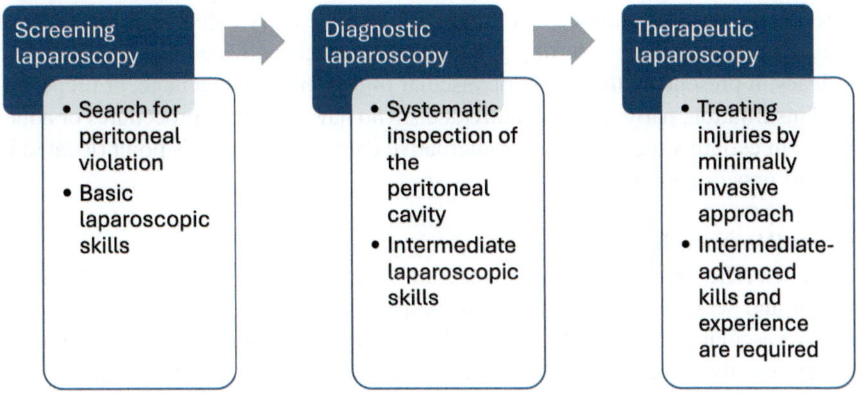

Fig. 7.2 Steps in the laparoscopic approach to trauma patients and required surgical skills [5]

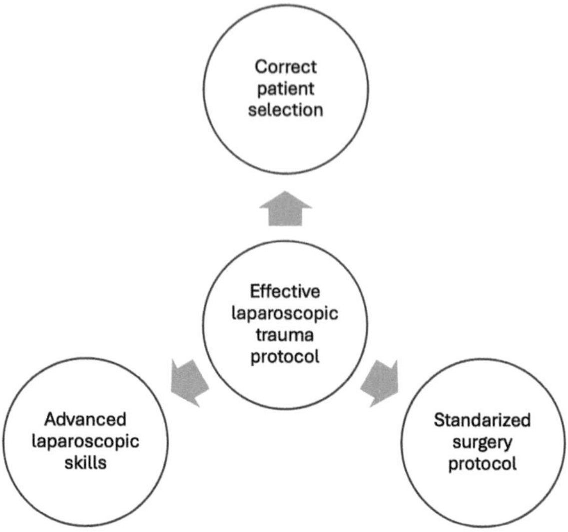

Fig. 7.3 Three pillars of an effective laparoscopic trauma protocol [5]

Trocar Placement Strategies

General Principles

A laparoscopy's first entry into the peritoneal space is still one of the most important parts, especially for trauma patients whose risk of complications may be increased by adhesions, concealed injuries, or anatomical distortion. The closed technique (Veress needle) and the open technique (Hasson) are the two main methods used.

Closed (Veress) Technique

The Veress needle technique is a minimally invasive entry aided by insufflation of the peritoneum before inserting the trocar. Although preferred for its speed and efficacy, it presents with the risk of vascular injury, intestinal damage, or preperitoneal insufflation, particularly in individuals who have had prior procedures or adhesions. In certain situations, a safer alternative entrance is Palmer's point (located in the left upper quadrant) [2].

Open (Hasson) Technique

The open (Hasson) technique involves a short incision at the umbilicus under direct vision and with blunt dissection into the peritoneal space. It reduces the risk of major vascular damage and is especially beneficial in patients who have already undergone abdominal surgery, are obese, or have adhesions. Most trauma surgeons use it on unstable or high-risk patients because it offers a very high degree of safety, even if it takes a little longer [1, 2].

Avoiding Vascular and Bowel Injury

To prevent vascular damage, transillumination and Doppler evaluation may be employed to detect and bypass epigastric vessels. The inferior epigastric arteries need to be detected, and ports placed a minimum of two fingerbreadths medial to the anterior superior iliac spine. Elevating the abdominal wall during Veress or trocar placement, as well as the use of optical trocars with direct visualization, also significantly reduces the risk of blind injuries to the bowel or retroperitoneal organs [2].

Port Placement by Injury Pattern

Port configuration and placement must be specifically made according to the probable injury pattern and requirements for maximum visualization and instrumentation.

- Blunt abdominal trauma: In patients with stable blunt trauma, laparoscopy is used to evaluate potential intra-abdominal injuries, especially diaphragm disruptions. One common configuration is a periumbilical camera port (10 mm) with functional ports in the left upper and right lower quadrants. This triangulated posture allows easy access to the pelvis, upper abdomen, and diaphragm [6].
- Penetrating trauma: In penetrating abdominal trauma, diagnostic laparoscopy is useful in establishing peritoneal violation, bowel injury, and diaphragmatic damage. Individualized placement of ports is performed based on wound location and direction. In anterior abdominal stab wounds, the ports are placed off the tract of injury to preserve working angles and avoid the zone of potential contamination [2].
- Diaphragmatic injuries: Laparoscopy is extremely useful for diagnosing diaphragmatic injuries, particularly those on the left side, where abdominal organ herniation might occur. A subxiphoid or epigastric port is used to see the diaphragm directly, while additional ports in the left upper quadrant are used for repair. Due to the presence of the liver, diaphragmatic injuries may need a combined thoracoscopic approach [7, 8].
- Pelvic trauma: In pelvic injury with potential bowel or bladder involvement, lower abdominal ports should be preferred. These must be placed medial to the anterior superior iliac spines and lateral to the inferior epigastric vessels. This allows both diagnostic and therapeutic access to the pelvic cavity without disturbing ongoing orthopedic stabilization [2].

Port Configuration Examples

- Upper quadrant trauma

  For upper abdominal injuries (liver, stomach, spleen, or diaphragm), port location should provide unrestricted access to the subphrenic region. A 10-mm camera port is often placed at the periumbilical or epigastric level, with two 5-mm working ports in the left and right upper quadrants, far enough apart for triangulation [2]

- Lower abdomen access
  Ports on the abdominal wall will be low and lateral when access to the lower quadrants is necessary, such as to check the sigmoid colon, bladder, or pelvic organs. A periumbilical camera port is used, with 5-mm working ports in the left and right lower quadrants and transillumination to avoid the inferior epigastric arteries [2].
- Combined thoracoabdominal access.
  In complex cases with trauma to both thoracic and abdominal cavities with high diaphragmatic rupture or transdiaphragmatic injury, a hybrid thoracoscopy-laparoscopy may be performed. A lateral working port, a subxiphoid camera port, and one or more thoracic ports provide safe visualization and repair of the peritoneal and pleural tissues [2, 9].

Ergonomics and Workflow Efficiency

Surgeon and Assistant Positioning

In trauma laparoscopy settings, the primary surgeon typically stands contralateral to the injury side of the patient, for example, on the left side for a right upper quadrant trauma. Meanwhile, the assistant or camera operator takes position opposite to or at the level of the caudal end for pelvic exploration. The table height is typically maintained at an elbow flexion of 90–110°. Whereas the monitor placement should be 10–25° below eye level, 1–3 m away and centered in order to reduce fatigue. These positioning practices follow established ergonomics principles adapted to emergency trauma settings and minimize strain and allow for smooth and rapid conversions if needed [10].

Scope Navigation

Smooth scope handling maintains field orientation and reduces disorientation in active bleeding or visually obstructed fields. A 30-degree laparoscope is preferred for its ability to visualize around organs and into recess without physically moving the camera. In trauma settings, this flexibility is critical during time constraints. The camera operator must coordinate with the surgeon's lead instrument to preserve the visual field, avoid nausea-inducing movement, and reduce operative delays [10].

Instrument Triangulation

Poor triangulation hinders reach, leads to internal collisions, and prolongs operative time during bleeding control or bowel examination. A triangular configuration should be formed by the ports, with the target organ about 15–20 cm from the camera port and the working instruments 5–7 cm apart at 60–90° angles. In trauma, this angulation ensures maximal dexterity, minimal torque at the abdominal wall, and readiness for rapid action [10].

Conversion Readiness

Trauma cases can decompensate rapidly; therefore, access planning must allow for seamless conversion to open surgery. Port placement should align with potential laparotomy incisions. The midline camera port is typically placed at or above the umbilicus for upper quadrant injuries and may be expanded into a midline incision if conversion is needed. Draping, staff roles, and instruments must be pre-assigned for immediate conversion if bleeding control or exposure fails laparoscopically [11].

Complications Related to Positioning and Access

Nerve Injuries

Even brief intraoperative nerve compression can cause lasting dysfunction, affecting rehabilitation in trauma survivors. Hence, trauma patients are particularly vulnerable due to prolonged operative times and emergency setups. Brachial plexus injuries may result from excessive arm abduction or shoulder braces. Femoral and peroneal nerves are compressed by stirrups or improper lower limb positioning. Stats indicate 12.9% nerve injury rate in prolonged laparoscopies, increasing with each additional operative hour [12].

Pressure Ulcers

In hypotensive and coagulopathic trauma patients, pressure injuries can develop quickly and lead to prolonged ICU stays. Gel pads, neutral positioning, and monitoring operative time are critical factors [13]. Even a period of 2–3 h of uninterrupted pressure in unstable patients can cause stage 1–2 ulcers, particularly over the sacrum, heels, and occiput [14].

Missed Injuries Due to Poor Exposure

Subtle injuries such as retroperitoneal hematomas, serosal tears, etc. can be missed if the field is inadequately exposed. Proper tilt (e.g., reverse Trendelenburg for upper quadrants, left tilt for splenic mobilization) enhances exposure. Repositioning for trauma exploration should be routinely done during surgery to ensure no quadrant is overlooked [15].

Trocar Site hernias and Vascular Injury

Long-term morbidity can result from trocar-site complications if not prevented during access. Optical trocar entry is safer than blind Veress insertion in trauma, where adhesions or bowel injury risk is high [16]. Vascular injuries, particularly to the inferior epigastric vessels, can be avoided with transillumination and careful lateral port planning. Fascial closure is mandatory for ports >10 mm [17].

Positioning and Port Placement in Damage Control Laparoscopy

Adaptations for Critically Ill Patients

Trauma patients are usually coagulopathic, hypothermic, and acidotic, which can worsen outcomes even from minor physiologic disturbances. To avoid hypotension, use a supine position with minimal reverse Trendelenburg to allow upper abdominal access. Pneumoperitoneum pressures should remain at or below 10–12 mm Hg. Steep Trendelenburg or prolonged tilt should be avoided. The operative team must prioritize time and limit unnecessary exploration and transition to open surgery at the first sign of compromise [17].

Positioning in ICU-Based Laparoscopy

Optimally, the ICU bed must be flattened and leveled. Port layout is simplified, often using just 2–3 trocars, with camera and working ports placed to allow focused intervention. Monitor height and lighting must be customized. Ventilator tubing, IV lines, and patient monitors should not obstruct movement [18].

Temporary Abdominal Closure Techniques

In trauma patients undergoing damage control laparoscopy, temporary abdominal closure (TAC) is necessary. This is to prevent swelling from causing pressure on organs, to avoid further bleeding or contamination, and to allow a second surgery once the patient is more stable. In such cases, the open abdomen should be covered temporarily using methods like a sterile plastic sheet, towel clips, or vacuum dressings (negative pressure wound therapy). These techniques help protect the internal organs, prevent infection, and make it easier to go back in for a second operation.

In rare cases, the abdomen may be temporarily closed using laparoscopy. This requires keeping the gas pressure inside the abdomen low (10–12 mm Hg) and is only done if the patient is stable. Mostly, open temporary closure is safer and more practical, especially in extremely sick patients. The goal is to protect the bowel, avoid consequences from high abdominal pressure, and make smooth and quick re-entry for another surgery if required [19].

Clinical Pearls and Pitfalls

Case-Based Tips

In hemodynamically stable patients with penetrating epigastric trauma, if there is damage to the diaphragm, it is recommended to place the camera port sufficiently lateral to allow upward angulation toward the diaphragm. A subxiphoid trocar can facilitate viewing of superior regions in upper abdominal injuries [20]. Additionally, in patients with obesity or high-riding diaphragms, it may be challenging to visualize the area of interest from an umbilical port, in which additional ports may be required for retraction or better view angle [21].

In patients with blunt abdominal trauma with suspected mesentery tears, prioritize a systematic approach to thoroughly inspect the abdomen. It is common to miss occult injuries if the camera port is too low. A supraumbilical port is ideal for bowel visualization [22].

Patients with prior midline or Pfannenstiel incisions have many adhesions, therefore avoid umbilical entry and use Palmer's point for trocar entry [23] (Table 7.4).

Troubleshooting Poor Exposure

Poor exposure results in a limited visual field, an increased risk of trocar-related injuries, or missed intra-abdominal pathologies, which is critical in trauma where rapid and accurate assessment is crucial. Common reasons for poor exposure are inadequate pneumoperitoneum, bowel distension, hemoperitoneum, and clouding of the visual field due to smoke and debris (Table 7.5).

Decision-Making for Alternative Approaches

Alternative approaches include: conversion to open laparotomy, hand-assisted laparoscopy, and robotic surgeries. The decision to alter the course requires sound judgment and should be in the best interest of the patient. Surgeons must weigh several factors like patient's overall health, complexity of surgery, and their experience with different techniques before making any decision.

Table 7.4 Clinical-based tips

Case	Clinical tips
Trauma to the diaphragm	Place the camera port sufficiently lateral, subxiphoid trocar for better visualization
Obese patients, thick abdominal wall	Additional ports for retraction and better view angle
Mesentery tear	Supraumbilical port for better bowel visualization
Adhesions post-trauma or surgery	Avoid umbilical entry and use Palmer's point for trocar entry

Table 7.5 Troubleshooting poor exposure

Causes of poor exposure	Solution
Inadequate pneumoperitoneum [24]	Increase intra-abdominal pressure to 15–18 mmHg, check for gas leaks around trocars
Bowel distension [25]	Insert orogastric tube, avoid using Trendelenburg positioning
Hemoperitoneum [26]	Ensure proper patient positioning (Trendelenburg, Reverse Trendelenburg or lateral tilt), use advanced visualization systems like Enhanced Laparoscopic Vision (ELV), 4K or 3D laparoscopes, and augmented reality systems
Smoke or clouding [27]	New technology which includes visual field clearing systems can be used

Conversion to open laparotomy is life-saving for patients with uncontrollable hemorrhage, inaccessible injury areas, or dense adhesions restricting the procedure [3].

Tactile feedback is essential in some complex and blunt trauma cases, and therefore switching to a hand-assisted laparoscopic procedure is ideal, which combines the benefits of both open and laparoscopic surgery [28].

While laparoscopy is widely used, it has limitations in trauma due to incomplete visibility, blind spots, potential missed injuries, and a steep learning curve for surgeons. Surgeons may opt to perform robotic surgery, which has enhanced precision and 3D visualization, and reduces surgeon fatigue. However, its lack of tactile feedback and high costs are disadvantages.

Ultimately, the choice depends on patient needs, complexity of the case, and availability of resources [29].

Future Directions and Innovations

3D Planning and Imaging-Based Positioning

3D modeling can influence laparoscopic planning. Preoperative identification of the extent of injury, like mapping the path of a stab wound through the abdominal wall, can help with camera orientation as well as patient positioning [30].

AI-Guided Trocar Planning

AI is being developed to analyze scans like CT scans, injury zone, and surgical intent to identify the best trocar positions tailored to individual patients to minimize injury. AI models can also propose real-time adjustments based on intraoperative data like hemoperitoneum and organ position.

Although the development is still in its early stages, AI can help revolutionize decision-making and improve outcomes in trauma laparoscopy. Integration of this model with an alarm system allows for timely reminders for surgeons to tilt the scope [31].

AI predictive models for potential exposure limitations may identify factors that increase the risk of complications or difficulty. These models may predict outcomes like duodenal stump leakage, hypothermia, or the need to convert to open surgery [32].

Positioning in Robotic Trauma Laparoscopy

Robotics in trauma is limited to selected patients, but the use is growing in complex cases. Key considerations for robotic positioning are:

1. Wider port spacing and longer docking arms.
2. More precise tilt and table positioning which may be automated in future systems.
3. AI enhanced vision and instrument control.

Proper patient positioning is important to allow access to the surgical field, robotic camera system, and working arms. Traditional da Vinci systems require final positioning before docking and once docked, repositioning is limited. However, newer robotic systems allow integrated table motions, which allow the table to tilt while the robot is docked [33].

Conclusion

Because of advances in imaging, instrumentation, and intraoperative planning, minimally invasive surgery in trauma has become a valuable resource in the management of hemodynamically stable trauma patients. Its successful application requires not only surgical skill but also comprehensive thinking that allows the integration of the patient's physiology, operative ergonomics, and careful procedural planning. This includes careful patient selection, along with a deep understanding of indications and potential complications. The correct management of pneumoperitoneum, trocar placement guided by injury patterns taking into consideration a correct triangulation, and adequate patient positioning are key elements that allow the surgeon to create a safe environment. However, adaptability remains essential, and every surgeon must be prepared to convert to open if clinical conditions demand it. In this chapter, it is well established that preparation is not only a technical step, but a fundamental component of operative success and patient safety.

References

1. Sermonesi G, Tian BW, Vallicelli C, et al. Cesena guidelines: WSES consensus statement on laparoscopic-first approach to general surgery emergencies and abdominal trauma. World J Emerg Surg. 2023;18:57. https://doi.org/10.1186/s13017-023-00520-9.
2. Madhok B, Nanayakkara K, Mahawar K. Safety considerations in laparoscopic surgery: a narrative review. World J Gastrointest Endosc. 2022;14(1):1–16. https://doi.org/10.4253/wjge.v14.i1.1.
3. Victory J, Golden A, Jaikaran O, Vu AH, Ferzli GS. Emergent trauma surgery: a narrative review of laparoscopy, thoracoscopy and robotics. Ann Laparosc Endosc Surg. 2025;8:18. https://doi.org/10.21037/ales-23-23. Published online 2025 Apr 14.
4. Lee-Ong A, Buenafe AA. Operating room setup and patient positioning in MIS. In: Lomanto D, Chen WTL, Fuentes MB, editors. Mastering Endo-laparoscopic and thoracoscopic surgery. Singapore: Springer; 2023. https://doi.org/10.1007/978-981-19-3755-2_10.
5. Ramos JP, Arenas CE, Zinco A, Lugo JA, Ottolino PR. Laparoscopy for penetrating trauma, protocol to avoid missing injuries during the learning curve. J Surg. 2022;7:1621. https://doi.org/10.29011/2575-9760.001621.
6. Martins R, dos Santos M, Revez T. Laparoscopy in blunt abdominal trauma: diaphragmatic and bladder lacerations repair. J Trauma Injury. 2019;32(3):176–80. https://doi.org/10.20408/jti.2019.019.
7. Shichiri K, Imamura K, Takada M, Anbo Y. Minimally invasive repair of right-sided blunt traumatic diaphragmatic injury. BMJ Case Rep. 2020;13(11):e235870. https://doi.org/10.1136/bcr-2020-235870.
8. Kesavaramanujam S, Morell MC, Harigovind D, et al. Total thoracic herniation of the liver: a case of delayed right-sided diaphragmatic hernia after blunt trauma. Surg Case Rep. 2020;6:178. https://doi.org/10.1186/s40792-020-00941-7.
9. Armstrong M, Moore RA. Anatomy, patient positioning [Internet]. In: StatPearls. Treasure Island (FL): StatPearls Publishing; 2025. [updated 2022 Oct 31; cited 2025 Jul 22]. Available from: https://www.ncbi.nlm.nih.gov/books/NBK513320/.
10. Yeola M, Gode D, Bora A. Ergonomics in laparoscopy. Int J Recent Surg Med Sci. 2017;03(02):102–8.
11. Matsevych O, Koto M, Balabyeki M, Aldous C. Trauma laparoscopy: when to start and when to convert? Surg Endosc. 2017;32(3):1344–52.
12. Zarandona Del Campo A, Herreros Marias N, Torvisco Macias A, Barandica Bilbao AM, Rodriguez Otazua L, Aguirre Larracoechea U, et al. Factors associated with peripheral nerve injury after pelvic laparoscopy: the importance of surgical positioning. J Nurs Res [Internet]. [cited 2022 Nov 23]; https://doi.org/10.1097/jnr.0000000000000530. Available from: https://journals.lww.com/jnr-twna/Fulltext/9900/Factors_Associated_With_Peripheral_Nerve_Injury.43.aspx.
13. Aldermen J. Risk factors for hospital-acquired pressure injury in surgical critical care patients [internet]. 2020. Available from: https://pmc.ncbi.nlm.nih.gov/articles/PMC8717926/.
14. Han MJ, Ko S. Comparison of interface pressures and subjective comfort of pressure-relieving overlays on the operating table for healthy volunteers. Int J Environ Res Public Health. 2021;18(5):2640.
15. Li Y, Xiang Y, Wu N, Wu L, Yu Z, Zhang M, et al. A comparison of laparoscopy and laparotomy for the management of abdominal trauma: a systematic review and meta-analysis. World J Surg. 2015;39(12):2862–71.
16. McKernan JB, Finley CR. Experience with optical trocar in performing laparoscopic procedures. Surg Laparosc Endosc Percutan Tech. 2002;12(2):96–9.
17. Kindel T, Latchana N, Swaroop M, Chaudhry UI, Noria SF, Choron RL, et al. Laparoscopy in trauma: an overview of complications and related topics. Int J Crit Illn Inj Sci [Internet]. 2015 [cited 2021 Jan 18];5(3):196–205. Available from: https://www.ncbi.nlm.nih.gov/pmc/articles/PMC4613419/.

18. Palladino A, Vallicelli C, Perrina D, Girolamo Convertini, Coccolini F, Luca Ansaloni, et al. Bedside laparoscopy in the critically ill: a review of the literature. J Clin Med [Internet]. 2024 Mar 7 [cited 2024 Aug 11];13(6):1530–0. Available from: https://www.mdpi.com/2077-0383/13/6/1530#:~:text=The%20present%20analysis%20shows%20that.
19. Mahoney EJ, Bugaev N, Appelbaum R, Goldenberg-Sandau A, Baltazar GA, Posluszny J, et al. Management of the open abdomen: a systematic review with meta-analysis and practice management guideline from the Eastern Association for the surgery of trauma. J Trauma Acute Care Surg [Internet]. 2022 Sep 1 [cited 2023 Jan 30];93(3):e110–8. Available from: https://pubmed.ncbi.nlm.nih.gov/35546420/.
20. [Author unknown]. Title unknown. Egypt J Surg. [cited 2025 Jul 22]. Available from: https://ejsur.journals.ekb.eg/article_387633_969a21217997f6821a7097635f5d4091.pdf.
21. Chow A, Purkayastha S, Paraskeva P. Single-incision laparoscopic surgery for cholecystectomy: a review. J Laparoendosc Adv Surg Tech A. 2009;19(6):669–74. Available from: https://pmc.ncbi.nlm.nih.gov/articles/PMC12112246/.
22. Abu Hilal M, Aldrighetti L, Dagher I, Edwin B, Troisi RI, Alikhanov R, et al. The second international consensus conference on laparoscopic liver resection: convened in Morioka. World J Emerg Surg. 2015;10:1. Available from: https://wjes.biomedcentral.com/articles/10.1186/s13017-015-0007-8.
23. Carroll BJ, Fallas MJ, Munro MG. The learning curve for laparoscopic myomectomy. Am J Obstet Gynecol. 1998;179(6 Pt 1):1475–9. Available from: https://pubmed.ncbi.nlm.nih.gov/9822474/.
24. Mellinger JD, Robbins K, Markwell S. Residency and fellowship training in advanced laparoscopy: defining the curriculum. Surg Endosc. 2017;31(1):219–26. Available from: https://pmc.ncbi.nlm.nih.gov/articles/PMC5477171/.
25. De Simone B, Sartelli M, Coccolini F, Biffl WL, Leppäniemi A, Moore EE, et al. Intra-abdominal infections: the role of the gut microbiota. Int J Environ Res Public Health. 2022;19(22):14708. Available from: https://www.mdpi.com/1660-4601/19/22/14708.
26. [Author unknown]. Title unknown. Surg J. [cited 2025 Jul 22]. Available from: https://pdf.sciencedirectassets.com/.../am.pdf (check full PDF for complete citation).
27. Society of American Gastrointestinal and Endoscopic Surgeons. Ultravision visual field clearing system. SAGES TAVAC Safety and Effectiveness Analysis. [cited 2025 Jul 22]. Available from: https://www.sages.org/publications/tavac/ultravision-visual-field-clearing-system/.
28. Aggarwal R, Ward J, Balasundaram I, Sains P, Athanasiou T, Darzi A. Proving the effectiveness of virtual reality simulation for training in laparoscopic surgery. Ann Surg. 2007;246(5):771–9. Available from: https://pmc.ncbi.nlm.nih.gov/articles/PMC3015515/.
29. Mishra RK. Laparoscopic surgery: limitations and challenges. World Laparoscopy Hospital. [cited 2025 Jul 22]. Available from: https://www.laparoscopyhospital.com/worldlaparoscopyhospital/index.php?pid=679&p=2.
30. Bai Y, Li W, Sun J, Wang Y, Wu H, Liu L, et al. Deep learning-based image segmentation improves laparoscopic view. J Imaging. 2024;10(8):180. Available from: https://www.mdpi.com/2313-433X/10/8/180.
31. Looijen A, Slooter GD, Kruyt PM, Bonjer HJ, Meijerink WJHJ. Real-time hypothermia monitoring during laparoscopic surgery. Surg Endosc. 2024;38(2):541–8. Available from: https://pubmed.ncbi.nlm.nih.gov/37558826/.
32. National Library of Medicine. A study of therapeutic hypothermia in trauma patients. ClinicalTrials.gov. [cited 2025 Jul 22]. Available from: https://clinicaltrials.gov/study/NCT05958550.
33. DA Surgical. Robotics in practice: new angles on safer positioning. DA Surgical News. 2024. Available from: https://da-surgical.com/2024/01/24/robotics-in-practice-new-angles-on-safer-positioning/.

Minimally Invasive Surgery Training Models

8

Marcus Cezillo, Robson Uwagoya, Bruno Tabajuihanski, and Bruna Amaral da Cruz

Introduction

The search for autonomy, especially in laparoscopy, is constant for every surgeon. This is because learning curves are slow [1, 2], resulting in prolonged operation time and reduced technical repertoire [3]. As open surgery skills are not transferable to laparoscopic and robotic surgery, evolution is, sometimes, not realized, and the difficulty with mastering minimally invasive surgery (MIS) is reported [4].

Several studies have related methods of training laparoscopic and robotic skills, using different types of simulation models. The use of simulation as a supplement to traditional training for the development of surgical skills enables learning curves to be shortened in a secure and controlled setting [5], without the need of practicing them for the first time in a patient [6]. These models include box training simulation with a camera—with adapted material or real equipment—practicing on synthetic materials or pieces of animal tissue (non-live tissue) and virtual reality.

These activities improve technical MIS skills and build confidence in a controlled condition, without environmental interaction. As a result, the surgeon could have a false sense of security when they enter the operating room because they think the method is easier than it actually is. Considering the aforementioned, simulation training on non-live tissue should never be used in place of live tissue training; rather, they should be added to it and be a necessary step prior to advanced laparoscopic skills on animals [7]. Following the complexity sequence, after non-live

M. Cezillo (✉)
Trauma Surgery Department, Hospital de Base do Distrito Federal (HBDF), Brasília, DF, Brazil

R. Uwagoya · B. A. da Cruz
Grupo de Pesquisa e Extensão em Cirurgia (GPEC), São Paulo, Brazil

B. Tabajuihanski
Hospital Municipal do Campo Limpo, São Paulo/SP, Brazil

© The Author(s), under exclusive license to Springer Nature Switzerland AG 2026
M. Cezillo, B. M. Pereira (eds.), *Minimally Invasive Surgery Trauma*,
https://doi.org/10.1007/978-3-032-28971-1_8

tissue training, practicing should be on live tissue (pig or other animal, depending on the local laws) and the last and most real and trustworthy training, the human cadaver.

Contemporary surgical practice increasingly demands a minimally invasive approach. Laparoscopy has become the gold standard for most procedures currently performed. As such, it is essential to provide adequate training in this skill set to surgeons in training. However, laparoscopic training is associated with a prolonged and steep learning curve, raising important concerns regarding patient safety during the acquisition of these technical competencies.

Artificial simulation models provide opportunities for training both basic and advanced laparoscopic skills by enabling the development of surgical psychomotor abilities in controlled environments. These settings can replicate a wide range of scenarios that allow for repeated practice and objective evaluation. Using virtual, synthetic, and biologic models, surgeons can develop cognitive, emotional, and psychomotor competencies by engaging in observation, imitation, deliberate practice with guided feedback, without any concerns with patient safety.

Several studies have related methods of training laparoscopic and robotic skills, using different types of simulation models. The use of simulation as a supplement to traditional training for the development of surgical skills enables learning curves to be shortened in a secure and controlled setting.

Types of Simulation

Inorganic Simulation

Laparoscopic Simulator (Box Trainers)

Knowledge and practical learning in surgical procedures are acquired during the surgeon's training. Generally, this training occurs through the transfer of knowledge from a more experienced professional to a less experienced surgeon [1].

Surgical procedures have their own specific learning curves, meaning that for a surgeon to become experienced depends on numerous factors. Minimally invasive procedures are increasingly becoming the first choice, such as cholecystectomies, appendectomies, and bariatric surgeries [8].

To improve laparoscopic surgical skills, we can make use of various equipment and methods, such as the use of live animals, cadavers, training boxes, and virtual reality. Throughout this chapter, we will address all these methods, but we must remember that each requires different structures and investments [8, 9].

Simulation boxes are not as expensive when compared to other methods, and they also do not require large structures or specific care for storage or disposal. These boxes may or may not have an anatomical shape of the abdomen or another part of the human body. They are generally composed of a fixed or mobile optic, endograsper, Maryland dissector, needle holder, and scissors [9].

There are countless exercises that can be performed in this type of simulator. Ideally, training should always start with manual coordination and depth perception exercises. The trainee surgeon is tasked with transferring objects from one container to another, performing calculations on a calculator. As skills advance, training can progress to techniques involving cutting, dissection, suturing, and clipping [9, 10].

The recommended step-by-step is to begin with basic procedures and progress as the trainee surgeon evolves. We can suggest the following steps [9, 10]:

Step 1—Navigation and adaptation with the instruments.
In this stage, the trainee surgeon will learn to handle the instruments and move them within a confined space. To do this, we can place a calculator inside the box and ask the trainee physician to use two graspers to perform calculations on the calculator.
Step 2—Coordination.
The second step aims to train the physician to work with both hands in coordination. For this, we can use a tube or rope with markings placed every 1 cm. The exercise consists of moving along the rope or tube using a pair of endograspers, with the requirement to position the graspers on the blue markings.
Step 3—Grasping, transferring, and manipulating.
Now, with navigation and coordination skills in place, training advances to the stage where procedures requiring finer movements begin. Grasping is the act of manipulating, holding, and transferring objects in laparoscopy. For this, the trainee surgeon will transfer beans or small bolts between containers. Preferably using four containers — two blue and two red, for example — with the objective of always transferring to the container of the same color.
Step 4—Cutting and sectioning.
With grasping skills firmly established, the junior surgeon is now ready to begin sectioning tasks. For this, we will use a spool of thread with markings every 1 cm. The task is to manipulate the thread with a grasper and cut at each marking using scissors.
Step 5—Precision and speed.
Videolaparoscopy requires precise movements, especially because its image lacks clearly defined depth perception. Therefore, in this step, the trainee physician will train both the precision and speed needed to separate beans or buttons into their corresponding containers. In a colored container, colored beans of two different colors—or buttons of two colors—will be mixed. The objective is to separate the colors into their respective containers, using one hand for each color. For example, blue buttons will be handled only with the right hand, while red buttons will be handled only with the left hand.
Step 6—Final challenge: dissection and suturing.
Now, with all the basic skills trained, we will move on to performing movements that simulate real procedures. At this stage, there are various possible exercises. Below, we will demonstrate two of these possibilities:

Dissection

Insert a thin tubular drain inside a procedural glove. This drain should have three markings. On the glove, at the level of the drain's markings, draw three circles: leave the first one empty, fill in the second one by coloring it with a pen, and leave the third, most external one, empty (Fig. 8.1).

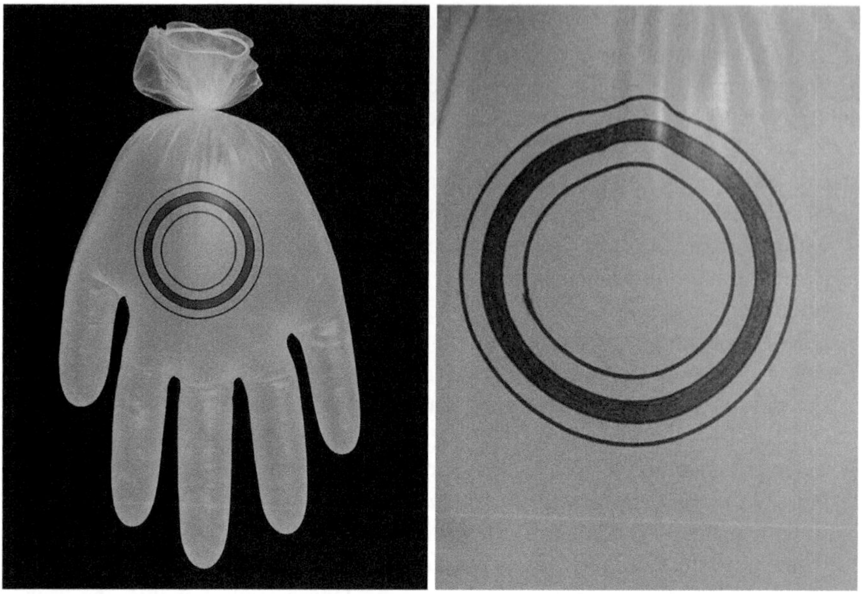

Fig. 8.1 Dissection training with gloves

The objective of this test is for the trainee physician, using an endograsper and scissors, to cut out the first (innermost) circle, fold it back, and access the inner part of the glove. Once inside, an endoclip should be placed at both the proximal and distal markings. To finish, the trainee must section the drain at the middle marking, between the two endoclips.

Suturing

One of the most well-known techniques for suturing training in box-type simulators is suturing on synthetic skin or grape peels (Fig. 8.2). As a first step, it is recommended to begin with synthetic skins, and with the trainee physician's favorable progression, gradually advance the training to more delicate objects.

Laparoscopic training is essential in modern surgical education, considering the growing demand for minimally invasive procedures across multiple specialties. As demonstrated throughout this chapter, the development of laparoscopic skills requires a logical, structured progression — starting from basic exercises such as navigation, coordination, and grasping, and advancing to more complex techniques involving dissection, clipping, suturing, and sectioning [11–15].

The use of box trainers has proven to be an accessible and effective tool for developing fundamental laparoscopic skills (Table 8.1). It offers a safe, low-cost, and reproducible environment that allows trainees to improve their psychomotor abilities and hand-eye coordination without risks to patients. Furthermore, as skills improve, these exercises can be intensified with tasks demanding greater precision, speed, and technical decision-making [16].

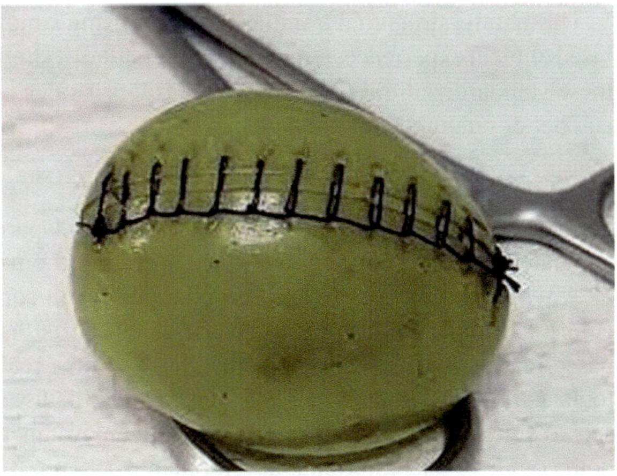

Fig. 8.2 Training suture in grape peels

Table 8.1 Low-cost laparoscopy simulators (2014–2025)

First author (Year)	Box material	Access hole design	Laparoscopic instruments	Imaging system	Estimated average cost
Martins et al. (2015) [17]	Plastic box with metal rods and rubber accessories	Cable grommets as trocars on the lid	Real laparoscopic instruments (grasper, trocar)	USB webcam attached to an aluminum rod	~US$ 90
Wong et al. (2015) [18]	Plastic/acrylic recycled box	Standard entry holes made with rotary tools	Basic or real laparoscopic kits	HD webcam connected to a PC/laptop	US$ 100–160
Peyton et al. (2019) [19]	Recycled IKEA-style trash bin	Manual drilled holes with reinforced borders	Donated or training instruments	HD USB webcam and laptop	~US$ 59
Cooper et al. (2023) [20]	Cardboard box with EVA foam panel	Cross-cut X-shape entry points in foam	3D-printed reusable instruments	Smartphone on flexible mount	~US$ 35
Soriero et al. (2020) [21]	Plywood frame with rigid rubber abdominal wall	Triangulated holes for realistic access	Simulated laparoscopic instruments	Bullet camera on TV connection	~US$ 85
Yeung et al. (2020) [22]	Transparent plastic storage box	Rubber sealing gaskets for tool insertion	Reused commercial laparoscopic kits	USB camera connected to computer	~US$ 55
Sutar et al. (2014) [23]	Metal or recycled plastic box	Drilled holes reinforced with rubber or foam	Real or simulated instruments	HD camera with laptop display	~US$ 50
Sellers (2019) [24]	Recycling bin	Drill a hole (with a 9/64″ drill bit) through the lid, covered by a mousepad	Borrowed or donated instruments	USB camera module with metal case for computer	~US$ 50
Duren (2014) [25]	Cardboard box	Simple hole in the box	Out-of-date equipment	A smart phone connected to a tablet computer	No data

Ultimately, structured training programs using simulation, combined with supervised clinical experience, remain the cornerstone of surgical education. Incorporating these standardized training protocols ensures a safer learning curve for the trainee and better outcomes for patients.

Virtual Reality Training

Virtual reality (VR) is an emerging technology in laparoscopic surgery which could simulate the virtual environment of an operating room in a secure setting.

A typical virtual reality (VR) simulation system consists of an enclosed console connected to a monitor, featuring instrument ports that interface with a software-based platform (Fig. 8.3). This setup allows for the realistic manipulation of virtual tools and tissues. More recent systems involve the use of virtual reality (VR) headsets to simulate a real-time operating room environment, creating opportunities for both cognitive and emotional development.

VR-based training allows learners to develop fundamental surgical skills such as eye-hand coordination, camera navigation, tissue grasping, cutting, and suturing. Importantly, it also provides exposure to the sequential phases of surgical procedures, fostering a better understanding of operative flow.

However, VR training is not without limitations. One of the major drawbacks of current virtual simulation platforms is the lack of tactile (haptic) feedback. This sensory input is essential for developing an accurate perception of the force required to manipulate tissues safely and effectively. To address this limitation, newer simulation devices are being developed to incorporate haptic feedback into the interaction with virtual instruments.

The literature presents inconclusive meta-analyses regarding the superiority of VR simulation over traditional training methods. Therefore, VR should be

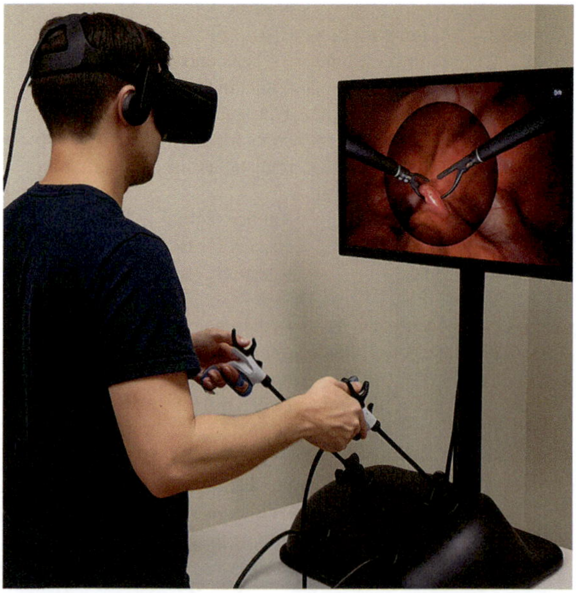

Fig. 8.3 VR simulation platform

considered a valuable supplemental tool rather than a replacement. Its integration with training models that provide tactile feedback appears to offer the most promising approach for improving surgical performance in real clinical settings.

Organic Simulation

Animal Tissues Parts in Laparoscopic Training

The use of animals and biological tissues has always been fundamental in the development of medicine. Since the earliest experiments that led to medical advancements, animals have played a central role in research. However, in recent years, new regulations have been imposed to reduce animal suffering in scientific studies. Some of these changes have restricted the use of biological tissues and live animals for medical research. Despite these limitations, there are still numerous possibilities for using animal parts in laparoscopic training and for improving the surgical learning curve [26].

The use of animal parts remains a key tool in surgical training, particularly because they provide realistic anatomical fidelity and tissue response. In laparoscopic surgery, animal tissues offer an accessible, high-fidelity opportunity for technical skill development and familiarization with tissue texture, tensile strength, and suturing behavior [27].

A variety of animal tissues can be used in laparoscopic simulation training, such as small intestine, liver, tongue, muscle, and skin. These tissues can be collected post-euthanasia and processed through cleaning and preservation techniques to maintain adequate quality for use [28]. Utilizing these tissues after euthanasia also reduces costs associated with synthetic models and promotes the development of both technical and non-technical skills, as their preparation and use require a multidisciplinary collaboration for collection, preparation, and training execution [27, 28].

In the context of laparoscopic training, organs from pigs, cattle, and sheep are the most commonly used due to their availability and relative anatomical similarity to human structures. These models provide excellent opportunities for practicing intracorporeal suturing, resections, and simulating intraoperative complications such as bleeding [27].

For simulation practices, animal parts are typically fixed inside laparoscopic training boxes, with trocars, laparoscopic instruments, a camera, and light source—allowing practice with real surgical instruments under spatial limitations and ergonomic constraints typical of laparoscopy (Fig. 8.4). Additionally, animal tissue training allows for the development of non-technical skills such as team coordination and communication in the operating room—aspects increasingly emphasized in recent literature [27].

There are already laparoscopic training boxes specifically designed for the use of prepared or fresh animal parts (Fig. 8.4). As described by Waseda in 2005, these boxes feature a built-in fluid collector to facilitate cleaning and safety during practice. Besides the fluid reservoir, the trainer incorporates a dorsal

Fig. 8.4 Laparoscopic training boxes for animal parts

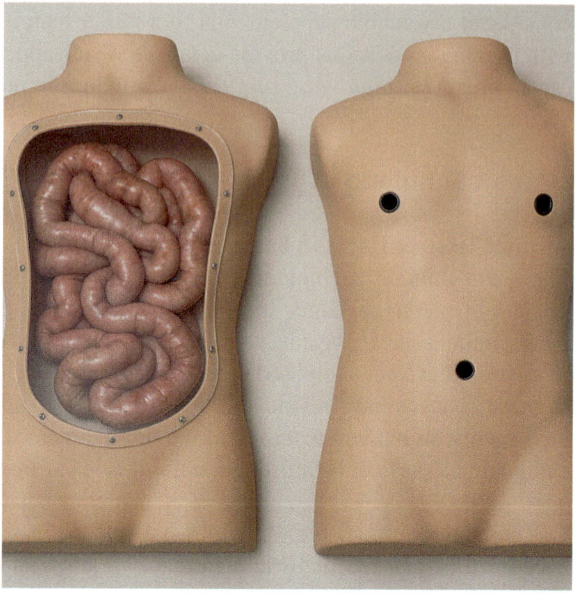

abdominal wall formed by a mesh structure to improve drainage, and an anterior wall covered with neoprene material to simulate the texture and resistance of the human abdominal wall [29].

Within this model, several procedures can be simulated, including appendectomy, cholecystectomy, fundoplication, colorectal surgeries, and transanal endoscopic procedures. Materials such as pig liver and gallbladder, calf colorectal tract, and bovine ileum and cecum are used. Suggested exercises include:

- Cholecystectomy
  This procedure is performed using a pig liver and gallbladder fixed in the upper quadrant of the simulator. The trainee should perform all the standard steps of laparoscopic cholecystectomy, including liver retraction, gallbladder dissection, identification of bile ducts and vessels, clipping, and gallbladder removal [30].
- Appendectomy
  The simulation uses bovine ileum and colon sutured together, positioned in the right iliac fossa. Participants practice identifying the appendix, dissecting the mesoappendix, and transecting the appendix. Cattle do not have a true appendix; however, we can create an appendix similar to the human one using the cecum and distal ileum of these animals [31].
- Fundoplication
  For this procedure, the simulator must have an opening at the level of the diaphragmatic hiatus to accommodate a porcine upper abdominal block containing the diaphragm, liver, spleen, and stomach. The esophagus is passed through the hiatus, and the procedure continues with dissection of the region, encircling of the distal esophagus and suturing of the gastric fundus to simulate a Nissen fundoplication [32].

- Colorectal

  It is possible to perform various colorectal training; for that, we need a calf colorectal tract with mesentery and peritoneum integrated into the pelvic cavity of the trainer. Peritoneum, mesentery, and the end of the rectum are fixed onto the trainer. It is possible to use a perfusion system if the box simulator is able to do so.

The use of animal parts remains an essential and effective approach for laparoscopic surgical training. Despite evolving ethical regulations that limit the use of live animals, the application of post-euthanasia tissues from pigs, cattle, and sheep continues to provide high-fidelity anatomical and tactile experiences critical for skill acquisition. These models enable the practice of complex procedures under realistic conditions, fostering both technical proficiency and non-technical skills such as team coordination. The integration of animal tissues in specialized laparoscopic trainers bridges the gap between simulation and real surgery, supporting safer and more efficient surgical education. Therefore, animal-based models retain significant value in advancing minimally invasive surgery training and should be considered a complementary resource alongside emerging synthetic and virtual simulation technologies [31, 33].

Cadaver Tissue Simulation

Fresh Frozen Cadaver

The fresh frozen cadavers (FFC), despite not being accessible in many institutions, are an intriguing resource for MIS training with good improvement in technical skills [33]. This method enables the instruction of both fundamental and sophisticated abilities while utilizing a simulation that more closely resembles reality thanks to access to real preserved anatomy [34]. According to studies, trainers are quite satisfied with FFCs because of their realistic texture, capacity to replicate real-world procedures, and anatomical placement accuracy. The significance and benefits of dissection courses in surgical training were also demonstrated by the outcomes [35] over other training models in laparoscopic surgery but are currently not widely used [36, 37].

The challenge of creating pneumoperitoneum to distend the abdominal wall and provide a suitable working space that mimics that of an anesthetized patient is one of the key barriers to using cadavers as teaching models. Some of the training centers use embalmed human cadavers, an expensive and complex preparation that is not available in low- and middle-income training centers [38, 39]. Some countries don't allow the use of the human body for study or training; others accept not only donated bodies but also unclaimed bodies. Depending on the law enforcement, the access to this training model can be limited or even unavailable in several countries [40]. Despite the cost involved in preparing the FFC, many universities prefer to invest in this training model; based on the fact, it's a beneficial option for schools that do not have as many opportunities for surgical skills training, where the added cost would be well spent for the additional experience [41].

Cadaver Tissue (Not Prepared)

Facing the barrier of a pneumoperitoneum creation, MAKUMA et al. (2016) proposed the laparoscopic training model using fresh human cadavers without the establishment of pneumoperitoneum with a system based on a synthetic "table station," avoiding direct vision, where it's possible to maintain the surgical material [4].

An alternative to this "table station" is a fake abdominal wall by using a pregnant belly dummy rather than pneumoperitoneum for simulating basic and advanced training (Fig. 8.5). With this device, it can be created a simple and practical pneumoperitoneum-like environment on the cadaver, properly opened. The cadaver is opened with a large abdominal incision, allowing for wide access to the abdominal cavity organs. The flaps are fixed with simple suture on the skin for full exposure of the abdominal contents (Fig. 8.6).

In order to insufflate the abdomen, the pregnant belly dummy creates a pneumoperitoneum-like environment where holes (trocar incisions) are distributed according to the procedures to be trained. A practical method is to divide into modules: biliopancreatic surgery, esophagogastric surgery, right and left colon procedures, and pelvic procedures. This device allows the insertion of

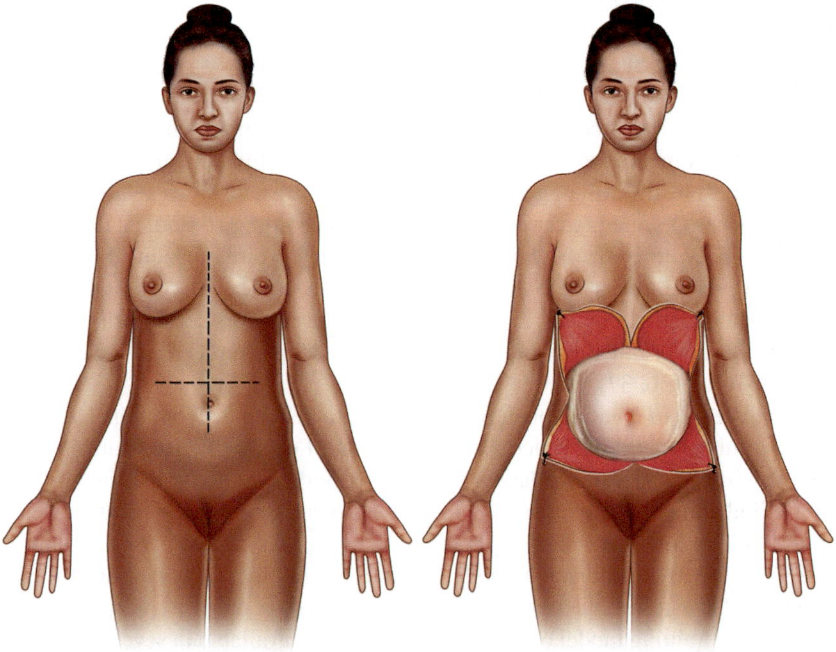

Fig. 8.5 Fake abdominal wall by using a pregnant belly dummy rather than pneumoperitoneum for simulating basic and advanced training

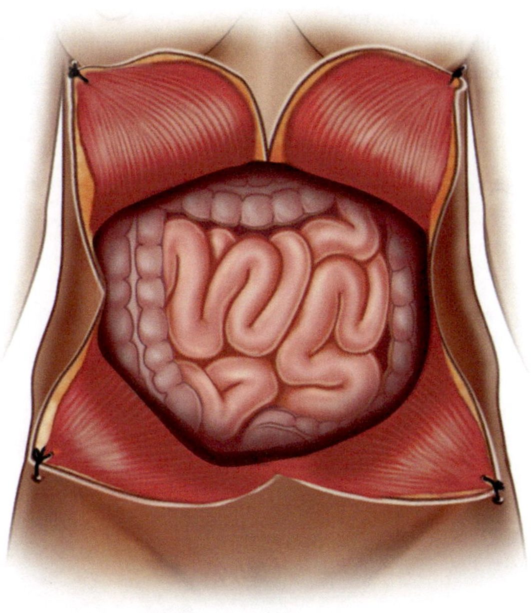

Fig. 8.6 Access to the abdominal cavity organs using large incisions and fixation of the flaps for full exposure of the abdominal content

different trocar sites or even the insertion of laparoscopic material directly. The holes need to be large enough for adequate adjustment and mobility of the equipment (Fig. 8.7).

When using a cadaver, prepared or not, the absence of a surgical table, which offers decubitus changes, can make the procedure more difficult and less realistic. To deal with this, it's possible to improve the exposure and the realism of the procedure by changing the decubitus, using an angled and entire piece of wood, metal, or hard plastic for positioning the cadaver, inserting it on the back side where the exposure is needed (Fig. 8.8). This "homemade device" can be put in different positions to produce different decubitus according to the procedure intended. This device is an affordable tool and a very valuable training model for laparoscopic advanced teaching because it can deal with space and exposure limitations, making it accessible for low-resource institutions.

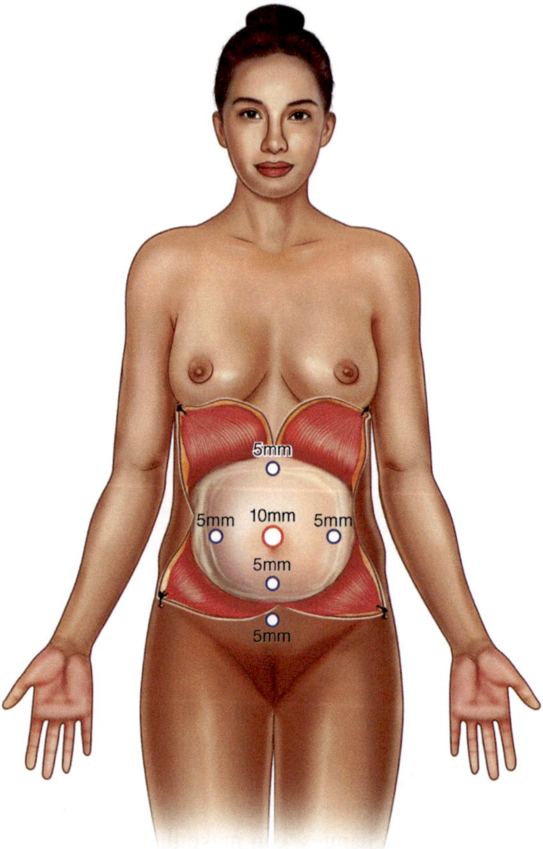

Fig. 8.7 Example of different trocar sites for use in the fake abdominal wall

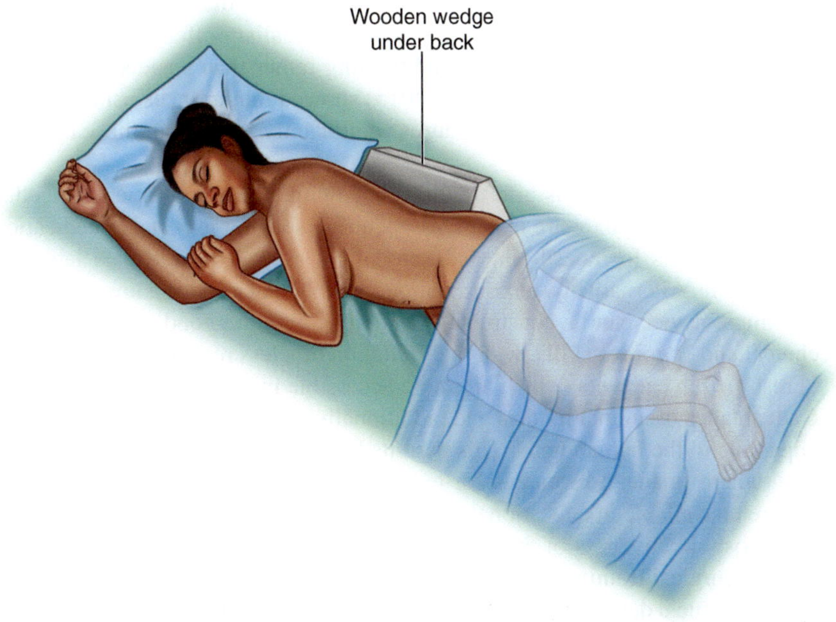

Fig. 8.8 Technique of the piece of wood, metal, or hard plastic for positioning the cadaver, inserting it on the back side where the exposure is needed

Discussion

The limited availability of laparoscopic training, combined with a steep learning curve, discourages many surgeons from adopting the minimally invasive surgery (MIS) approach. In general, laparoscopic simulators—whether using live or synthetic tissue—are not affordable for low- and middle-income surgical residency programs. For this reason, this chapter presents alternative devices and methods for adapting materials to achieve the most realistic training possible.

Box training simulation with a camera—using adapted materials or real equipment—allows practice on synthetic materials or animal tissue (non-live tissue), as well as virtual reality simulators, each with their own advantages and disadvantages.

There is a trend to use synthetic devices; however, these do not reproduce real tissue handling, anatomical positioning, or the relationship between structures because they use synthetic materials instead of live tissue [42]. Similar limitations are found in virtual simulators. Besides being expensive and complex, they lack tissue handling feedback and spatial navigation. While these limitations are not critical for basic skills exercises, they are essential for advanced procedures [43].

No study has conclusively compared the efficacy of different simulation methods. However, Leblanc et al. (2010) demonstrated that the human cadaver model was technically more challenging but better appreciated than simulators for laparoscopic sigmoid colectomy training. Due to the realism offered by the cadaver model, it is more suitable for advanced training rather than basic skills development [42]. Similarly, Bruwaene et al. (2015) showed that trainees using a porcine (live tissue) model performed procedures significantly faster than those using virtual trainers [43].

Although animal models offer realistic breathing, bowel movements, bleeding, and tissue handling, they are expensive, requiring specific materials, medications, and professionals for anesthesia and ventilation, as well as adequate laboratory infrastructure. Alternatively, box simulation (dry lab) can provide a low-cost option. This simple device can be constructed at home and allows good training for basic technical and cognitive skills, with the limitation of a less realistic scenario [17].

Fresh frozen cadavers, which are more accessible in many institutions, offer all the advantages of animal models and, additionally, provide a high-fidelity resource comparable to the human body. This permits laparoscopic training within the local reality where financial resources for expensive simulators or laparoscopic equipment are unavailable in educational hospitals.

The cost-effectiveness of this suggested model makes it feasible to incorporate advanced surgical training courses into structured postgraduate curricula, meeting both the technical demands of minimally invasive surgery and patient safety requirements. In developing countries, seeking alternatives is reasonable given the lack of equipment and experience [44]. The non-embalmed cadaver offers a professional and realistic training scenario with materials commonly available and is often preferred by experienced trainees when performing advanced techniques, progressing from basic to complex skills [45].

Under these circumstances, it is reasonable to infer that these countries face severe difficulties in training surgeons in laparoscopy, especially when using low-cost gasless models or artificial abdominal walls.

The model described here may be more accessible for institutions in developing countries with budget constraints seeking to establish laparoscopic training programs. By substituting costly equipment with cheaper and more readily available materials, this method provides a realistic tool that enables reproduction of operative steps, recognition of real anatomical structures in a 2D view, and teamwork—fundamental for both individual and group improvement [46].

Conclusion

A non-embalmed cadaver with a non-pneumoperitoneum cavity seems to be an affordable and feasible laparoscopic training model. An improved exposure to fundamental maneuvers, greater confidence in trainee capabilities, and early operative independence are all benefits of cadaver-based simulation training. The low-cost model is presented in this study. Simulator training (before) followed by cadaver training can appropriately integrate simulators into the learning curve and maintain the benefits of both training methodologies.

References

1. Graham LA, Hawn MT. Learning curves and the challenges of adopting new surgical techniques. JAMA Netw Open. 2019;2(10):e1913569.
2. Valsamis EM, Chouari T, O'Dowd-Booth C, Rogers B, Ricketts D. Learning curves in surgery: variables, analysis and applications. Postgrad Med J. 2018;94(1115):525–30.
3. Hardon F, Van Gastel LA, Horeman T, Daams F. Assessment of technical skills based on learning curve analyses in laparoscopic surgery training. Surgery. 2021;170(3):831–40.
4. Makuma ES, Ussami EY, Meyer A. Laparoscopic training model using fresh human cadavers without establishment of pneumoperitoneum. J Minim Access Surg. 2016;12(2):190–3.
5. Aggarwal R, Darzi A. Simulation to enhance patient safety: why aren't we there yet? Chest. 2011;140:854–8.
6. Brindley PG, Jones DB, Grantcharov T, de Gara C. Surgical simulation: the solution to safe training or a promise unfulfilled? Can J Surg. 2012;55:S200–6.
7. Ferrufino FL, Cohen JV, Schaffner EB, Eulufi FC, Muller FP, Castillo JM, et al. Simulación en cirugía laparoscópica. Cir Esp. 2015;93:4–11.
8. Gurusamy KS, Nagendran M, Toon CD, Davidson BR. Laparoscopic surgical box model training for surgical trainees with limited prior laparoscopic experience. Cochrane Database Syst Rev. 2014;3:CD010478.
9. Anastakis DJ, Regehr G, Reznick RK, Cusimano M, Murnaghan J, Brown M, et al. Assessment of technical skills transfer from bench training model to the human model. Am J Surg. 1999;177(2):167–70.
10. Munz Y, Kumar BD, Moorthy K, Bann S, Darzi A. Laparoscopic virtual reality and box trainers: is one superior to the other? Surg Endosc. 2004;18:485–94.
11. Derossis AM, Fried GM, Abrahamowicz M, Sigman HH, Barkun JS, Meakins JL. Development of a model for training and evaluation of laparoscopic skills. Am J Surg. 1998;175:482–7.
12. Reznick R, Regehr G, MacRae H, Martin J, McCulloch W. Testing technical skill via an innovative "bench station" examination. Am J Surg. 1996;173:226–30.
13. Torkington J, Smith SG, Rees BI, Darzi A. The role of simulation in surgical training. Ann R Coll Surg Engl. 2000;82:88–94.
14. Guerrero-Hernández AJ, et al. Laparoscopic training by use of a physical simulator and its application in general surgery residency. Med Univ. 2016;18(73):189–93.
15. Montoya-Chinchilla R, et al. Low-cost laparoscopic training: necessary time for acquiring expertise. Cir Cir. 2012;80(3):253–60.
16. Łysak JM, Lis M, Więckowski PR. Low-cost laparoscopic simulator: enabling access to laparoscopic training for medical students. Surgeon. 2023;21(6):351–5.
17. Martins JMP, Ribeiro RVP, Cavazzola LT. White box: low-cost box for laparoscopic training. Arq Bras Cir Dig. 2015;28(3):204–6.
18. Wong J, Bhattacharya G, Vance SJ, Bistolarides P, Merchant AM. Construction and validation of a low-cost laparoscopic simulator. J Surg Educ. 2013;70(4):443–50.
19. Peyton C, Hogg M, McKechnie T, et al. Development and validation of an inexpensive homemade laparoscopic trainer. J Surg Simul. 2019;7:1–8.
20. Pakataridis P, Daskalov M, Khan M, Chelmis F, Sorotou IN, Neeli A, Sivridis A, Naseva E, Valle V. Low-cost biodegradable 3-dimensional-printed laparoscopic simulator: A sustainable alternative for surgical training. Surgery. 2025;187:109624. https://doi.org/10.1016/j.surg.2025.109624. Epub 2025 Aug 25. PMID: 40857976.
21. Soriero D, et al. Development and validation of a homemade laparoscopic simulator. Int J Environ Res Public Health. 2020;17:1–14.
22. Yeung T, et al. Building a low-cost laparoscopic box trainer for surgical practice. MedEdPORTAL. 2020;16:10947.
23. Sutar S, et al. Design and development of a low-cost laparoscopic trainer. J Clin Diagn Res. 2014;8:NC01–3.

24. Sellers T, Ghannam M, Asantey K, Roach VA. Low-cost laparoscopic skill training for medical students using homemade equipment. MedEdPORTAL. 2019;15:10826. https://doi.org/10.15766/mep_2374-8265.10826.
25. van Duren BH, van Boxel GI. Use your phone to build a simple laparoscopic trainer. J Minim Access Surg. 2014;10(4):219–220. https://doi.org/10.4103/0972-9941.141534.
26. Koscielny A. What is the value of animal models in laparoscopic surgery?—a systematic review. Ann Laparosc Endosc Surg. 2022;7:37. https://doi.org/10.21037/ales-21-52.
27. Davidson EL, et al. Advancements in surgical education: exploring animal and simulation models in fetal and neonatal surgery training. Front Pediatr. 2024;12:1402596.
28. Ladowski JM, et al. Animal models within surgical simulation: a novel approach to the 3Rs. J Surg Res. 2024;303:275.
29. Waseda M, et al. Innovative trainer for surgical procedures using animal organs. Minim Invasive Ther Allied Technol. 2005;14:262–6.
30. Bailey RW, Imbembo AL, Zucker KA. Establishment of a laparoscopic cholecystectomy training program. Am Surg. 1991;57:231–6.
31. Lasley DS, Seth SR, Yancey MK. Porcine laparoscopy training for surgeons. J Am Assoc Gynecol Laparosc. 1995;2:24.
32. Yokoyama M, Mailaender L, Raestrup H, Buess G. Training system for laparoscopic fundoplication. Minim Invasive Ther Allied Technol. 2003;12:143–50.
33. Sharma M, Macafee D, Horgan AF. Laparoscopic skills training using fresh frozen cadaver: randomized trial. Am J Surg. 2013;206(1):23–31.
34. Pattanshetti VM, Pattanshetti SV. Laparoscopic surgery on cadavers: teaching tool for residents. ANZ J Surg. 2010;80:676–8.
35. Song YK, Jo DH. Use of fresh frozen cadaver in surgical training and anatomical education. Anat Sci Educ. 2022;15(5):957–69.
36. Lloyd GM, Maxwell-Armstrong C, Acheson AG. Fresh frozen cadavers in laparoscopic colorectal training. Color Dis. 2011;13:e303–4.
37. Giger U, Frésard I, Häfliger A, Bergmann M, Krähenbühl L. Laparoscopic training on Thiel human cadavers. Surg Endosc. 2008;22:901–6.
38. Brenner E, Bleys RLAW, de Caro R, et al. Legal and ethical framework governing body donation in Europe. Ann Anat. 2024;252:152195.
39. Qualls AC, Fox WB, Merchant A. Comprehensive review on the use of fresh frozen cadavers in procedural skill training of medical students. Int J Surg Educ. Published online 2024 Nov 12. https://doi.org/10.5281/zenodo.14838174.
40. James HK, Pattison GTR, Griffin DR, Fisher JD. Influence of cadaveric simulation on orthopedic residents learning. J Surg Educ. 2020;77:671–82.
41. Sharma M, Horgan A. Comparison of cadaver and virtual reality laparoscopic training. World J Surg. 2012;36:1732–7.
42. LeBlanc F, Champagne BJ, Augestad KM, et al. Cadaver vs augmented reality simulator in laparoscopic training. J Am Coll Surg. 2010;211:250–5.
43. Van Bruwaene S, Schijven MP, Napolitano D, De Win G, Miserez M. Porcine cadaver organ vs virtual simulation training. J Surg Educ. 2015;72:483–90.
44. Kim SC, Fisher JG, Delman KA, Hinman JM, Srinivasan JK. Cadaver-based simulation increases resident confidence. J Surg Educ. 2016;73:e33–41.
45. Ackermann J, Wedel T, Hagedorn H, et al. Advanced laparoscopic training based on human body donors. Surg Endosc. 2021;35:1385–94.
46. Emken JL, McDougall EM, Clayman RV. Training and assessment of laparoscopic skills. JSLS. 2004;8:195–9.

Technical Aspects of the Minimally Invasive Surgery in a Teaching Hospital

9

Carlos Yánez Benítez and Jody Miller

Introduction

Minimally invasive surgery has undergone a remarkable evolution and is now widely available in many hospitals worldwide. This advanced surgical approach is not limited to elective procedures; it is also effectively utilized in managing numerous acute care conditions, demonstrating its versatility and relevance across various clinical scenarios [1–3]. The widespread adoption of these techniques has opened doors for many young surgeons to engage in hands-on training early in their careers. This early exposure to minimally invasive surgical techniques plays a crucial role in enhancing their surgical skills and confidence, enabling them to tackle complex and challenging cases with precision and expertise, and with assurance [4].

Furthermore, in addition to the technical training, young surgeons are benefiting from significant technological advancements. The development of sophisticated and simple-to-use mono and bipolar vessel sealing energy devices, specifically designed for dissection and hemostasis, has transformed the way trauma surgeries are performed, enhancing both efficiency and safety [5]. These innovations also include the introduction of endostaplers, which are essential for navigating more complex surgical scenarios, including those encountered in trauma surgery. They enable faster, safer, and easier management of hollow viscus injuries commonly encountered in trauma surgery. The combination of advanced techniques and cutting-edge technology in MIS not only has contributed to elevating the standard of trauma surgical care but has also inspired a new generation of surgeons to continually push the boundaries of minimally invasive techniques, ultimately leading to improved patient outcomes.

C. Y. Benítez (✉)
Mediclinic Parkview Hospital, Dubai, UAE

J. Miller
Department of Trauma and Acute Care Surgery, Mediclinic Parkview Hospital, Dubai, UAE

© The Author(s), under exclusive license to Springer Nature Switzerland AG 2026

M. Cezillo, B. M. Pereira (eds.), *Minimally Invasive Surgery Trauma*,
https://doi.org/10.1007/978-3-032-28971-1_9

In surgical trauma care, technological advancements in imaging and resuscitation have transformed practice, enabling early and more precise diagnosis along with improved patient outcomes. Better imaging quality from both ultrasound and CT scans allows for quicker and more accurate detection of traumatic injuries, assisting trauma teams in making timely decisions [6–8]. Similarly, resuscitation techniques have seen significant changes over the past decade, with the early application of massive transfusion protocols, balanced and hemostatic resuscitation, and the use of whole blood showing clear benefits [9–11]. Likewise, minimally invasive surgery (MIS) has been widely adopted by the trauma surgery community and is now accepted for selected patients [12–16]. However, its implementation has been, in the author's view, slower and not universally adopted by trauma teams due to inconsistencies in its indications and global availability. The successful adoption of minimally invasive surgery (MIS) in trauma care relies on the availability of resources and effective collaboration among the surgical team. Managing trauma with MIS requires careful patient selection, accurate diagnosis, effective team coordination, and surgical expertise, making teamwork essential in every case [17–19]. A competent trauma team must excel in prompt resuscitation, patient selection, and effectively integrating laparoscopic and open surgical techniques. Together, they ensure that patient outcomes can improve even amidst the chaos of trauma. This exemplifies the intersection of technology and teamwork in the surgical environment.

In addition to equipment and skills, team dynamics play a crucial role in the success of minimally invasive surgery (MIS) implementation in trauma [20, 21]. Effective communication is essential and encompasses various elements such as task allocation, leadership roles, distribution of responsibilities, and thorough debriefing sessions after procedures [21]. Each of these components significantly enhances the team's performance and ensures optimal patient outcomes. Therefore, careful consideration of team dynamics, particularly in terms of communication and operational strategies, is vital in the context of minimally invasive trauma surgery. This chapter will explore the current role of MIS in trauma care, the specific indications and contraindications, the challenges of implementing these techniques in emergency settings, and the educational strategies necessary to ensure safe and effective training in academic institutions. By examining real-world integration, simulation-based training, competency assessment, and the expansion of MIS indications, this chapter aims to provide a practical and forward-looking framework for trauma surgeons and educators alike.

The Role of the Trauma Surgeon in Minimally Invasive Trauma Surgery

Laparoscopic surgery, also known as minimally invasive surgery (MIS), is becoming an increasingly specialized field within general surgery. Surgeons today often develop advanced expertise tailored to specific fields, including acute care surgery, abdominal wall surgery, upper gastrointestinal (GI) surgery, colorectal procedures, and hepatobiliary and pancreatic (HBP) surgery [22–26]. Each subspecialty necessitates a unique combination of techniques, anatomical knowledge, and operative strategies. However, MIS in the context of trauma presents a markedly different identity, one that is dynamic, time-sensitive, and driven by high-stakes decision-making processes.

The trauma surgeon, a vital member of the trauma team, must cultivate a unique surgical mindset [27]. Unlike elective surgery, trauma surgery does not focus on perfect dissection planes or extensive operative planning. Instead, it emphasizes swift and accurate judgment under pressure. The trauma laparoscopist must excel at identifying sources of bleeding, efficiently exposing injured structures, and promptly controlling life-threatening injuries. This requires not only technical skills but also the ability to maintain situational awareness and prioritize interventions within the broader context of the critically injured patient [28].

The trauma surgeon must determine which patients are suitable candidates for a minimally invasive approach [29]. This decision needs to be made quickly, often within minutes, based on the patient's hemodynamic status, mechanism of injury, radiological findings, and the potential for rapid deterioration. The threshold for converting to an open procedure should remain low; there is no room for ego or unnecessary delays in the trauma bay or operating room. The focus must always be on patient survival and damage control.

To acquire, maintain, and teach laparoscopic proficiency, trauma surgeons must engage in a continuous process of training and skill refinement. This often involves performing elective laparoscopic procedures such as cholecystectomies, appendectomies, or diagnostic explorations, both independently and as part of multidisciplinary teams. Elective cases provide not only technical practice but also an opportunity to develop depth perception, instrument handling, and familiarity with minimally invasive equipment and energy devices.

Furthermore, the successful implementation of laparoscopic trauma techniques does not rely solely on the surgeon. Trauma care is inherently multidisciplinary. The trauma surgeon must prepare the entire operative team to work together effectively in minimally invasive situations. This requires close collaboration with anesthesiologists to manage ventilation and fluid status in patients with abdominal trauma, engaging scrub nurses skilled in the instrumentation and workflow of laparoscopy, and consulting with other surgical subspecialties, such as colorectal, hepatobiliary, or vascular surgery, when complex injuries necessitate shared expertise. Simulation-based training, intraoperative video reviews, and structured team briefings can enhance preparedness and foster a culture of safety [30–33]. The trauma team must develop the agility to switch between open and laparoscopic modalities based on patient response and intraoperative findings. This team-based readiness ensures that minimally invasive trauma surgery is not only technically feasible but also safe, reproducible, and outcome-driven.

Key Learning Points:

- Trauma MIS demands a unique mindset that focuses on swift decision-making, rapid assessment of hemodynamic stability, and willingness to transition to open surgery without hesitation.

- Patient selection is crucial and depends on the mechanism of injury, imaging, and clinical status to identify candidates who may benefit from a minimally invasive approach.
- Maintaining laparoscopic proficiency through elective procedures is crucial for trauma surgeons, as it supports skill retention and enhances technical refinement.
- Care, enhancing readiness, adaptability, and consistent outcomes in high-risk situations.

Team Composition and Dynamics in Laparoscopic Trauma Surgery

The successful application of minimally invasive techniques in trauma surgery depends not only on the surgeon's skills but also on the functionality and preparedness of a cohesive, multidisciplinary team. Trauma care is inherently collaborative and time-sensitive; in the context of laparoscopic interventions, where equipment, visualization, and coordination are critical, team composition becomes even more vital. A well-prepared trauma team for laparoscopic surgery typically includes:

1. Trauma Surgeons and Surgical Residents

   At the center of the team is the trauma surgeon, who must possess strong laparoscopic skills, sound judgment, and leadership abilities [34]. The trauma surgeon directs the resuscitation and operative plan, prioritizing trauma care based on hemodynamic status and response to resuscitation [35]. They also select the required equipment, deliver instructions for patient positioning, determine the initial port disposition and surgical approach, and coordinate intraoperative decisions. In academic hospitals, surgical residents play a vital supporting role, assisting with visualization, retraction, and occasionally performing portions of the procedure under supervision. Laparoscopic trauma cases provide a valuable teaching opportunity for residents to understand the indications, limitations, and strategies of minimally invasive surgery in trauma settings. However, resident involvement must always be balanced with patient safety and procedural efficiency, especially in patients with unstable conditions.
2. Anesthesiologists

   The anesthesiology team is a crucial partner in trauma laparoscopy. Pneumoperitoneum affects hemodynamics, venous return, and respiratory physiology parameters that must be carefully managed in trauma patients, many of whom are already compromised. The surgical team may need to adjust the patient's position to either Trendelenburg or Fowler's position, which may further complicate physiology and ventilation. Anesthesiologists should be ready to maintain balanced resuscitation and implement permissive hypotension strategies. They must also adjust ventilation techniques, particularly in cases of chest trauma and active bleeding. Additionally, they need to manage blood pressure and provide real-time feedback to the surgical team regarding the patient's physiological response. Communication between the surgeon and anesthesiologist is crucial, particularly when considering the risks associated with proceeding with laparoscopy versus converting to an open approach.

3. Scrub Nurses and Surgical Technicians

   Experienced scrub nurses and laparoscopic technicians play a crucial role in the successful execution of trauma laparoscopy. They must be well-versed in the setup and operation of laparoscopic towers, light sources, insufflation systems, energy devices, and advanced tools such as suction-irrigation systems and vascular clips. In trauma cases, where timing is critical, any delays caused by unfamiliarity or technical errors can be detrimental. Thus, training and regular drills for the scrub team are essential, especially in institutions where trauma laparoscopy occurs infrequently.

4. Circulating Nurses and OR Support Staff

   Efficient coordination outside the sterile field is crucial to the overall success of surgical operations. Circulating nurses must anticipate the diverse equipment needs throughout the procedure and ensure the immediate availability of essential blood products, which can be critical during ongoing massive transfusion protocols. Additionally, they are responsible for assisting the surgical team with screen positioning and quickly converting setups if adjustments are necessary during the operation. Their heightened situational awareness, combined with their exceptional ability to multitask in high-pressure environments, is vital for supporting the workflow of the sterile team, ultimately enhancing patient safety and ensuring that the entire surgical process runs smoothly and efficiently. By maintaining clear communication, preemptively addressing potential issues, and remaining alert to developments within the operating room, circulating nurses significantly enhance the effectiveness of surgical procedures, resulting in improved patient outcomes.

5. Other Surgical Subspecialists

   In complex trauma cases, the trauma surgeon may require intraoperative consultation or collaboration with other specialists, including colorectal, hepatobiliary, urology, or vascular surgeons. Institutions with structured trauma pathways should facilitate rapid intraoperative support from these teams when injuries go beyond the trauma surgeon's expertise. Prior simulation training and joint cases can improve coordination and mutual understanding of roles in the laparoscopic environment.

The Need for Predefined Roles and Training

To enhance both efficiency and safety in laparoscopic trauma care, every member of the surgical team needs to have well-defined roles and responsibilities. This clarity streamlines workflow and minimizes potential confusion during high-pressure situations, ultimately leading to better patient outcomes. One of the most effective methods to achieve this is through comprehensive simulation-based training, which includes various components such as laparoscopic drills, video debriefings, and multidisciplinary trauma simulations [36]. These methods serve a dual purpose:

they not only improve interprofessional communication among team members but also promote a greater understanding of each role within the procedure. Given the complexity of trauma scenarios, such preparation is invaluable, as it equips the team with the necessary skills and coordination required to manage urgent and challenging cases effectively. Furthermore, trauma centers aiming to integrate MIS should develop standard procedures and checklists tailored for laparoscopic surgery and trauma interventions [37, 38]. These protocols ensure that all team members are aligned and can anticipate each phase of the procedure, from induction and positioning to trocar placement, exploration, and potential conversion.

Key Learning Points:

- *Multidisciplinary collaboration is crucial* in laparoscopic trauma surgery, demanding seamless coordination among surgeons, anesthesiologists, nurses, and support staff.
- *Surgeon leadership and resident involvement* must balance operative efficiency, educational value, and patient safety, particularly in unstable patients.
- *Anesthesiology plays a vital role* in managing altered physiology during pneumoperitoneum and in maintaining real-time communication with the surgical team.
- *Trained and prepared scrub and circulating staff* are essential to prevent delays, meet equipment needs, and enable quick responses during high-stakes procedures.

Decision-Making and Coordination: Triage, Case Selection, and Intraoperative Teamwork

The integration of laparoscopic surgery into trauma care reflects the evolution of minimally invasive techniques in acute surgical settings. However, its success relies not only on the surgeon's technical expertise but also on the trauma team's ability to execute timely, coordinated decision-making. From triage to intraoperative collaboration, each step requires clear communication, situational awareness, and dynamic leadership [39].

Triage and Case Selection

In trauma settings, triage and case selection for laparoscopy require rapid clinical judgment. The trauma team must identify which patients are candidates for a minimally invasive approach based on hemodynamic stability, the mechanism of injury, and the availability of imaging. Laparoscopy is generally reserved for, but not limited to, hemodynamically stable patients with penetrating abdominal trauma, suspected hollow viscus injury, or uncertain abdominal findings [40–44]. Interdisciplinary communication at this stage is crucial, often involving trauma surgery, radiology, and anesthesia in joint assessments.

Key Considerations for Case Selection Include:

- *Stability of the patient*: Unstable patients with ongoing hemorrhage are not candidates for laparoscopy and should go directly to laparotomy.
- *Injury pattern*: Isolated injuries (e.g., diaphragmatic tears, suspected bowel perforations, or localized peritonitis) may respond well to laparoscopy.
- *Availability of resources:* A complete laparoscopic setup, experienced laparoscopic trauma surgeons, advanced equipment, and a skilled anesthesia team are critical (Figs. 9.1 and 9.2).
- *Diagnostic uncertainty*: Laparoscopy serves a crucial role in both diagnosis and management, thus preventing unnecessary laparotomies.

Intraoperative Teamwork

Once the decision for laparoscopy is made, intraoperative coordination is crucial. The trauma environment varies significantly from elective surgical settings, and successful minimally invasive trauma surgery demands a trauma team that is well-trained in (Fig. 9.3):

- *Roles*: Clearly defining roles for each team member (e.g., camera operator, assistant, scrub nurse, circulator) ensures smooth operation and readiness for rapid conversion if necessary.
- *Crisis anticipation*: The entire team must be prepared for swift conversion. Instruments for open conversion, vascular control, and major bleeding should be easily accessible.
- *Real-time communication*: The lead surgeon must communicate findings and changes in strategy promptly. Feedback from anesthesia regarding the patient's status, especially during pneumoperitoneum, informs intraoperative decisions.

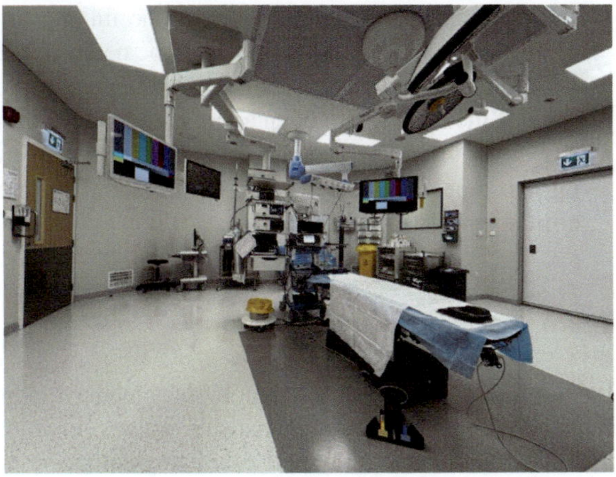

Fig. 9.1 A modern operating room prepared for laparoscopic trauma surgery setup: a fully equipped operating theater featuring a central surgical table, a laparoscopy tower, multiple screen suspended from the ceiling, allowing view from different angles of the surgical field, insufflation, energy devices, and trauma instruments ready for rapid intervention. The setup highlights readiness for a surgical procedure, emphasizing hygiene, advanced technology, and efficient space use

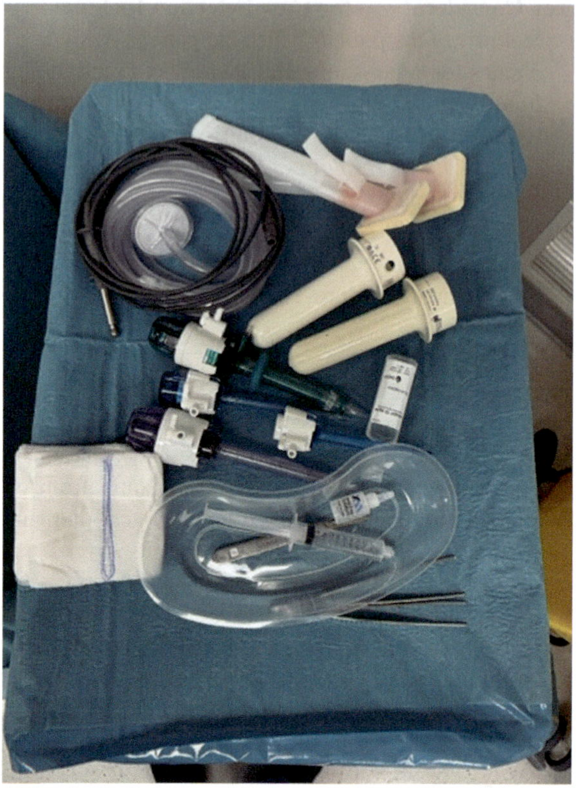

Fig. 9.2 Basic laparoscopic set for initial laparoscopic approach including clorhexidine sponges, insufflation tubing, monopolar energy cable, different sizes of laparoscopic ports (5 and 10 mm), local anesthesia, antifog solution, and scaple with forceps for port site placement

- *Systematic approach*: Trauma laparoscopy, like open trauma laparotomy, must be a well-planned and structured procedure in which all intra-abdominal structures are examined systematically to prevent missing injuries.
- *Early decision-making*: During the exploratory laparoscopy, the surgical team should promptly determine whether the findings allow for a definitive laparoscopic approach or if conversion will be necessary. The team should avoid wasting time and should discontinue the laparoscopic approach if any findings suggest the need for an open approach to ensure proper injury management.
- *Backup plans*: A pre-established protocol for converting to open surgery, including the preparation of the surgical field and equipment, reduces delays during critical moments.

Team Leadership and Dynamics

Laparoscopic trauma surgery emphasizes leadership and non-technical skills. The trauma surgeon must lead decisively while remaining open to input from team members. A flat hierarchy and psychological safety encourage team members to voice their concerns in the event of a deteriorating patient status or technical issues.

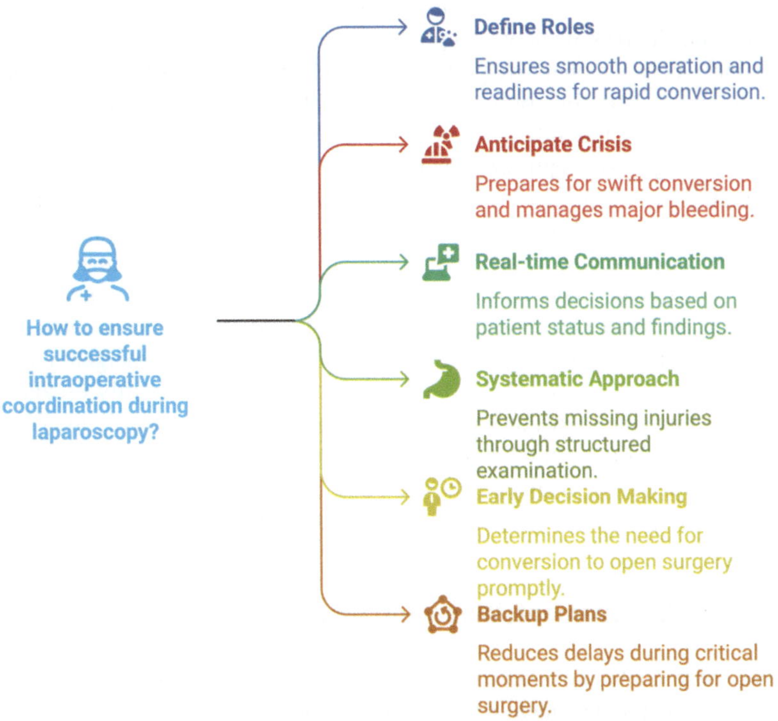

Fig. 9.3 For a successful intraoperative coordination, the surgical team must define clear roles (e.g., camera operator, scrub nurse) for efficient trauma laparoscopy. They should prepare for rapid conversion to open surgery with accessible instruments and maintain real-time communication about the patient. A systematic examination of all intra-abdominal structures is crucial, and timely decisions on conversion are key for effective injury management. Pre-established protocols for conversion and surgical preparation minimize delays in critical moments

Effective coordination among team members during laparoscopic trauma procedures reduces operative time, minimizes complications, and facilitates a smooth transition from diagnosis to therapy. Simulation-based training, along with trauma-specific laparoscopic drills and protocols, can further enhance team readiness and performance [45, 46].

Training and Supervision Challenges in Trauma Laparoscopy: Balancing Efficiency with Resident Learning

The trauma bay and operating room during severe trauma are complex and noisy environments; there is a sense of controlled chaos, with all team members actively working together to deliver quality care. Intra-abdominal access, adequate injury identification, exposure time to the bleeding site, and hemorrhage control can all determine survivability [47]. In this demanding setting, the introduction of laparoscopic surgery presents unique challenges: how to effectively train surgical residents and fellows without compromising patient safety or surgical efficiency. The balance between operative performance and education is particularly challenging in trauma, where time pressure, unpredictable pathology, and limited teaching opportunities converge [48].

Trauma surgery often presents the most formative learning moments for surgical trainees due to unexpected findings, critical decision-making, and high-intensity teamwork. However, it frequently requires procedures led by attending surgeons, which are time-efficient interventions that limit hands-on involvement for those who are not trained. This tension is heightened in laparoscopy, where technical skills such as depth perception, camera control, and ambidextrous maneuvering demand deliberate practice and time, both of which are scarce in emergency settings.

In trauma laparoscopy, where diagnostic uncertainty can swiftly escalate into life-threatening conditions, the attending surgeon often must act with precision and speed. This limits opportunities for residents to "struggle" through tasks such as trocar placement, initial diagnostic exploration, or careful dissection, which are vital for developing competence but may delay crucial decisions.

Structured Involvement: When and What to Delegate

Despite these challenges, key opportunities exist within trauma laparoscopy for integrating structured resident involvement without compromising care (Fig. 9.4).

- *Access and setup*: Residents may be assigned to perform safe Veress needle or optical trocar placement under supervision, as well as camera insertion and the initial exploration of the peritoneal cavity.
- *Camera navigation*: Controlled camera operation during the diagnostic phase helps learners develop hand-eye coordination while engaging in critical intraoperative steps.
- *Targeted dissections*: Under stable conditions (e.g., diaphragm evaluation, minor mesenteric bleeding, or omental assessment), junior surgeons can carry out specific steps with direct guidance.

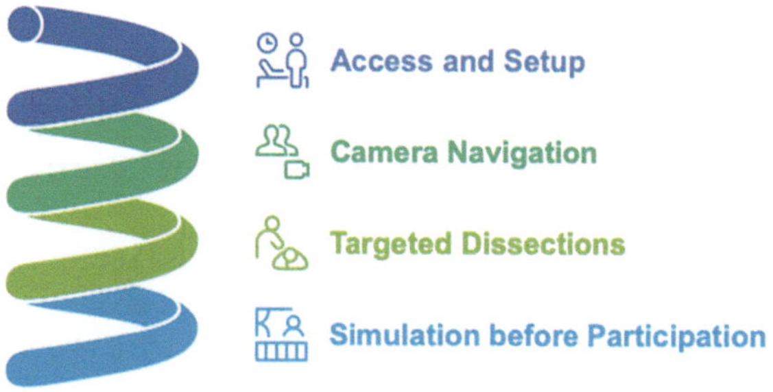

Fig. 9.4 Key elements that support the integration of team members during formation and structured resident involvement, all without compromising care during laparoscopic surgery in trauma

- *Simulation before participation*: Prior experience with simulation-based training, including laparoscopic trauma modules, can equip residents to perform specific intraoperative tasks, thereby increasing both confidence and safety [31, 32].

This "selective delegation" approach maximizes learning within clinically acceptable time frames, upholding the educational mission while acknowledging the urgency of trauma.

Key Learning Points:
- *Effective triage and case selection* for trauma laparoscopy require quick evaluation of patient stability, injury patterns, and available resources.
- *Intraoperative teamwork and clear role definitions* are essential for ensuring safety, efficiency, and preparedness during open conversion.
- *Real-time communication and leadership* by the trauma surgeon ensure adaptive responses and informed decisions during surgery.
- *Resident training needs to be designed* to ensure safe, supervised participation without compromising patient outcomes or efficiency.
- *Simulation and selective task delegation* enhance resident preparedness and team performance in high-pressure trauma scenarios.

Supervision Models in Trauma Laparoscopy

Different models of supervision have emerged to accommodate both safety and learning (Fig. 9.5):

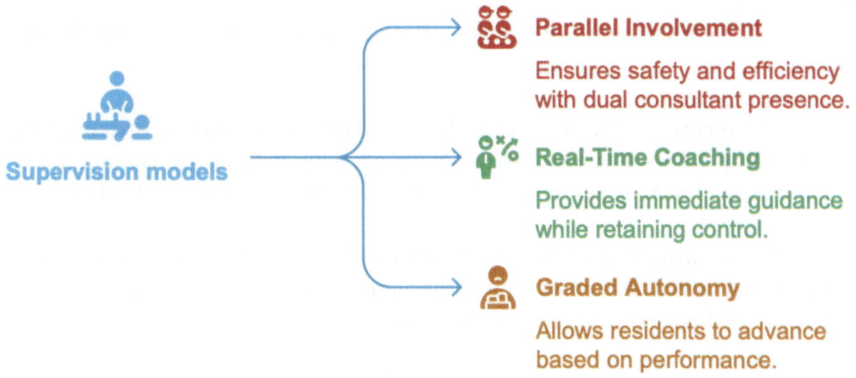

Fig. 9.5 The benefits of different supervision models that enable residents and novice team members to develop skills and enhance autonomy during the learning curve of laparoscopic surgery for trauma

- *Parallel involvement*: In situations with dual consultant presence, one senior surgeon can guide the resident while the other maintains safety and efficiency, especially in tertiary centers or teaching hospitals.
- *Real-time coaching*: An attending physician can assume a coaching role for segments of the case while retaining the authority to take control if clinical conditions change.
- *Graded autonomy*: Through structured assessments (e.g., Objective Structured Assessment of Technical Skills [OSATS]), residents can advance to higher levels of responsibility in selected trauma cases based on their previous performance [49].

Adequate supervision in trauma laparoscopy is not passive observation; it is deliberate, context-sensitive coaching in which autonomy is earned, and risks are actively mitigated.

Indications and Contraindications in Trauma Laparoscopy

Trauma laparoscopy occupies a unique and evolving role within the acute care surgeon's technical arsenal. Once deemed too slow and unreliable for trauma, minimally invasive techniques are now widely accepted in selected trauma scenarios. However, the safe and effective use of laparoscopy depends on two fundamental elements: appropriate patient selection, primarily influenced by hemodynamic status and the mechanism of injury [50–52].

Hemodynamic Stability

The primary consideration in trauma laparoscopy is maintaining *hemodynamic stability*.

- *Stable patients* are the most suitable candidates for diagnostic or therapeutic laparoscopy. This group includes individuals with isolated abdominal injuries, ambiguous imaging findings, or suspected hollow viscus or diaphragmatic injuries.
- *In contrast, unstable patients* are seldom candidates for laparoscopy because of the time-sensitive nature of their resuscitation and the physiological effects of pneumoperitoneum, which can reduce venous return and worsen shock.

In practical terms, laparoscopy is contraindicated in any patient requiring active, ongoing resuscitation or showing signs of hemorrhagic shock (e.g., systolic BP <90 mmHg, lactate >4 mmol/L, need for massive transfusion).

Mechanism of Injury: Blunt vs. Penetrating Trauma

Penetrating Trauma

Laparoscopy is especially effective for penetrating anterior abdominal injuries, where the aim is to:

- *Evaluate peritoneal penetration* (especially with stab wounds).
- *Avoid non-therapeutic laparotomies* in stable patients without peritoneal signs.
- *Assess diaphragm integrity*, particularly in left-sided thoracoabdominal injuries.

Multiple studies have confirmed the high negative predictive value of laparoscopy in stable penetrating trauma, making it an effective diagnostic tool for avoiding unnecessary laparotomies [12, 19, 53].

Caution Deep penetrating injuries with a suspected trajectory through solid organs or central vasculature still require caution; even in stable patients, a low threshold for laparotomy should be maintained when visualization is limited.

Blunt Trauma

Blunt trauma poses a unique challenge. The role of laparoscopy in this context is less established, although it is evolving [54–56]. Possible indications include:

- *Suspected hollow viscus injury* with equivocal CT findings.
- *Diaphragmatic injury* (especially after high-velocity motor vehicle collisions).
- *Assessment of hemoperitoneum* in stable patients where the source is unclear.

However, laparoscopy is relatively contraindicated in blunt trauma patients with:

- *Multiple injuries* and unclear sources of bleeding.
- *Evolving instability*, even if initial vital signs are acceptable.
- *Extensive intra-abdominal contamination* or concern for major retroperitoneal bleeding, which may be missed laparoscopically.

Relative Contraindications and Limitations

Beyond stability and mechanism, other essential contraindications include:

- *Severe cardiopulmonary compromise*: Pneumoperitoneum can impair ventilation and venous return.
- *Extensive intra-abdominal adhesions or prior surgery*: Increases the risk of iatrogenic injury and limits visualization.

- *Need for rapid exposure and access*: If time to control bleeding or contamination is critical, open surgery remains the superior option.

Challenges and Solutions in Implementing Minimally Invasive Surgery (MIS) in Trauma Teams

The adoption of minimally invasive surgery (MIS) in trauma care presents unique opportunities for improving outcomes, but its integration is not without significant challenges. Trauma surgery, by its nature, demands rapid decision-making, cross-specialty coordination, and high technical proficiency, which can strain the incorporation of minimally invasive surgery (MIS) techniques. This section of the chapter addresses targeted solutions concerning the MIS learning curve and institutional resource limitations.

Learning Curve and Skill Acquisition: From Diagnostic to Therapeutic Laparoscopy

Unlike elective minimally invasive surgery (MIS), where the learning curve can be gradual and mentored over time, trauma laparoscopy often thrusts young surgeons into high-stakes, high-pressure environments. While diagnostic laparoscopy for peritoneal violation or diaphragmatic injury serves as a feasible entry point, the transition to therapeutic interventions (e.g., bowel resection, bleeding control) requires significant expertise.

Specific Issues

- Inconsistent exposure to laparoscopic trauma during residency or fellowship.
- Risk of prolonged operative time or iatrogenic injury in the hands of inexperienced surgeons.
- Hesitation to attempt laparoscopy in trauma due to fear of complications.

Solutions:

- Stepwise skill development, beginning with diagnostic laparoscopy and gradually incorporating advanced therapeutic steps.
- Mentor-guided intraoperative teaching, using dual-console platforms or structured delegation of tasks.
- Standardized curricula and competency checklists for trauma MIS, linked to simulation labs, cadaver training, and supervised live surgery.
- Establishing “low-risk high-yield” cases (e.g., stable patients with suspected bowel injury or retained hemoperitoneum) as training opportunities.

Resource Limitations: Equipment, Costs, and Hospital Policy Barriers

While the clinical benefits of MIS are well-documented, such as faster recovery, fewer wound complications, and reduced length of stay, upfront implementation costs can be a barrier, particularly for trauma systems operating with limited budgets or within public healthcare structures.

Specific Issues:

- High initial costs for towers, instrumentation, and energy devices.
- Maintenance burdens and sterilization logistics for delicate MIS tools.
- Lack of inclusion of trauma MIS in hospital protocols or billing codes.
- Limited access in rural or under-resourced trauma centers.

Solutions:

- Cost-benefit analysis studies specific to trauma populations to justify capital investment.
- Use of reusable instruments and low-cost trainers for skills acquisition.
- Collaboration with industry partners to provide training equipment and support.
- Incorporation of MIS into trauma protocols and pathways (e.g., "laparoscopy-first" for stable abdominal trauma).
- Advocacy for policy inclusion at national and hospital levels, with emphasis on long-term savings via reduced complications and LOS.

Key Learning Points:

- *Penetrating trauma* is better suited for laparoscopy than blunt trauma, which has more relative contraindications and diagnostic limitations.
- *Training must tackle the steep learning curve* of trauma MIS through simulation, mentor-guided procedures, and structured curricula that progress from diagnostic to therapeutic skills.
- *Institutional barriers*, such as equipment costs and a lack of protocol integration, must be addressed through cost-benefit analyses, reusable tools, and policy advocacy to support the broader adoption of laparoscopic surgery in trauma.

Expanding Indications for Minimally Invasive Surgery (MIS) in Trauma Care: Vascular, Thoracic, and Pelvic Trauma

Historically, trauma surgery has been synonymous with open procedures, including rapid laparotomy and thoracotomy, which provide wide exposure to control hemorrhage and repair injuries. However, advancements in technology, surgical techniques, and imaging have expanded the role of minimally invasive surgery (MIS) in trauma settings to include select cases of thoracic and pelvic trauma, reflecting a paradigm shift toward precision, reduced morbidity, and enhanced recovery [57–59].

Thoracic Trauma: VATS for Hemothorax and Lung Injury

The use of video-assisted thoracoscopic surgery (VATS) in trauma has rapidly increased, especially in tertiary trauma centers. While it was traditionally applied in elective thoracic surgery, VATS now plays a critical role in both diagnosis and treatment. The timing of VATS is crucial, as it is often most effective when performed within 48–72 h post-injury to prevent clot organization and inflammation [60]. VATS also enables the visualization of lung parenchyma, control of bleeding, and repair of lacerations with minimal invasiveness. However, hemodynamic instability, massive hemothorax (greater than 1500 mL), or complex hilar injuries still require traditional thoracotomy.

Indications for VATS in Trauma

- Retained hemothorax after chest tube insertion.
- Persistent air leaks or suspected bronchopleural fistulas.
- Diaphragmatic injuries (especially left-sided blunt trauma).

Advantages

- Decreased pain and pulmonary complications.
- Shorter hospital stays and quicker mobilization.
- Better cosmesis, particularly in young trauma patients.

Pelvic Trauma Laparoscopy

Pelvic trauma often involves a mix of orthopedic, vascular, genitourinary, and gastrointestinal injuries. Open procedures have traditionally been the standard for diagnostic clarity and access. However, in a select group of stable patients, laparoscopy and endoscopic techniques now provide diagnostic precision and therapeutic options with less invasiveness [61, 62]. Multidisciplinary collaboration during trauma surgery, involving urology, orthopedics, and interventional radiology, is crucial for effective minimally invasive surgery integration in pelvic trauma.

Current Indications of MIS in Pelvic Trauma

- Diagnostic laparoscopy for peritoneal violation in stab wounds.
- Assessment and repair of bladder injuries (combined cystoscopy and laparoscopy).
- Repair of extraperitoneal rectal injuries (in conjunction with diverting ostomy).
- Guidance for pelvic hematoma drainage or packing in hybrid ORs.

Training and Education in a Teaching Hospital Setting

Developing skills in trauma laparoscopic surgery care relies not only on experienced faculty but also on structured training and the progressive growth of surgical residents. Teaching hospitals fulfill a dual mission: providing timely, safe patient care while preparing the next generation of surgeons through hands-on experience, theoretical instruction, and simulation. In an era where patient safety, efficiency, and accountability are facing increasing scrutiny, trauma training must strike a balance between educational depth and operational demands. The three core components of trauma laparoscopic training are simulation-based training, intraoperative teaching, and competency assessment [63–66].

Simulation-Based Training

- Dry simulation has revolutionized surgical education by enabling learners to acquire and refine skills in a safe, reproducible environment. In laparoscopic trauma surgical care, where decisions often need to be made quickly and under pressure, simulation provides a structured method for teaching uncommon, complex, or technically challenging procedures.
- Cadaver labs, when available, offer the highest level of anatomical realism. However, this model is rarely used for laparoscopic training scenarios due to the quality and availability of tissue.
- The use of animals in wet lab settings offers the valuable advantage of live tissue, enhancing the development and refinement of advanced laparoscopic skills.
- Box trainers and task simulators are often used to teach essential laparoscopic and suturing skills. These tools help residents develop hand-eye coordination, instrument handling, and bimanual dexterity. They are particularly beneficial for acquiring basic laparoscopic training and are primarily utilized by junior residents. Their advantages include low cost and the ability to be reused for specific tasks, such as knot tying, precision cutting, and intracorporeal suturing.
- Virtual Reality (VR) and Augmented Reality (AR) can simulate trauma laparoscopic procedures. These tools may incorporate simulations that include hemodynamic instability, decision trees, and technical tasks, providing feedback on performance and timing for crucial decisions during the scenario.

Intraoperative Teaching Techniques

- The operating room acts as both a learning environment and a clinical practice scenario. Teaching in real time must strike a balance between patient safety, operational efficiency, and resident development. In trauma surgery, where time is often critical and surgical findings are unpredictable, this balance is particularly delicate.
- Gradual participation under the supervision and guidance of a consultant is one of the most effective teaching strategies. Early in their training, residents observe and assist. As they progress, they are assigned parts of procedures, such as bowel anastomosis, eventually advancing to full procedural responsibility under supervision. The gradual model allows for real-time feedback and promotes autonomy without compromising safety.
- In laparoscopic trauma surgery, mentor-guided participation is a common practice worldwide. Senior surgeons often stand across from the resident and provide vocal and manual guidance throughout the procedure. This method is especially effective in laparoscopic trauma, where tactile feedback is limited, and visual cues must be interpreted quickly.

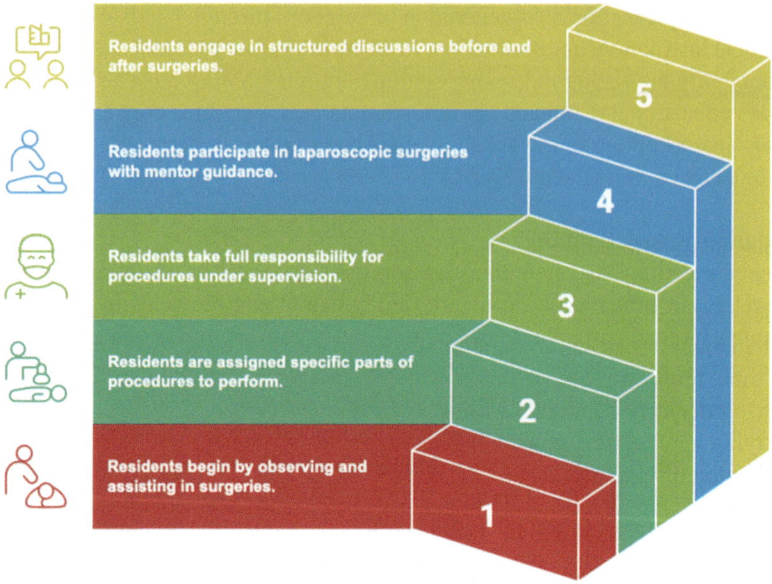

Fig. 9.6 Structured intraoperative teaching techniques in laparoscopic trauma surgery: balancing patient safety with resident autonomy through progressive participation, mentor-guided instruction, and reflective pre- and postoperative learning

- Preoperative and postoperative discussions, along with reflective learning, are key components of laparoscopic trauma management training. Structured preoperative planning and postoperative debriefings are essential. Discussing indications, anatomy, risks, and contingencies before entering the operating room (OR) and reviewing outcomes and complications afterward ensures that residents contextualize their experiences, transforming them into valuable learning opportunities for knowledge (Fig. 9.6).

Competency Assessment

As surgical education shifts toward competency-based training, structured assessment tools are essential. Trauma programs must ensure that progression through training is linked to observed proficiency rather than merely procedural counts.

- Many trauma services utilize validated tools, such as the Objective Structured Assessment of Technical Skill (OSATS) or specific procedure checklists, to assess technical skills [49, 67]. These tools enable supervisors to assess residents on aspects such as instrument handling, workflow, and decision-making. Checklists can be used during simulations or live procedures.
- Milestone-based evaluation is another tool used for competency assessment [68]. In alignment with frameworks such as the ACGME Milestones Project, surgical

residency programs are increasingly adopting tiered competency frameworks that range from novice to expert. Trauma-specific milestones may include managing hemorrhagic shock, performing damage control laparotomy, or safely leading a multidisciplinary trauma resuscitation. Feedback and reflective learning are essential components of competency acquisition in any laparoscopic trauma program. Assessment without feedback holds limited value. Structured debriefs improve reflective learning, a powerful method for enhancing both technical and cognitive skills.

Summary

Laparoscopy in trauma is a valuable tool when used thoughtfully. Patient stability and the mechanism of injury are essential for decision-making. In skilled hands and appropriate settings, minimally invasive techniques can reduce morbidity, shorten hospital stays, and improve diagnostic accuracy. However, improper use of laparoscopy can lead to delays, missed injuries, and negative outcomes. Ultimately, clinical judgment, prompt triage, and team preparedness must direct its application.

Training trauma surgeons in laparoscopic surgery at a teaching hospital requires structured educational strategies that extend beyond simple exposure to high-volume emergencies. Simulation improves preparedness, intraoperative teaching develops real-world skills, and competency assessments ensure progress. Together, these elements lay the groundwork for cultivating skilled, confident trauma surgeons who are ready for the challenges posed by the laparoscopic surgical approach.

Balancing efficiency with resident learning in trauma laparoscopy involves an ongoing negotiation between the urgency of patient care and the pedagogy of training. By carefully structuring participation, adopting flexible supervision models, and investing in simulation-based training, trauma programs can support both patient safety and surgical education. The key lies not in choosing between speed and learning but in strategically integrating the two, transforming every trauma case into both a lifesaving intervention and a teaching opportunity.

The expansion of MIS into vascular, thoracic, and pelvic trauma reflects a shift toward precision, enhanced recovery, and tailored surgical care. While patient selection remains critical—favoring hemodynamically stable individuals—the growing accessibility of hybrid operating environments, advanced imaging, and simulation-based training is bridging the gap between traditional and modern trauma care.

Integrating MIS into trauma care requires a deliberate, systemic effort that spans clinical, educational, and institutional domains. Although time constraints, training deficiencies, and equipment costs present significant challenges, they are not insurmountable. With multidisciplinary planning, dedicated faculty mentorship, and an institutional commitment to modernizing trauma surgery, MIS can be safely and effectively implemented even in high-acuity environments.

In the long term, trauma centers that invest in minimally invasive surgery (MIS) will improve clinical outcomes and help nurture a new generation of surgeons trained in minimally invasive, multidisciplinary trauma care. This model embodies the future of high-quality surgical intervention.

Future directions may include robotic-assisted trauma surgery for challenging anatomical areas, AI-guided intraoperative imaging for vascular injuries, and portable endovascular capabilities in military and prehospital settings. As trauma surgery evolves, the training and infrastructure that support the integration of minimally invasive surgery (MIS) must also advance. This includes simulation labs, cadaver training, and cross-disciplinary fellowships to ensure that trauma surgeons remain at the forefront of minimally invasive innovation.

Chapter Key Messages

Use laparoscopy in trauma carefully: Patient hemodynamic stability and the mechanism of injury must guide the decision to utilize laparoscopy. When applied thoughtfully and by skilled teams, it reduces morbidity and improves outcomes, but improper use can cause harm.

Training must be structured and ongoing: Developing trauma laparoscopic skills requires more than clinical exposure. Simulation, intraoperative coaching, and competency assessments are essential for developing safe and confident surgeons.

Balance efficiency with education: Trauma cases should be designed to meet both clinical needs and training opportunities. Supervision models and team coordination must effectively integrate patient care with surgical teaching.

Institutional commitment is essential for the successful integration of MIS: Overcoming challenges such as costs, training deficits, and equipment limitations requires coordinated efforts that involve faculty mentorship, simulation resources, and protocol development. Investing in MIS today establishes a foundation for the future of trauma surgery.

References

1. Mandrioli M, Inaba K, Piccinini A, Biscardi A, Sartelli M, Agresta F, Catena F, Cirocchi R, Jovine E, Tugnoli G, Di Saverio S. Advances in laparoscopy for acute care surgery and trauma. World J Gastroenterol. 2016;22(2):668–80. https://doi.org/10.3748/wjg.v22.i2.668. PMID: 26811616; PMCID: PMC4716068.
2. Perri SG, Altilia F, Pietrangeli F, Dalla Torre A, Gabbrielli F, Amendolara M, Nicita A, Nardi M Jr, Lotti R, Citone G. La laparoscopia nelle urgenze addominali. Indicazioni e limiti [Laparoscopy in abdominal emergencies. Indications and limitations]. Chir Ital. 2002;54(2):165–78. Italian. PMID: 12038107.
3. Ietto G, Amico F, Pettinato G, Iori V, Carcano G. Laparoscopy in emergency: why not? Advantages of laparoscopy in major emergency: a review. Life (Basel). 2021;11(9):917. https://doi.org/10.3390/life11090917. PMID: 34575066; PMCID: PMC8470929.
4. Malangoni MA, Biester TW, Jones AT, Klingensmith ME, Lewis FR Jr. Operative experience of surgery residents: trends and challenges. J Surg Educ. 2013;70(6):783–8. https://doi.org/10.1016/j.jsurg.2013.09.015. Epub 2013 Sep 26. PMID: 24209656.

5. Harrell AG, Kercher KW, Heniford BT. Energy sources in laparoscopy. Semin Laparosc Surg. 2004;11(3):201–9. https://doi.org/10.1177/107155170401100310. PMID: 15510316.
6. Wolmarans A, Fru PN, Moeng MS. Accuracy of CT scan for detecting hollow viscus injury in penetrating abdominal trauma. World J Surg. 2023;47(6):1457–63. https://doi.org/10.1007/s00268-023-06954-1. Epub 2023 Mar 1. PMID: 36859569; PMCID: PMC10156834.
7. Thorisdottir S, Oladottir GL, Nummela MT, Koskinen SK. Diagnostic performance of CT and the use of GI contrast material for detection of hollow viscus injury after penetrating abdominal trauma. Experience from a level 1 Nordic trauma center. Acta Radiol. 2020;61(10):1309–15. https://doi.org/10.1177/0284185120902389. Epub 2020 Feb 11. PMID: 32046497.
8. Richards JR, Knopf NA, Wang L, McGahan JP. Blunt abdominal trauma in children: evaluation with emergency US. Radiology. 2002;222(3):749–54. https://doi.org/10.1148/radiol.2223010838. PMID: 11867796.
9. Van Gent JM, Clements TW, Cotton BA. Resuscitation and Care in the Trauma bay. Surg Clin North Am. 2024;104(2):279–92. https://doi.org/10.1016/j.suc.2023.09.005. Epub 2023 Oct 20. PMID: 38453302.
10. Vulliamy P, Thaventhiran AJ, Davenport RA. What's new for trauma haemorrhage management? Br J Hosp Med (Lond). 2019;80(5):268–73. https://doi.org/10.12968/hmed.2019.80.5.268. PMID: 31059346.
11. Tosounidis TH, Giannoudis PV. Paediatric trauma resuscitation: an update. Eur J Trauma Emerg Surg. 2016;42(3):297–301. https://doi.org/10.1007/s00068-015-0614-9. Epub 2015 Dec 22. PMID: 26696087; PMCID: PMC4886151.
12. Uranues S, Popa DE, Diaconescu B, Schrittwieser R. Laparoscopy in penetrating abdominal trauma. World J Surg. 2015;39(6):1381–8. https://doi.org/10.1007/s00268-014-2904-5. PMID: 25446491.
13. Cocco AM, Bhagvan S, Bouffler C, Hsu J. Diagnostic laparoscopy in penetrating abdominal trauma. ANZ J Surg. 2019;89(4):353–6. https://doi.org/10.1111/ans.15140. Epub 2019 Mar 14. PMID: 30873735.
14. Buisset C, Mazeaud C, Postillon A, Nominé-Criqui C, Fouquet T, Reibel N, Brunaud L, Perez M. Evaluation of diagnostic laparoscopy for penetrating abdominal injuries: about 131 anterior abdominal stab wound. Surg Endosc. 2022;36(5):2801–8. https://doi.org/10.1007/s00464-021-08566-z. Epub 2021 Jun 2. PMID: 34076764.
15. Wu C, Lin KL, Chang YJ, Lin HF. Role of laparoscopy in management of patients with anterior abdominal stab wounds. Surg Endosc. 2023;37(12):9173–82. https://doi.org/10.1007/s00464-023-10487-y. Epub 2023 Oct 14. PMID: 37833508.
16. Justin V, Fingerhut A, Uranues S. Laparoscopy in blunt abdominal trauma: for whom? when? and why? Curr Trauma Rep. 2017;3(1):43–50. https://doi.org/10.1007/s40719-017-0076-0. Epub 2017 Jan 28. PMID: 28690974; PMCID: PMC5477632.
17. Bouzat P, Valdenaire G, Gauss T, Charbit J, Arvieux C, Balandraud P, Bobbia X, David JS, Frandon J, Garrigue D, Long JA, Pottecher J, Prunet B, Simonnet B, Tazarourte K, Trésallet C, Vaux J, Viglino D, Villoing B, Zieleskiewicz L, Gil-Jardiné C, Weiss E. Early management of severe abdominal trauma. Anaesth Crit Care Pain Med. 2020;39(2):269–77. https://doi.org/10.1016/j.accpm.2019.12.001. Epub 2019 Dec 13. PMID: 31843714.
18. Siriratsivawong K, Kang J, Riffenburgh R, Hoang TN. Immersion team training in a realistic environment improves team performance in trauma resuscitation. Surgery. 2016;160(3):586–90. https://doi.org/10.1016/j.surg.2016.03.029. Epub 2016 May 24. PMID: 27233635.
19. Ahmed N, Whelan J, Brownlee J, Chari V, Chung R. The contribution of laparoscopy in evaluation of penetrating abdominal wounds. J Am Coll Surg. 2005;201(2):213–6. https://doi.org/10.1016/j.jamcollsurg.2005.04.021. PMID: 16038818.
20. Gjeraa K, Spanager L, Konge L, Petersen RH, Østergaard D. Non-technical skills in minimally invasive surgery teams: a systematic review. Surg Endosc. 2016;30(12):5185–99. https://doi.org/10.1007/s00464-016-4890-1. Epub 2016 Apr 11. PMID: 27066972.
21. Alexandrino H, Martinho B, Ferreira L, Baptista S. Non-technical skills and teamwork in trauma: from the emergency department to the operating room. Front Med (Lausanne).

2023;10:1319990. https://doi.org/10.3389/fmed.2023.1319990. PMID: 38116034; PMCID: PMC10728672.
22. Blackmore AE, Wong MT, Tang CL. Evolution of laparoscopy in colorectal surgery: an evidence-based review. World J Gastroenterol. 2014;20(17):4926–33. https://doi.org/10.3748/wjg.v20.i17.4926. PMID: 24803804; PMCID: PMC4009524.
23. Suda K, Nakauchi M, Inaba K, Ishida Y, Uyama I. Minimally invasive surgery for upper gastrointestinal cancer: our experience and review of the literature. World J Gastroenterol. 2016;22(19):4626–37. https://doi.org/10.3748/wjg.v22.i19.4626. PMID: 27217695; PMCID: PMC4870070.
24. Olmi S, Uccelli M, Cesana GC, Oldani A, Giorgi R, De Carli SM, Ciccarese F, Villa R. Laparoscopic abdominal wall hernia repair. JSLS. 2020;24(1):e2020.00007. https://doi.org/10.4293/JSLS.2020.00007. PMID: 32265582; PMCID: PMC7112985.
25. Caruso F, Ciccarese F, Cesana G, Uccelli M, Castello G, Olmi S. Massive incisional hernia repair with Parietex: monocentric analysis on 500 cases treated with a laparoscopic approach. J Laparoendosc Adv Surg Tech A. 2017;27(4):388–92. https://doi.org/10.1089/lap.2016.0623. Epub 2017 Mar 1. PMID: 28249126.
26. Ban D, Kudo A, Irie T, Ochiai T, Aihara A, Matsumura S, Tanaka S, Tanabe M. Advances in reduced port laparoscopic liver resection. Asian J Endosc Surg. 2015;8(1):11–5. https://doi.org/10.1111/ases.12164. Epub 2014 Dec 15. PMID: 25510567.
27. Johnsen BH, Westli HK, Espevik R, Wisborg T, Brattebø G. High-performing trauma teams: frequency of behavioral markers of a shared mental model displayed by team leaders and quality of medical performance. Scand J Trauma Resusc Emerg Med. 2017;25(1):109. https://doi.org/10.1186/s13049-017-0452-3. PMID: 29126452; PMCID: PMC5681813.
28. Briggs A, Raja AS, Joyce MF, Yule SJ, Jiang W, Lipsitz SR, Havens JM. The role of non-technical skills in simulated trauma resuscitation. J Surg Educ. 2015;72(4):732–9. https://doi.org/10.1016/j.jsurg.2015.01.020. Epub 2015 Mar 26. PMID: 25817012.
29. Jastaniah A, Grushka J. The role of minimally invasive surgeries in trauma. Surg Clin North Am. 2024;104(2):437–49. https://doi.org/10.1016/j.suc.2023.10.003. Epub 2023 Nov 22. PMID: 38453312.
30. Lang F, Gerhäuser AS, Wild C, Wennberg E, Schmidt MW, Wagner M, Müller-Stich BP, Nickel F. Video-based learning of coping strategies for common errors improves laparoscopy training-a randomized study. Surg Endosc. 2023;37(5):4054–64. https://doi.org/10.1007/s00464-023-09969-w. Epub 2023 Mar 21. PMID: 36944741; PMCID: PMC10156798.
31. Dehabadi M, Fernando B, Berlingieri P. The use of simulation in the acquisition of laparoscopic suturing skills. Int J Surg. 2014;12(4):258–68. https://doi.org/10.1016/j.ijsu.2014.01.022. Epub 2014 Feb 4. PMID: 24503123.
32. Stefanidis D, Hope WW, Korndorffer JR Jr, Markley S, Scott DJ. Initial laparoscopic basic skills training shortens the learning curve of laparoscopic suturing and is cost-effective. J Am Coll Surg. 2010;210(4):436–40. https://doi.org/10.1016/j.jamcollsurg.2009.12.015. PMID: 20347735.
33. Segalini E, Khan M, Podda M, Gallo G, Morello A, Marziali I, DI Saverio S. The role of laparoscopic splenectomy in traumatic splenic injury: a narrative review. Minerva Surg. 2023;78(1):76–80. https://doi.org/10.23736/S2724-5691.22.09799-4. Epub 2022 Nov 30. PMID: 36448883.
34. Maarseveen OECV, Ham WHW, Huijsmans RLN, Leenen LPH. The pace of a trauma resuscitation: experience matters. Eur J Trauma Emerg Surg. 2022;48(3):2503–10. https://doi.org/10.1007/s00068-021-01838-2. Epub 2022 Feb 9. PMID: 35141771; PMCID: PMC9192480.
35. Quon S, Riddell J, Bench KF, Roepke C, Burner E. Training leaders in trauma resuscitation: teacher and learner perspectives on ideal methods. West J Emerg Med. 2022;23(2):192–9. https://doi.org/10.5811/westjem.2021.5.51428. PMID: 35302453; PMCID: PMC8967462.
36. Alaker M, Wynn GR, Arulampalam T. Virtual reality training in laparoscopic surgery: a systematic review & meta-analysis. Int J Surg. 2016;29:85–94. https://doi.org/10.1016/j.ijsu.2016.03.034. Epub 2016 Mar 15. PMID: 26992652.

37. Romain B, Chemaly R, Meyer N, Brigand C, Steinmetz JP, Rohr S. Value of a preoperative checklist for laparoscopic appendectomy and cholecystectomy. J Visc Surg. 2012;149(6):408–11. https://doi.org/10.1016/j.jviscsurg.2012.10.001. Epub 2012 Nov 17. PMID: 23164526.
38. Verdaasdonk EGG, Stassen LPS, Hoffmann WF, et al. Can a structured checklist prevent problems with laparoscopic equipment? Surg Endosc. 2008;22:2238–43. https://doi.org/10.1007/s00464-008-0029-3.
39. Bento A, Ferreira L, Yánez Benitez C, Koleda P, Fraga GP, Kozera P, Baptista S, Mesquita C, Alexandrino H. Worldwide snapshot of trauma team structure and training: an international survey. Eur J Trauma Emerg Surg. 2023;49(4):1771–81. https://doi.org/10.1007/s00068-022-02166-9. Epub 2022 Nov 21. PMID: 36414695.
40. Cabrera Vargas LF, Pedraza M, Rincon FA, Pulido JA, Mendoza-Zuchini A, Gomez D, Moreno-Villamizar MD, Ferrada P, Lopez P, Di Saverio S. Fully therapeutic laparoscopy for penetrating abdominal trauma in stable patients. Am J Surg. 2022;223(1):206–7. https://doi.org/10.1016/j.amjsurg.2021.07.008. Epub 2021 Jul 17. PMID: 34294385.
41. Trejo-Ávila ME, Valenzuela-Salazar C, Betancourt-Ferreyra J, Fernández-Enríquez E, Romero-Loera S, Moreno-Portillo M. Laparoscopic versus open surgery for abdominal trauma: a case-matched study. J Laparoendosc Adv Surg Tech A. 2017;27(4):383–7. https://doi.org/10.1089/lap.2016.0535. Epub 2017 Mar 2. PMID: 28253051.
42. Chakravartty S, Sarma DR, Noor M, Panagiotopoulos S, Patel AG. Laparoscopy has a therapeutic role in the management of abdominal trauma: a matched-pair analysis. Int J Surg. 2017;44:21–5. https://doi.org/10.1016/j.ijsu.2017.05.035. Epub 2017 May 18. PMID: 28529193.
43. Matsevych OY, Koto MZ, Motilall SR, Kumar N. The role of laparoscopy in management of stable patients with penetrating abdominal trauma and organ evisceration. J Trauma Acute Care Surg. 2016;81(2):307–11. https://doi.org/10.1097/TA.0000000000001064. PMID: 27032004.
44. Matsevych OY, Koto MZ, Aldous C. Laparoscopic-assisted approach for penetrating abdominal trauma: a solution for multiple bowel injuries. Int J Surg. 2017;44:94–8. https://doi.org/10.1016/j.ijsu.2017.06.040. Epub 2017 Jun 16. PMID: 28629766.
45. Doumouras AG, Hamidi M, Lung K, Tarola CL, Tsao MW, Scott JW, Smink DS, Yule S. Non-technical skills of surgeons and anaesthetists in simulated operating theatre crises. Br J Surg. 2017;104(8):1028–36. https://doi.org/10.1002/bjs.10526. Epub 2017 Apr 4. PMID: 28376246.
46. Feliciano DV. Abdominal trauma revisited. Am Surg. 2017;83(11):1193–202. PMID: 29183519.
47. O'Malley E, Boyle E, O'Callaghan A, Coffey JC, Walsh SR. Role of laparoscopy in penetrating abdominal trauma: a systematic review. World J Surg. 2013;37(1):113–22. https://doi.org/10.1007/s00268-012-1790-y. PMID: 23052797.
48. Sidwell R, Matar MM, Sakran JV. Trauma education and prevention. Surg Clin North Am. 2017;97(5):1185–97. https://doi.org/10.1016/j.suc.2017.06.010. PMID: 28958365.
49. Martin JA, Regehr G, Reznick R, MacRae H, Murnaghan J, Hutchison C, Brown M. Objective structured assessment of technical skill (OSATS) for surgical residents. Br J Surg. 1997;84(2):273–8. https://doi.org/10.1046/j.1365-2168.1997.02502.x. PMID: 9052454.
50. Poole GV, Thomae KR, Hauser CJ. Laparoscopy in trauma. Surg Clin North Am. 1996;76(3):547–56. https://doi.org/10.1016/s0039-6109(05)70461-8. PMID: 8669014.
51. Cirocchi R, Birindelli A, Inaba K, Mandrioli M, Piccinini A, Tabola R, Carlini L, Tugnoli G, Di Saverio S. Laparoscopy for trauma and the changes in its use from 1990 to 2016: a current systematic review and meta-analysis. Surg Laparosc Endosc Percutan Tech. 2018;28(1):1–12. https://doi.org/10.1097/SLE.0000000000000466. PMID: 28915204
52. Berg RJ, Karamanos E, Inaba K, Okoye O, Teixeira PG, Demetriades D. The persistent diagnostic challenge of thoracoabdominal stab wounds. J Trauma Acute Care Surg. 2014;76(2):418–23. https://doi.org/10.1097/TA.0000000000000120. PMID: 24458047.
53. Kim DH, Kim M, Lee DS, Hong TH, Park H, Cho H. Role of laparoscopic surgery in managing hemodynamically stable abdominal trauma patients: a single level I trauma center, propensity score matching study. Eur J Trauma Emerg Surg. 2024;50(5):2517–25. https://doi.org/10.1007/s00068-024-02642-4. Epub 2024 Sep 3. PMID: 39225806; PMCID: PMC11599316.

54. Lin HF, Chen YD, Lin KL, Wu MC, Wu CY, Chen SC. Laparoscopy decreases the laparotomy rate for hemodynamically stable patients with blunt hollow viscus and mesenteric injuries. Am J Surg. 2015;210(2):326–33. https://doi.org/10.1016/j.amjsurg.2014.11.009. Epub 2015 Apr 14. PMID: 25963637.
55. Lee PC, Lo C, Wu JM, Lin KL, Lin HF, Ko WJ. Laparoscopy decreases the laparotomy rate in hemodynamically stable patients with blunt abdominal trauma. Surg Innov. 2014;21(2):155–65. https://doi.org/10.1177/1553350612474496. Epub 2013 Jan 28. PMID: 23361491.
56. Lin HF, Chen YD, Chen SC. Value of diagnostic and therapeutic laparoscopy for patients with blunt abdominal trauma: a 10-year medical center experience. PLoS One. 2018;13(2):e0193379. https://doi.org/10.1371/journal.pone.0193379. PMID: 29470527; PMCID: PMC5823439.
57. Schreyer C, Eckermann C, Neudecker J, Becker L, Schulz-Drost S. Videoassistierte Thorakoskopie (VATS) beim Thoraxtrauma [VATS in thorax trauma]. Zentralbl Chir. 2023;148(1):74–84. https://doi.org/10.1055/a-1957-5511. German. Epub 2022 Dec 5. PMID: 36470290.
58. Manlulu AV, Lee TW, Thung KH, Wong R, Yim AP. Current indications and results of VATS in the evaluation and management of hemodynamically stable thoracic injuries. Eur J Cardiothorac Surg. 2004;25(6):1048–53. https://doi.org/10.1016/j.ejcts.2004.02.017. PMID: 15145008.
59. David G, Giorgi M, Bernard F, Di Francia R, Mauffrey C, Rony L. Enhanced bone exposure via laparoscopy in acetabulum and pelvic ring surgeries. Int Orthop. 2025;49(6):1275–81. https://doi.org/10.1007/s00264-025-06515-2. Epub 2025 Mar 31. PMID: 40163078; PMCID: PMC12075018.
60. Chou YP, Lin HL, Wu TC. Video-assisted thoracoscopic surgery for retained hemothorax in blunt chest trauma. Curr Opin Pulm Med. 2015;21(4):393–8. https://doi.org/10.1097/MCP.0000000000000173. PMID: 25978625; PMCID: PMC5633323.
61. Arnold MR, Lu CD, Thomas BW, Sachdev G, Cunningham KW, Vaio R, Heniford BT, Sing RF. Advancing the use of laparoscopy in trauma: repair of intraperitoneal bladder injuries. Am Surg. 2019;85(12):1402–4. PMID: 31908226.
62. AlJumaiah S, AlAthel A, AlBabtain I, AlShalfan R. Laparoscopic intraperitoneal bladder injury repair of a trauma patient: a case report. Urol Case Rep. 2022;42:102044. https://doi.org/10.1016/j.eucr.2022.102044. PMID: 35530557; PMCID: PMC9073284.
63. Goldenberg MG, Fok KH, Ordon M, Pace KT, Lee JY. Simulation-based laparoscopic surgery crisis resource management training-predicting technical and nontechnical skills. J Surg Educ. 2018;75(4):1113–9. https://doi.org/10.1016/j.jsurg.2017.11.011. Epub 2017 Dec 19. PMID: 29273339.
64. Balcombe J. Medical training using simulation: toward fewer animals and safer patients. Altern Lab Anim. 2004;32(Suppl 1B):553–60. https://doi.org/10.1177/026119290403201s90. PMID: 23581135.
65. Hamid M, Siddiqui Z, Joiya SA. Recovery of surgical training through extended laparoscopic simulation training. Cureus. 2021;13(10):e18695. https://doi.org/10.7759/cureus.18695. PMID: 34786267; PMCID: PMC8581952.
66. Ortiz C, Vela J, Contreras C, Belmar F, Paul I, Zinco A, Ramos JP, Ottolino P, Achurra P, Jarufe N, Alseidi A, Varas J. A new approach for the acquisition of trauma surgical skills: an OSCE type of simulation training program. Surg Endosc. 2022;36(11):8441–50. https://doi.org/10.1007/s00464-022-09098-w. Epub 2022 Mar 2. PMID: 35237901; PMCID: PMC8890468.
67. Schmidt MW, Haney CM, Kowalewski KF, Bintintan VV, Abu Hilal M, Arezzo A, Bahra M, Besselink MG, Biebl M, Boni L, Diana M, Egberts JH, Fischer L, Francis N, Hashimoto DA, Perez D, Schijven M, Schmelzle M, Soltes M, Swanstrom L, Welsch T, Müller-Stich BP, Nickel F. Development and validity evidence of an objective structured assessment of technical skills score for minimally invasive linear-stapled, hand-sewn intestinal anastomoses: the A-OSATS score. Surg Endosc. 2022;36(6):4529–41. https://doi.org/10.1007/s00464-021-08806-2. Epub 2021 Nov 9. PMID: 34755235; PMCID: PMC9085690.
68. Edgar L, Fig LM. ACGME Milestone Project. J Nucl Med. 2012;53(4):15N. PMID: 22473531.

Involving the Trauma Team: Technical Aspects of Minimally Invasive Surgery in a Teaching Hospital

10

Rafael Dib Possiedi, Syed Fouzaan Albeez, Faaleha Heba Fakruddin, Sophie Tran, and Marcelo Augusto Fontenelle Ribeiro Jr

Introduction

In recent years, minimally invasive surgery (MIS) has transformed general surgery, offering benefits over traditional open procedures. These benefits include improved patient outcomes, reduced surgical risks, and more efficient use of healthcare resources. While initially designed for elective treatments, its adoption in trauma surgery has progressed gradually. This change, influenced by clinical experience, hospital resources, better surgical training, and technology, shows a growing understanding of how effective minimally invasive surgery techniques are in trauma care, particularly for injuries in the abdomen and chest. A concise timeline of this gradual transition is presented in Table 10.1 to illustrate the evolution of MIS in trauma care. Nacul has drawn a useful historical parallel between the gradual maturation of laparoscopy and the more recent emergence of robotic surgery, underscoring how each successive minimally invasive technology has progressively reshaped operative practice [17].

Despite its growing use in elective and urgent situations, MIS is still not widely adopted in trauma care due to concerns about technology limitations, the urgency of decision-making, and the skill level of surgeons during emergencies.

R. D. Possiedi
R Adams Cowley Shock Trauma Center, University of Maryland, Baltimore, MD, USA

S. F. Albeez · F. H. Fakruddin
Batterjee Medical College, Jeddah, Saudi Arabia

S. Tran
School of Medicine, University of Maryland, Baltimore, MD, USA
e-mail: stran@som.umaryland.edu

M. A. F. Ribeiro Jr (✉)
R Adams Cowley Shock Trauma Center, University of Maryland, Baltimore, MD, USA

© The Author(s), under exclusive license to Springer Nature Switzerland AG 2026

M. Cezillo, B. M. Pereira (eds.), *Minimally Invasive Surgery Trauma*,
https://doi.org/10.1007/978-3-032-28971-1_10

Table 10.1 Timeline of key milestones in the adoption of MIS in trauma care

Year/period	Development milestone
1980s–1990s	MIS introduced for elective surgeries
Early 2000s	Diagnostic laparoscopy in selective trauma cases
Mid 2000s	Early studies on trauma laparoscopy published
2010s	Growing evidence of safety and efficacy in stable trauma patients
2020s	Structured MIS training programs (e.g., WSES guidelines)

Early attempts at trauma laparoscopy faced skepticism because of missed injuries and a limited range of treatments. However, improvements in MIS techniques, along with better training and patient selection, have increased its safety and effectiveness, especially for hemodynamically stable patients with penetrating abdominal trauma (PAT). In these cases, diagnostic laparoscopy has lowered the need for unnecessary laparotomies [1]. Recognizing the need for organized education, de'Angelis et al. [10] proposed a step-by-step MIS curriculum in their 2022 WSES position paper. The program includes simulation, supervised clinical experience, proctoring, and certification. It shows that MIS training should include not only surgeons but also the whole perioperative team, including anesthesiologists, nurses, and technicians, to improve team performance and prepare for emergencies [10].

Furthermore, Sermonesi et al. describe the WSES Cesena Guidelines [11], which offer consensus-based recommendations for a laparoscopic-first approach in emergency abdominal surgery and trauma, especially for hemodynamically stable patients. The guidelines emphasize that adopting minimally invasive surgery in trauma should not rely only on surgical enthusiasm; it must also include clear institutional protocols, well-defined inclusion criteria—such as the absence of shock and controlled bleedingand structured team roles [11]. As minimally invasive surgery continues to develop in trauma care, particularly in academic centers, it calls for coordinated, multidisciplinary implementation backed by solid training frameworks and system-wide readiness.

Indications and Limitations of MIS in Trauma

Clinical Scenarios and Patient Selection

Over the past 20 years, minimally invasive surgery (MIS) has evolved from being primarily used in elective procedures to becoming a valuable option in selected trauma cases. Its greatest benefit is seen in hemodynamically stable patients with isolated abdominal injuries, where MIS can help avoid unnecessary laparotomies, shorten hospital stays, and reduce postoperative complications [1, 10]. The most frequent indication for MIS in trauma is penetrating abdominal injury, particularly stab wounds. Diagnostic laparoscopy is useful for assessing peritoneal violation and intra-abdominal injuries, and it is especially effective in identifying diaphragmatic tears at the thoracoabdominal junction—injuries that are often missed on imaging. In contrast, MIS is less commonly employed in blunt trauma due to its multisystem nature and the potential for occult bleeding [11]. Koto et al. similarly characterized laparoscopy in blunt abdominal trauma as a particularly challenging endeavor, requiring rigorous patient selection, advanced laparoscopic expertise, and a low threshold for conversion to open exploration when occult or multi-cavitary injuries are suspected [20].

Safety Criteria and Institutional Readiness

The cornerstone of minimally invasive surgery (MIS) safety in trauma is *hemodynamic stability*. MIS is contraindicated in patients with peritonitis, ongoing hemorrhage, or shock, as these conditions require immediate intervention often beyond the capabilities of laparoscopy. The WSES Cesena Guidelines recommend MIS only for stable patients with a clear operative indication and always with readiness to convert to open surgery [11]. Equally critical is institutional capacity: many facilities lack 24/7 access to equipment, trained staff, or established protocols. Alfa-Wali and Osaghae [6] have documented how limitations in low- and middle-income countries (LMICs), including unreliable energy sources and poor equipment maintenance, hinder safe MIS implementation. Wilkinson et al. further highlight barriers such as inadequate curricula, poor interdepartmental communication, and limited access to simulation, which reduce the effective use of laparoscopy even when equipment is available [7].

Training, Technical Demands, and Practical Integration

Trauma MIS requires careful preparation in both infrastructure and training. Decision-making in trauma surgery is rapid, and laparoscopy must be performed efficiently. To support this, the WSES position paper outlines a step-by-step training framework that includes simulation, supervised hands-on cases, proctoring, and structured evaluation [10]. Team training is equally essential, involving anesthesiologists and scrub staff working in coordinated roles. In practice, MIS is effective for treating diaphragmatic injuries, hollow organ perforations, and selected solid organ procedures such as splenic salvage [13]. However, these cases test a surgeon's judgment, adaptability, and communication skills. MIS in trauma should not be viewed as a routine solution; it is a specialized approach that requires clear protocols and institutional readiness (Fig. 10.1). Its role will likely expand as technology and training improve, but only in systems that acknowledge and manage its limitations responsibly.

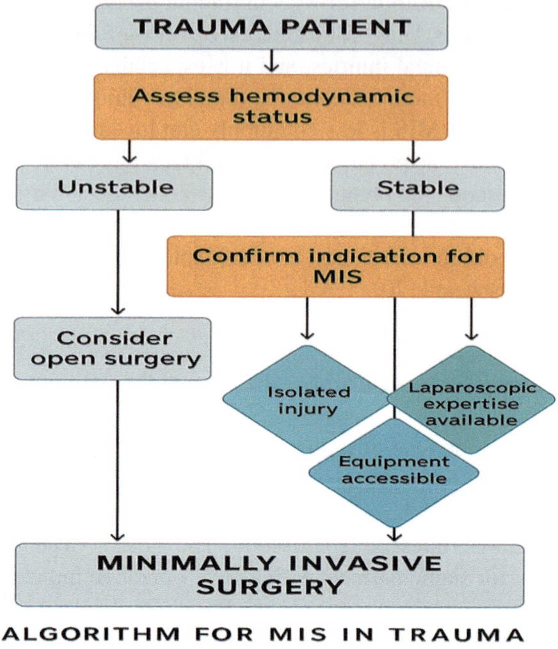

Fig. 10.1 Clinical algorithm for the use of MIS in trauma

Specific Methodologies and Strategies

The application of minimally invasive surgery (MIS) in trauma is increasingly common for both diagnostic and therapeutic purposes. Its integration into trauma protocols within academic medical centers requires definitive decision-making regarding technique, timing, and patient selection to maintain a balance between safety and efficacy. The use of MIS in trauma depends primarily on the patient's hemodynamic stability and the extent of injury [11, 12]. MIS is employed in both penetrating and blunt trauma involving the abdominal and thoracic cavities.

Diagnostic Laparoscopy in Abdominal Trauma

Diagnostic laparoscopy has proven to be a valuable tool in evaluating hemodynamically stable patients with penetrating abdominal trauma, particularly when physical examination or imaging findings are inconclusive. It is considered the diagnostic test of choice in abdominal trauma caused by stabbing or gunshot wounds, as it effectively rules out fascial penetration and intra-abdominal organ injury [12]. By enabling direct visualization of peritoneal violations, diaphragmatic injuries, and intra-abdominal trauma, diagnostic laparoscopy reduces the incidence of unnecessary laparotomies associated with significant morbidity [14, 18, 19]. It also permits thorough assessment of the diaphragm, solid organs such as the liver and spleen, and the entire length of the small and large intestines—especially in cases of suspected anterior abdominal wall trauma where local wound exploration may be insufficient.

Therapeutic Laparoscopy: Surgeries Involving the Diaphragm, Bowel, Liver, and Spleen

Laparoscopy has been used in the form of irrigation, hemostasis, and the application of hemostatic agents in low-grade liver or splenic laceration [14, 18, 19]. Successful laparoscopic splenectomy has been performed in high-volume centers for high-grade splenic injury when conservative management was not appropriate [13]. Laparoscopic repair of perforations of the stomach, colon, or bowel has been increasingly successful in well-selected patients [14]. Diaphragmatic rupture, often missed in thoracoabdominal penetrating trauma, can be accurately diagnosed and successfully treated with laparoscopy [21]. Laparoscopic techniques have also been used successfully in pediatric trauma, decreasing long-term morbidity from extensive incisional trauma by a considerable amount [15]. Dedicated pediatric MIS training pathways—described by Balogh and Kovács as a structured "through-the-keyhole" curriculum—have been advocated to ensure that pediatric surgeons attain the technical proficiency needed for safe laparoscopy in this delicate population, an approach equally relevant to pediatric trauma teams in academic centers [9].

Thoracoscopy in Hemothorax and Diaphragmatic Injury

Video-assisted thoracoscopic surgery (VATS) is a basic and widely accepted approach for trauma surgeons managing thoracic trauma in hemodynamically stable patients. Beyond mere chest-tube insertion, VATS is the gold standard for retained hemothorax management, permitting direct visualization and mechanical debridement of clots and debris to prevent trapped lung and empyema [22]. VATS also provides high diagnostic accuracy in stable patients with penetrating injuries near the heart or great vessels—confirming injury tracts, ruling out active hemorrhage, and detecting pericardial tamponade that may require emergent thoracotomy. It is also essential in the management of left-sided diaphragmatic rupture with herniated bowel, as thoracoscopic reduction and secure repair can be performed safely [23].

Hybrid Approaches and Conversion Indications

With acknowledgment that MIS is suboptimal for the management of complex or extensive injury, hybrid techniques are being accepted. These include starting procedures laparoscopically to evaluate injury and, when necessary, converting to open access to accomplish definitive repair. The hypothesis is that the advantages of MIS, such as less postoperative pain and more rapid recovery, are preserved with the assurance of timely open intervention, as necessary. Conversion to open operation is not a failure but an intraoperative decision necessary for safety. Indications are usually poor visualization, uncontrollable bleeding, or complex injury necessitating tactile exploration or suturing. Teaching when and how to convert is a valuable skill that underscores the need for coordinated trauma teams [24, 25, 29].

Integration of the Trauma Team

Coordination Among Trauma Surgeons, Residents, and MIS Specialists

Before beginning a case, each member of the trauma team, including the training resident, should know their role. It is the attending surgeon's responsibility to actively mentor and supervise residents, while also facilitating teaching opportunities provided by the MIS specialists. To ensure a smooth transition to hands-on practice, trauma surgeons should take advantage of simulations, footage review, and case discussions prior to the procedure to minimize confusion and increase resident confidence in the acute setting [24].

Multidisciplinary Collaboration

Effective trauma care relies not only on technical skills but also on seamless collaboration between surgical, anesthesia, radiology, and nursing teams, particularly during the "golden hour" [25]. A culture of mutual respect, pre-procedural briefings, and intraoperative checklists enhance coordination [26]. Briefly reviewing team roles, procedural plans, and expectations before incision improves safety, provided that such tools remain concise and context appropriate [27].

Communication During Urgent Intraoperative Decision-Making

Given the high-stakes and time-sensitive nature of trauma surgery, clear intraoperative communication is essential. Studies report that nearly 50% of communication-related errors at trauma centers occur during resuscitation [28]. To address this, trauma simulations increasingly incorporate non-technical skills training, emphasizing structured communication tools [29]. Official schemas like the Non-Technical Skills for Surgeons (NOTSS) and TeamSTEPPS that outline specific approaches to better situational management are used to streamline urgent decision-making and reduce cognitive overload during crises [30, 31].

Teaching Environment and Technical Training

Challenges of Resident Training in Trauma MIS

There are a host of challenges associated with resident training in trauma MIS, ranging from case volume to patient safety. One study found that the average surgical resident at a trauma center participates in only 15 trauma laparotomies, 6 diagnostic peritoneal lavages, and 45 ultrasound examinations per year, assuming 1 night of 4 on call [32]. Surgical residents on the trauma service often have more exposure to nonoperative management as opposed to procedures, and therefore struggle with learning and having confidence in performing surgical procedures due to limited case exposure [33]. A recent cross-continental assessment of surgical training in the Americas by Cassidy et al. likewise documented persistent disparities in trainee exposure to minimally invasive versus open techniques, with many residents reporting insufficient operative volume in advanced laparoscopy by graduation—an imbalance that has direct implications for the readiness of future trauma surgeons to perform MIS in emergent settings [5].

Case Selection and Ethics in Academic Centers

Especially in emergent trauma cases where MIS is required, attendings must not compromise patient safety in exchange for providing residents hands on training. However, there have been studies showing that the implementation of a surgical training program at a trauma center does not reveal any significant change in mortality before and after resident intraoperative participation [34].

Simulation Preparation

To address patient safety and limited case exposure in the trauma setting, academic centers turn to simulation-based education to allow residents to practice minimally invasive surgeries in a safe, controlled environment [29]. The repeatability and accessibility of simulations also reduce the expense risk of training residents in the already costly OR [29]. The following section outlines the three main modes of laparoscopic training that have been validated based on several variables established by Gallagher et al. and Javid et al., including how well the simulator feels and looks like the real-life scenario (face) or whether the outcomes in the simulator replicate real-life responses (content) [35–37].

Wet Lab

While human cadavers have served as the traditional model for surgical skill training, most minimally invasive procedures are performed on cadaveric or anesthetized small animals like rabbits or larger specimens like pigs, dogs, and sheep. Using larger anesthetized animals has proven to be especially beneficial in improving total procedure time and overall performance scores and adheres closest to performing full operations compared to other training methods [33, 34]. However, live animal models are more expensive and do require hands on surveillance by technicians and veterinary anesthetists [34].

Box Trainers

Box trainers are considered the first laparoscopic-specific simulators. The device is either a table or model torso with ports connected to laparoscopic instruments (Maryland Dissector, Metzenbaum, Modular needle holder, etc.), which have access to a platform underneath with different tasks [34]. A camera displays the platform onto a visual screen so that trainees can laparoscopically practice skills such as bead transfer, bowel tracing, and suture drills [34]. Reduced operative time following box trainer simulations has been proven for both total extraperitoneal hernia repair and laparoscopic cholecystectomy [29, 38, 39]. Video box trainers are advantageous in refining dexterity and psychomotor skills and offer an affordable alternative to virtual reality, especially with more basic, simplified equipment like the mirrored box simulator [34, 40]. Even resource-constrained programs have benefited from this approach: Mir et al. demonstrated that a structured curriculum built around an inexpensive endotrainer produced measurable improvements in the laparoscopic performance of trainee surgeons, supporting the integration of low-cost box-trainer modules into trauma MIS education when high-fidelity platforms are not available [8].

Virtual/Augmented Reality

A more recent advancement in laparoscopic simulation is virtual or augmented reality [29]. Along with high-definition visualization of the anatomical field, touch feedback to maneuvers allows for a realistic, responsive environment that can emulate whole cases that cannot be achieved with box trainers [32]. VR simulation is especially beneficial when used as supplementary material to traditional apprenticeship or when teaching novice learners at the introductory level [41]. That said, Munz et al. found that virtual reality has not shown improved operational outcomes when compared to box training alone, and the technology is on the more costly side [34, 42].

Equipment and Logistics

Preparedness in High-Stakes Trauma Environments

MIS in trauma care is not merely about using advanced tools; it is about coordinating swift decisions, clinical precision, and seamless teamwork under immense pressure. Unlike planned elective surgeries, trauma cases unfold suddenly, with little warning and high stakes. This unpredictability makes it essential that everything, from the operating room setup to the surgical instruments, is not just available but instantly usable. In such high-stress environments, the real value of MIS emerges only when modern equipment is supported by systems that enable rapid activation, safe handling, and seamless integration into the trauma team's workflow [6].

Core Equipment and Setup Requirements

Laparoscopic procedures require several essential tools, including a laparoscopic tower, an insufflation system, a light source, and a camera unit. Additionally, various surgical instruments, such as graspers, scissors, dissectors, and needle holders, are necessary. Each tool serves a specific purpose, ensuring safe and efficient access to the abdominal cavity through minimally invasive techniques. Before the trauma patient arrives in the operating room, the equipment must be available, functional, sterile, and correctly set up. For example, the insufflator needs to maintain pneumoperitoneum by delivering high-flow CO. At the same time, the camera system should give clear and stable images without requiring frequent adjustments during the procedure. If any parts are missing, damaged, or put together incorrectly because of poor teamwork, the setup's effectiveness will be compromised.

Global Disparities and Systemic Challenges

In high-resource environments, specialized MIS teams and operating rooms with established protocols help ensure they are well-prepared. However, many low- and middle-income countries (LMICs) face logistical challenges that make it hard to implement trauma MIS. Problems like inconsistent equipment availability, unreliable energy supplies, a shortage of trained personnel, and supply-chain disruptions slow down progress. Alfa-Wali and Osaghae identified the lack of high-definition monitors and maintenance systems as key barriers, resulting in sporadic rather than routine MIS use [6]. Similarly, Wilkinson et al. highlighted systemic shortcomings, including unstructured training, limited routine MIS exposure, and a lack of team readiness that result in underuse of laparoscopic setups even when they exist [7]. A broader systematic review by Chao et al. corroborated these findings while also outlining pragmatic strategies—including locally adapted training initiatives, cooperative equipment-sharing arrangements, and context-specific protocols—that have enabled selected LMIC centers to expand the safe use of laparoscopic surgery, lessons that are equally applicable to trauma MIS programs in resource-limited environments [16].

Successful MIS in trauma relies on both operational logistics and surgical skills. A well-organized trauma center understands that the choice to perform laparoscopy does not happen in a vacuum. It depends on the entire system being ready to support that choice from the start of the procedure to its completion. So, bringing MIS into trauma surgery requires more than just enthusiasm. It also requires clear protocols that prioritize preparation over improvisation. It requires investments in infrastructure and training across different fields. Table 10.2 gives a summary of these key requirements for successful MIS integration in trauma settings.

Table 10.2 Core institutional requirements for implementing MIS in trauma care

Element	Requirement
Specialized trauma MIS team	Inclusion of a trained surgeon, anesthesiologist, scrub nurse, and support staff
Laparoscopic equipment	Availability of tower, CO insufflator, HD camera system, light source, and instruments
Trauma-specific protocols	Clearly defined guidelines for selecting MIS candidates among trauma patients
Simulation-based training	Ongoing simulation programs for multidisciplinary emergency team coordination
Round-the-clock accessibility	24/7 readiness of sterile, functional laparoscopic equipment
Conversion readiness	Protocols in place for timely switch to open surgery if needed
Team communication systems	Predefined communication strategies and role allocations for trauma scenarios

Outcomes and Supporting Evidence

Comparative Benefits: Pain, Recovery, and Morbidity

Laparoscopic management in trauma care has proven beneficial when compared to open surgery. A notable 2015 meta-analysis by Li et al. comparing laparotomy vs. laparoscopy across 64 studies in 9058 abdominal trauma patients found significant advantages with the MIS approach [43]. Improved outcomes along with the listed mean difference include:

Decreased postoperative pain duration (−21.34 h), decreased intraoperative blood loss (−141.33 mL), decreased operation time (−19.93 min), decreased length of hospital stay (−5.15 days), decreased time in the ICU (−1.89 days), and time to regular diet (−3.46 h) [39].

Not only does laparoscopy reduce pain duration, but it also reduce pain intensity; as studies also reported reduced use of narcotics [43]. Minimally invasive management also results in decreased wound infection compared to open surgery, as evidenced by decreased postoperative pneumonia and accesses [44].

Comparative Costs and Diagnostic Laparoscopy

Given the decreased operation time and length of ICU stay, laparoscopy in the trauma setting also significantly reduces hospital costs [43]. Especially when used diagnostically for hemodynamically stable abdominal trauma patients, the MIS approach saves expenses by minimizing the use of unnecessary exploratory laparotomies that would otherwise lengthen hospital stay and operation time [45]. The large incision required for exploratory laparotomies also increases risk and morbidity, particularly when 45% of suspected diaphragmatic injury cases potentially end in non-therapeutic laparotomies [46]. Laparoscopy, on the other hand, has shown high sensitivity and specificity for suspected thoracoabdominal penetrating injuries, which is highly advantageous when ultrasound and CT imaging can only detect diaphragmatic and occult small bowel injuries with a sensitivity of approximately 26% [46].

Balancing Training and Patient Care

In training hospitals where new doctors are learning, it is necessary to train them properly while still offering the best possible care to patients. Resident learning of MIS is essential, but patients must not be put at extra risk because of this. A 2008 study noted that incorporating laparoscopic training into busy residency programs can be challenging, particularly when adequate supervision is lacking [2]. A 2017 study demonstrated that early use of simulation devices allows trainees to develop their skills more rapidly and reduces the likelihood of errors [3]. A fifteen-year experience from a Brazilian tertiary teaching hospital reported by Damous et al. further illustrates how educational, institutional, and logistical barriers can delay the routine adoption of laparoscopy even for common emergency procedures such as appendectomy, reinforcing the need for sustained institutional commitment, dedicated curricula, and protected operative time when integrating MIS—including trauma MIS—into academic surgical practice [4].

In high-resource environments, specialized MIS teams and operating rooms with established protocols help ensure readiness. However, in low- and middle-income countries (LMICs), logistical challenges—including inconsistent equipment availability, unreliable energy supplies, shortages of trained personnel, and supply-chain disruptions—hinder the implementation of trauma MIS [6]. Alfa-Wali and Osaghae identified the absence of high-definition monitors and robust maintenance systems as key barriers, resulting in sporadic rather than routine MIS use [6]. Similarly, Wilkinson et al. highlighted systemic shortcomings, unstructured training, limited routine MIS exposure, and insufficient team readiness that lead to underutilization of laparoscopic setups even when equipment is available [7].

Conclusion

Minimally invasive surgery (MIS) has emerged as a transformative approach in trauma care within academic hospitals, offering improved patient outcomes through reduced morbidity, shorter recovery times, and fewer complications, particularly for hemodynamically stable patients with penetrating or select blunt injuries. Its integration into trauma protocols demands meticulous coordination, robust institutional infrastructure, and comprehensive training programs. Structured curricula, incorporating simulation-based learning and adherence to guidelines like the WSES Cesena recommendations [11], are critical for equipping surgical residents and trauma teams with the necessary technical proficiency and decision-making acumen. Effective multidisciplinary collaboration, clear communication, and readiness to convert to open surgery when needed ensure patient safety remains paramount. As advancements in technology and training continue to refine MIS applications, teaching hospitals must balance educational goals with clinical excellence, fostering skilled surgeons while upholding the highest standards of care through disciplined, evidence-based practice.

Acknowledgments The author acknowledges the trauma faculty and minimally invasive surgery mentors at the R Adams Cowley Shock Trauma Center for their clinical insights and support. No AI tools were used in the writing of this chapter beyond standard grammar and reference checks.

Competing Interests The author declares no competing interests.

Ethics Approval Not applicable for this narrative chapter.

References

1. Nacul MP. Laparoscopy & robotics: a historical parallel. Rev Col Bras Cir. 2020;47:e20202811. https://doi.org/10.1590/0100-6991e-20202811. English, Portuguese
2. Matsevych OY, Koto MZ, Aldous C. Trauma laparoscopy: A prospect of skills training (cohort study). Int J Surg. 2018;55:117–23. https://doi.org/10.1016/j.ijsu.2018.05.033.
3. de'Angelis N, Marchegiani F, Schena CA, Khan J, Agnoletti V, Ansaloni L, Barría Rodríguez AG, Bianchi PP, Biffl W, Bravi F, Ceccarelli G, Ceresoli M, Chiara O, Chirica M, Cobianchi L, Coccolini F, Coimbra R, Cotsoglou C, D'Hondt M, Damaskos D, De Simone B, Di Saverio S, Diana M, Espin-Basany E, Fichtner-Feigl S, Fugazzola P, Gavriilidis P, Gronnier C, Kashuk J, Kirkpatrick AW, Ammendola M, Kouwenhoven EA, Laurent A, Leppaniemi A, Lesurtel M, Memeo R, Milone M, Moore E, Pararas N, Peitzmann A, Pessaux P, Picetti E, Pikoulis M, Pisano M, Ris F, Robison T, Sartelli M, Shelat VG, Spinoglio G, Sugrue M, Tan E, Van Eetvelde E, Kluger Y, Weber D, Catena F. Training curriculum in minimally invasive emergency digestive surgery: 2022 WSES position paper. World J Emerg Surg. 2023;18(1):11. https://doi.org/10.1186/s13017-023-00476-w.
4. Sermonesi G, Tian BWCA, Vallicelli C, Abu-Zidan FM, Damaskos D, Kelly MD, Leppäniemi A, Galante JM, Tan E, Kirkpatrick AW, Khokha V, Romeo OM, Chirica M, Pikoulis M, Litvin A, Shelat VG, Sakakushev B, Wani I, Sall I, Fugazzola P, Cicuttin E, Toro A, Amico F, Mas FD, De Simone B, Sugrue M, Bonavina L, Campanelli G, Carcoforo P, Cobianchi L, Coccolini F, Chiarugi M, Di Carlo I, Di Saverio S, Podda M, Pisano M, Sartelli M, Testini M, Fette A, Rizoli S, Picetti E, Weber D, Latifi R, Kluger Y, Balogh ZJ, Biffl W, Jeekel H, Civil I, Hecker A, Ansaloni L, Bravi F, Agnoletti V, Beka SG, Moore EE, Catena F. Cesena guidelines: WSES consensus statement on laparoscopic-first approach to general surgery emergencies and abdominal trauma. World J Emerg Surg. 2023;18(1):57. https://doi.org/10.1186/s13017-023-00520-9.
5. Koto MZ, Matsevych OY, Mosai F, Patel S, Aldous C, Balabyeki M. Laparoscopy for blunt abdominal trauma: a challenging endeavor. Scand J Surg: SJS. 2019;108(4):273–9. https://doi.org/10.1177/1457496918816927.
6. Alfa-Wali M, Osaghae S. Practice, training and safety of laparoscopic surgery in low and middle-income countries. World J Gastrointest Surg. 2017;9(1):13–8. https://doi.org/10.4240/wjgs.v9.i1.13.
7. Wilkinson E, Aruparayil N, Gnanaraj J, Brown J, Jayne D. Barriers to training in laparoscopic surgery in low- and middle-income countries: A systematic review. Trop Dr. 2021;51(3):408–14. https://doi.org/10.1177/0049475521998186.
8. Birindelli A, Martin M, Khan M, Gallo G, Segalini E, Gori A, Yetasook A, Podda M, Giuliani A, Tugnoli G, Lim R, TraumaLap Study Group, Di Saverio S. Laparoscopic splenectomy as a definitive management option for high-grade traumatic splenic injury when non operative management is not feasible or failed: a 5-year experience from a level one trauma center

with minimally invasive surgery expertise. Updat Surg. 2021;73(4):1515–31. https://doi.org/10.1007/s13304-021-01045-z.
9. Di Saverio S, Birindelli A, Podda M, Segalini E, Piccinini A, Coniglio C, Frattini C, Tugnoli G. Trauma laparoscopy and the six w's: why, where, who, when, what, and how? J Trauma Acute Care Surg. 2019;86(2):344–67. https://doi.org/10.1097/TA.0000000000002130.
10. Cirocchi R, Birindelli A, Inaba K, Mandrioli M, Piccinini A, Tabola R, Carlini L, Tugnoli G, Di Saverio S. Laparoscopy for trauma and the changes in its use from 1990 to 2016: A current systematic review and meta-analysis. Surg Laparosc Endosc Percutan Tech. 2018;28(1):1–12. https://doi.org/10.1097/SLE.0000000000000466.
11. Lim KH, Chung BS, Kim JY, Kim SS. Laparoscopic surgery in abdominal trauma: a single center review of a 7-year experience. World J Emerg Surgery: WJES. 2015;10:16. https://doi.org/10.1186/s13017-015-0007-8.
12. Villavicencio RT, Aucar JA. Analysis of laparoscopy in trauma. J Am Coll Surg. 1999;189(1):11–20. https://doi.org/10.1016/s1072-7515(99)00052-6.
13. Campos Costa F, Cardoso V, Monteiro AM, Guerreiro J. Laparoscopic repair of an acute traumatic diaphragmatic hernia: clinical case. Cureus. 2020;12(10):e11082. https://doi.org/10.7759/cureus.11082.
14. Marwan A, Harmon CM, Georgeson KE, Smith GF, Muensterer OJ. Use of laparoscopy in the management of pediatric abdominal trauma. J Trauma Injury Infect Crit Care. 2010;69(4):761–4. https://doi.org/10.1097/TA.0b013e3181c816a8.
15. Balogh B, Kovács T. Gyermeksebészeti szakképzés kulcslyukon keresztül [Training for pediatric surgeons through the keyhole]. Orv Hetil. 2018;159(43):1747–53. Hungarian. https://doi.org/10.1556/650.2018.31189.
16. Meyer DM, Jessen ME, Wait MA, Estrera AS. Early evacuation of traumatic retained hemothoraces using thoracoscopy: a prospective, randomized trial. Ann Thorac Surg. 1997;64(5):1396–401. https://doi.org/10.1016/S0003-4975(97)00899-0.
17. Radjou AN, Uthrapathy M. Video-assisted thoracoscopy in trauma: case report and review of literature. Lung India. 2011;28(2):142–4. https://doi.org/10.4103/0970-2113.80335.
18. Miyasaka KW, Martin ND, Pascual JL, Buchholz J, Aggarwal R. A simulation curriculum for management of trauma and surgical critical care patients. J Surg Educ. 2015;72(5):803–10. https://doi.org/10.1016/j.jsurg.2015.03.001.
19. Adedeji OA, Driscoll PA. The trauma team–a system of initial trauma care. Postgrad Med J. 1996;72(852):587–93. https://doi.org/10.1136/pgmj.72.852.587.
20. Seeger P, Kaldis N, Nickel F, Hackert T, Lykoudis PM, Giannou AD. Surgical training simulation modalities in minimally invasive surgery: how to achieve evidence-based curricula by translational research. Am J Surg. 2025;242:116197. https://doi.org/10.1016/j.amjsurg.2025.116197.
21. Lingard L, Espin S, Rubin B, Whyte S, Colmenares M, Baker GR, Doran D, Grober E, Orser B, Bohnen J, Reznick R. Getting teams to talk: development and pilot implementation of a checklist to promote interprofessional communication in the OR. Qual Saf Health Care. 2005;14(5):340–6. https://doi.org/10.1136/qshc.2004.012377.
22. Steinemann S, Bhatt A, Suares G, Wei A, Ho N, Kurosawa G, Lim E, Berg B. Trauma team discord and the role of briefing. J Trauma Acute Care Surg. 2016;81(1):184–9. https://doi.org/10.1097/TA.0000000000001024.
23. Bergs EA, Rutten FL, Tadros T, Krijnen P, Schipper IB. Communication during trauma resuscitation: do we know what is happening? Injury. 2005;36(8):905–11. https://doi.org/10.1016/j.injury.2004.12.047.
24. Yule S, Flin R, Paterson-Brown S, Maran N, Rowley D. Development of a rating system for surgeons' non-technical skills. Med Educ. 2006;40(11):1098–104. https://doi.org/10.1111/j.1365-2929.2006.02610.x.
25. Davis DA, Mazmanian PE, Fordis M, Van Harrison R, Thorpe KE, Perrier L. Accuracy of physician self-assessment compared with observed measures of competence: a systematic review. JAMA. 2006;296(9):1094–102. https://doi.org/10.1001/jama.296.9.1094.

26. Fakhry SM, Watts DD, Michetti C, Hunt JP. MD for the EAST multi-institutional blunt hollow viscous injury research group. The resident experience on trauma: declining surgical opportunities and career incentives? Analysis of data from a large multi-institutional study. J Trauma Injury Infect Crit Care. 2003;54(1):1–8.
27. Kuhlenschmidt KM, Houshmand N, Bisgaard E, Grant J, Dumas R, Park C, Cripps MW. Simulation-based skill training in trauma: A much needed confidence boost. J Am Coll Surg. 2020;231(4):256 10.1016/j.jamcollsurg.2020.07.394.
28. Cassidy BP, Stingl CS, Méndez N, Machain GM, Vega-Rivera F, Ribeiro MAF Jr, Sacoto H, Ottolino P, Beitia SK, Quiodettis M, Rodas EB, Mallah MM. Surgical training trends in the Americas: A cross-continental assessment of minimally invasive surgery and open surgery among surgical trainees. World J Surg. 2024;48(11):2686–96. https://doi.org/10.1002/wjs.12378.
29. Raval MV, Wang X, Cohen ME, Ingraham AM, Bentrem DJ, Dimick JB, Flynn T, Hall BL, Ko CY. The influence of resident involvement on surgical outcomes. J Am Coll Surg. 2011;212(5):889–98. https://doi.org/10.1016/j.jamcollsurg.2010.12.029.
30. Dhariwal AK, Prabhu RY, Dalvi AN, Supe AN. Effectiveness of box trainers in laparoscopic training. J Minim Access Surg. 2007;3(2):57–63. https://doi.org/10.4103/0972-9941.33274.
31. Gallagher AG, Ritter EM, Satava RM. Fundamental principles of validation, and reliability: rigorous science for the assessment of surgical education and training. Surg Endosc. 2003;17(10):1525–9. https://doi.org/10.1007/s00464-003-0035-4.
32. Javid P, Aydın A, Mohanna PN, Dasgupta P, Ahmed K. Current status of simulation and training models in microsurgery: a systematic review. Microsurgery. 2019;39(7):655–68. https://doi.org/10.1002/micr.30513.
33. Zendejas B, Cook DA, Bingener J, Huebner M, Dunn WF, Sarr MG, Farley DR. Simulation-based mastery learning improves patient outcomes in laparoscopic inguinal hernia repair: a randomized controlled trial. Ann Surg. 2011;254(3):502–9; discussion 509–11. https://doi.org/10.1097/SLA.0b013e31822c6994.
34. Bansal VK, Raveendran R, Misra MC, Bhattacharjee H, Rajan K, Krishna A, Kumar P, Kumar S. A prospective randomized controlled blinded study to evaluate the effect of short-term focused training program in laparoscopy on operating room performance of surgery residents (CTRI/2012/11/003113). J Surg Educ. 2014;71(1):52–60. https://doi.org/10.1016/j.jsurg.2013.06.012.
35. Keyser EJ, Derossis AM, Antoniuk M, Sigman HH, Fried GM. A simplified simulator for the training and evaluation of laparoscopic skills. Surg Endosc. 2000;14(2):149–53. https://doi.org/10.1007/s004649900088.
36. Mir IS, Mohsin M, Malik A, Shah AQ, Majid T. A structured training module using an inexpensive endotrainer for improving the performance of trainee surgeons. Trop Dr. 2008;38(4):217–8. https://doi.org/10.1258/td.2008.070359.
37. Jin C, Dai L, Wang T. The application of virtual reality in the training of laparoscopic surgery: a systematic review and meta-analysis. Int J Surg. 2021;87:105859. https://doi.org/10.1016/j.ijsu.2020.11.022.
38. Munz Y, Kumar BD, Moorthy K, Bann S, Darzi A. Laparoscopic virtual reality and box trainers: is one superior to the other? Surg Endosc. 2004;18:485–94. https://doi.org/10.1007/s00464-003-9043-7.
39. Chao TE, Mandigo M, Opoku-Anane J, Maine R. Systematic review of laparoscopic surgery in low- and middle-income countries: benefits, challenges, and strategies. Surg Endosc. 2016;30(1):1–10. https://doi.org/10.1007/s00464-015-4201-2.
40. Li Y, Xiang Y, Wu N, Wu L, Yu Z, Zhang M, Wang M, Jiang J, Li Y. A comparison of laparoscopy and laparotomy for the Management of Abdominal Trauma: a systematic review and meta-analysis. World J Surg. 2015;39(12):2862–71. https://doi.org/10.1007/s00268-015-3212-4.
41. Hajibandeh S, Hajibandeh S, Gumber AO, Wong CS. Laparoscopy versus laparotomy for the management of penetrating abdominal trauma: a systematic review and meta-analysis. Int J Surg. 2016;34:127–36. https://doi.org/10.1016/j.ijsu.2016.08.524.

42. Taner AS, Topgul K, Kucukel F, Demir A, Sari S. Diagnostic laparoscopy decreases the rate of unnecessary laparotomies and reduces hospital costs in trauma patients. J Laparoendosc Adv Surg Tech A. 2001;11(4):207–11. https://doi.org/10.1089/109264201750539718.
43. Uranues S, Popa DE, Diaconescu B, Schrittwieser R. Laparoscopy in penetrating abdominal trauma. World J Surg. 2015;39(6):1381–8. https://doi.org/10.1007/s00268-014-2904-5.
44. Stefanidis D, Acker CE, Swiderski D, Heniford BT, Greene FL. Challenges during the implementation of a laparoscopic skills curriculum in a busy general surgery residency program. J Surg Educ. 2008;65(1):4–7. https://doi.org/10.1016/j.jsurg.2007.11.009.
45. Cullinan DR, Schill MR, DeClue A, Salles A, Wise PE, Awad MM. Fundamentals of laparoscopic surgery: not only for senior residents. J Surg Educ. 2017;74(6):e51–4. https://doi.org/10.1016/j.jsurg.2017.07.017.
46. Damous SHB, Menegozzo CAM, Rocha MC, Collet-E-Silva FS, Utiyama EM. Challenges to implement laparoscopic appendectomy as the first-line treatment for acute appendicitis: a fifteen-year experience in a tertiary hospital in Brazil. Rev Col Bras Cir. 2023;50:e20233527. https://doi.org/10.1590/0100-6991e-20233527-en.

Laparoscopy in Penetrating Injuries: When and How?

11

Selman Uranues, Viktor Frieders-Justin, and Philipp Stiegler

Introduction

Penetrating abdominal trauma remains a frequent cause of emergency surgical admissions worldwide, especially in younger populations. Historically, patients with suspected intra-abdominal injury underwent mandatory laparotomy, with a high rate of unnecessary explorations; non-therapeutic laparotomy rates up to 21–41% have been observed and were associated with non-neglectable postoperative morbidity in up to 20% of cases [1, 2].

The advent of selective non-operative management (NOM) in combination with improved imaging and the introduction of laparoscopy into trauma surgery have dramatically reduced the need for routine laparotomy in penetrating trauma. However, in their analysis of over 25,000 thousand cases, Zafar et al. reported a failure of NOM in 20.8% of gunshot wounds and 15.2% stab wounds leading to an increased mortality risk (4.48 and 9.83 fold increase, respectively; adjusted for demographics, injury severity, and clinical variables) [3]. Especially, lacerations of the hollow viscera pose a challenge to clinicians as these injuries often present a certain delay until peritonitis can clinically be suspected.

Laparoscopy can solve this *diagnostic uncertainty*: it bridges the gap between NOM and exploratory laparotomy with the intent to minimize any delay in diagnosing potentially life-threatening injuries and unnecessary morbidity associated with

S. Uranues (✉) · P. Stiegler
Department of Surgery, Section for Surgical Research, Medical University of Graz, Graz, Austria
e-mail: selman.uranues@medunigraz.at; philipp.stiegler@medunigraz.at

V. Frieders-Justin
Department of Surgery, Section for Surgical Research, Medical University of Graz, Graz, Austria

Department of Surgery, Klinik Donaustadt, Vienna Healthcare Group, Vienna, Austria
e-mail: viktor.frieders-justin@gesundheitsverbund.at

© The Author(s), under exclusive license to Springer Nature Switzerland AG 2026

M. Cezillo, B. M. Pereira (eds.), *Minimally Invasive Surgery Trauma*,
https://doi.org/10.1007/978-3-032-28971-1_11

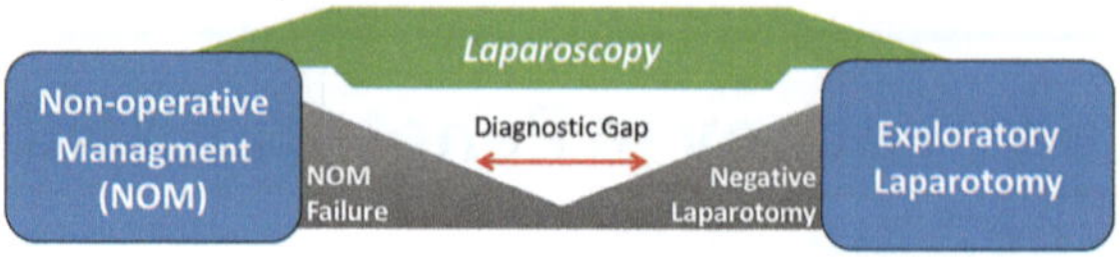

Fig. 11.1 Laparoscopy bridges the gap!

negative laparotomy (Fig. 11.1). Diagnostic laparoscopy offers both diagnostic clarity and the opportunity for therapeutic intervention, if applicable by the patient's condition. Especially in low-volume trauma centers with laparoscopic expertise but little experience in NOM for penetrating trauma, it marks an ideal tool to minimize the risk of missed injuries with delayed repair.

The primary aim of laparoscopy is to assess peritoneal penetration and organ injury to guide subsequent laparoscopic or open treatment. When the patient's condition and the expertise of the surgical team allow, it also offers the potential for minimally invasive management of the injuries.

A significant concern, particularly during the early days of laparoscopy, was the risk of overlooking injuries. Advances in equipment, expertise, and implementation of standardized systematic exploration, however, have led to a significant improvement in diagnostic accuracy up to 100% [4–7].

More recent data show low missed injury rates while reducing the need for unnecessary laparotomy, postoperative complications, and hospital stay [7–9]. In addition to diagnosis, laparoscopy allows for therapeutic interventions, including diaphragmatic, bowel and gastric repair as well as control of mesenteric bleeding, and prevention of contamination [3, 6, 10–12]. Several international guidelines incorporate the use of laparoscopy in penetrating trauma, however emphasizing the importance of correct patient selection and a laparoscopic skill set [1, 13, 14].

Interestingly, a 2024 Trauma Quality Improvement Program database analysis of over 5900 hemodynamically stable patients undergoing surgical exploration for penetrating trauma found that laparoscopy was only used 15.5% [15]. The authors concluded that there is a potential for a *"6 to 45 % increased usage of laparoscopy for stabbing abdominal trauma."* This observation alone lets us thank you for reading this book!

When to Consider Laparoscopy?

When considering a patient for laparoscopy, it is of utmost importance to confirm the eligibility and to exclude possible contraindications. *A minimally invasive approach in the wrong patient will do more harm than good!*

Prerequisites and Contraindications

At the time of surgery, the patient must be hemodynamically stable and remain stable. While several definitions for hemodynamic stability exist, the Advanced Trauma

Life Support (ATLS) Classification of blood loss (Table 11.1) is useful for an informed decision. ATLS Class I and—if responding to fluid resuscitation—Class II are suitable candidates. Laparoscopy is contraindicated in the more severe classes of shock.

Further (relative) contraindications include:

- Severe head trauma: Intraperitoneal carbon dioxide insufflation and positioning during laparoscopy may increase intracranial pressure, thus significant trauma to the head should be considered as a contraindication for pneumoperitoneum and Trendelenburg positioning.
- History of prior abdominal surgery anticipating extensive adhesions.
- Large evisceration.
- Overt peritonitis.
- Lack of expertise in advanced laparoscopic techniques.

It is crucial to understand that in trauma surgery, time from initial presentation to bleeding control is the most important factor. That means the primary treatment goal is to stop potentially life-threatening bleeding and prevent contamination. Definitive repair of all injuries may only be attempted if the patient's condition allows and reconstruction is adapted to the patient's needs. Losing too much time—for the sake of personal ego—performing a complex minimally invasive repair may worsen the outcome and even risk the patient's survival. In collaboration with the anesthesiologist, the best surgical technique—open or minimally invasive—should be chosen for the most efficient lifesaving procedure.

Table 11.1 ATLS classification of blood loss

	I	II	III	IV
Blood loss	<750 mL	750–1500 mL	1500–2000 mL	>2000 mL
% Blood volume lost	<15%	15–30%	30–40%	>40%
Heart rate	<100 bpm	>100 bpm	>120 bpm	>140 bpm
Blood pressure (systolic)	Normal	Normal	Decreased	Markedly decreased
Pulse pressure	Normal	Decreased	Decreased	Very narrow/ absent
Respiratory rate	14–20	20–30	30–40	>35
Mental status	Alert	Anxious	Confused	Lethargic/ unconscious
Urine output	>30 mL/h	20–30 mL/h	5–15 mL/h	Negligible
Hemodynamic stability	**Stable**	**Borderline**	**Unstable**	**Severely unstable**
Laparoscopy?	**YES**	**Potentially, if patient responds adequately to resuscitation**	**NO**	**NO**

Adapted from Spahn et al. [16]

Laparoscopy for Whom?

The diagnostic aim of laparoscopy is to exclude or confirm peritoneal violation. Depending on the findings, surgery can be stopped (if no penetration has been found), a laparoscopic exploration +/– repair can be performed (if injury severity and minimally invasive comfort level of the surgeon allow for it) or the operation can be converted to open surgery.

Indications for Laparoscopic Exploration in Penetrating Trauma

- *Stab wounds* to the (anterior) abdomen: when fascial breach can't be excluded with local wound exploration and/or free fluid (blood) is confirmed by ultrasound or CT-scan, laparoscopy is warranted. Stable stab wounded patients without signs of peritonitis should laparoscopically be explored if hematoperitoneum is confirmed. In high volume centers with optimal observation, NOM might be an option for these patients. In select cases, however, NOM can also be an option, in isolated stab wound with low-grade injury to the liver and spleen.
- *Tangential gunshot wounds* (GSW) with unclear trajectory: due to the velocity of the projectile, GSW and other similar injuries (like shrapnel etc.) tend to have larger injury extend than stab wounds. Even if the entry point may seem small, intrabdominal lacerations can be devastating due to cavitation and "tumbling" of the bullet. When a direct GSW to the abdomen occurs, laparoscopic treatment often is too complex and time-consuming and should therefore be avoided. However, if peritoneal penetration is not clear, it is a great diagnostic tool to minimize surgery related morbidity.
- *Thoracoabdominal Injuries*: Stab wounds at the thoracoabdominal border may injure both the pleural and the peritoneal spaces. Often, diaphragmatic perforations can be better visualized with laparoscopy, than in open surgery. However, the risk of tension pneumothorax should be considered in these patients.

Imaging Studies

Choice of imaging modalities in penetrating trauma depends on the state of the patient, local resources, and institutional policies. In unstable patients, not adequately responding to resuscitation, eFAST (extended Focused Assessment Sonography in Trauma) alone is the only diagnostic tool before performing trauma laparotomy and/or thoracotomy. Hemodynamically stable patients may undergo further investigations after eFAST. In these cases, computed tomography (CT) is the investigational method of choice. While eFAST has both high sensitivity and specificity (90% and 95%, respectively) for the detection of intraperitoneal free fluid, CT even yields a higher sensitivity of 94% and a specificity of 95% to detect intra-abdominal fluid *and* organ injuries [17]. However, injuries to the small bowel, the mesentery, and the diaphragm remain weak spots of imaging [14, 17, 18]. Especially in diaphragmatic injuries, multidetector CT scan only has a pooled sensitivity rate of 74% and a specificity rate of 92%, a substantial diagnostic weakness given the high complication rate after these injuries [18, 19].

How Do We Perform Trauma Laparoscopy?

Operation Room Setup

The patient is positioned supine, with both arms tucked. Spread legs facilitate better access around the patient and enhance visualization of all quadrants, particularly for repairing diaphragmatic injuries. Positioning should allow the surgeon to operate from all sides easily. A 30° laparoscope, two atraumatic laparoscopic bowel graspers, and a laparoscopic suction device should be at hand.

Access to the Abdomen and Trocar Placement

Trocar placement should follow a standardized method to gain safe and quick access to the abdomen. Never place a trocar through the penetrating wound, you aim to explore—this might change the intraperitoneal situation and mask the peritoneal penetration site. Additionally, it may increase the infection risk.

For exploration, usually a 10–12 mm camera port and two 5 mm working ports are recommended. However, additional ports or upsizing the 5 mm to 10–12 mm ports may be necessary to improve visualization and/or exposure.

For the first trocar, we advocate for an open placement previously described by our group [20]. This open approach, preferably at the superior border of the umbilicus, has been proven to be safe and quick as the subcutaneous layer is at its' thinnest even in obese patients. Although our primary choice for the first trocar is the umbilicus and periumbilical area, in penetrating injuries, the trocar site always depends on the location of the skin injury. If the injury happens to be at the umbilicus, the first trocar should be placed at least about 10 cm away. The working trocars should be positioned at both flanks establishing a good triangulation (exemplary positioning shown in Fig. 11.2). Capnoperitoneum should be set between 10 and 14 mmHg according to patient's tolerance level.

Systematic Intra-abdominal Exploration

Once access to the abdomen has been obtained, a microbial sample should be taken and a structured exploration should be performed; the threshold to convert should be low:

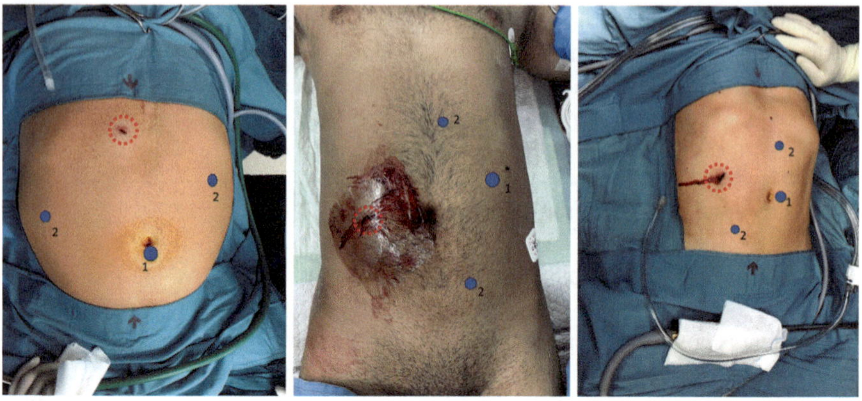

Fig. 11.2 Potential trocar setups (**1** = 10–12 mm optical trocar; **2** = 5 mm working trocar) depending on injury site (red circle)

1. Check for accidental injuries during entry and overt contraindications to laparoscopy (e.g., significant amount of feces).
2. Visualize the part of the parietal peritoneum corresponding to the skin laceration and check for active bleeding from abdominal wall.
3. If the peritoneum is intact, end the procedure—you have prevented an unnecessary laparotomy! If the peritoneum has been penetrated, further exploration (of all quadrants) is warranted. When in doubt conversion is a wise decision.
4. In contrast to blunt abdominal trauma, *exploration* in penetrating trauma should *start in that area where the injuries are expected*. Evacuate any blood clots in the potential area to inspect the probably affected organs:
   (a) Flowing blood or any kind of fluid might be a leading sign to the injury site. Hematoma of the corresponding omentum or mesentery might be leading signs for small bowel injuries. Hematoma in the bowel wall or in the corresponding retroperitoneum is suspicious for injuries. While without mobilization only the intraperitoneal part of large bowel can be visualized, potentially injured parts of the colon should be mobilized and explored profoundly.
   (b) Ongoing bleeding from the abdominal wall can mostly be controlled laparoscopically by coagulation or tamponade with a swab. In case of laceration of the epigastric vessels, transfascial sutures (e.g., using a suture passer) are highly recommended.
5. Once the suspected impact area (close to the peritoneal laceration) has been examined and any encountered injuries have been repaired, further exploration of the remaining abdominal cavity is warranted. Perform a systematic examination of all quadrants including large and small bowel, mesenteries, lesser sac, and retroperitoneum. Opening the retroperitoneum is only in selected patients indicated. Tilting the table to one or other side may help to move the bowel loops and omentum, enabling better visualization of both sides and the corresponding mesentery.

6. Any additional time-consuming procedures, adhesiolysis of unrelated areas, or incidentally detected pathologic findings (e.g., gallstones, inguinal- or umbilical hernias, fibromas, etc.) should be disregarded.
7. *Drains*: There is no data supporting the routine use of intraperitoneal drains after diagnostic and therapeutic laparoscopy. The decision, thus, has to be based on the intraoperative findings, performed procedure, and expected complications like fistula in pancreatic lacerations.

Uncertain findings, poor visualization, inadequate access to a suspected injury site, or the need for time-consuming procedures call for immediate conversion.

Therapeutic Laparoscopy

Several penetrating injuries can be dealt with laparoscopically:

- *Hollow viscus injuries*: Isolated and small injuries (Figs. 11.3 and 11.4) can be sutured preferably with a 4-0 monofilament absorbable suture. Management of larger defects requiring resection may be also managed laparoscopically given the necessary expertise. However, due to the increased complexity, it may be prudent to perform a laparoscopically assisted mini-laparotomy at the nearest point of injury. In hollow viscus injuries, especially anterior gastric wall injuries, the opposite wall should always be checked as well, particularly in vascular injuries. This may require mobilization, e.g., entering the lesser sac when the stomach is involved or detachment of the omentum in transverse colon injuries.
- *Diaphragmatic injuries*: Laparoscopy is highly useful in diagnosing and treating diaphragmatic injuries. Small lacerations can be sutured laparoscopically usually using a 2-0 to 3-0 non-absorbable suture. Use of a mesh might rarely be indicated. The fixation should be hand-sutured and not with tacks or clips. Larger defects requiring complex repair should be converted. We do *not* recommend laparoscopic mobilization of the liver to expose the right portion of the diaphragm.

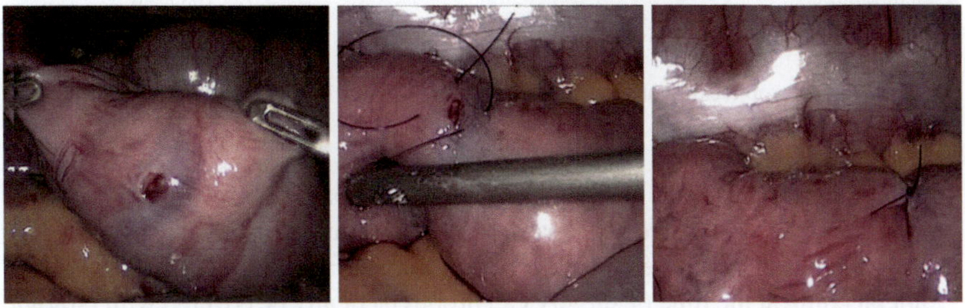

Fig. 11.3 Laparoscopic management of an isolated stab wound to the small bowel

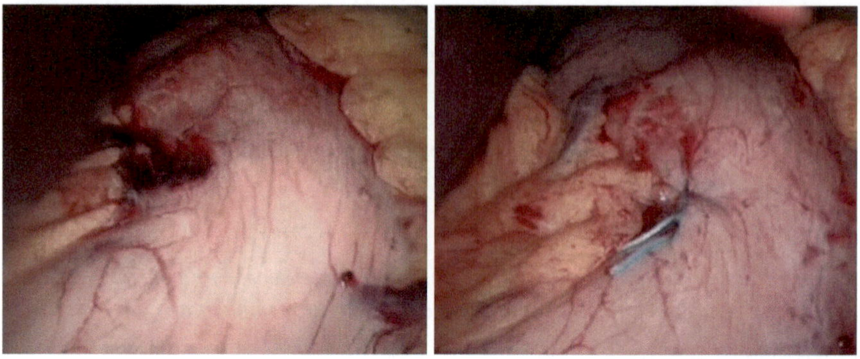

Fig. 11.4 Stab injury to the stomach

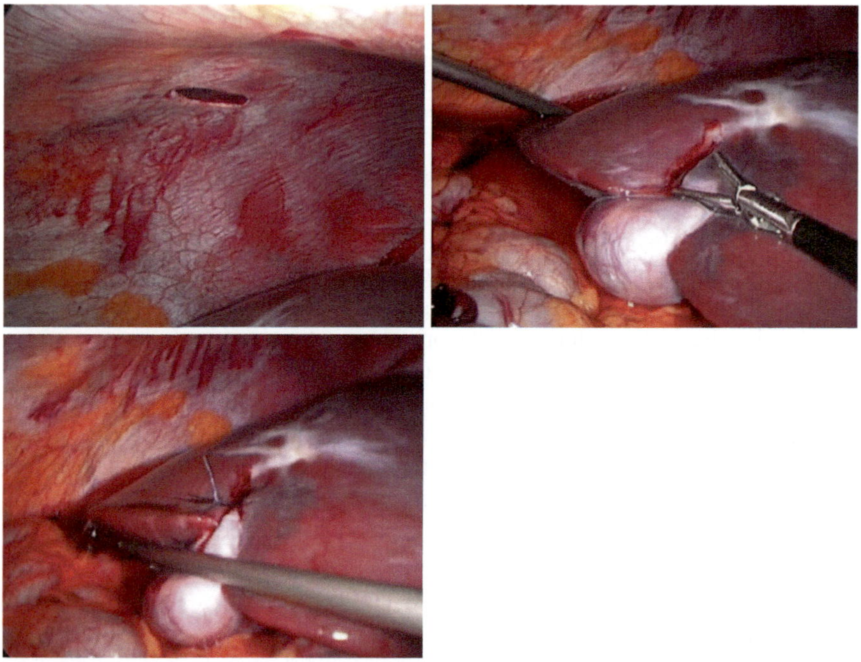

Fig. 11.5 laparoscopic exploration and suture closure of liver laceration without removal of the gallbladder

- *Solid organ injuries* in hemodynamically stable patients are usually managed non-operatively. However, if laparoscopy is indicated for other reasons, minor lacerations can be sutured or sealed with biomaterials (Fig. 11.5). Also, injuries not bleeding at the time of surgery can prophylactically be covered with biologic materials (FloSeal^{R}, Hemopatch^{R}, Tisseel^{R}, Baxter Company, USA). Liver lacerations may be sutured, sealed with a fleece or, if there is bleeding from the injury tract, tamponade with fluid hemostatic agents like FloSeal^{R}.

Conclusion

Laparoscopy for penetrating trauma is a useful tool to improve outcomes and reduce morbidity in carefully selected patients. It has both diagnostic and therapeutic potential depending on the trauma mechanism, injury pattern, and patient status as well as the expertise of the surgeon in both trauma and advanced laparoscopic techniques.

References

1. Como JJ, Bokhari F, Chiu WC, et al. Practice management guidelines for selective non-operative management of penetrating abdominal trauma. J Trauma. 2010;68:721–33. https://doi.org/10.1097/TA.0b013e3181cf7d07.
2. Renz BM, Feliciano DV. Unnecessary laparotomies for trauma: a prospective study of morbidity. J Trauma. 1995;38:350–6. https://doi.org/10.1097/00005373-199503000-00007.
3. Zafar SN, Onwugbufor MT, Hughes K, et al. Laparoscopic surgery for trauma: the realm of therapeutic management. Am J Surg. 2015;209:627–32. https://doi.org/10.1016/j.amjsurg.2014.12.011.
4. Dorricott AR, Dickinson A, McNickle AG, et al. Trauma laparoscopy: time efficient, cost effective, and safe. J Surg Res. 2024;301:455–60. https://doi.org/10.1016/j.jss.2024.06.045.
5. Kawahara NT, Alster C, Fujimura I, et al. Standard examination system for laparoscopy in penetrating abdominal trauma. J Trauma. 2009;67:589–95. https://doi.org/10.1097/ta.0b013e3181a60593.
6. Uranues S, Popa DE, Diaconescu B, et al. Laparoscopy in penetrating abdominal trauma. World J Surg. 2015;39:1381–8. https://doi.org/10.1007/s00268-014-2904-5.
7. Wu C, Lin K-L, Chang Y-J, et al. Role of laparoscopy in management of patients with anterior abdominal stab wounds. Surg Endosc. 2023;37:9173–82. https://doi.org/10.1007/s00464-023-10487-y.
8. Hajibandeh S, Hajibandeh S, Gumber AO, et al. Laparoscopy versus laparotomy for the management of penetrating abdominal trauma: a systematic review and meta-analysis. Int J Surg. 2016;34:127–36. https://doi.org/10.1016/j.ijsu.2016.08.524.
9. Li Y, Xiang Y, Wu N, et al. A comparison of laparoscopy and laparotomy for the management of abdominal trauma: a systematic review and meta-analysis. World J Surg. 2015;39:2862–71. https://doi.org/10.1007/s00268-015-3212-4.
10. Chestovich PJ, Browder TD, Morrissey SL, et al. Minimally invasive is maximally effective: diagnostic and therapeutic laparoscopy for penetrating abdominal injuries. J Trauma Acute Care Surg. 2015;78:1076–83; discussion 1083-5. https://doi.org/10.1097/TA.0000000000000655.
11. Menegozzo CAM, Damous SHB, Sabioni GR, et al. Could trauma laparoscopy be the standard of care for hemodynamically stable patients? A retrospective analysis of 165 cases. Surg Endosc. 2023;37:6727–35. https://doi.org/10.1007/s00464-023-10121-x.
12. O'Malley E, Boyle E, O'Callaghan A, et al. Role of laparoscopy in penetrating abdominal trauma: a systematic review. World J Surg. 2013;37:113–22. https://doi.org/10.1007/s00268-012-1790-y.
13. Martin MJ, Brown CVR, Shatz DV, et al. Evaluation and management of abdominal stab wounds: a Western Trauma Association critical decisions algorithm. J Trauma Acute Care Surg. 2018;85:1007–15. https://doi.org/10.1097/TA.0000000000001930.
14. Sermonesi G, Tian BWCA, Vallicelli C, et al. Cesena guidelines: WSES consensus statement on laparoscopic-first approach to general surgery emergencies and abdominal trauma. World J Emerg Surg. 2023;18:57. https://doi.org/10.1186/s13017-023-00520-9.
15. Campbell BR, Rooney AS, Krzyzaniak A, et al. To the point: utility of laparoscopy for operative management of stabbing abdominal trauma. Am J Surg. 2024;231:125–31. https://doi.org/10.1016/j.amjsurg.2024.01.028.

16. Spahn DR, Bouillon B, Cerny V, et al. Management of bleeding and coagulopathy following major trauma: an updated European guideline. Crit Care. 2013;17:R76. https://doi.org/10.1186/cc12685.
17. Ozkan OV, Justin V, Fingerhut A, Uranues S. Laparoscopy in Abdominal Trauma. Curr Trauma Rep. 2016;2:238–46. https://doi.org/10.1007/s40719-016-0067-6.
18. Hassankhani A, Amoukhteh M, Valizadeh P, et al. Diagnostic utility of multidetector CT scan in penetrating diaphragmatic injuries: a systematic review and meta-analysis. Emerg Radiol. 2023;30:765–76. https://doi.org/10.1007/s10140-023-02174-1.
19. Degiannis E, Levy RD, Sofianos C, et al. Diaphragmatic herniation after penetrating trauma. Br J Surg. 1996;83:88–91. https://doi.org/10.1002/bjs.1800830128.
20. Uranues S, Ozkan OV, Tomasch G. Safe and easy access technique for the first trocar in laparoscopic surgery. Langenbeck's Arch Surg. 2016;401:909–12. https://doi.org/10.1007/s00423-016-1474-4.

Thoracoscopy for Thoracic Traumatic Injuries: Procedure Systematization

12

Luiz von Lohrmann Cruz Arraes
and Ricardo Kalaf Mussi

Introduction

Definition and Context

Chest trauma is an important cause of morbidity and mortality in multiple trauma patients, accountable for a significant number of deaths resulting from traffic accidents, urban violence, and falls from great heights [1–3]. Thoracic involvement may include a variety of injuries, such as hemothorax, pneumothorax, lung contusions, rib fractures, and vascular and diaphragmatic lesions. Furthermore, chest trauma is frequently associated with injuries in other systems, requiring a multidisciplinary approach and well-established protocols to ensure the best care possible.

In this context, videothoracoscopy (Video-Assisted Thoracic Surgery—VATS) has emerged in the last decades as a minimally invasive alternative to traditional surgical techniques, such as thoracotomy [4–6]. VATS allows access to the pleural space through small incisions, using high-definition cameras and specialized instruments, enabling both the diagnosis and treatment of diverse intrathoracic conditions with less morbidity. As a result, the patient has a significant reduction in postoperative pain, a shorter hospitalization period, a smaller rate of infectious complications, and a more rapid return to daily activities [7–9].

L. von Lohrmann Cruz Arraes (✉)
State University of Campinas (UNICAMP-SP), Campinas, São Paulo, Brazil

Hospital Ophir Loyola (HOL-Belem/PA), Belém, Brazil

R. K. Mussi
State University of Campinas (UNICAMP-SP), Campinas, São Paulo, Brazil

© The Author(s), under exclusive license to Springer Nature Switzerland AG 2026

M. Cezillo, B. M. Pereira (eds.), *Minimally Invasive Surgery Trauma*,
https://doi.org/10.1007/978-3-032-28971-1_12

History and Evolution of Videothoracoscopy in Trauma

Thoracoscopy was introduced in the beginning of the twentieth century, when Hans Christian Jacobaeus used a modified cystoscope to visualize the pleural cavity of patients affected by tuberculosis [10]. Although rudimentary, this technique established the fundamental principles behind the use of optical instruments in the chest. Throughout the following decades, advances in optical technology, light sources, and endoscopic instruments enabled the expansion of thoracoscopy. Initially, thoracoscopy was used mainly for diagnostic purposes, along with pleural biopsy and effusion evaluation.

From the 1980s, with the consolidation of minimally invasive surgery, laparoscopy served as an inspiration for the development of similar approaches in the chest. In the 1990s, with the development of imaging methods, such as optical fibers, miniaturization of electronic components, and popularization of videosurgery systems, videothoracoscopy has been cemented as a robust surgical technique for elective procedures, including pulmonary lobectomies and nodule resections [11–13]. Gradually, its application was extended to trauma scenarios, timidly at the beginning and restricted to top medical centers. With increasing clinical evidence, multicenter studies and technological improvements, VATS was integrated into protocols of surgical societies, such as the Eastern Association for the Surgery of Trauma (EAST) and the European Society of Trauma and Emergency Surgery (ESTES), and has become a recognized option in selected chest trauma cases [9, 14, 15].

Importance in the Current Context

A global increase in trauma related to road accidents, armed conflicts, and urban violence demands efficient and safe intervention techniques [16–18]. In this scenario, VATS offers substantial benefits, permitting more accurate diagnoses, less aggressive surgical interventions, and lower hospital costs in long term [19–22]. By reducing complications, length of hospital stay, and morbidity, videothoracoscopy corresponds to the contemporary trends in medicine that attempt to optimize clinical, economic, and social results.

Thoracic Anatomy

Mastering thoracic anatomy is fundamental for the surgeon who employs VATS in trauma surgery. The thoracic cavity contains vital organs: lungs, heart, great vessels (aorta, superior and inferior vena cava), in addition to mediastinal structures (trachea, esophagus) and diaphragm [23, 24]. Chest contusions may provoke rib fractures, pulmonary contusion, hemothorax, and pneumothorax. In contrast, penetrating chest injuries may affect the vessels, bronchi, pulmonary parenchyma, and diaphragm, producing complex and potentially fatal lesions.

VATS has the capacity to access the pleural cavity directly, which enables the identification of retained clots, bronchopleural fistula, lung lacerations, and diaphragmatic ruptures. Visualization is direct and less invasive. Detailed knowledge of the topographical relations between the ribs, intercostal muscles, and parietal and visceral pleura, in addition to lung segmentation, is essential for safe manipulations [25–27]. Trained surgeons can approach complex lesions, avoiding iatrogenic damage and optimizing therapeutic effectiveness.

Fundamentals of Videothoracoscopy (VATS)

Equipment and Instruments Used

The following equipment is required for videothoracoscopy: video towers, high-definition cameras (HD or 4K), cold light sources, insufflation pumps (if necessary), and specific surgical instruments, such as grasping forceps, endoscopic scissors, vessel staplers, and endoscopic sutures [19, 25, 28]. In the context of trauma, the availability of vessel sealers and hemostatic instruments is crucial for rapid bleeding control. The current trend is to miniaturize and improve the performance of instruments, allowing smaller incisions and less tissue trauma.

The uniportal approach (a single port access) has gained prominence in some centers, notably in Spain, China, and Latin America, providing less postoperative pain and better cosmetic results [29–32]. In the United States, Canada, and part of Europe, the multiportal approach is still dominant, especially in complex trauma, since it offers a greater freedom of movement and facilitates the simultaneous use of diverse instruments [33, 34].

Advantages and Limitations

Compared to the open surgical techniques, VATS results in less pain, a shorter hospital stay, a lower rate of lung complications and infections, and lower hospital costs [35–37]. In functional terms, studies have demonstrated that patients experience a better preservation of respiratory function and a more rapid return to habitual activities.

Nevertheless, there are some limitations. The learning curve is an important factor. Surgeons require training in specialized centers, simulators for thoracoscopic surgery, and proctoring. The shortage of advanced equipment in smaller hospitals or in developing countries limits a wider use of the technique [21, 38]. Furthermore, hemodynamically unstable patients or those presenting with complex vascular injuries may demand emergency thoracotomy, due to lack of suitable time to prepare for VATS.

Indications for Videothoracoscopy in Trauma

Blunt and Penetrating Trauma

In trauma, VATS may be performed with diagnostic and/or therapeutic purposes. However, in the majority of cases, VATS combines both indications in hemodynamically stable patients who are not immediate candidates for thoracotomy. The most common diagnostic indications for VATS are suspected diaphragmatic injuries, suspected pericardial and cardiac injuries, and visualization of the trajectory of mediastinal wounds (vessels, esophagus) (Fig. 12.1). Therapeutic indications are presence of residual collection (retained hemothorax or empyema), diaphragmatic suture, suture and/or hemostasis of the lung parenchyma, and removal of foreign bodies (projectiles, bone fragments, medical devices, etc.).

VATS is particularly useful in cases of retained hemothorax (Fig. 12.2), when clotted blood in the pleural cavity cannot be adequately drained by the chest tube [9, 14, 39]. Early intervention (within 24–72 hours of injury) prevents infections, empyema, and adhesions, improving clinical outcome. The technique is also useful for the management of a persistent pneumothorax, identifying the site of air escape and correcting it directly.

In cases of active bleeding or bleeding >200 ml/h for more than three hours after chest tube drainage, the hemodynamically stable patient can be a candidate for videosurgery for bleeding control, using endoclips, cauterization, pressure tamponade for eventual intercostal artery injuries, internal thoracic artery injuries, or even pulmonary lesions, or it is defined that a thoracotomy is necessary [40, 41].

In penetrating trauma (due to gunshot or stab wounds), VATS can evaluate the integrity of the diaphragm better than laparoscopy, particularly when the injuries are small, lateral, or posterior. Laparoscopy is more commonly indicated when simultaneous abdominal injuries require treatment. In this condition, the occurrence of hypertensive pneumothorax through the eventual pleuroperitoneal communication is always a possibility that should be borne in mind. Countries with a high

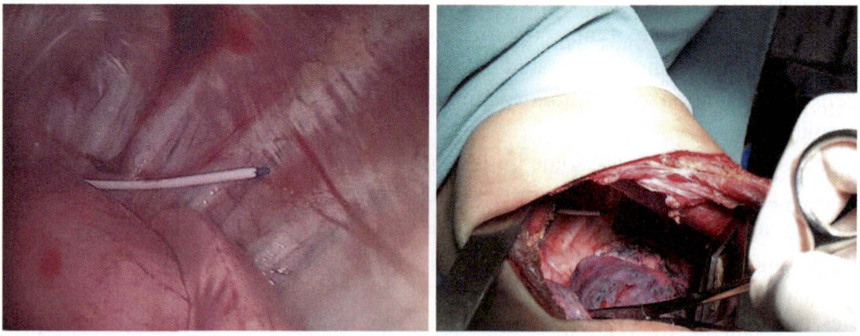

Fig. 12.1 (**a**) Treatment of hemothorax by thoracoscopy after central access. (**b**) Treatment of hemothorax by thoracotomy after central access

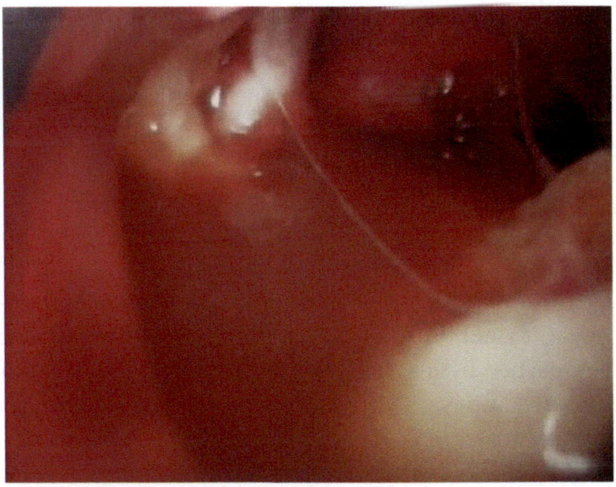

Fig. 12.2 Presence of blood and clots in the pleural cavity, still without infection or empyema

Table 12.1 Contraindications for laparoscopy procedure

Absolute	Relative
Hemodynamic instability	Coagulation alterations
Lateral decubitus impossible	High pressure mechanical ventilation
Selective ventilation (unilateral) impossible	Obliterated pleural space
Clear indication for thoracotomy or laparotomy	Injuries to large airways and esophagus

prevalence of penetrating wounds, such as South Africa and some Latin American regions, have reported successful experiences with VATS, and the use of more invasive interventions has decreased [28, 29].

In injuries with the possibility of transfixing the diaphragm, the diagnosis may be underestimated in 30% of the cases at the time of early evaluation, despite the use of methods such as computed tomography and echography, and some doubts still remain in the literature:

(a) Should all patients systematically undergo diagnostic surgical procedures for a possible diaphragmatic injury?
(b) Should every diaphragmatic wound be sutured?
(c) Can patients be under observation and operated only if they develop diaphragmatic hernia, mainly on the right side?

Contraindications are described in the following Table 12.1.

Patient Selection Criteria

Perhaps the most important concept to emphasize in this chapter is the fact that VATS is not a substitute for thoracotomy, although it is a safe and efficient form of access in selected chest trauma patients, considering the logistics available at the location.

Patient selection is fundamental for the success of VATS in trauma. Classical indications for VATS include hemodynamically stable patients, without apparent catastrophic vascular injuries at imaging tests. High-resolution computed tomography (CT) and FAST ultrasound can help define possible lesions that are liable to be approached by invasive techniques [43–45]. North-American and European guidelines recommend that VATS should be considered in patients with retained hemothorax greater than 500 mL, unresolved pneumothorax after drainage, suspicion of diaphragmatic injury, or assessment of intrathoracic foreign bodies [11, 46, 47].

Practical Systematization for the Performance of VATS in Trauma

A. Initial Patient Evaluation:

- Hemodynamic stability (unstable patients indicate thoracotomy).
- Imaging tests (CT, FAST ultrasound) to identify hemothorax, pneumothorax, or diaphragmatic injuries. In precordial and transmediastinal wounds, transthoracic echocardiogram (TTE) is considered a first-line test by the majority of surgeons. TTE may be performed in the emergency room or operating room. The use of VATS as a diagnostic method in suspected cardiac injury is controversial.
- Exclusion of major vascular injuries.

B. Patient selection:

- Indications: Retained hemothorax (>500 mL), persistent pneumothorax, suspected diaphragmatic injury.
- Ideally, intervention should occur within 72 hours of trauma for optimal results.

C. Preoperative preparation:

- Laboratory tests, blood typing, coagulation test.
- General anesthesia with selective intubation; in the lack of an available or trained anesthesiologist, the use of endobronchial blockers under guidance of fiberoptic bronchoscopy may be very helpful.
- Patient placed in the lateral decubitus position.

D. Teams and materials:

- Surgeon and assistant with expertise in VATS.

- Video tower, HD/4 K camera, appropriate videosurgical tweezers, electrocautery, endoscopic staplers, and vessel sealers (these are the most widely recommended items for a safe surgery).
- Monitoring should include direct measurements of venous and arterial pressure, capnography, oximetry, and electrocardiography.

E. Procedure execution:

- Uniportal or multiportal access according to experience. Regardless of the choice, incisions should be made thinking of a possible conversion from a VATS procedure to thoracotomy. In case of a multiportal access, the trocars should be positioned in a triangular distribution to avoid collision between the optical trocar and the instruments.
- Cavity exploration, removal of clots, suture of lung or diaphragmatic injuries.
- Chest drainage at the end.
- The surgeon who opts for videosurgery must have a full grasp of both the endoscopic and open technique, which may be necessary in various patients. The surgical team responsible for the execution of the procedure should understand the contraindications and potential need for conversion.

F. Postoperative:

- Monitoring pulmonary function, pain control, and radiological evaluation.
- Drain removal according to lung expansion, quality and amount of fluid output, and cessation of air escape.
- Outpatient follow-up to evaluate functional recovery.

Surgical Technique and Practical Approaches

Procedure Steps

The patient is usually placed in the lateral decubitus position, under general anesthesia and selective intubation, permitting the creation of a stable surgical field. Trocars are strategically inserted to optimize the angle of vision and freedom of movements. The uniportal approach, using an incision of approximately 3–4 cm, has become increasingly more common in specialized centers, while multiportal approaches (2–3 incisions) of 0.5–1.0 cm offer more versatility [24, 31].

After entrance into the pleural space, the surgeon examines the cavity thoroughly, identifying clots, lung lesions, lacerations, perforations, spikes/bone fragments, or foreign material. Smaller lung lesions may be sealed with mechanical staplers, while bleeding is controlled with an electric scalpel or vessel sealer [28, 39]. Diaphragmatic injuries are sutured, frequently with continuous suture, ensuring a long-lasting repair [48].

Specific Cases

Retained hemothorax: An Israeli multicenter study points to a significant decrease in infections and conversion to thoracotomy with early use of VATS in retained hemothorax. Blood clot removal under direct vision reduces the risk of fibrothorax and lung complications [7, 20, 35].

Diaphragmatic injuries: VATS is considered a reliable method for the evaluation and repair of diaphragmatic rupture, avoiding unnecessary laparotomies. British and German guidelines reinforce the importance of diaphragmatic inspection in penetrating wounds in the lower hemithorax [3, 6, 49].

Benefits of VATS in Trauma

Clinical Results

Comparative studies between VATS and thoracotomy show a clear advantage of the minimally invasive technique in terms of reduction in mortality, decreased length of hospitalization, lower incidence of empyema, and better postoperative pulmonary function [22, 25, 44, 49]. Hospital centers in Asia report mean hospital stays of less than 5 days, reflecting the efficiency of the method [42].

Economic and Logistical Impact

From an economic viewpoint, VATS reduces costs by decreasing the length of hospital stay, use of antibiotics, use of ICU resources, and need for multiple procedures [27, 50, 51]. European studies have demonstrated that the routine adoption of VATS may generate a 10 to 20% cost saving in comparison to open surgical approaches [26, 52]. Furthermore, less surgical trauma benefits patients, who return sooner to their usual activities, reducing the socioeconomic impact of trauma.

Limitations and Challenges

Learning Curve and Human Resources

The technical complexity of VATS demands specific training. Simulation programs and guided tutoring by experienced surgeons have been implemented in countries such as the North America, aimed at shortening the learning curve [52–55]. However, the availability of training centers and the initial resistance of surgical teams accustomed to open techniques may delay a large-scale incorporation of VATS.

Low-Income Context

In low-income and middle-income countries, the acquisition of equipment, maintenance of equipment, and lack of trained teams make the dissemination of VATS difficult [28–30]. Initiatives of international cooperation, remote capacitation (telemedicine), and equipment donations may contribute to overcome these hurdles, expanding access to a technique that can offer effective benefits to patients.

Current Scenario, Global Experience, and Regional Protocols

Global experience with VATS in trauma varies according to resources and local epidemiology. In the United States, the integration of VATS to ATLS protocols and EAST guidelines is well-established. In Europe: Germany, the United Kingdom, and Spain stand out for the production of regional guidelines and multicenter researches, strengthening the adoption of the technique. In Japan and South Korea, the incorporation of advanced technologies, such as robotic-assisted surgery and 3D systems, has improved accuracy and safety. Developing countries advance according to their ability to overcome technological and training barriers, benefitting from professional partnerships and exchanges [3, 4, 28–30].

Experience in Brazil and Latin America

In Latin America, the dissemination of VATS in trauma has faced economic and structural barriers, although centers in countries such as Brazil, Chile, Colombia, and Argentina have experienced a gradual advance [28–30]. In Brazil, university hospitals and trauma centers have incorporated VATS, promoted by medical societies such as the Brazilian Society of Thoracic Surgery (SBCT) and the Brazilian Society of Integrated Care of Trauma Patient (SBAIT), that promote courses, training, and scientific discussions.

Strengthening of cooperation networks, scientific exchange, use of telemedicine, and regional training programs are contributing to expand the access and quality of VATS in trauma throughout Latin America, improving trauma patient care.

Innovation and Technology in Videothoracoscopy

Technological advance drives the expansion of VATS in trauma. High-definition cameras, 3D systems, augmented reality, and artificial intelligence help identify structures and lesions, increasing safety and decreasing surgical time [56, 57]. Robotic-assisted surgery permits more precise maneuvers, reducing tremors and facilitating suture of complex lesions [58, 59]. Furthermore, telemedicine and distant teaching platforms expand access to continuing education, enabling surgeons from remote regions to acquire current skills and knowledge.

Conclusions

Videothoracoscopy is not a replacement for thoracotomy, although it is an important addition in the surgical arsenal. It currently occupies a prominent position in the management of chest trauma, combining the advances of minimally invasive technology with the clinical need for safer, more efficient and cost-effective interventions. The technique permits more accurate diagnoses reducing the incidence of subclinical lesions, less aggressive treatment, reduction of complications, and improvement in functional outcomes.

Although challenges still remain, such as the learning curve, equipment costs, and unequal access among countries, the global scenario is in continuous expansion. Investment in training, research, and the incorporation of new technologies, associated with evidence-based clinical protocols, strengthens the role of VATS in the management of chest trauma. By prioritizing patient safety and the efficiency and quality of results, videothoracoscopy is consolidated as a useful tool in contemporary surgical practice, contributing to the constant evolution of trauma patient care.

References

1. American College of Surgeons. Advanced Trauma Life Support (ATLS®): student course manual. 10th ed. Chicago: ACS; 2018.
2. Bulger EM, Arneson MA, Mock CN, Jurkovich GJ. Rib fractures in the elderly. J Trauma. 2000;48(6):1040–6.
3. Ludwig C, Koryllos A. Management of chest trauma. J Thorac Dis. 2017;9(Suppl 3):S172–7. https://doi.org/10.21037/jtd.2017.03.52.
4. Ahmed N, Jones D. Video-assisted thoracic surgery: state of the art in trauma care. Injury. 2004;35(5):479–89. https://doi.org/10.1016/S0020-1383(03)00289-4. PMID: 15081325.
5. Landreneau RJ, Mack MJ, Hazelrigg SR, et al. Video-assisted thoracic surgery: basic technical concepts and applications. Ann Thorac Surg. 1992;54(4):800–7.
6. Ben-Nun A, Orlovsky M, Best LA. Video-assisted thoracoscopic surgery in the treatment of chest trauma: long-term benefit. Ann Thorac Surg. 2007;83(2):383–7. https://doi.org/10.1016/j.athoracsur.2006.09.082. PMID: 17257954.
7. Badkur M, Baskaran S, Prakash S, Kishore L, Lodha M, Rodha M, Chaudhary R, Puranik A. Traumatic retained hemothorax: is it time for video assisted thoracoscopic surgery? Int Surg J. 2020;7(11):3880–3884.
8. Rossmann M, Altomare M, Pezzoli I, Abruzzese A, Spota A, Vettorello M, Cioffi SPB, Virdis F, Bini R, Chiara O, Cimbanassi S. Risk factors for retained hemothorax after trauma: a 10-years monocentric experience from first-level trauma center in Italy. J Pers Med. 2022;12(10):1570. https://doi.org/10.3390/jpm12101570.
9. Radjou AN, Uthrapathy M. Video-assisted thoracoscopy in trauma: case report and review of literature. Lung India. 2011;28:142–4.
10. Jacobaeus HC. Über die Möglichkeit die Zystoskopie bei Untersuchung seröser Höhlungen anzuwenden. Munch Med Wochenschr. 1910;57:2090–2.
11. Swierzy M, Faber S, Nachira D, Günsberg A, Rückert JC, Ismail M. Uniportal video-assisted thoracoscopic surgery for the treatment of thoracic emergencies. J Thorac Dis. 2018;10(Suppl 31):S3720–5. https://doi.org/10.21037/jtd.2018.08.126. PMID: 30505557; PMCID: PMC6258644.
12. Graeber GM, Jones DR. The role of thoracoscopy in thoracic trauma. Ann Thorac Surg. 1993;56(3):646–8. https://doi.org/10.1016/0003-4975(93)90939-f. PMID: 8379761.

13. Mack MJ, Aronoff RJ, Acuff TE, Douthit MB, Bowman RT, Ryan WH. Present role of thoracoscopy in the diagnosis and treatment of diseases of the chest. Ann Thorac Surg. 1992;54(3):403–8; discussion 407–9. https://doi.org/10.1016/0003-4975(92)90428-7. PMID: 1510505.
14. Schreyer C, Schulz-Drost S, Markewitz A, et al. Surgical management of chest injuries in patients with multiple and/or severe trauma– a systematic review and clinical practice guideline update. Eur J Trauma Emerg Surg. 2024;50:2061–71. https://doi.org/10.1007/s00068-024-02556-1.
15. Alwatari Y, Simmonds A, Ayalew D, et al. Early video-assisted thoracoscopic surgery (VATS) for non-emergent thoracic trauma remains underutilized in trauma accredited centers despite evidence of improved patient outcomes. Eur J Trauma Emerg Surg. 2022;48:3211–9. https://doi.org/10.1007/s00068-022-01881-7.
16. WHO. Global status report on road safety. Geneva: World Health Organization; 2018.
17. Navsaria PH, Nicol AJ. Video-assisted thoracoscopic pericardial window for penetrating cardiac trauma. S Afr J Surg. 2006;44(1):18–20.
18. Sikander N, Ahmad T, Shaikh KA Sr, Abid A, Mazcuri M, Nasreen S. Analysis of injury patterns and outcomes of blunt thoracic trauma in elderly patients. Cureus. 2020;12(8):e9974. https://doi.org/10.7759/cureus.9974. PMID: 32850270; PMCID: PMC7445091.
19. Duggan J, Rodriguez G, Peters A, Antevil J, Trachiotis G. Video-assisted thoracoscopic surgery (VATS) in trauma: a narrative review. Video-assist Thorac Surg. 2024;9:8.
20. Patel NJ, Dultz L, Ladhani HA, Cullinane DC, Klein E, McNickle AG, Bugaev N, Fraser DR, Kartiko S, Dodgion C, Pappas PA, Kim D, Cantrell S, Como JJ, Kasotakis G. Management of simple and retained hemothorax: a practice management guideline from the Eastern Association for the Surgery of Trauma. Am J Surg. 2021;221(5):873–84. https://doi.org/10.1016/j.amjsurg.2020.11.032. Epub 2020 Nov 17. PMID: 33487403.
21. Lundin A, Akram SK, Berg L, et al. Thoracic injuries in trauma patients: epidemiology and its influence on mortality. Scand J Trauma Resusc Emerg Med. 2022;30:69. https://doi.org/10.1186/s13049-022-01058-6.
22. Chen W, Yu Z, Zhang Y, Liu H. Comparison of cost effectiveness between video-assisted thoracoscopic surgery (VATS) and open lobectomy: a retrospective study. Cost Eff Resour Alloc. 2021;19(1):55. https://doi.org/10.1186/s12962-021-00307-2. PMID: 34454507; PMCID: PMC8400899.
23. Pearson F, Cooper J, Deslauriers J, Ginsberg R, Hiebert C, Patterson A, Urschel, H. Thoracic surgery. 2nd ed. Illustrated. Edinburgh: Churchill Livingstone; 2002. British Journal of Surgery.
24. Uribe RA, Pachon CE, Frame SB, Enderson BL, Escobar F, Garcia GA. A prospective evaluation of thoracoscopy for the diagnosis of penetrating thoracoabdominal trauma. J Trauma. 1994;37(4):650–4. https://doi.org/10.1097/00005373-199410000-00020. PMID: 7932898.
25. Oparka JD, Yan TD, Walker WS. Twenty years of video-assisted thoracoscopic surgery: the past, present, and future. Thorac Cancer. 2013;4(2):91–4. https://doi.org/10.1111/1759-7714.12017. PMID: 28920195.
26. Mancini M, Smith LM, Nein A, Buechter KJ. Early evacuation of clotted blood in hemothorax using thoracoscopy: case reports. J Trauma. 1993;34(1):144–7. https://doi.org/10.1097/00005373-199301000-00028. PMID: 8437182.
27. Dare A, Grimes C, Gillies R, et al. Global surgery: defining an emerging global health field. Lancet. 2014;384(9961):2245–7.
28. Cetindag IB, Neideen T, Hazelrigg SR. Video-assisted thoracic surgical applications in thoracic trauma. Thorac Surg Clin. 2007;17(1):73–9. https://doi.org/10.1016/j.thorsurg.2007.02.007. PMID: 17650699.
29. Vannucci F, de Castro CCB. Thoracic surgery in Brazil: an overview. J Thorac Dis. 2022;14:3083–90. https://doi.org/10.21037/jtd-21-1809.
30. Lambert H, Oliu N, Dolz A, Curbelo O. Uniportal Video-Assisted Thoracic Surgery (U-VATS): experiences and challenges in oncologic patients in The Dominican Republic. Open J Thorac Surg. 2024;14:55–67.
31. Gonzalez-Rivas D, de la Torre M, Fernandez R, Delgado M. Single-port video-assisted thoracoscopic left upper lobectomy. Interact Cardiovasc Thorac Surg. 2011;13(4):539–41.

32. Guido-Guerrero W, Bolaños-Cubillo A, González-Rivas D. Single-port video-assisted thoracic surgery (VATS)-advanced procedures & update. J Thorac Dis. 2018;10(Suppl 14):S1652–61. https://doi.org/10.21037/jtd.2018.05.43. PMID: 30034831; PMCID: PMC6035913.
33. Lewis RJ, Caccavale RJ, Bocage JP, Widmann MD. Video-assisted thoracic surgical non-rib spreading simultaneously stapled lobectomy: a more patient-friendly oncologic resection. Chest. 1999;116(4):1119–24. https://doi.org/10.1378/chest.116.4.1119. PMID: 10531183.
34. Burfeind WR Jr, D'Amico TA. Thoracoscopic lobectomy. Oper Tech Thorac Cardiovasc Surg. 2004;9(2):98–114.
35. Tong BC, Hanna J, Toloza EM, et al. Outcomes of video-assisted thoracoscopic decortication. Ann Thorac Surg. 2010;89(1):220–5.
36. Zeiler J, Idell S, Norwood S, Cook A. Hemothorax: a review of literature. Clin Pulm Med. 2020;27(1):1–12. https://doi.org/10.1097/CPM.0000000000000343. Epub 2020 Jan 10. PMID: 33437141; PMCID: PMC7799890.
37. Billeter AT, Druen D, Franklin GA, Smith JW, Wrightson W, Richardson JD. Video-assisted thoracoscopy as an important tool for trauma surgeons: a systematic review. Langenbeck's Arch Surg. 2013;398(4):515–23. https://doi.org/10.1007/s00423-012-1016-7. Epub 2013 Apr 4. PMID: 23553352.
38. Jeon JH, Kang CH, Kim HS, Seong YW, Park IK, Kim YT, Kim JH. Video-assisted thoracoscopic lobectomy in non-small-cell lung cancer patients with chronic obstructive pulmonary disease is associated with lower pulmonary complications than open lobectomy: a propensity score-matched analysis. Eur J Cardiothorac Surg. 2014;45(4):640–5. https://doi.org/10.1093/ejcts/ezt460. Epub 2013 Sep 19. PMID: 24052605.
39. Villavicencio RT, Aucar JA, Wall MJ Jr. Analysis of thoracoscopy in trauma. Surg Endosc. 1999;13(1):3–9. https://doi.org/10.1007/s004649900886. PMID: 9869678.
40. Darlong LM. Thoracoscopy for trauma. Lung India. 2011;28(2):87–8. https://doi.org/10.4103/0970-2113.80313. PMID: 21712937; PMCID: PMC3109850.
41. Reddy VS. Minimally invasive techniques in thoracic trauma. Semin Thorac Cardiovasc Surg. 2008;20(1):72–7. https://doi.org/10.1053/j.semtcvs.2008.01.008. PMID: 18420131.
42. Kurimoto Y, Watanabe A, Koyanagi T, Ito T, Higami T, Maekawa K, Tanno K, Asai Y. Video-assisted thoracic surgery as a less-invasive management for acute Hhemothorax in blunt trauma. Surg Sci. 2012;3(3):136–40.
43. Hashimoto DA, Rosman G, Rus D, Meireles OR. Artificial intelligence in surgery: promises and perils. Ann Surg. 2018;268(1):70–6.
44. Lang-Lazdunski L, Mouroux J, Pons F, Grosdidier G, Martinod E, Elkaïm D, Azorin J, Jancovici R. Role of videothoracoscopy in chest trauma. Ann Thorac Surg. 1997;63(2):327–33. https://doi.org/10.1016/s0003-4975(96)00960-5. PMID: 9033295.
45. Wanek S, Mayberry JC. Blunt thoracic trauma: flail chest, pulmonary contusion, and blast injury. Crit Care Clin. 2004;20(1):71–81.
46. Dennis BM, Bellister SA, Guillamondegui OD. Thoracic trauma. Surg Clin North Am. 2017;97(5):1047–64.
47. Dijkink S, Nederpelt C, Krijnen P, Velmahos G, Schipper I. Trauma systems around the world: a systematic overview. J Trauma Acute Care Surg. 2017;83:1.
48. Yanık F, Karamustafaoğlu YA, Yörük Y. The role of VATS in the diagnosis and treatment of diaphragmatic injuries after penetrating thoracic traumas. Ulus Travma Acil Cerrahi Derg. 2020;26(3):469–74. English. https://doi.org/10.14744/tjtes.2019.02682. PMID: 32436965.
49. Walker WS. Video-assisted thoracoscopic surgery (VATS) lobectomy: the Edinburgh experience. Semin Thorac Cardiovasc Surg. 1998;10(4):291–9.
50. Leppäniemi A, Haapiainen R. Diagnostic laparoscopy in abdominal stab wounds: a prospective, randomized study. J Trauma. 2003;55(4):636–45.
51. DuBose J, Inaba K, Demetriades D, Scalea TM, O'Connor J, Menaker J, Morales C, Konstantinidis A, Shiflett A, Copwood B; AAST Retained Hemothorax Study Group. Management of post-traumatic retained hemothorax: a prospective, observational, multicenter AAST study. J Trauma Acute Care Surg. 2012;72(1):11–22; discussion 22–4; quiz 316. https://doi.org/10.1097/TA.0b013e318242e368. PMID: 22310111.

52. Lemaire A, Burfeind WR Jr, Toloza E, D'Amico TA, Harpole DH Jr. Minimally invasive thoracic surgery: evaluation of learning curve for diagnosis and treatment of chest disease. Semin Thorac Cardiovasc Surg. 2005;17(2):126–35.
53. Igai H, Kamiyoshihara M, Furusawa S, Ohsawa F, Yazawa T, Matsuura N. The learning curve of thoracoscopic surgery in a single surgeon and successful implementation of uniportal approach. J Thorac Dis. 2021;13(7):4063–71. https://doi.org/10.21037/jtd-21-500. PMID: 34422336; PMCID: PMC8339743.
54. Lodhia JV, Konstantinidis K, Papagiannopoulos K. Video-assisted thoracoscopic surgery in trauma: pros and cons. J Thorac Dis. 2019;11(4):1662–7.
55. Caputo G, Meda S, Piccioni A, Saviano A, Ojetti V, Savioli G, Piccini GB, Ferrari C, Voza A, Pellegrini L, Ottaviani M, Spadazzi F, Volonnino G, La Russa R. Thoracic trauma: current approach in emergency medicine. Clin Pract. 2024;14(5):1869–85. https://doi.org/10.3390/clinpract14050148. PMID: 39311298; PMCID: PMC11417912.
56. Arjomandi Rad A, Vardanyan R, Thavarajasingam SG, Zubarevich A, Van den Eynde J, Sá MPBO, Zhigalov K, Sardiari Nia P, Ruhparwar A, Weymann A. Extended, virtual and augmented reality in thoracic surgery: a systematic review. Interact Cardiovasc Thorac Surg. 2022;34(2):201–11. https://doi.org/10.1093/icvts/ivab241. PMID: 34542639; PMCID: PMC8766198.
57. Davis MC, Can DD, Pindrik J, Rocque BG, Johnston JM. Virtual interactive presence in global surgical education: International collaboration through augmented reality. World Neurosurg. 2016;86:103–11. https://doi.org/10.1016/j.wneu.2015.08.053. Epub 2015 Sep 3. PMID: 26342783; PMCID: PMC5476961.
58. Cerfolio RJ, Cichos KH, Wei B, Minnich DJ. Robotic lobectomy can be taught while maintaining quality patient outcomes. J Thorac Cardiovasc Surg. 2016;152(4):991–7. https://doi.org/10.1016/j.jtcvs.2016.04.085. Epub 2016 May 10. PMID: 27292875.
59. Gharagozloo F, Margolis M, Tempesta B, Strother E, Najam F. Robot-assisted lobectomy for early-stage lung cancer: report of 100 consecutive cases. Ann Thorac Surg. 2009;88(2):380–4.

Laparoscopy for Abdominal Traumatic Injuries: Procedure Systematization

13

Marcus Cezillo, Robson Uwagoya, Hugo Gregoris de Lima, and Bruno Monteiro Pereira

Deciding to Do Laparoscopy in Trauma

Standardized rules are present in some procedures and are well accepted in the literature because of their positive consequences for patient safety, learning facility, and reproducibility of the method. These "how-to-do" procedures are found in laparoscopic cholecystectomy [1], laparoscopic inguinal hernia repair [2], laparoscopic deep endometriosis treatment [3], and others, but there are few mentions of a step-by-step diagnostic laparoscopy. The literature offers scarce material regarding standardized laparoscopic examination for the evaluation of the peritoneal cavity. Kawahara (2009) [4] published one of the first articles to describe a systematic standardized laparoscopic approach, which objective was to correctly identify missed occult small bowel injuries (SBI) in the peritoneal cavity for penetrating abdominal trauma (PAT). Later, in 2018, Koto (2018) [5] published a standardized diagnostic laparoscopy (DL) for PAT and described the strategies on how to avoid missed injuries.

Besides this evidence of a tool for guiding trauma surgeons, there is still a lack of consensus regarding the use of laparoscopy in abdominal trauma. The trauma surgeon's main concern is about missing injuries and the possibility of exploring the

M. Cezillo (✉)
Trauma Surgery Department, Hospital de Base do Distrito Federal (HBDF), Brasília, DF, Brazil

R. Uwagoya
Grupo de Pesquisa e Extensão em Cirurgia (GPEC), São Paulo, Brazil

H. G. d. Lima
Hospital Municipal Antônio Giglio (HMAG), Osasco, Brazil

B. M. Pereira
University of Vassouras, Surgical Group® President, Campinas Brazil. World Society of the Abdominal Compartment Past-President, Campinas, Brazil

© The Author(s), under exclusive license to Springer Nature Switzerland AG 2026

M. Cezillo, B. M. Pereira (eds.), *Minimally Invasive Surgery Trauma*,
https://doi.org/10.1007/978-3-032-28971-1_13

entire abdomen, pelvis, and retroperitoneum to exclude injuries or diagnose them for further decision between laparoscopic treatment and non-operative treatment (NOT) in blunt or penetrating trauma when there is diagnostic doubt or probable injury that needs surgical treatment (or that cannot be treated non-operatively) [6]. Another indication for this method is the NOM failing due to recurrent bleeding of the solid organs, or any probably missed injury to the hollow viscus. For this important decision, the trauma surgeon must be confident with the method, with the team, with the equipment, and mainly with the way he/she manages it using methods that guide a safe and effective procedure [7, 8].

Evidence of the establishment of a solid concept of systematization in diagnostic laparoscopy can be found in important recent contributions that have proposed standardized sequential procedures. By matching both important publications associated with concepts of trauma cavity exploration and laparoscopic exposure, it was possible to establish a new concept of standardized diagnostic laparoscopy known as the 7-rule technique, which describes a new way of understanding the assessment of the abdominal, pelvic, and retroperitoneal spaces, offering better practice in looking for possible injuries, according to the trauma mechanism, effectively and safely [9, 10].

Technical Aspects

Observation of technical aspects is essential to the procedure's feasibility. It comprehends minimum requirements such as an aspirator, bowel traction (bowel grasper), a dissecting device (electrocautery, scissors, and Maryland dissector), trained personnel with experience in trauma and routine laparoscopic procedures, camera-video system with a clear image, and a surgical table with mobility [11]. The non-observation of these aspects can make the procedure stressful, elevating the number of conversions or even increasing the rates of iatrogenic and missed injuries [12]. Limitations imposed by material and personnel need to be tailored to the surgeon's perception of the moment to stop laparoscopy.

Prior publication describes techniques for assessment of the four quadrants: (1) observation of damage to massive viscera (liver, spleen, and kidney); (2) evaluation of the gastrointestinal tract, including anterior and posterior stomach and pancreas; (3) evaluation of small loops from the angle of Treitz to the cecal ileum valve; and (4) observation of the portion from the colon to the rectum and then retro uterine pouch [13, 14].

The exploration of the cavity by laparoscopy, considering careful selection of patients, should include exploration techniques mentioned in previous studies and other auxiliary tasks that are critical to the success of the procedure. These tasks involve positioning and moving the surgical table and choosing the location of the punctures for better evaluation of the organs in the search for injuries and sources of bleeding.

The uncertain scenario in trauma needs a perfect investigation of the cavity, explored indirectly by a hand camera, with main and assistant trocars placed in different manners depending on the explored region. Each surgeon has a personal technique and trocar placement, but, in general, it is advisable to use an umbilical port for the laparoscope (10 mm/30°), a working port in the right paraumbilical region (5 mm or 12 mm), and another paraumbilical left assist port (5 mm or 12 mm) [15]. This distribution, allied to decubitus changes, allows better visualization and manipulation of the entire abdomen with the necessary accessibility. Some conditions, like obesity, adherence, or congenital diseases, may require other puncture sites depending on the trauma surgeon's judgment.

The camera port (10, 11, or 12 mm) can be placed for pneumoperitoneum using the open (Hasson) technique or Veress technique (periumbilical). Palmer's point and Lee Huang Point (epigastrium) are options, and eventually, the injury site can be used. The choice for peritoneal access should be individualized based on factors such as patient sex, clinical diagnosis, and most importantly, the surgeons' experience and preference [16]. Carbon dioxide pneumoperitoneum can vary from 8 to 15 mmHg with a standard value of 12 mmHg [17]. For better ergonomics and exposure for cavity investigation, working ports (10, 11, or 12 mm trocar) can be placed on each side at the umbilicus level. According to the findings, after DL, the positioning of the trocars can be moved for adequate exposure for the treatment.

In addition, the variation in the patient's decubitus must be constant according to the region of the abdomen to be explored and the patient's profile (obesity or pregnancy) [18]. Furthermore, the surgeon, assistants, and the video monitor must be repositioned for better exposure and presentation of regions to be assessed. The ergonomics of the surgical team are essential for this technique and directly affect the surgical time and the procedure outcome [19].

In laparoscopic surgery, especially for trauma surgery, it's essential to position the patient, ensure trauma team experience, and have a mobile surgical table and specific materials. The patient's position should vary according to the region of the abdomen to be explored. Although the position promotes the displacement of mobile viscera and fluids, aspiration may be necessary for better visualization of each region. For this purpose, we suggest the trauma surgeon work with the aspirator in one trocar and grasping forceps in another, holding a gauze ball for better manipulation (displacement) of the organs and to act as a "filter" on which the aspirator will act, reducing the aspiration of gas from the cavity and concentrating it on the fluid with which it is in contact. In addition, the surgeon, assistants, and video monitor should be repositioned for better exposure and presentation of the regions to be evaluated. The ergonomics of the surgical team are essential for this technique and directly affect the surgical time and the outcome of the procedure [19, 20]. Therefore, it is necessary for the patient to be fixed to the surgical bed with their arms at their sides and the monitor always in a position that requires the least movement of the surgeon's gaze, in an ergonomic manner [21].

A smooth intentional intra-abdominal hypertension is created and must be as low as possible, considering the pneumoperitoneum in the laparoscopic procedure needs to be constantly evaluated, looking for possible early physiologic consequences on the ventilation and hemodynamic status. Pneumoperitoneum can be created by puncture after evaluation of previous imaging exams and by using confirmation techniques prior to the insufflation; however, the open technique (Hasson) is preferable, producing grade I intra-abdominal hypertension (IAH) (12–15 mmHg), without major systemic repercussions. However, in the case of a polytrauma patient, the intra-abdominal pressure (IAP) created must be constantly evaluated, looking for possible early physiologic consequences on ventilation and hemodynamic status [22].

Besides that, each team has its particular way of performing a diagnostic laparoscopy, but all of them are based on a practical systematization according to personal experience. The present step-by-step technique is a result of different systematization suggestions organized into a 7-rule procedure to be an effective and didactic option for a total investigation of the abdominal cavity.

Operative Technique

The first thing we do is look for active bleeding and injuries with contamination potential. Active bleeding can be safely treated following a sequence proposed by Vega (2022) based on communication, control, exposure, and repair. This sequence starts when the trauma surgeon faces bleeding and immediately informs the entire operation room team of the event, initiates an organized response, lays out a management strategy, delegates roles to all personnel, and minimizes the emotional toll of this crisis on performance. Bleeding control is necessary when there is active bleeding and aims at minimizing blood loss. It includes primary methods for bleeding control, such as compression with gauze, hemostatic agents, temporary clips, and clamps, and using specific maneuvers (Pringle's maneuver). After bleeding control, ensure all equipment and surgical materials are available. Depending on the selected repairing technique (clipping, energy source, hemostatic agent or stapler, manual suture, or ligation), additional ports must be considered to improve visualization or it must be safer to consider conversion if exposure is not possible or exposure of the bleeding area can lead to additional or worsening bleeding [23, 24].

Despite the lack of articles discussing laparoscopic infection control, studies have shown some approaches to the contaminated abdomen targeting the control of the infection source. Early treatment of the injury with the most severe contamination potential is crucial during trauma laparoscopy. During the DL, the procedure must follow its path (7-rule technique). Contamination must be controlled (clipping, stapler, manual suture, or ligation); it is indicated for simple bowel perforations, reserving immediate repair only for moments of controlling failure or gross contamination [25] such as large colon perforations.

Right Upper Quadrant

To explore the upper quadrants, we can use the reverse Trendelenburg position, allowing all the mobile hollow viscera to move downward to the pelvic region and making the region "clearer" for exploratory maneuvers (in obese patients or in patients with distended intestines, it may be necessary to combine the lateral decubitus position according to the side to be evaluated). In this position, the evaluation of the diaphragm on the right and the liver surface begins. If a diaphragmatic lesion is identified, its treatment should be postponed until the cavity evaluation is completed, except in cases where the lesion is causing significant changes in the ventilatory dynamics, a fact that should be discussed with the anesthesiologist during the evaluation. Deeper lesions, with active bleeding in the liver, should be filled with gauze or, preferably, with hemostatic agents. Less severe and superficial bleeding can be compressed in the same way as before or cauterized. It is not advisable to explore lesions due to the risk of additional lesions and bleeding, less manipulation, and less trauma.

The lower surface of the liver can be exposed by pulling the round ligament toward the diaphragm after sectioning or by gently pushing the liver with a pair of forceps wrapped in gauze. We do not recommend pulling the gallbladder, as this may cause inadvertent injury and require iatrogenic cholecystectomy, except in cases where there is already gallbladder injury or suspected bile duct injury that requires transcystic intraoperative cholangiography (IOC). In these situations, both procedures (cholecystectomy or IOC) are postponed until the complete evaluation of the abdomen is complete [26].

Left Upper Quadrant

The diaphragm on the left and the spleen are then evaluated. Lacerations in the spleen are evaluated in a similar way to those in the liver, with additional attention paid to exposing the spleen by sectioning its ligaments if necessary, seeking to examine the anterior and posterior regions and its hilum with little mobilization due to the friability of the spleen, and giving preference to conservative treatment. In cases of uncontrollable active bleeding requiring immediate splenectomy, an aspirator or gauze should be used so that the structures can be visualized, and clips or even a stapler can be used for hemostasis. Experienced surgeons can achieve control without the need for an extra portal for assistance; however, in the event of the slightest difficulty, an extra trocar to assist should be added for the safety and benefit of the procedure, which may also be necessary in cases of hemostasis with the use of ligatures with surgical threads.

Epigastrium Assessment

Through direct visualization, it is possible to assess the anterior surface of the stomach. Its posterior surface can be accessed through the gastrocolic ligament, in the greater curvature of the stomach. Through this maneuver, it is also possible to assess the body of the pancreas in search of hematomas, which can be treated conservatively or surgically, depending on the trauma mechanism and the preoperative imaging exam. The definitive treatment of perforations in the stomach may be postponed until the end of the evaluation, especially with the use of a nasogastric tube.

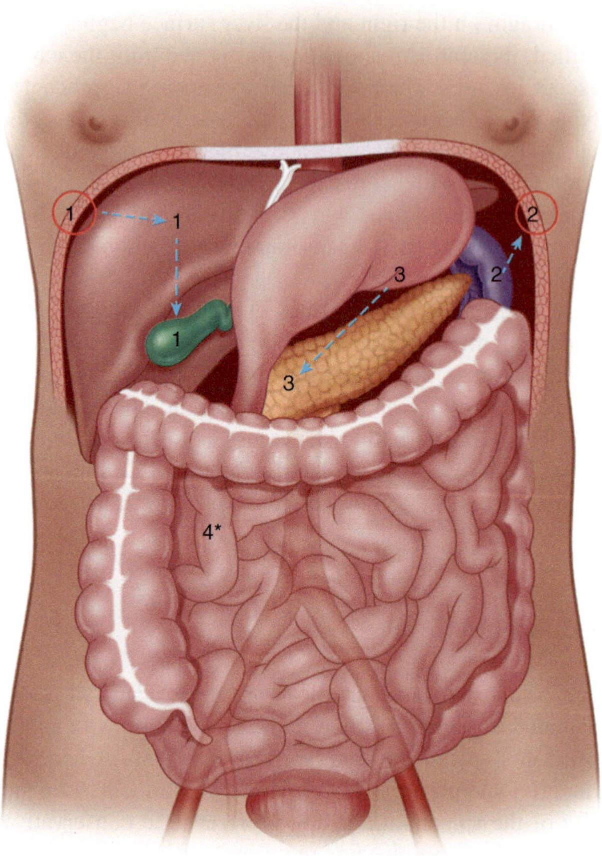

Fig. 13.1 Steps 1, 2, and 3 showing, respectively, right upper quadrant, left upper quadrant, and epigastrium assessment

Duodenal injuries are uncommon in blunt abdominal trauma; however, we reserve access to the first portions of the duodenum (duodenal arch and head of the pancreas) during colon mobilization. At this time of evaluation of the epigastrium, we assess the small intestine from the duodenojejunal angle, obtained after mobilization of the transverse colon and mesocolon in the cranial direction.

Steps 1, 2, and 3 are illustrated below (Fig. 13.1). Step 4 is more detailed in Fig. 13.2.

Running Bowel

After locating the fixed loop, it is possible to inspect the small intestine starting at the duodenojejunal angle (DJ) and moving up to the ileocecal valve (IVC). In some

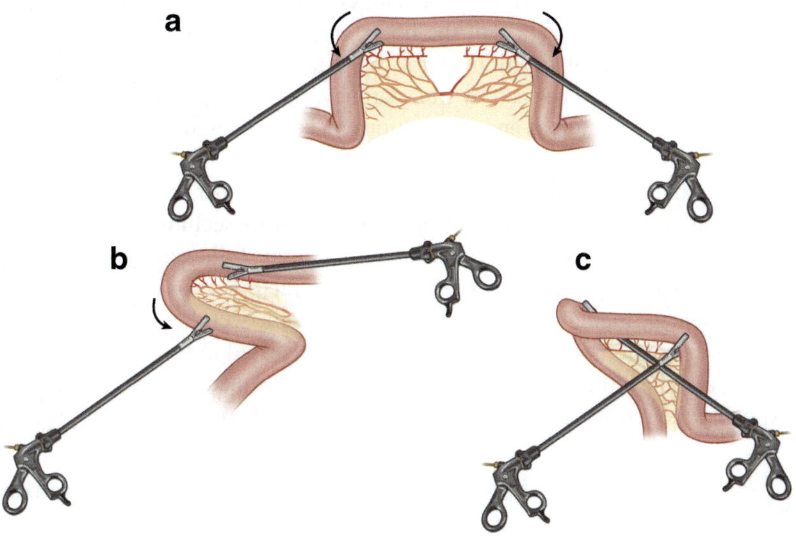

Fig. 13.2 Running bowel sequence A-B-C

situations, such as adhesions, obesity, or distension of the loops, it may be necessary to evaluate in the opposite direction, starting from the IVC and moving up to the DJ.

When using two atraumatic forceps, the small intestine should be presented with a slight enough grip so that it can be pulled without causing excessive paleness or injury to the serosa. The antimesenteric border is the site of choice for traction, reducing the chance of vascular injury to the mesentery. The forceps present an intestinal portion of approximately 10 cm (anterior face). To visualize the posterior face of this same segment, the most proximal part of the forceps crosses the front of the portion where the most distal forceps are presenting, "folding" the small intestine over itself and revealing the posterior part following the sequence A-B-C of Fig. 13.2. After this movement, the most distal clamp is released and fixed immediately before the site where the distal clamp is fixed in the duodenum, allowing the distal clamp to be moved 10 cm forward, advancing the evaluation process. As the VIC is approached, it may be necessary to use the Trendelenburg position, with the table tilted to the left.

Hematomas in the mesentery should be cleaned and evaluated for vascularization and appearance of the mesentery. Suspicious lesions may be marked for later reevaluation and decision on conservative treatment or not.

Colon Assessment

When assessing the pelvis, a change in position is necessary, and the Trendelenburg position is indicated to the desired side as the assessment progresses. This positioning exposes a great part of the right colon and left colon (Fig. 13.3). Obese patients may require manual mobilization of the bowel or great omentum, but, in general, despite the retroperitoneal position of the right and left colon, their location is superficial and mostly can be seen by transparency, without assessing the retroperitoneum. Therefore, hematomas and perforation can be diagnosed directly or through medial rotation of both colons using Toldt's fascia.

The colon can be grasped with an atraumatic bowel grasper and retracted medially. The colon is mobilized off the retroperitoneum by dissecting through the thin white line (avascular Toldt's line) with scissors or energy, followed by blunt dissection with the grasper or gauze or even by energy. Lateral dissection can go on rolling the colon mesentery medially away from Gerota's fascia over the kidney [27].

The transverse colon, due to its mobility, can be assessed in the same way as the small colon, and the left and sigmoid colon can be rotated medially (Mattox maneuver), exposing the retroperitoneal organs on that side if there is suspicion of injury

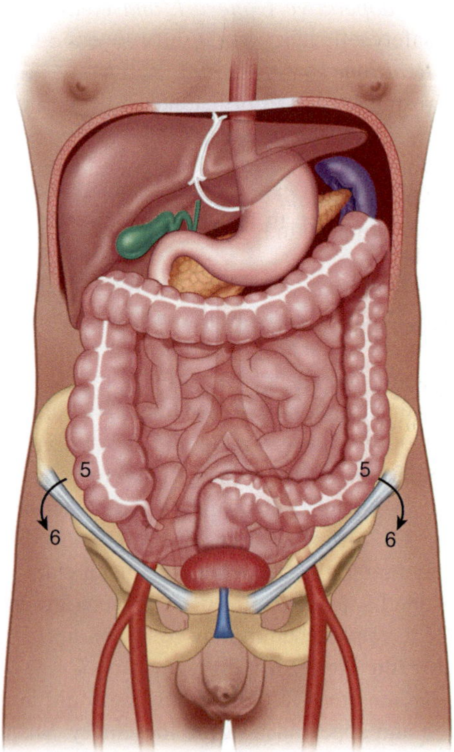

Fig. 13.3 Step 5 showing the assessment of the transverse colon, anterior portion of the right and left colon and sigmoid, preparing for the retroperitoneal spaces assessment by mobilizing the colon medially

or diagnostic doubt. For these maneuvers, when there is a strong suspicion of retroperitoneal injury, entry into the retroperitoneum of small and thin patients can be performed using the configuration of trocars used in diagnostic laparoscopy. However, it may be necessary to change the position of the trocars for better execution in some more obese patients, placing a suprapubic or epigastric working trocar, which allows the surgeon to operate facing the colon.

Retroperitoneum Assessment

As the colon is assessed, it is possible to rotate the colon medially (Cattell-Braasch maneuver—right medial rotation and Mattox's maneuver—left medial rotation) and expose the posterior region of the colon, the ureter, kidney, and its hilum. However, with the assessment of the trauma mechanism, imaging examination, and surgeon experience, access to the retroperitoneum on both sides may be an optional step in case of doubt or high suspicion. This maneuver can be performed by using the position on the opposite side in relation to the side of the maneuver, pulling the colon from the Taenia—with atraumatic forceps or moving it away by laying the grasper on the colon or using a folded gauze—using the most distal trocar, while the closest trocar performs the section with scissors, simple or advanced electrocautery on the avascular line of Toldt. Using two forceps, it can be created dissection spaces by placing them at the same point of loose connective tissue (after opening the Toldt's fascia) and moving the forceps in opposite directions, creating an opening in the space (Figs. 13.4 and 13.5). This maneuver can be done with gauze and allows exposure of the retroperitoneal structures without significant bleeding. Any diagnosed colon lesion should be marked in the same way as the small intestine so that it can be treated at the end of the evaluation (diagnostic laparoscopy).

Pelvic Floor Assessment

The rectum can be examined directly, with the patient in the Trendelenburg position, allowing access to its intraperitoneal portion (Fig. 13.3). Rectum mobilization can be performed using two atraumatic forceps, grasping the structure smoothly, or moving it away by laying the grasper on the rectum or using a folded gauze. Dissection generally is not necessary during the diagnostic investigation, unless there is an indication for colectomy and rectum mobilization, which is necessary most of the time for anastomosis. Blunt abdominal trauma rarely produces injuries to this organ, but evaluation is necessary and the conduct upon finding an injury is the same as for the colon.

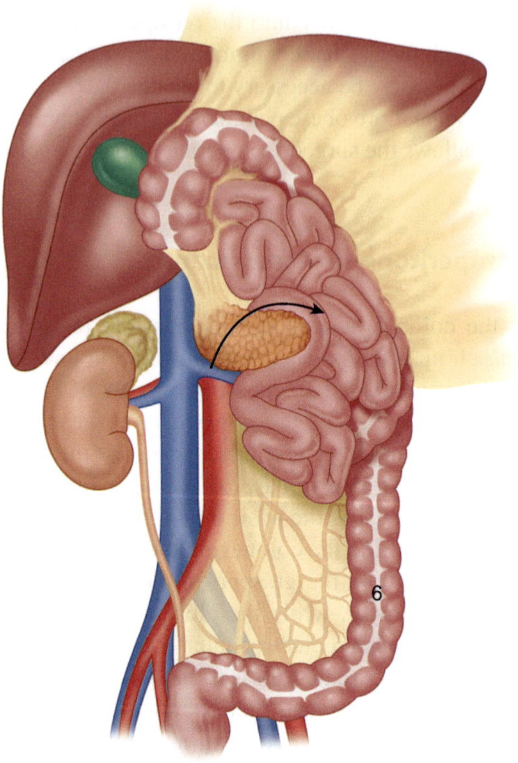

Fig. 13.4 Medial rotation of the right colon, throughout Toldt's fascia exposing right retroperitoneal structures

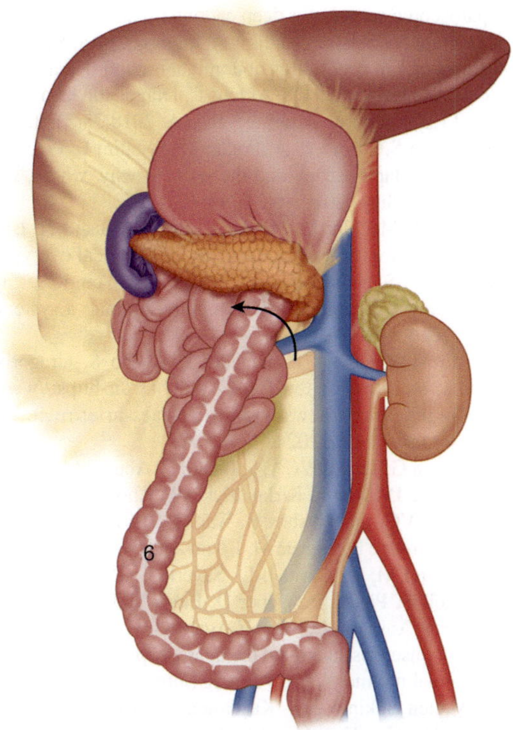

Fig. 13.5 Medial rotation of the left colon, throughout Toldt's fascia exposing left retroperitoneal structures

Conclusion

Trauma surgery frequently is not reproducible due to the difficulty of standardizing techniques, so the "how to do" way makes possible the sharing of experiences, offering a step-by-step technique that makes the procedure safe, reducing the risk of conversion, iatrogenic injuries, missing injuries, and saving time. This 7-rule technique presents an option of DL for the support systematization procedure, serving as a basis for other step-by-step procedures that need to be adapted to any other reality and reach the main goal, increase trauma laparoscopy among trauma surgeons, demystify fears and doubts related to it, and offer better care to trauma patients.

References

1. Vettoretto N, Saronni C, Harbi A, Balestra L, Taglietti L, Giovanetti M. Critical view of safety during laparoscopic cholecystectomy. JSLS. 2011;15(3):322–5.
2. Claus C, Furtado M, Malcher F, Cavazzola LT, Felix E. Ten golden rules for a safe MIS inguinal hernia repair using a new anatomical concept as a guide. Surg Endosc. 2020;34(4):1458–64.

3. Casagrande L, Avella MS, De Deus AM, Campos P, Maia A, Duarte A. Systematization of laparoscopic surgery for deep endometriosis. J Minim Invasive Gynecol. 2021;28(11):S145.
4. Kawahara NT, Alster C, Fujimura I, Poggetti RS, Birolini D. Standard examination system for laparoscopy in penetrating abdominal trauma. J Trauma. 2009;67(3):589–95.
5. Koto MZ, Matsevych OY, Aldous C. Diagnostic laparoscopy for trauma: how not to miss injuries. J Laparoendosc Adv Surg Tech A. 2018;28(5):506–13.
6. Di Saverio S, Birindelli A, Podda M, Segalini E, Piccinini A, Coniglio C, Frattini C, Tugnoli G. Trauma laparoscopy and the six w's: why, where, who, when, what, and how? J Trauma Acute Care Surg. 2019;86(2):344–67.
7. Alkatout I, Mechler U, Mettler L, Pape J, Maass N, Biebl M, Gitas G, Laganà AS, Freytag D. The development of laparoscopy-A historical overview. Front Surg. 2021;8:799442.
8. Hajibandeh S, Hajibandeh S, Gumber AO, Wong CS. Laparoscopy versus laparotomy for the management of penetrating abdominal trauma: a systematic review and meta-analysis. Int J Surg. 2016;34:127–36.
9. Cezillo M, Uwagoya R, Panadés P, Bueno S, Gregoris H. Laparoscopy in the context of trauma: too slow or too fast? Available on https://www.facs.org/for-medical-professionals/news-publications/news-and-articles/acs-brief/reviews/laparoscopy-in-context-of-trauma. Accessed on 11 Dec 2024.
10. Sermonesi G, Tian BWCA, Vallicelli C, Abu-Zidan FM, Damaskos D, Kelly MD, Leppäniemi A, Galante JM, Tan E, Kirkpatrick AW, Khokha V, Romeo OM, Chirica M, Pikoulis M, Litvin A, Shelat VG, Sakakushev B, Wani I, Sall I, Fugazzola P, Cicuttin E, Toro A, Amico F, Mas FD, De Simone B, Sugrue M, Bonavina L, Campanelli G, Carcoforo P, Cobianchi L, Coccolini F, Chiarugi M, Di Carlo I, Di Saverio S, Podda M, Pisano M, Sartelli M, Testini M, Fette A, Rizoli S, Picetti E, Weber D, Latifi R, Kluger Y, Balogh ZJ, Biffl W, Jeekel H, Civil I, Hecker A, Ansaloni L, Bravi F, Agnoletti V, Beka SG, Moore EE, Catena F. Cesena guidelines: WSES consensus statement on laparoscopic-first approach to general surgery emergencies and abdominal trauma. World J Emerg Surg. 2023;18(1):57.
11. van Veelen, Jakimowicz, Kazemier. Improved physical ergonomics of laparoscopic surgery. Minim Invasive Ther Allied Technol. 2004;13(3):161–6.
12. Liu J, Qiao X, Xiao Y, Deng Z, Cui J, Wu M, Zhang H, Ran K, Luo H, Tang B. Physical and mental health impairments experienced by operating surgeons and camera-holder assistants during laparoscopic surgery: a cross-sectional survey. Front Public Health. 2023;11:1264642.
13. Ribeiro MAF Jr, Tebar GK, Salgueiro JLR, Galindo GFC, Hughes JD, Sayari AA, Soucy ES, Mohseni S. Role and limitations of laparoscopy in abdominal trauma. Med Res Arch. 2023;[S.l.](11):8.
14. Hancheol J, Kim DH. Diagnostic and therapeutic laparoscopy for abdominal trauma: a single surgeon's experience at a level I trauma center. J Trauma Injury. 2021;34(4):248–56.
15. Lim KH, Chung BS, Kim JY, Kim SS. Laparoscopic surgery in abdominal trauma: a single center review of a 7-year experience. World J Emerg Surg. 2015 Mar;12(10):16.
16. Alhajress GI, Al Babtain I, Alsaghyir A, Arishi H. Complications of veress needle versus open technique in abdominal surgeries. Cureus. 2021;13(5):e14926.
17. Umano GR, Delehaye G, Noviello C, Papparella A. The "Dark Side" of pneumoperitoneum and laparoscopy. Minim Invasive Surg. 2021;2021:5564745.
18. Damous SHB, Utiyama EM. Laparoscopy in trauma: can Brazil fit into the global trend? Rev Col Bras Cir. 50:e20233602EDIT01.
19. Matern U. Ergonomic deficiencies in the operating room: examples from minimally invasive surgery. Work. 2009;33(2):165–8.
20. Aitchison LP, Cui CK, Arnold A, Nesbitt-Hawes E, Abbott J. The ergonomics of laparoscopic surgery: a quantitative study of the time and motion of laparoscopic surgeons in live surgical environments. Surg Endosc. 2016;30(11):5068–76.
21. Supe AN, Kulkarni GV, Supe PA. Ergonomics in laparoscopic surgery. J Minim Access Surg. 2010;6(2):31–6.
22. Ott DE. Abdominal compliance and laparoscopy: a review. JSLS. 2019;23(1).:e2018.00080.

23. Vega EA, Salehi O, Loewenthal JV, Kutlu OC, Vellayappan U, Freeman R, Pomposelli F, Asbun HJ, Gayet B, Conrad C. Strategic response to bleeding in laparoscopic hepato-pancreato-biliary surgery: an intraoperative checklist. HPB (Oxford). 2022;24(4):452–60.
24. You N, Li J, Zheng L. Bleeding control during complex laparoscopic surgeries of the spleen: current status and challenges. Chin Med J. 2022;135(24):2938–40.
25. Coccolini F, Tranà C, Sartelli M, Catena F, Di Saverio S, Manfredi R, Montori G, Ceresoli M, Falcone C, Ansaloni L. Laparoscopic management of intra-abdominal infections: systematic review of the literature. World J Gastrointest Surg. 2015;7(8):160–9.
26. Kim J, Choi J. Round ligament traction method during laparoscopic hemihepatectomy. J Gastrointest Surg. 2021;25(3):861–5.
27. Morris MC, Paquette IM. Laparoscopic left colectomy: surgical technique. Ann Laparosc Endosc Surg. 2019;4:18.

Part II

Diagnosing and Treating Traumatic Injuries Through Laparoscopy

14 Minimally Invasive Approaches in Cardiac Injuries

Patrizio Petrone, José A. Pezati Tenani, Bruno Monteiro Pereira, John McNelis, and Corrado P. Marini

Introduction

Cardiac injuries, blunt, penetrating, or iatrogenic, pose significant challenges due to their life-threatening nature and potential to rapidly compromise cardiovascular function. Traditional management involves sternotomy or thoracotomy procedures that, while effective, are associated with considerable morbidity, extended recovery times, and increased risks of complications such as infection and prolonged hospital stays.

Early History and Boerhaave's Contribution

Herman Boerhaave (1727–1734), a Dutch physician and professor of medicine at Leiden University, is remembered as a pioneering figure in medical history, particularly for his contributions to the study of human anatomy and physiology. Boerhaave was

The original version of the chapter has been revised. A correction to this chapter can be found at https://doi.org/10.1007/978-3-032-28971-1_35

P. Petrone (✉)
NYU Grossman Long Island School of Medicine, Mineola, NY, USA

Chairman, Research Committee, Panamerican Trauma Society, Mineola, NY, USA

J. A. Pezati Tenani
Unidade de Emergencia, Hospital das Clinicas of Ribeirão Preto, Faculdade de Medicina de Ribeirão Preto, University of São Paulo, Ribeirão Preto, Brazil

B. M. Pereira
University of Vassouras, Surgical Group® President, Campinas Brazil. World Society of the Abdominal Compartment Past-President, Campinas, Brazil

J. McNelis · C. P. Marini
Department of Surgery, Albert Einstein College of Medicine, Jacobi Medical Center, Bronx, NY, USA

© The Author(s), under exclusive license to Springer Nature Switzerland AG 2026, corrected publication 2026

M. Cezillo, B. M. Pereira (eds.), *Minimally Invasive Surgery Trauma*, https://doi.org/10.1007/978-3-032-28971-1_14

one of the earliest to describe a traumatic injury to the heart with a therapeutic focus in his writings, though he was not the first to recognize the heart as a critical organ in trauma care. His work during the early eighteenth century predated significant advancements in surgical techniques, particularly for conditions involving the heart [1].

At the time Boerhaave was active, the heart was still seen as a mysterious and untouchable organ. Early medical practitioners, deeply influenced by ancient beliefs, considered surgery on the heart (and other vital organs) almost sacrilegious, and the heart itself was considered off-limits for any intervention. If someone suffered a traumatic injury to the heart, it was usually considered fatal. Surgery was viewed as dangerous, and even the anatomical dissection of the heart was a delicate and sometimes frowned-upon practice.

Boerhaave's involvement in the treatment of traumatic cardiac injury stemmed from his own work in observing and documenting medical cases, particularly those involving blunt and penetrating chest trauma. His key observation was that a traumatic injury to the heart could be survivable if treated carefully, which was a novel perspective at the time.

Boerhaave's Notable Case

The specific case that cemented Boerhaave's role in the history of cardiac injury involved penetrating trauma to the chest, which led to a pericardial injury. Boerhaave documented the surgical repair of a heart wound in 1727 after a patient was pierced by a spear. Despite the traumatic nature of the injury, Boerhaave successfully conducted the repair, making a careful incision into the thorax to gain access to the heart. Though this early form of surgery was rudimentary by today's standards, it marked a significant departure from the belief that the heart was "untouchable."

At that time, surgery for heart trauma was extremely risky, and Boerhaave's success was more about demonstrating that careful intervention could save lives than about precise technical methods. His approach to dealing with such injuries was groundbreaking, and his careful handling of the heart was seen as almost miraculous. Boerhaave's clinical writings would inspire later surgeons to push the boundaries of surgery further.

The "Sacred Heart" and Surgical Taboo

In Boerhaave's era, many believed that opening the thorax and touching the heart was akin to an irreverent or fatal act, even though the patient had no other options for survival. The "sacred heart" was regarded with a combination of reverence and fear. This reverence, however, gradually faded as surgeons recognized the potential for life-saving interventions in the case of heart trauma.

Prior to Boerhaave, there was little to no surgical intervention for patients with traumatic heart injuries. The medical approach was largely palliative—attempting to manage pain and prevent suffocation or hemorrhage through basic wound care and chest dressing. Trauma to the chest or heart almost always resulted in death, especially if the injury involved a puncture or significant blunt force.

Boerhaave's approach marked the beginning of systematic attempts to treat cardiac trauma surgically. His clinical successes, however, didn't immediately erase the prevailing taboo surrounding heart surgery. Surgeons after Boerhaave still largely avoided direct intervention on the heart, relying on conservative measures or, when necessary, attempting external chest compressions or surgical interventions on the pericardium rather than the heart itself [1].

Advances in Cardiac Surgery: From Boerhaave to the Twentieth Century

Following Boerhaave's early attempts, the development of cardiac surgery remained slow and cautious for many years. Major advancements only occurred much later in history, particularly with the development of open-heart surgery and the establishment of cardiopulmonary bypass in the mid-twentieth century.

1. The nineteenth century: Surgeons like William Halsted and John Hunter would take significant steps in advancing surgical techniques, but heart trauma remained largely beyond their reach. Cardiac surgery, in general, was not a widely accepted practice, as mortality rates were high and there was little understanding of the heart's anatomy or physiology.
2. Early twentieth century: In the early 1900s, advances in surgical techniques, anesthesia, and antiseptic methods began to make more complex surgeries feasible. Even so, heart injuries were still treated with caution, and many patients who suffered cardiac trauma did not survive long enough to be candidates for surgery.
3. The mid-twentieth century and beyond: With the advent of cardiopulmonary bypass in the 1950s, open-heart surgery became a routine procedure. Surgeons gained the ability to directly repair heart injuries, and the field of cardiac surgery evolved dramatically. However, the minimal invasive approaches, including laparoscopy and robotic surgery, did not come into practice until the late twentieth and early twenty-first centuries, offering new avenues for repairing cardiac trauma with fewer complications and quicker recovery times.

Key Figures Who Followed Boerhaave's Lead

Though Boerhaave made early strides in cardiac trauma treatment, it wasn't until the late nineteenth and early twentieth centuries that other pioneering figures began to push the boundaries of surgery to directly intervene in cardiac trauma. Some key figures include:

- Dr. Dwight Harken (1940s–50s): Often considered one of the founders of modern cardiac surgery, Harken made significant contributions to the field by performing the first successful heart surgery to treat trauma patients during World War II.

- Dr. Michael DeBakey and Dr. Denton Cooley (1950s–60s): These cardiac surgeons performed pioneering work in heart surgery, including the repair of traumatic injuries and the development of techniques for coronary artery bypass surgery.
- Dr. Paul M. Zoll: In the 1950s, Dr. Zoll developed the first cardiac pacemaker, marking a critical breakthrough in understanding cardiac injuries and treatments.

Boerhaave's work in treating cardiac trauma was groundbreaking, occurring in a time when heart surgery was viewed as a near-impossibility. His careful approach to cardiac injury—coupled with his recognition of the potential for survival with intervention—laid the groundwork for future advances in the field. Though heart surgery would not become widespread until the twentieth century, Boerhaave's treatment of traumatic cardiac injuries remains a cornerstone of surgical history.

From Boerhaave's "touching" of the heart to the modern minimally invasive cardiac surgery we see today, the treatment of traumatic cardiac injuries has evolved significantly. Today, the heart is no longer regarded as an untouchable organ, and the advancements Boerhaave set in motion continue to save countless lives.

In recent years, the emergence of minimally invasive techniques has revolutionized the treatment of cardiac injuries, enabling precise interventions with reduced physiological stress. These strategies include a variety of approaches, such as percutaneous interventions, video-assisted thoracoscopic surgery (VATS), and catheter-based repairs. These techniques prioritize smaller incisions and minimal tissue disruption, providing enhanced precision and leveraging advancements in imaging, instrumentation, and procedural methodologies [2].

Minimally invasive methods are increasingly employed to treat conditions such as superficial and full-thickness myocardial lacerations, ventricular septal defects, coronary artery injuries, and pericardial effusions. By reducing the invasiveness of these procedures, patients benefit from faster recovery times, shorter hospital stays, and an improved overall quality of life. The primary goal is to optimize outcomes by balancing reduced physiological impact with the effectiveness of the intervention.

This book chapter delves into the principles, techniques, and clinical outcomes associated with minimally invasive approaches to cardiac injury management. It provides a comprehensive overview of their role in modern cardiac care, with a focus on their clinical applications, advantages, and limitations.

Pathophysiology and Types of Cardiac Injuries

Cardiac injuries can be classified into three main categories: blunt trauma, penetrating trauma, and iatrogenic injuries.

Blunt cardiac injuries, often resulting from motor vehicle accidents, may lead to myocardial contusion, chamber rupture, or valvular damage [3]. Penetrating injuries, caused by projectiles or sharp objects, are more likely to result in life-threatening complications such as cardiac tamponade or exsanguination. Iatrogenic injuries, including catheter-induced perforations, have become increasingly prevalent due to the rising use of interventional cardiology procedures.

Minimally Invasive Diagnosis and Treatment of Cardiac Injuries

Minimally invasive approaches have significantly advanced the diagnosis and treatment of cardiac injuries, providing effective alternatives to traditional open surgical methods. These strategies utilize state-of-the-art imaging technologies, catheter-based interventions, and precision instruments to enhance patient outcomes. By reducing the invasiveness of procedures, these techniques minimize physiological stress, shorten recovery times, and decrease the risk of complications, thereby optimizing care for patients with a wide range of cardiac injuries.

A. *Diagnosis*

Commonly employed diagnostic methods include the following:

1. *Echocardiography*
    - Transthoracic Echocardiography (TTE): A non-invasive ultrasound procedure that provides real-time imaging of cardiac structures. TTE is particularly effective in detecting injuries such as pericardial effusion or myocardial contusion.
    - Transesophageal Echocardiography (TEE): By positioning a probe in the esophagus with lack of intervening lung and bone, TEE offers superior visualization of the posterior cardiac structures and smaller cardiac injuries, making it especially valuable in complex cases.
2. *Computed Tomography (CT) and CT Angiography*
    - High-resolution imaging modalities facilitate the evaluation of structural damage, assessment of coronary artery injuries, and detection of complications such as aortic dissection or cardiac tamponade.
3. *Magnetic Resonance Imaging (MRI)*
    - Cardiac MRI provides detailed soft-tissue contrast, making it a powerful tool for assessing myocardial integrity and identifying scar tissue or other sequelae of trauma.
4. *Cardiac Catheterization and Angiography*
    - A minimally invasive technique allows direct visualization of coronary arteries and cardiac chambers. This method is particularly useful in cases of suspected vascular injury.

B. *Treatment*

Advancements in minimally invasive treatments for cardiac injuries aim to reduce recovery time, lower infection risk, and improve overall outcomes. These treatments are particularly beneficial for patients with severe trauma or multi-cavitary injuries. Key modalities include:

1. Percutaneous Coronary Interventions (PCI)
    - Techniques such as balloon angioplasty and stent placement are employed to treat coronary artery injuries or blockages resulting from trauma [4].
2. *Catheter-Based Pericardiocentesis*
    - A guided procedure to drain pericardial fluid or blood accumulation caused by injury, preventing cardiac tamponade.
3. *Endovascular Repair*
    - For vascular injuries, such as aortic tears, endovascular stent-graft placement provides a life-saving, minimally invasive alternative to open repair [5].
4. *Transcatheter Valve Repair and Replacement*
    - Injuries involving heart valves can sometimes be addressed with transcatheter approaches, such as Transcatheter Aortic Valve Replacement (TAVR) or edge-to-edge mitral valve repair [6].
5. *Electrophysiological Interventions*
    - Minimally invasive procedures, including catheter ablation and the implantation of pacemakers or defibrillators, are used to treat arrhythmias caused by trauma.

C. *Advantages of Minimally Invasive Techniques*

- *Reduced morbidity:* Smaller incisions and less disruption to surrounding tissues lead to faster recovery.
- *Lower risk of infection:* Avoiding open surgical exposure minimizes the risk of postoperative infections.
- *Shorter hospital stays:* Many procedures can be performed on an outpatient basis or with brief hospitalizations.
- *Enhanced precision:* Advanced imaging and tools enable precise targeting of injuries.

D. *Challenges and Considerations*

- *Patient selection:* Not all cardiac injuries are suitable to minimally invasive techniques. Severe, complex, or unstable cases may still require open surgery.
- *Specialized training:* Physicians must possess advanced training in the use of advanced tools and imaging modalities.
- *Access to technology:* The availability of minimally invasive techniques may be limited in resource-constrained settings.

Minimally invasive approaches are revolutionizing the management of cardiac injuries, offering safe and effective alternatives to traditional methods. Ongoing advancements in imaging, tools, and techniques promise to further expand the scope and efficacy of these methods, paving the way for improved patient outcomes in the future [7].

Contraindications for the Use of Minimally Invasive Techniques in Cardiac Injuries

Minimally invasive techniques (such as thoracoscopy or percutaneous procedures) are increasingly utilized in managing cardiac injuries [8]. However, their application is limited by specific contraindications, which can be categorized into absolute and relative contraindications:

Absolute Contraindications

1. *Hemodynamic Instability*
   - Patients in cardiogenic shock or with ongoing massive hemorrhage requiring immediate open surgical intervention.
   - Inability to maintain stable vital signs despite resuscitation.
2. *Penetrating Cardiac Trauma with Hemopericardium*
   - Risk of cardiac tamponade, which may require rapid open thoracotomy for decompression.
3. *Complex Cardiac or Great Vessel Injuries*
   - Injuries to the aorta, pulmonary artery, or coronary arteries requiring direct visualization and repair.
4. *Severe Pericardial Adhesions*
   - Resulting from prior surgeries or chronic inflammatory conditions, making minimally invasive access technically infeasible.
5. *Large Foreign Bodies*
   - Retained objects like knives or projectiles that may necessitate controlled extraction and open visualization to prevent further damage.

Relative Contraindications

1. *Coagulopathy or Anticoagulant Use*
   - Increased risk of bleeding, making precise minimally invasive control challenging.
2. *Severe Obesity (Morbid Obesity)*
   - Difficulties in accessing the thoracic cavity or pericardium through minimally invasive approaches.
3. *Limited Expertise or Resources*
   - Facilities or surgical teams lacking adequate training or specialized equipment for minimally invasive cardiac surgery.
4. *Extensive Chest Trauma*
   - Rib fractures or flail chest complicating the use of thoracoscopic method.
5. *Concurrent Injuries*
   - Polytrauma involving abdominal or cranial injuries requiring open access for comprehensive management.

6. *Previous Thoracic Surgeries*
   - Scar tissue or altered anatomy may impede the safe introduction of minimally invasive instruments.
7. *Suspected Intracardiac Lesions*
   - Complex intracardiac damage requiring direct tactile evaluation or complex repairs.

Minimally Invasive Diagnosis and Treatment of Cardiac Injuries

Minimally invasive techniques for managing cardiac injuries offer significant benefits, such as reduced surgical trauma, shorter recovery times, and decreased hospital stays. However, they come with potential complications that need to be carefully considered. Here are the main complications associated with these techniques:

1. *Incomplete repair:* Difficulty visualizing the full extent of the cardiac injury can lead to incomplete repair, resulting in persistent bleeding, ongoing hemodynamic instability, or poor functional outcomes.
2. *Bleeding and hemorrhage:* Despite the minimally invasive approach, manipulation of cardiac structures can cause vascular injury or inadequate control of the bleeding site, leading to hemorrhage. There are also challenges in achieving hemostasis compared to open techniques.
3. *Infection:* Although smaller incisions reduce infection risk, improper handling of instruments or inadequate sterilization can still lead to localized or systemic infections.
4. *Technical limitations:* Limited workspace and visibility can hinder precise repair of complex cardiac injuries, especially in emergency settings. Reliance on advanced imaging and instrumentation increases the procedure's complexity and susceptibility to technical failure.
5. *Conversion to open surgery:* In cases of unexpected complications or inability to achieve adequate repair, conversion to open surgery may be necessary, which increases surgical time and complexity.
6. *Residual defects:* Incomplete closure of cardiac lacerations, improperly repaired valves, or residual septal defects can occur, potentially leading to long-term functional impairment.
7. *Hemodynamic instability:* Inadequate decompression of cardiac tamponade or delayed diagnosis of complications like pericardial effusion may worsen hemodynamics. Air embolism or accidental injury to major vessels can also precipitate instability.
8. *Arrhythmias:* Manipulation of cardiac structures can irritate the myocardium, leading to arrhythmias such as atrial fibrillation or ventricular tachycardia.
9. *Limited applicability:* Not all patients with cardiac injuries are suitable candidates for minimally invasive approaches. Attempting these techniques in unsuitable cases can exacerbate complications.

10. *Learning curve and operator dependence:* Outcomes are highly dependent on the surgeon's expertise with minimally invasive tools and techniques. An inexperienced operator may have a higher risk of complications.
11. *Delayed diagnosis of complications:* Postoperative complications, such as pericardial effusion or pseudoaneurysm, may not be immediately evident and require careful postoperative monitoring and imaging.
12. *Cost and accessibility:* These techniques often require specialized equipment and training, which may not be readily available in resource-limited settings.

By weighing these potential complications against the benefits, the decision to use minimally invasive techniques should be tailored to each patient's specific needs and clinical scenario. To avoid these potential complications, there are several preventive measures that can be implemented, such as [9]:

- *Preoperative planning:* Comprehensive imaging and case evaluation to assess feasibility.
- *Surgeon training:* Ensuring that the surgical team is skilled in minimally invasive techniques.
- *Intraoperative monitoring:* Use of advanced imaging modalities (e.g., echocardiography) to ensure precise repair.
- *Postoperative care:* Vigilant monitoring for signs of complications like bleeding, arrhythmias, or infection.

Minimally Invasive Cardiac Injury Management via Thoracoscopy: How We Do It

Cardiac injuries, though rare, are a significant cause of morbidity and mortality in trauma patients. Historically, the management of these injuries involved open surgical procedures, which, while effective, carried high risks due to the invasive nature of the intervention. Over the past few decades, minimally invasive approaches, including laparoscopy and robotic surgery [10], have revolutionized the way we manage blunt and penetrating cardiac trauma. These techniques allow for reduced surgical morbidity, shorter recovery times, and improved cosmetic outcomes, all while maintaining high efficacy in addressing minor cardiac injuries.

In this chapter, we will explore the step-by-step process of managing minor cardiac injuries using laparoscopy, focusing on the application in stable patients with blunt or penetrating trauma. We will also discuss the AAST Cardiac Injury Grade and its relevance to the surgical decision-making process.

AAST Cardiac Injury Grading System

The American Association for the Surgery of Trauma (AAST) grading system provides a standardized way of categorizing cardiac injuries, which guides both the diagnostic and therapeutic approach to these injuries. The system categorizes injuries from Grade I (minor) to Grade V (severe) based on the extent of tissue damage, from superficial contusions to full-thickness myocardial lacerations [11].

AAST Cardiac Injury Grades

- *Grade I:* Contusion or minor hematoma of the myocardium, pericardium, or epicardium.
- *Grade II:* Myocardial laceration without significant damage to the heart's functional structure.
- *Grade III:* Severe myocardial contusion or laceration with damage to the heart's functional anatomy, including the conduction system.
- *Grade IV:* Injury involving the coronary vessels with possible compromise of myocardial perfusion or heart function.
- *Grade V:* Complete rupture of the heart or major coronary artery, often requiring open-heart surgery or other immediate interventions.

For this chapter, we will focus primarily on Grade I to Grade II injuries, which can be treated effectively through minimally invasive techniques such as laparoscopy. These injuries are typically characterized by myocardial contusions or small lacerations that do not cause major hemodynamic compromise but still require surgical intervention to prevent further complications.

Thoracoscopic Approach to Cardiac Injury in Stable Patients

In the context of blunt and penetrating cardiac trauma, stable patients can often benefit from a minimally invasive approach, provided the injury is not severe enough to necessitate immediate open surgery. The goals of thoracoscopy in these cases are to stabilize the patient, prevent complications, and allow for a thorough exploration of the injury with minimal tissue disruption.

Preoperative Assessment

Before proceeding with thoracoscopic intervention, a thorough clinical evaluation is essential:

1. *Initial trauma assessment:*

    - Perform a primary survey according to ATLS (Advanced Trauma Life Support) protocols.
    - Assess the patient for signs of shock, tamponade, or massive hemorrhage that would preclude a minimally invasive approach.
    - If the patient is stable with no signs of hemorrhagic shock, further evaluation via imaging (CT, echocardiography) is essential to determine the extent of the injury.

2. *Imaging:*
   - *CT chest with contrast:* To assess for pericardial effusion, myocardial injury, and damage to major coronary vessels.
   - *Echocardiogram:* To evaluate cardiac function and exclude significant injury to heart chambers or valves.
   - *Focused Assessment with Sonography in Trauma (FAST):* To detect free fluid in the pericardium and abdominal cavity.
3. *Indications for thoracoscopy:*
   - Stable patients with Grade I to Grade II injuries (as per AAST classification).
   - No signs of active bleeding or hemodynamic instability.
   - Small, isolated injuries with no involvement of the major coronary vessels.

Surgical Procedure: Thoracoscopy for Cardiac Injury

Once the decision to proceed with laparoscopy is made, the following steps outline the approach for stable patients:

1. *Preparation:*
   - *Positioning:* The patient is placed in the supine position on the operating table, with arms extended and a slight tilt toward the left side to avoid pressure on the heart.
   - *Anesthesia:* General anesthesia with endotracheal intubation is required to ensure full control of the airway. The patient should be placed under adequate muscle relaxation to facilitate access to the pericardium.
   - *Sterilization and Draping:* The abdominal and thoracic regions should be cleaned and draped in a sterile fashion to provide a broad surgical field.
2. *Port placement:*
   - *Primary access:* A 10-mm thoracoscope is inserted via a subxiphoid or infraumbilical approach. The subxiphoid incision offers better visualization of the heart and pericardium without disrupting the diaphragm.
   - *Secondary ports:* A 5-mm working port is placed at the left lower quadrant to facilitate the manipulation of instruments.
   - *Pneumoperitoneum:* CO_2 is insufflated to create space for visualization. The pressure is usually set at 10–12 mmHg to maintain optimal operative conditions.
3. *Initial exploration:*
   - Using the thoracoscope, the surgeon inspects the pericardium, looking for signs of injury, such as hemorrhage or tamponade.
   - If injury is identified, careful inspection is done to determine the extent of myocardial injury or vessel damage. In cases of minor contusion (Grade I), the myocardial tissue may appear bruised but not lacerated.

4. *Cardiac repair:*

   - *Minor contusions (Grade I):* In the case of myocardial contusions, the surgeon may not need to perform any direct repair. Instead, the injury is monitored closely for signs of worsening.
   - *Small myocardial lacerations (Grade II):* These injuries may require suturing. The surgeon can use fine, non-absorbable sutures to approximate the myocardial edges, ensuring no significant tension on the heart wall.
   - *Hemostasis:* If there is active bleeding, cauterization or suture ligation may be employed to control the hemorrhage.
   - *Pericardial drainage:* If a pericardial effusion is present, the pericardium may be drained using a catheter inserted via the laparoscope, or a small incision can be made for drainage.

5. *Final steps:*

   - After performing the necessary repairs, the surgeon carefully inspects the heart and surrounding structures for any remaining injuries or potential sources of bleeding.
   - The peritoneal cavity is carefully inspected to rule out any abdominal injuries that may have been overlooked.
   - *Drainage:* A small drain may be left in place in the pericardium or abdominal cavity if there is concern for continued effusion or bleeding.
   - The thoracoscopic ports are removed, and the incisions are closed with absorbable sutures.

6. *Postoperative care:*

   - *Monitoring:* Patients should be closely monitored in an intensive care unit for the first 24–48 h, with frequent echocardiographic evaluations to ensure that no significant pericardial effusion or myocardial dysfunction develops.
   - *Follow-up Imaging:* A follow-up CT or echocardiogram is often performed to assess the healing process.

Laparoscopic management of minor cardiac injuries offers a promising, less invasive alternative to traditional open cardiac surgery, particularly for stable patients with Grade I or II injuries. The benefits of laparoscopy include reduced recovery times, smaller scars, and minimized risk of infection [12, 13]. However, it requires meticulous attention to detail and appropriate patient selection to ensure optimal outcomes.

Clinical Case

To better illustrate the management of these types of injuries, we present a clinical case of an 18-year-old patient who presented to the emergency department following an accidental short-range shot wound from a low-caliber air gun to the left precordial region, along the midclavicular line at the fifth intercostal space, approximately 6 h before admission. The patient complained of mild left-sided chest discomfort, without dyspnea, and showed no signs of respiratory insufficiency, hemodynamic shock, and no clinical signs of pericardial tamponade. A bedside E-FAST was performed, revealing a pericardial effusion of approximately 1 cm and a small-volume pleural effusion on the left side. Laboratory tests showed a base deficit of 4.1, lactate at 2 mmol/L, hemoglobin at 12.6 g/dL, and normal coagulation profile, troponin, and electrocardiogram.

Based on the patient's stability, a contrast-enhanced chest CT was performed, which showed a minimal pneumothorax on the left, pleural effusion, blurring of pericardial fat, pericardial effusion, and a metallic-density foreign body in the pericardium (Figs. 14.1 and 14.2). It was decided to place a 28 FR chest tube on the left side, which drained 600 ml of blood, and the patient was kept under clinical observation. A repeat E-FAST after 6 h showed an increase in pericardial effusion to 1.95 cm (Fig. 14.3) and a chest tube output of approximately 300 ml over 6 h.

Given the suggestion of a projectile in the pericardial sac on CT and an increase in pericardial effusion volume on serial point-of-care ultrasound (POCUS), a decision was made to perform a VATS to assess the potential presence of a cardiac injury, despite the patient suffering only mild chest pain.

The patient was then taken to the operating room, intubated with selective pulmonary intubation and left lung blockade, positioned supine with left scapular elevation using a dorsal cushion, with the left arm abducted and the right arm along the body, and the surgical table tilted approximately 20° to the right. The thoracotomy tray was open and ready to use in case of VATS failure. The chest tube was removed, and a 10 mm trocar was inserted, followed by a 30° scope. Inspection of the cavity

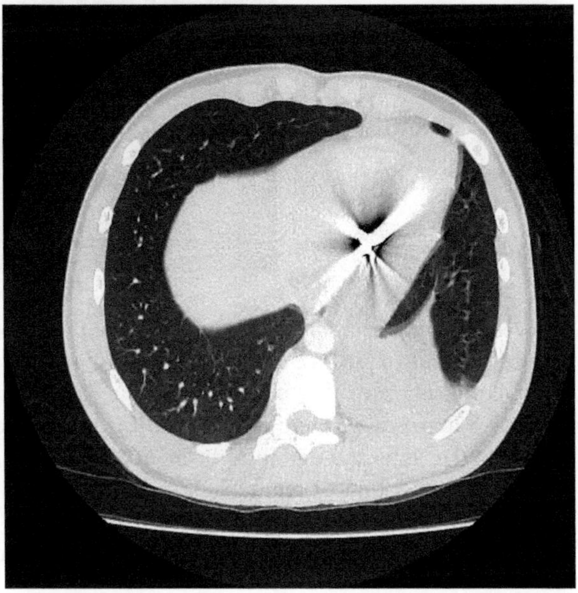

Fig. 14.1 Contrast-enhanced chest CT image shows a minimal pneumothorax on the left and pleural effusion

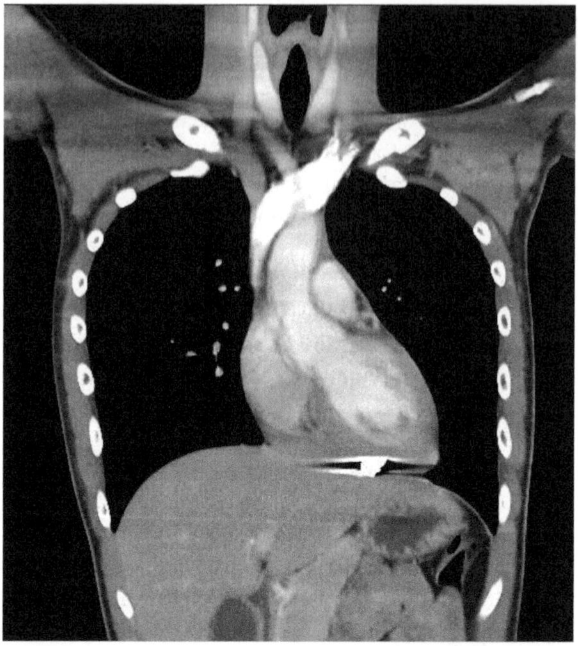

Fig. 14.2 Contrast-enhanced chest CT image shows blurring of pericardial fat, pericardial effusion, and a metallic-density foreign body in the pericardium

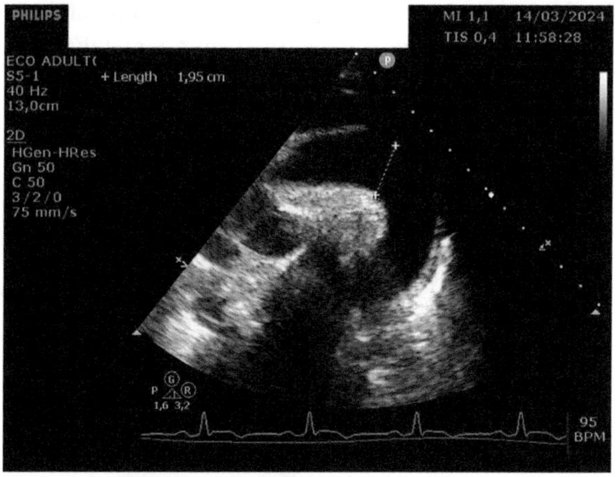

Fig. 14.3 E-FAST image after 6 h shows an increase in pericardial effusion to 1.95 cm

showed a minimal amount of coagulated hemothorax posteriorly, a laceration in the lingula without air leakage and a small local hematoma, and a non-constrictive pericardial effusion.

Two 5-mm trocars were then placed in the anterior axillary line under direct vision in the third and eighth right intercostal spaces, followed by pleural cavity lavage and aspiration of retained clots. A pericardial window was created with a pericardiotomy parallel and anterior to the left phrenic nerve (Fig. 14.4), providing good exposure of the myocardium and exposing a moderate amount of coagulated

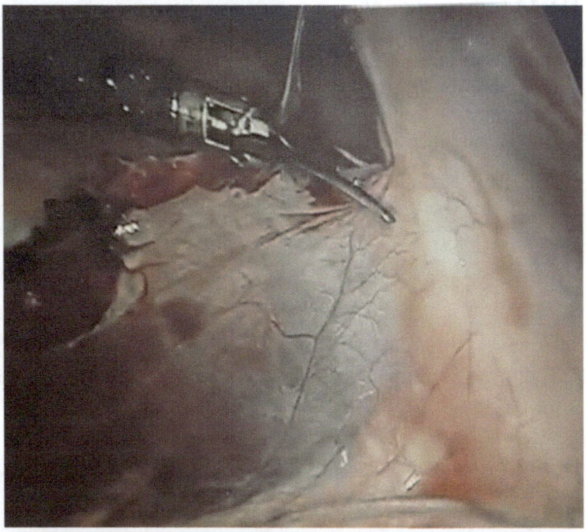

Fig. 14.4 Pericardial window was created with a pericardiotomy parallel and anterior to the left phrenic nerve, providing good exposure of the myocardium

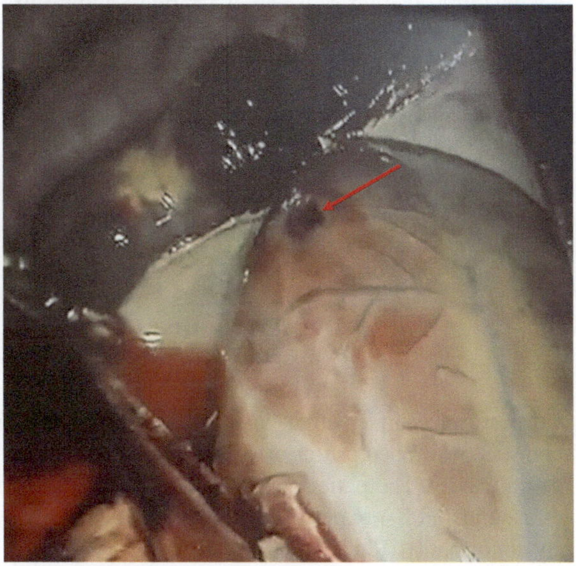

Fig. 14.5 Exposure of the myocardium showing a moderate amount of coagulated blood in the pericardium

blood in the pericardium (Fig. 14.5). Lavage and aspiration of the clots in the pericardial sac were performed, with no evidence of active myocardial bleeding. During this process, a projectile was found posterior to the myocardium, within the pericardial sac, and removed. Inspection of the myocardium revealed a pinpoint hole in the anterior inferior region of the left ventricle and another in the posterosuperior region of the left ventricle, both without signs of active bleeding (Fig. 14.6). The patient's hemodynamic stability throughout the procedure in the setting of absence of bleeding led to the decision for continued clinical observation. An intercostal nerve block

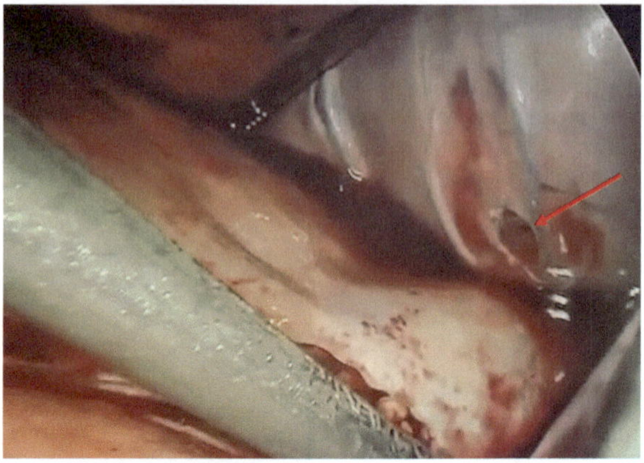

Fig. 14.6 Inspection of the myocardium revealed a pinpoint hole in the anterior inferior region of the left ventricle (red arrow) and another in the posterosuperior region of the left ventricle

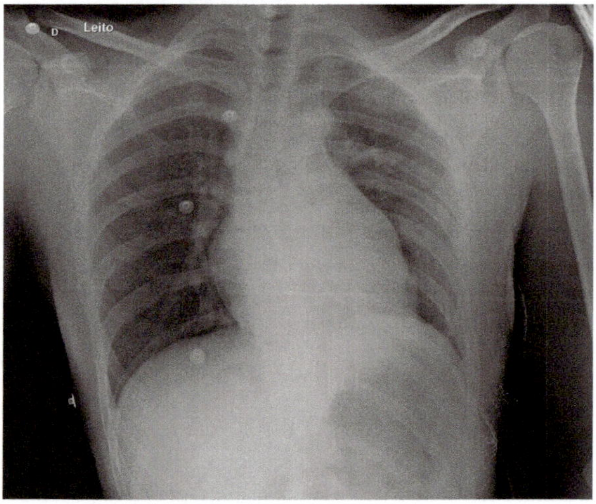

Fig. 14.7 X-ray image performed at post-op visit on days 15 without any abnormality

was performed under direct vision for postoperative analgesia, and a 28 FR chest tube was positioned posteriorly, leaving the pericardium open for drainage into the pleural cavity. The patient was successfully discharged on post-op day 4. POCUS ultrasound and X-ray performed at post-op visits on days 15 and 60 did not identify any abnormality (Fig. 14.7).

Conclusion

While minimally invasive techniques offer reduced morbidity, faster recovery, and smaller scars, their use must be carefully evaluated on a case-by-case basis. Absolute contraindications demand open surgical intervention to ensure patient safety, whereas relative contraindications require the surgeon to weigh the risks and benefits of the approach. A multidisciplinary team discussion is crucial for optimal decision-making.

References

1. Pereira BM, Nogueira VB, Calderan TR, Villaça MP, Petrucci O, Fraga GP. Penetrating cardiac trauma: 20-y experience from a university teaching hospital. J Surg Res. 2013;183(2):792–7. https://doi.org/10.1016/j.jss.2013.02.015.
2. He J. History and current status of mini-invasive thoracic surgery. J Thorac Dis. 2011;3(2):115–21. https://doi.org/10.3978/j.issn.2072-1439.2010.03.01.
3. EL-Andari R, O'Brien D, Bozso SJ, Nagendran J. Blunt cardiac trauma: a narrative review. Mediastinum. 2021;5:28. https://doi.org/10.21037/med-21-19.
4. Ursoleo JD, Losiggio R, Licheri M, Licheri M, Barucco G, Lazzari S, et al. Minimal invasive extracorporeal circulation: A bibliometric network analysis of the global scientific output. Perfusion. 2024:2676591241269729. https://doi.org/10.1177/02676591241269729.
5. Tinelli G, Minelli F, Sica S, De Nigris F, Massetti M, Tshomba Y. TEVAR for traumatic thoracic injury with the first-generation stent graft. J Vasc Surg Cases Innov Tech. 2020;7(1):16–20. https://doi.org/10.1016/j.jvscit.2020.08.035.
6. Misfeld M, Ehlermann P, Sievers HH. Transaortic repair of blunt traumatic cardiac wall and papillary muscle rupture. J Thorac Cardiovasc Surg. 2001;122(4):834–5. https://doi.org/10.1067/mtc.2001.115154.
7. Lewis MR, Georgoff P. Minimally invasive management of thoracic trauma: current evidence and guidelines. Trauma Surg Acute Care Open. 2024;9(Suppl 2):e001372. https://doi.org/10.1136/tsaco-2024-001372.
8. Reddy VS. Minimally Invasive Techniques in Thoracic Trauma. Semin Thorac Cardiovasc Surg. 2008;20(1):72–7. https://doi.org/10.1053/j.semtcvs.2008.01.008.
9. Maj G, Regesta T, Campanella A, Cavozza C, Parodi G, Audo A. Optimal management of patients treated with minimally invasive cardiac surgery in the era of Enhanced Recovery After Surgery and fast-track protocols: A narrative review. J Cardiothorac Vasc Anesth. 2022;36(3):766–75. https://doi.org/10.1053/j.jvca.2021.02.035.
10. Cerny S, Oosterlinck W, Onan B, Singh S, Segers P, Bolcal C, et al. Robotic cardiac surgery in Europe: Status 2020. Front Cardiovasc Med. 2021;8:827515. https://doi.org/10.339/fcvm.2021.827515.
11. American Association for the Surgery of Trauma (AAST) (2020). The AAST Organ Injury Scale: A Review of the Cardiac Injury Grading System. https://www.aast.org/resources-detail/injury-scoring-scale.
12. Claessens J, Rottiers R, Vandenbrande J, Gruyters I, Yilmaz A, Kaya A, Stessel B. Quality of life in patients undergoing minimally invasive cardiac surgery: a systematic review. Indian J Thorac Cardiovasc Surg. 2023;39(4):367–80. https://doi.org/10.1007/s12055-023-01501-y.
13. Ilcheva L, Risteski P, Tudorache I, Häussler A, Papadopoulos N, Odavic D, et al. Beyond conventional operations: Embracing the era of contemporary minimally invasive cardiac surgery. J Clin Med. 2023;12(23):7210. https://doi.org/10.3390/jcm12237210.

Lung Injuries and Laparoscopy: When and How?

15

Paula Duarte D'ambrosio, Jaqueline Schaparini Fonini, and Gabriel Lunardi Aranha

Introduction

Trauma to the thoracic wall may involve skin, muscle, ribs, intercostal neurovascular bundles, and underlying thoracic and abdominal organs. In penetrating thoracoabdominal trauma—defined as injuries below the nipple line anteriorly and the scapular tip posteriorly—there is a significant risk of transdiaphragmatic injury and associated intra-abdominal trauma, even in the absence of overt signs.

Historically, exploratory laparotomy was the standard approach in such scenarios, frequently resulting in non-therapeutic procedures. The evolution of minimally invasive techniques, particularly laparoscopy, has provided trauma surgeons with a valuable diagnostic and therapeutic tool. When appropriately indicated, laparoscopy or VATS offers excellent visualization of the diaphragm and upper abdominal organs and facilitates direct repair of injuries with reduced morbidity.

Thoracoabdominal Anatomy and Mechanism of Injury

The diaphragm, a musculotendinous structure separating the thoracic and abdominal cavities, spans from the xiphoid process and lower six ribs to the lumbar vertebrae. Penetrating injuries to the lower chest (4th–12th intercostal spaces anteriorly, 6th–9th posteriorly) risk traversing the diaphragm, leading to diaphragmatic tears and potential herniation of abdominal contents.

P. D. D'ambrosio (✉) · G. L. Aranha
InCor - Instituto do Coração do Hospital das Clínicas da FMUSP, São Paulo, SP, Brazil
e-mail: paula.dambrosio@hc.fm.usp.br; gabriel.aranha@hc.fm.usp.br

J. S. Fonini
Instituto do Cancer do estado de São Paulo, São Paulo, SP, Brazil
e-mail: j.fonini@hc.fm.usp.br

© The Author(s), under exclusive license to Springer Nature Switzerland AG 2026

M. Cezillo, B. M. Pereira (eds.), *Minimally Invasive Surgery Trauma*,
https://doi.org/10.1007/978-3-032-28971-1_15

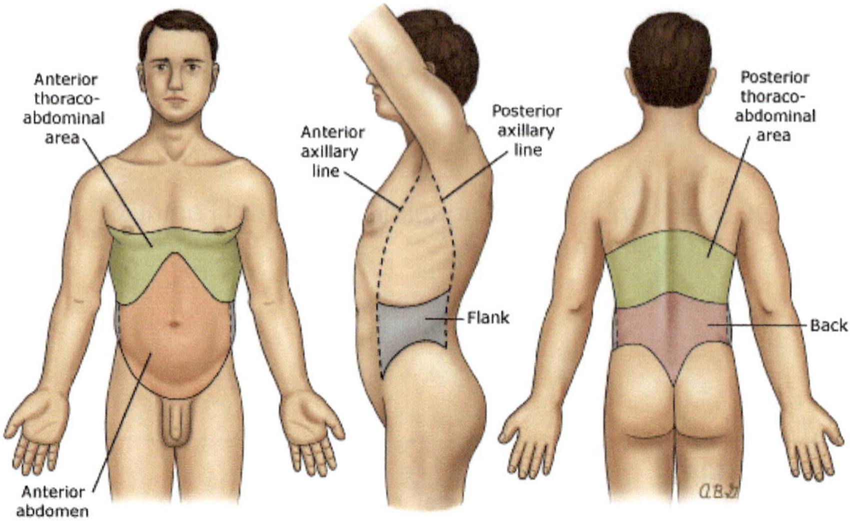

Fig. 15.1 Zones of thoracoabdominal trauma (anterior, lateral, and posterior views). (Genz et al. [8])

Blunt trauma may also cause diaphragmatic rupture due to sudden increases in intra-abdominal pressure. Left-sided injuries are more common due to the protective effect of the liver on the right (Fig. 15.1).

Indications for Laparoscopy and VATS in Thoracic Wall Trauma

Laparoscopy is particularly beneficial in the following scenarios:

- Penetrating injuries to the lower thoracic wall with unclear trajectory
- Suspected diaphragmatic injuries, especially on the left side
- Hemodynamically stable patients with thoracoabdominal trauma and equivocal Imaging
- Evaluation of peritoneal violation in transdiaphragmatic wounds
- Assessment and repair of solid or hollow organ injury in conjunction with thoracic wall trauma
- Early and complete evacuation of hemothorax, reducing empyema, respiratory failure, and hospital length of stay.
- Control of associated intrathoracic injuries
- Rib fracture repair

Contraindications include hemodynamic instability, suspected high-grade intra-abdominal hemorrhage, and lack of laparoscopic expertise.

Diagnostic Value of Laparoscopy and VATS

Computed tomography (CT) has limited sensitivity for small diaphragmatic defects. Diagnostic laparoscopy is superior for direct visualization and dynamic assessment of diaphragmatic integrity.

Key Diagnostic Advantages

- Detection of occult diaphragmatic injuries missed on imaging
- Real-time identification of active bleeding or peritoneal breach
- Evaluation of trajectory in penetrating trauma
- Assessment of adjacent intra-abdominal organs (liver, spleen, stomach, colon)

In a systematic review, diagnostic laparoscopy demonstrated a sensitivity of 96–100% and specificity of 98–100% for diaphragmatic injuries in penetrating thoracoabdominal trauma [1].

Therapeutic Applications

Beyond diagnosis, laparoscopy and VATS enable minimally invasive repair of injuries:

- Primary repair of diaphragmatic tears using intracorporeal suturing (nonabsorbable monofilament or barbed sutures)
- Hemostasis of minor solid organ lacerations
- Evacuation of hemoperitoneum or hemothorax via peritoneal or pleural breach
- Adhesiolysis and hernia reduction, if delayed diagnosis occurs
- Placement of intra-abdominal, subdiaphragmatic, and pleural drains under direct vision
- Early and complete evacuation of hemothorax, reducing empyema, respiratory failure, and hospital length of stay.
- Rib fracture repair

In experienced hands, laparoscopic or VATS repair is feasible even for large defects and may include prosthetic mesh if necessary.

Laparoscopic Surgical Technique

Patient Positioning

- Supine with reverse Trendelenburg to facilitate visualization of the upper abdomen
- Arms abducted; shoulder roll may aid exposure of left diaphragm
- In left-sided injuries, right tilt facilitates gastric mobilization

Port Placement (Fig. 15.2)

- 10-mm umbilical port (optical trocar)
- Two 5-mm working ports in bilateral lower quadrants
- Accessory subxiphoid port if needed for high anterior injuries

Exploration Sequence (Figs. 15.3 and 15.4)

1. Survey of entire peritoneal cavity
2. Liver retraction and inspection of right diaphragm
3. Mobilization of stomach and inspection of left diaphragm
4. Dynamic testing using positive pressure ventilation (bubbling with saline)
5. Identification and repair of injury
6. Consider VATS if diaphragmatic visualization remains inadequate

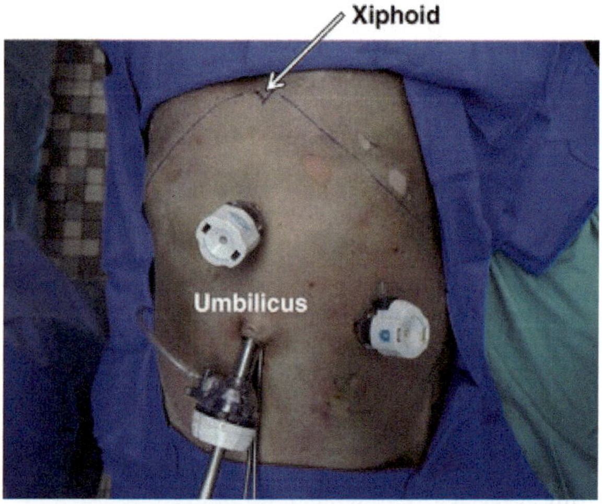

Fig. 15.2 Port placement in laparoscopy. (Lam and Tadlock [9])

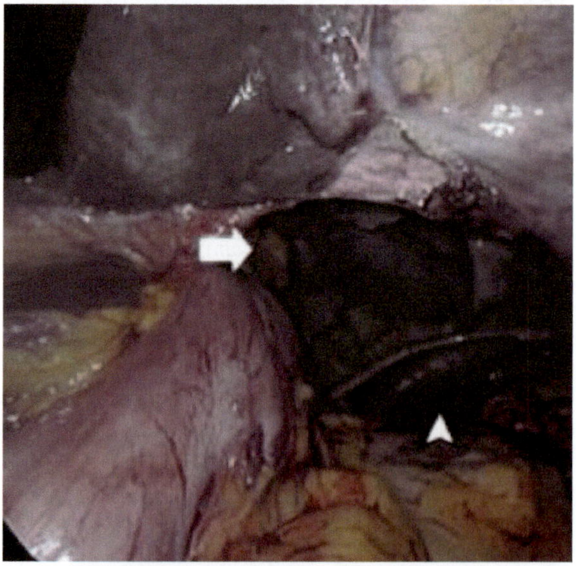

Fig. 15.3 Intraoperative image of left diaphragmatic defect. (Lam and Tadlock [9])

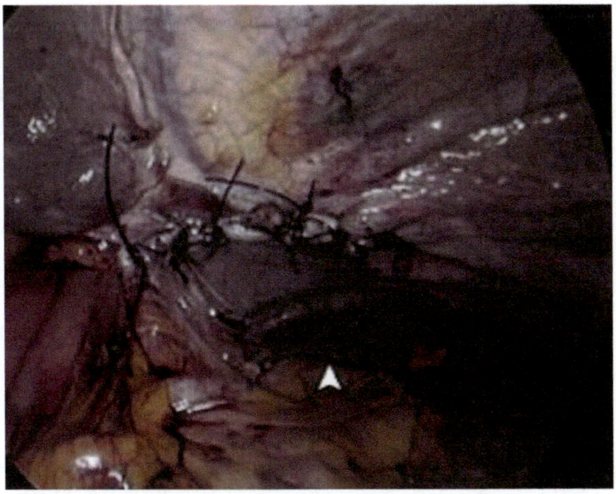

Fig. 15.4 Intracorporeal repair of diaphragm with running nonabsorbable suture. (Erdas et al. [10])

Vats Surgical Technique

Effective VATS in trauma necessitates optimal anesthetic management and patient positioning to facilitate surgical access and visualization.

- *Anesthesia:* "Intubation with a double-lumen tube or bronchial blocker for single-lung ventilation." This allows for selective collapse of the ipsilateral lung, creating working space within the thoracic cavity.
- *Positioning:* "Lateral decubitus position with elevation of the affected hemithorax; meticulous padding." Proper positioning ensures the affected side is optimally exposed, and meticulous padding prevents pressure injuries during prolonged procedures.

Access and Ports

The selection and placement of VATS ports are crucial for safe and efficient intervention.

- *First port placement:* Safe first port (generally seventh to eighth intercostal space (ICS) mid-axillary line/posterior) with an open "Hassan" technique when adhesions are suspected. The open Hassan technique is particularly important in trauma patients who may have underlying adhesions from previous injuries or inflammation, minimizing the risk of iatrogenic visceral injury upon entry.
- *CO2 insufflation:* Low CO2 insufflation (optional) to facilitate lung collapse in difficult cases. While not always necessary, gentle CO2 insufflation can help expand the pleural space and push the lung away, improving visibility and working room, especially in cases with partial lung collapse or adhesions.

- *Additional ports:* Additional ports as needed for instruments, 30° optics, clot-grasping forceps, and aspirator. The number and placement of subsequent ports are tailored to the specific pathology, allowing triangulation of instruments for effective dissection, hemostasis, and debris removal. A 30° angled scope is often preferred for better panoramic vision.

Therapeutic Steps

Once access is established, a systematic approach to intrathoracic exploration and management is followed:

1. *Systematic inspection:* The initial step involves a thorough assessment of the thoracic cavity. Systematic inspection: apex → base, anterolateral → posterior; pleura, diaphragmatic dome, pericardium, and hilum. This ensures no associated injuries are missed and allows for mapping of the extent of trauma, including any active bleeding, air leaks, or foreign bodies.
2. *Hemothorax/clot evacuation:* A common finding in thoracic trauma is hemothorax. The technique involves, evacuation of hemothorax/clots: suction and colon clamp/endobagger; warm irrigation; adhesion lysis with cold energy/Metzenbaum scissors. This process aims for complete removal of blood and clots, which is critical to prevent complications like empyema and fibrothorax. Warm irrigation helps break down clots and facilitates their removal.
3. *Bleeding control:* Addressing active hemorrhage is paramount. Bleeding control: sutures, clips, energy devices, hemostatic agents; conversion to thoracotomy in case of significant arterial bleeding. VATS can manage low to medium intensity bleeding; however, prompt conversion to an open thoracotomy is indicated for significant arterial bleeding that cannot be controlled minimally invasively, prioritizing patient safety.
4. *Associated repairs: lung injuries:* Lung: sutures over pledgets, sealants, atypical segmentectomy if necessary. This covers the repair of parenchymal lacerations, control of air leaks, and management of contused or devitalized lung tissue.
5. *Diaphragmatic injuries:* For diaphragmatic defects, "Diaphragm: non-absorbable suture in two layers; evaluate small hidden defects." This highlights the importance of thorough inspection and meticulous repair to prevent herniation of abdominal contents into the chest.
6. *Assistance to surgical stabilization of rib fractures (SSRF):* VATS plays a crucial role as an adjunct to SSRF, allowing for internal visualization and manipulation.
7. *Final aspiration, lung re-expansion under direct vision*, Valsalva maneuver for leak tests, and ideal drain placement. This comprehensive final check ensures lung re-expansion, integrity, and proper drain placement.

Table 15.1 Criteria for laparoscopy vs VATS decision

Criteria	Laparoscopy	VATS
Best for	Abdominal side of diaphragm	Thoracic cavity and pleura
Position	Supine	Lateral decubitus
Access to intra-abdominal organs	Yes	Limited
Use in hemodynamically stable	Yes	Yes
Port placement	Lower abdomen	Thoracic wall

Integration into Trauma Algorithms

In many trauma centers, laparoscopy has replaced mandatory laparotomy in stable patients with penetrating thoracoabdominal injuries. A protocolized approach includes:

1. Initial evaluation with EFAST and CT
2. Laparoscopy X Vats for indeterminate or positive peritoneal signs
3. Conversion to laparotomy only when required (therapeutic laparoscopy failure)

This strategy has been shown to reduce unnecessary laparotomies, hospital stay, and complication rates [2, 3].

While thoracoscopy (VATS) is ideal for intrathoracic assessment, laparoscopy provides superior access to the abdominal aspect of the diaphragm. Table 15.1 provides characteristics of each technique for specific condition.

Combined use may be necessary in complex injuries or when injuries traverse both cavities [4].

Outcomes

- Reduced non-therapeutic laparotomy rate: 60–70% to <10% in some series [5]
- Shorter hospital stay and faster return to baseline activity [6]
- Low complication rates when performed by trained surgeons
- High diagnostic accuracy for diaphragmatic and solid organ injury

Prospective studies continue to support the role of laparoscopy as both a diagnostic and therapeutic modality in trauma [7].

VATS as an Adjunct in the Management of Rib Fractures

Video-assisted thoracic surgery (VATS) has evolved from a diagnostic tool into a key therapeutic component in the modern management of rib fractures, especially in cases of retained hemothorax, persistent air leak, extensive pulmonary contusions, suspected diaphragmatic injury, and when surgical stabilization of rib fractures (SSRF) is planned. In selected patients, VATS allows for:

- Early and complete evacuation of hemothorax, reducing empyema, respiratory failure, and hospital length of stay.
- Control of associated intrathoracic injuries (lung parenchyma, pleura, diaphragm, pericardium).
- Direct assistance to SSRF (intrathoracic visualization, extrapleural "buttress," parenchymal protection during drilling, drain placement, and immediate outcome evaluation).
- Analgesia and pain modulation via regional techniques and direct vision of neurovascular bundle

Better outcomes are achieved with appropriate patient selection, early timing (48–72 hours when possible), an experienced team, and multimodal analgesia and rehabilitation protocols.

Indications for VATS in the Context of Rib Fractures

Common and well-accepted indications include:

1. *Suspected/confirmed retained or clotted hemothorax*
   - Persistent opacification, chest tube drainage failure, fever, pain, decreased compliance, leukocytosis, or signs of impending empyema.
   - Maximum benefit when performed early (typically 24–72 hours) after trauma and failure of the chest tube to completely drain.
2. *Persistent air leak (≥3–5 days) or unresolved lung collapse*
   - Allows identification and segmental/subsegmental repair of parenchymal injuries or traumatic subpleural bullae; seals sutures with reinforcement (e.g., sealants/pleurodesis, when appropriate).
3. *Suspected diaphragmatic injury in low thoracic or thoracoabdominal trauma*
   - Diagnosis and repair with continuous/"figure-of-eight" suture, with or without reinforcement.
4. *Therapeutic assessment in massive hemothorax/stable penetrating injury*
   - In hemodynamically stable patients without immediate indication for thoracotomy, VATS can control low/medium intensity bleeding and remove clots.
5. *Assistance to SSRF*
   - Intrathoracic visualization for:
     - Releasing adhesions and protecting the lung during bicortical drilling/perforations.
     - Guiding screw placement, evaluating dynamic alignment ("breath-hold tests"), and removing blunt intrathoracic fragments.

       Positioning drains under direct vision and confirming re-expansion.

   Relative contraindications:

- Hemodynamic instability requiring resuscitative thoracotomy.
- Massive adhesions "inaccessible" by VATS and/or arterial bleeding not controllable by minimally invasive technique.
- Respiratory insufficiency that cannot tolerate single-lung ventilation (to be evaluated with anesthesia).

Patient Selection and Timing

Hemodynamically stable patients capable of single-lung ventilation are the best candidates.

- "Opportunistic timing" is critical:
  - *Retained hemothorax:* Ideally within 48–72 hours of trauma (before dense fibrinous organization).
  - *Persistent air leak:* Consider VATS on day 3–5 if no trend towards resolution. *SSRF assistance:* Perform VATS during the same operative time as fixation, preferably within the first 72 hours, when edema and pain allow for safer manipulation and reduced complications.
- In elderly and multimorbid patients, early VATS can shorten mechanical ventilation and reduce pneumonia compared to expectant management of retained hemothorax.

Operative Technique (Key Points)

Anesthesia and Positioning

- Intubation with a double-lumen tube or bronchial blocker for single-lung ventilation.
- Lateral decubitus position with elevation of the affected hemithorax; meticulous padding.

Access and Ports

- Safe first port (generally seventh to eighth intercostal space (ICS) mid-axillary line/posterior) with an open "Hassan" technique when adhesions are suspected.
- Low CO_2 insufflation (optional) to facilitate lung collapse in difficult cases.
- Additional ports as needed for instruments, 30° optics, clot-grasping forceps, and aspirator.

Therapeutic Steps

1. *Systematic Inspection:* Apex → base, anterolateral → posterior; pleura, diaphragmatic dome, pericardium, hilum.
2. *Hemothorax/Clot Evacuation:* Suction and colon forceps/"endobagger"; warm irrigation; lysis of adhesions with cold energy/Metzenbaum scissors.

3. *Bleeding Control:* sutures, clips, energy, hemostatic agents; conversion to thoracotomy if significant arterial bleeding.
4. *Associated Repairs:*
   - *Lung:* Sutures over pledgets, sealants, atypical segmentectomy if necessary.
   - *Diaphragm:* Nonabsorbable suture in two layers; evaluate small hidden defects.
5. *SSRF Assistance:*
   - Identify from inside-out fractures with paradoxical mobility/overriding that correlate with external findings.
   - Safe passage of drills/bicortical perforations with intrathoracic "buttress" (e.g., mandrel, rasp, spatula) protecting the parenchyma.
   - Confirmation of screw length and plate position; avoid prominent pleural violation.
   - Final aspiration, lung re-expansion under direct vision, Valsalva maneuver for leak tests, drain placement in optimal position.
6. *Direct Vision Analgesia*

Future Directions

- Training in advanced trauma laparoscopy should be incorporated into trauma fellowships
- Robotic-assisted laparoscopy may expand applicability, particularly for complex diaphragmatic repairs
- Augmented imaging (e.g., indocyanine green, intraoperative ultrasound) may improve detection of vascular injuries

Conclusion

Laparoscopy and VATS are essential tools in the management of thoracic wall injuries, particularly those involving the thoracoabdominal region. It offers high diagnostic accuracy, therapeutic capabilities, and reduced morbidity when compared to open approaches. Trauma centers should adopt a protocolized, minimally invasive approach in stable patients, with proper training and infrastructure to optimize outcomes.

References

1. Murray JA, Demetriades D, Cornwell EE 3rd, et al. Penetrating left thoracoabdominal trauma: the role of laparoscopy. J Trauma. 1998;44(4):633–8.
2. O'Malley E, Boyle E, O'Callaghan A, et al. The utility of laparoscopy in penetrating abdominal trauma: a systematic review. Eur J Trauma Emerg Surg. 2021;47(4):1087–96.
3. Villavicencio RT, Aucar JA. Analysis of laparoscopy in trauma. J Am Coll Surg. 1999;189(1):11–20.

4. Petrone P, Asensio JA. Diaphragmatic injuries and post-traumatic diaphragmatic hernias. Curr Probl Surg. 2017;54(1):11–32.
5. Smith JW, Vassiliu P, Degiannis E. Laparoscopy in trauma. In: Mattox KL, Feliciano DV, Moore EE, editors. Trauma. 9th ed. New York: McGraw-Hill; 2020. p. 751–60.
6. Clarke DL, Bekker W, Hardcastle TC. Laparoscopy in trauma: pitfalls and promises. Br J Surg. 2014;101(2):e24–9.
7. Bala M, Kashuk J, Abu Gazala M, et al. Selective nonoperative management of abdominal gunshot wounds: a paradigm shift. J Trauma Acute Care Surg. 2016;80(1):15–21.
8. Genz M, Childress J III, Augenstein VA. Thoracoabdominal hernia. In: Docimo Jr S, Blatnik JA, Pauli EM, editors. Fundamentals of hernia radiology. Cham: Springer; 2023. https://doi.org/10.1007/978-3-031-21336-6_23.
9. Lam L, Tadlock MD. Diaphragm injury. In: Demetriades D, Inaba K, Velmahos G, editors. Atlas of surgical techniques in trauma. Cambridge University Press; 2015. p. 162–4.
10. Erdas E, Canu GL, Gordini L, Mura P, Laconi G, Pisano G, et al. Emergency laparoscopic repair of giant left diaphragmatic hernia following minimally invasive esophagectomy: description of a case and review of the literature. Case Rep Surg. 2018;

Retained Hemothorax Treatment with VATS (Video-Assisted Thoracoscopic Surgery)

16

Jorge Luiz Carnesecca Sobrinho
and Rafael Izar Domingues da Costa

Introduction

Retained hemothorax (RH) is a common and significant complication following thoracic trauma, with an incidence of up to 18% after initial tube thoracostomy [1]. It results from the incomplete evacuation of intrapleural blood, leading to the persistence of clotted collections in the pleural cavity (Fig. 16.1). If not promptly addressed, RH may progress to empyema, fibrothorax, or trapped lung, resulting in impaired pulmonary mechanics and prolonged hospital stay [2–4].

The Eastern Association for the Surgery of Trauma (EAST) guidelines emphasize early identification and management to avoid complications [2, 5]. Among the therapeutic options, video-assisted thoracoscopic surgery (VATS) has emerged as the preferred method due to its minimally invasive nature, superior visualization, and favorable outcomes. VATS enables effective evacuation of clotted blood, debridement of fibrinous adhesions, and full lung re-expansion [6–8]. It is particularly advantageous when performed within the first 4–7 days after trauma, before dense adhesions develop [9, 10]. This proactive approach has gained acceptance across trauma centers worldwide, particularly in resource-limited settings [11].

J. L. C. Sobrinho
Department of Surgery, Ribeirão Preto Medical School, University of São Paulo (USP), Ribeirão Preto, SP, Brazil
e-mail: jcarnesecca@hcrp.usp.br

R. I. D. da Costa (✉)
Department of Medicine, Federal University of São Carlos (UFSCar), São Carlos, SP, Brazil
e-mail: rafaelcosta@ufscar.br

© The Author(s), under exclusive license to Springer Nature Switzerland AG 2026

M. Cezillo, B. M. Pereira (eds.), *Minimally Invasive Surgery Trauma*,
https://doi.org/10.1007/978-3-032-28971-1_16

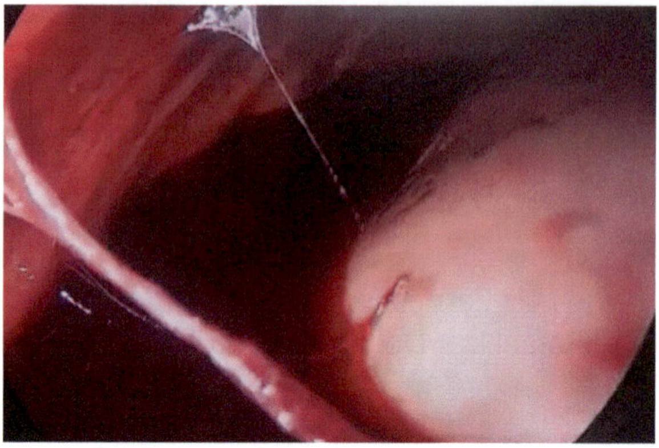

Fig. 16.1 Thoracoscopic view of retained hemothorax. The pleural cavity reveals organized clotted blood and fibrinous septations, consistent with retained hemothorax. These findings illustrate the need for surgical evacuation to restore lung expansion and prevent chronic complications. (Image from the author's personal archive)

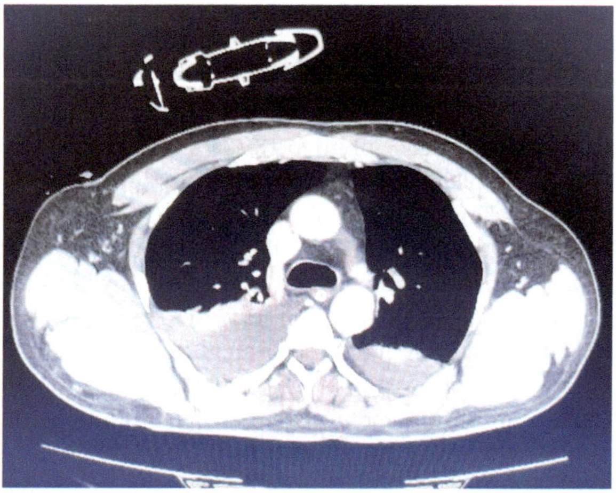

Fig. 16.2 Axial chest computed tomography demonstrating bilateral retained hemothoraces. Well-defined hyperdense collections are noted in both pleural cavities, compatible with organized hemothorax (measured attenuation between 35 and 70 Hounsfield units). Bilateral compressive atelectasis is evident, particularly in the dependent regions. Early thoracic imaging plays a crucial role in identifying patients who may benefit from surgical intervention. (Image from the author's personal archive)

Diagnostic Approach

Accurate diagnosis of retained hemothorax (RH) is fundamental for guiding timely intervention and minimizing morbidity. Initial evaluation typically involves chest radiography; however, its sensitivity is limited, especially in supine patients or in early post-trauma settings [2, 4]. Chest X-rays often underestimate the presence and volume of pleural collections [3].

Computed tomography (CT) has become the imaging modality of choice for diagnosing RH, offering superior sensitivity and anatomical detail (Fig. 16.2). RH is radiologically defined as a pleural fluid collection with attenuation values between

35 and 70 Hounsfield units (HU), consistent with clotted blood, and usually exceeding 300 mL in volume [3, 12]. CT also allows assessment of lung compression, loculations, and associated injuries [4, 7, 13].

Thoracic ultrasound may be used at the bedside for rapid detection of pleural fluid, particularly in unstable patients. While useful, it lacks specificity in distinguishing between liquid and clotted components, and is operator-dependent [5, 14].

In rare cases, diagnostic thoracentesis may be performed to analyze pleural fluid and differentiate RH from empyema or other effusions, though this is uncommon in trauma protocols [3]. Repeat imaging, especially CT within 48–72 hours of tube thoracostomy, is advised for patients with persistent opacities or clinical deterioration [9, 10].

Surgical Technique

The surgical management of retained hemothorax (RH) with video-assisted thoracoscopic surgery (VATS) has revolutionized thoracic trauma care. The procedure is typically performed under general anesthesia with single-lung ventilation to provide a clear operative field [6, 15]. The patient is positioned in lateral decubitus with the affected hemithorax facing upward to optimize exposure (Fig. 16.3) [15].

One to three ports are usually created—typically including a 10-mm camera port in the seventh or eighth intercostal space at the midaxillary line, and one or two working ports based on anatomical needs [7, 12]. The pleural cavity is inspected, clotted blood is evacuated, and copious lavage is performed. Adhesions and fibrin membranes are lysed to restore lung mobility and facilitate re-expansion [3, 10].

Intraoperative bleeding from intercostal or parenchymal vessels can be managed using electrocautery, clips, or endoscopic staplers. If active bleeding or extensive

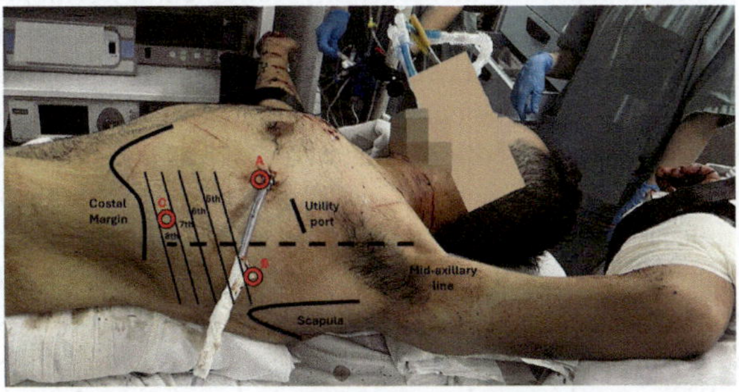

Fig. 16.3 Surgical positioning for video-assisted thoracoscopic surgery (VATS). The patient is placed in lateral decubitus with the affected hemithorax facing upward. This position allows for optimal exposure of the pleural cavity, facilitates gravitational retraction of the lung, and provides adequate space for port placement. The image demonstrates an example of portal configuration: A and B represent working ports, while C corresponds to the camera port. Portal planning varies by surgeon preference and case complexity, ranging from single-port approaches to the more common use of two to three auxiliary ports. (Image from the author's personal archive)

adhesions preclude safe thoracoscopic management, conversion to open thoracotomy may be necessary [13, 16].

One or more chest tubes are placed at the end of the procedure to ensure continued drainage and lung re-expansion. These are typically connected to low suction and removed once output decreases and imaging confirms resolution [5, 17].

Benefits of VATS

Multiple studies and guidelines support the early use of video-assisted thoracoscopic surgery (VATS) in the treatment of retained hemothorax (RH). When performed within 3–5 days after trauma, VATS is associated with significantly reduced morbidity, shorter hospital length of stay, and fewer postoperative complications compared to delayed or non-surgical interventions [2, 7, 8].

Meta-analyses have demonstrated that early VATS can reduce the need for thoracotomy by up to 70%, lower infection rates, and improve long-term pulmonary function [9–11]. Additionally, early evacuation of clotted blood before the formation of dense pleural adhesions results in shorter operative times and reduced technical complexity [15].

From a health economics perspective, early VATS reduces intensive care unit (ICU) stay, facilitates earlier ambulation, and promotes quicker return to baseline activity, thereby reducing overall healthcare costs [3, 14, 18]. These benefits make VATS the preferred strategy in appropriately selected patients.

Comparison with Other Approaches

Several therapeutic options are available for the management of retained hemothorax (RH), including repeat tube thoracostomy, intrapleural fibrinolytics, and open thoracotomy. However, among these strategies, video-assisted thoracoscopic surgery (VATS) demonstrates superior outcomes across multiple parameters, particularly when performed early in the course of treatment [2, 7, 8].

Repeat tube thoracostomy is often attempted as a less invasive alternative, especially in resource-constrained settings or in patients deemed unfit for surgery. However, multiple studies report low success rates due to the inability of chest tubes to evacuate organized clots or fibrinous material effectively [1, 3, 5]. This can delay definitive management, increase infection risk, and prolong hospital stay [4].

Intrapleural fibrinolytic therapy, typically with agents such as tissue plasminogen activator (tPA) or urokinase, has shown some benefit in selected cases. It may be considered in patients with minimal adhesions or as a bridge to surgery. Nonetheless, its efficacy is inconsistent, especially in cases with large or loculated collections. There are also potential risks, including hemorrhagic complications and allergic reactions [16, 17].

In contrast, VATS provides direct visualization of the pleural cavity, enables complete clot evacuation, and allows for targeted adhesiolysis. It has been associated with significantly fewer reinterventions, lower complication rates, and better pulmonary recovery compared to conservative methods [6, 10, 15].

Thoracotomy remains a viable and effective option, particularly in complex or late-presenting cases. However, it is more invasive, associated with greater postoperative pain, longer recovery, and higher morbidity. Therefore, thoracotomy is generally reserved for situations where VATS is not feasible, such as in cases of extensive fibrothorax, hemodynamic instability, or failed minimally invasive attempts [7, 13, 18].

Overall, the current evidence supports VATS as the optimal first-line strategy for the management of post-traumatic RH, striking a favorable balance between invasiveness and therapeutic efficacy [9, 11, 14].

Complications and Limitations

Although video-assisted thoracoscopic surgery (VATS) is widely regarded as a safe and effective method for the management of retained hemothorax (RH), it is not without potential complications. These can vary based on patient-specific factors, timing of the procedure, and surgeon experience [2, 4, 7].

Prolonged air leak is one of the most commonly reported complications, especially in patients with underlying lung injury, adhesions, or parenchymal fragility [1, 15]. Bleeding can occur intraoperatively during adhesiolysis, particularly when dissecting fibrous tissue or when vascular structures are obscured by clotted blood [9, 12]. Postoperative infections such as empyema or wound infection, though less frequent with early intervention, remain a concern in delayed or incomplete evacuation cases [3, 10, 13].

Conversion to open thoracotomy is required in a minority of cases, particularly when dense fibrothorax or uncontrolled bleeding prevents safe continuation via thoracoscopy. Reported conversion rates range from 5% to 15%, and are influenced by the duration of hemothorax retention and degree of pleural organization [7, 8, 18].

A key limitation of VATS lies in its dependency on specialized equipment and surgical expertise. The learning curve for VATS is significant, and optimal outcomes are typically achieved in centers with established thoracoscopic programs and multidisciplinary trauma care [6, 11, 17]. In low-resource settings, limited availability of instruments and trained personnel may delay definitive management or necessitate alternative approaches.

Furthermore, patient factors such as morbid obesity, severe cardiopulmonary disease, or multiple concurrent injuries may pose additional risks or contraindications to the thoracoscopic approach [5, 14, 16].

Despite these considerations, the overall safety and efficacy profile of VATS remains highly favorable. Early surgical consultation, careful patient selection, and adherence to institutional protocols are critical to minimizing complications and optimizing clinical outcomes.

Conclusion

Video-assisted thoracoscopic surgery (VATS) has proven to be a highly effective, safe, and minimally invasive technique for the management of retained hemothorax (RH) in trauma patients. Supported by numerous clinical studies and guideline recommendations, VATS offers significant advantages over alternative approaches, particularly when performed within the first 3–5 days following injury [2, 7, 8].

Early thoracoscopic intervention facilitates complete evacuation of clotted blood, prevention of fibrothorax, and restoration of lung function, thereby reducing the incidence of infectious complications, minimizing the need for open thoracotomy, and shortening hospital and ICU stays [6, 9, 10].

In hemodynamically stable patients with persistent pleural collections after chest tube drainage, VATS should be strongly considered as the first-line surgical strategy. Its effectiveness is further enhanced in institutions with trained thoracic surgeons and access to thoracoscopic equipment [3, 11, 15].

Ultimately, the implementation of early VATS protocols within trauma systems contributes not only to improved patient outcomes but also to more efficient use of healthcare resources. It represents the current standard of care in RH management and continues to gain traction as surgical experience and technology evolve. Below is a suggested algorithm for the management of retained hemothorax using VATS (Fig. 16.4).

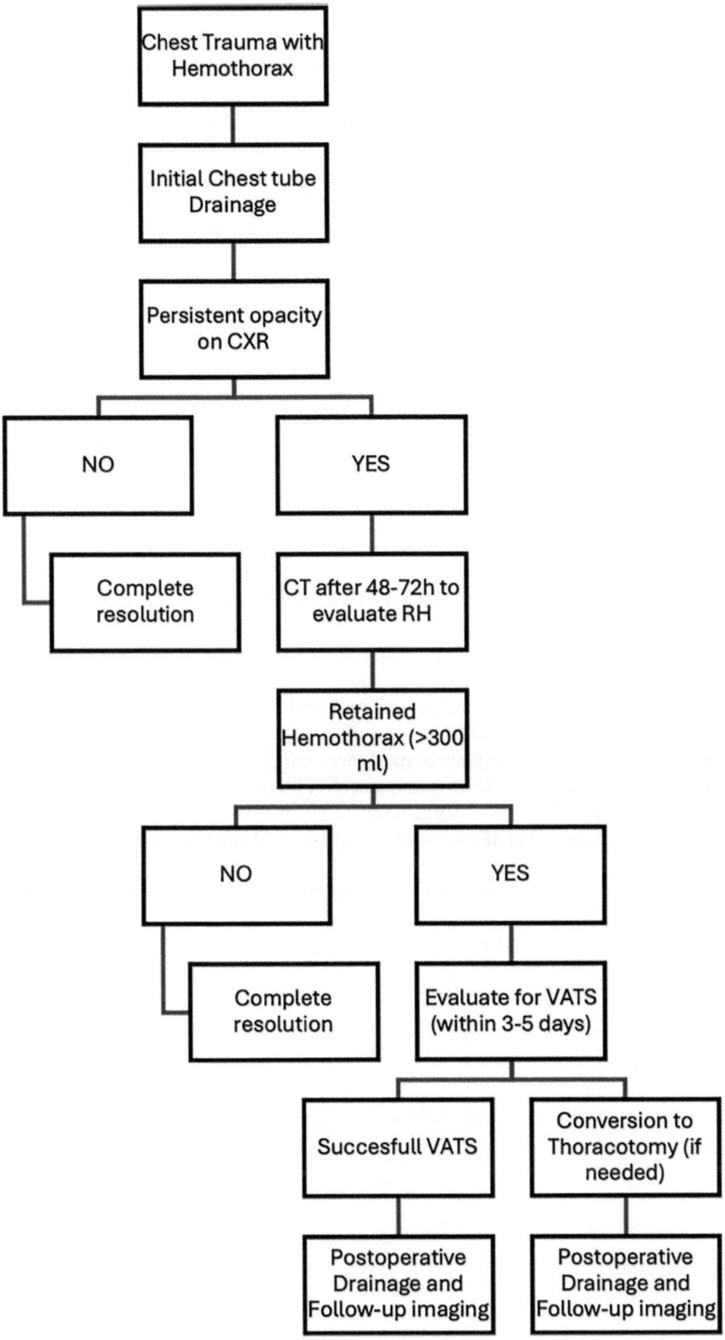

Fig. 16.4 Suggested algorithm for the management of retained hemothorax (RH) using video-assisted thoracoscopic surgery (VATS). The flowchart outlines the recommended diagnostic and therapeutic steps in the management of RH following thoracic trauma. It emphasizes early imaging, timely surgical intervention, and consideration of alternative strategies when VATS is not feasible. (Developed by the chapter author based on current literature)

References

1. Kulshrestha P, et al. Profile of chest trauma patients at level 1 trauma center and incidence of retained hemothorax. Int J Crit Illn Inj Sci. 2011;
2. Patel NJ, et al. Management of simple and retained hemothorax: a practice management guideline from the Eastern Association for the Surgery of Trauma. Am J Surg. 2020;
3. Yu H, Isaacson AJ, Burke CT. Management of traumatic hemothorax, retained hemothorax, and other thoracic collections. Curr Trauma Rep. 2017;
4. Beyer CA, et al. Management of traumatic pneumothorax and hemothorax. Curr Probl Surg. 2025;63:101707.
5. Mowery NT, et al. Practice management guidelines for management of hemothorax: Eastern Association for the Surgery of Trauma. J Trauma Acute Care Surg. 2020;
6. Lodhia JV, et al. Video-assisted thoracoscopic surgery in trauma: pros and cons. J Thorac Dis. 2019;11(4):1662–7.
7. Scarci M, et al. Video-assisted thoracoscopic surgery for post-traumatic retained hemothorax. Ann Thorac Surg. 2012;
8. Meyer DM, et al. Early evacuation of retained hemothoraces using thoracoscopy: a prospective, randomized trial. Ann Thorac Surg. 1997;64(5):1396–400.
9. Solaini L, et al. Minimally invasive surgery for post-traumatic retained hemothorax: early experience. Surg Endosc. 2006;
10. Kim YT, et al. Efficacy of early thoracoscopic evacuation for retained hemothorax. Ann Thorac Surg. 2002;
11. Brazilian Journal of Development. Early VATS approach to hemothorax: a review. Braz J Dev. 2022;8(12):80300–17.
12. Rzyman W, et al. VATS in thoracic trauma: retrospective analysis. Interact Cardiovasc Thorac Surg. 2013;
13. Ball CG, et al. A decade of experience with post-traumatic hemothorax management: time for a new guideline. Can J Surg. 2005;
14. Gordon NT, et al. Delayed hemothorax: incidence, management, and outcomes. J Trauma. 2015;
15. Mandal AK, et al. Role of VATS in management of blunt chest trauma with retained hemothorax. Indian. J Thorac Cardiovasc Surg. 2007;
16. Viana FL, et al. Retained hemothorax: comparison of fibrinolysis and surgery. Rev Col Bras Cir. 2014;
17. Morales Uribe CH, et al. Intrapleural fibrinolytics vs VATS for retained hemothorax. J Trauma. 2008;
18. Kim KS, et al. Use of VATS for hemothorax in elderly trauma patients. J Cardiothorac Surg. 2013;

Role of Laparoscopy on Esophageal Injuries

17

Sameh Abogabal, Zain Ali Khan, and Mansoor Ali Khan

Introduction

Esophageal injuries are relatively rare but highly complex traumas [1], often resulting from blunt or penetrating trauma, foreign body ingestion, iatrogenic perforation, or caustic ingestion. These injuries pose significant challenges for trauma surgeons due to the esophagus's anatomical positioning and the high risk of complications if treatment is delayed. The esophagus lies near several vital structures within the chest and abdomen, including the trachea, aorta, and vena cava, and it lacks the protective serosal covering that many other gastrointestinal organs have, making it particularly vulnerable to perforations and subsequent infections. When an esophageal injury occurs, timely diagnosis and repair are critical to prevent life-threatening complications, such as mediastinitis, empyema, sepsis, and multi-organ failure.

Historically, esophageal injuries have been managed with open thoracotomy or laparotomy [2], both of which involve large incisions and extended recovery times. These open approaches allow surgeons direct access to the esophagus, making it possible to thoroughly inspect the injury, control bleeding, and conduct repairs. However, open surgery carries its own set of risks, including prolonged hospitalization, postoperative pain, high infection rates, and respiratory complications due to the invasiveness of the procedure [3]. For many years, these trade-offs were deemed necessary, as the risks associated with untreated esophageal injuries were deemed too high to warrant alternative, less invasive approaches.

S. Abogabal
Hull University Teaching Hospitals, Hull, UK

Z. A. Khan
Nottingham University Medical School, Lincoln and Nottingham University Campus, Nottingham, UK

M. A. Khan (✉)
Iqarus Gulf FZ LLC, Dubai, UAE
e-mail: manskhan@doctors.org.uk; mansoorkhan@nhs.net

© The Author(s), under exclusive license to Springer Nature Switzerland AG 2026

M. Cezillo, B. M. Pereira (eds.), *Minimally Invasive Surgery Trauma*,
https://doi.org/10.1007/978-3-032-28971-1_17

With advancements in minimally invasive surgery, however, the field of trauma surgery has increasingly looked toward laparoscopy as a potential method for managing certain types of esophageal injuries [4]. Laparoscopy involves using a laparoscope—a small, flexible tube with a camera—to visualize the internal organs through small incisions, often less than a centimeter. This approach has proven beneficial in many abdominal and thoracic surgeries, leading to quicker recovery, reduced postoperative pain, and a lower incidence of complications. In trauma cases involving the esophagus, laparoscopic techniques are now being explored as an alternative to open surgery [5], particularly for injuries located in the lower third of the esophagus and at the gastroesophageal junction, where the abdominal approach provides good access.

The development of laparoscopic techniques for esophageal injuries has been gradual. Initially, these techniques were used primarily for diagnostic purposes. When surgeons encountered situations where imaging, such as CT or endoscopy, was inconclusive, laparoscopy allowed them to directly visualize the esophagus and assess any damage without committing to a full thoracotomy or laparotomy. This diagnostic use of laparoscopy has proven to be particularly helpful in cases of suspected lower esophageal perforations and gastroesophageal junction injuries. Over time, as experience grew, surgeons began to recognize the potential for laparoscopy to go beyond diagnosis and to also provide therapeutic solutions for certain esophageal injuries. Today, laparoscopy is increasingly used not only to diagnose but also to treat small perforations, contained leaks, and certain foreign body penetrations in hemodynamically stable patients with injuries to the lower esophagus [6].

Despite these advancements, laparoscopy in esophageal trauma remains highly selective, as it is only feasible in particular types of injuries [7]. The use of laparoscopy is currently most appropriate for hemodynamically stable patients with injuries confined to the lower esophagus and gastroesophageal junction. In contrast, upper and middle esophageal injuries, which require access to the thoracic cavity, are often inaccessible through a laparoscopic approach due to their anatomical location and the risks associated with reaching them through the abdomen. Moreover, cases with extensive damage or significant contamination are generally managed via open surgery, as this allows for more comprehensive debridement and repair [7]. The choice to use laparoscopy is thus contingent on several factors, including the patient's stability, the injury's location, and the surgeon's experience with minimally invasive techniques for thoracoabdominal injuries.

Laparoscopy offers several potential benefits when used in the appropriate trauma cases [8]. Minimally invasive techniques allow surgeons to access the injury site with less trauma to surrounding tissues, reducing the risk of respiratory complications and other postoperative issues that are common after thoracotomy or laparotomy. For patients, this means a shorter recovery period, reduced pain, and faster mobilization, often leading to shorter hospital stays. Additionally, laparoscopic techniques minimize the risk of infection, particularly in cases where the injury is small and contained. By avoiding large incisions, the chances of wound infection and surgical site complications are significantly reduced, which is particularly beneficial for trauma patients who may already be in a weakened or compromised state [8].

However, laparoscopy in esophageal trauma is not without limitations. The steep learning curve for complex laparoscopic procedures, coupled with the anatomical challenges presented by the esophagus's location, makes this approach challenging. Furthermore, unlike routine elective laparoscopic procedures, esophageal trauma cases require rapid decision-making, as delays in treatment can have serious consequences. For this reason, surgeons who attempt laparoscopic management of esophageal injuries must possess advanced skills and experience in both trauma surgery and minimally invasive techniques. Additionally, the technology and specialized instruments required for effective laparoscopic repair of esophageal injuries may not be available in all trauma centers, particularly those in low-resource settings.

Despite these challenges, the role of laparoscopy in esophageal injuries is likely to expand as technology and techniques continue to advance. Innovations such as high-definition imaging, robotic assistance, and improved surgical instruments are making it possible to conduct more complex repairs laparoscopically, even in hard-to-reach areas. Fluorescence imaging, for example, offers enhanced visualization, allowing surgeons to identify tissue damage and contamination more effectively, which could be invaluable in managing subtle or partial esophageal injuries. Robotic systems, though still costly and primarily available in well-funded hospitals, provide enhanced dexterity and control, making it easier to navigate the delicate structures surrounding the esophagus. As these technologies become more accessible, they hold the potential to make laparoscopic management of esophageal injuries more feasible in a broader range of cases.

In summary, laparoscopy in esophageal trauma is an emerging approach that offers a minimally invasive alternative to traditional open surgery for select patients. While it is not suitable for all cases, when applied appropriately, laparoscopy can reduce recovery times, lower the risk of complications, and improve patient outcomes. The decision to use laparoscopy requires careful evaluation of the injury, the patient's stability, and the available resources. As techniques and technologies continue to improve, laparoscopy is likely to play an increasingly important role in esophageal trauma management, paving the way for safer, more efficient care for these complex and high-risk injuries.

Indications for Laparoscopy in Esophageal Injuries

The decision to use laparoscopy in cases of esophageal injury is guided by a series of specific clinical indications and considerations. Given the delicate and complex anatomy of the esophagus and its proximity to vital structures, any intervention must be carefully planned. The primary goals of laparoscopy in esophageal trauma are twofold: accurate diagnosis and, where feasible, therapeutic management. While not every esophageal injury can or should be managed laparoscopically, certain indications provide a clear rationale for its use. These indications largely depend on the location of the injury, the patient's stability, the extent of contamination or perforation, and the overall experience of the surgical team with advanced laparoscopic techniques.

Hemodynamically Unstable Patients

A cornerstone of laparoscopic management in trauma surgery, including esophageal trauma, is the hemodynamic stability of the patient [9]. Laparoscopy requires a carefully controlled environment and typically takes longer to initiate compared to an open thoracotomy or laparotomy, making it suitable primarily for stable patients. Hemodynamically unstable patients with significant blood loss or shock may not tolerate the insufflation and increased intra-abdominal pressure that laparoscopy requires, and the time required to establish a laparoscopic view may delay necessary interventions. Therefore, laparoscopic exploration and repair are most appropriate in hemodynamically stable patients where the urgency is high but does not demand immediate open access. In these cases, laparoscopy provides a less invasive route for exploration and intervention, thereby reducing morbidity without compromising patient safety.

Injuries to the Lower Esophagus and Gastroesophageal Junction

One of the most important indications for laparoscopy in esophageal trauma is an injury located in the lower third of the esophagus, particularly near the gastroesophageal junction (GEJ). The lower esophagus is anatomically accessible through the abdominal cavity, making it easier for laparoscopic instruments to reach and visualize. Injuries at this site can often be identified, assessed, and managed laparoscopically, provided they are contained or limited in scope. This access point near the GEJ is particularly advantageous in cases where injuries are suspected to involve the stomach or proximal stomach as well, as laparoscopic techniques can facilitate the inspection of both structures in a single operation.

For example, lower esophageal perforations due to penetrating trauma, iatrogenic injury, or blunt trauma resulting in esophageal tearing may be addressed laparoscopically. By avoiding an open thoracotomy or laparotomy, which can be associated with high rates of respiratory complications and prolonged recovery, laparoscopy allows for a targeted approach that minimizes trauma to surrounding tissues. Injuries in this location can be inspected laparoscopically to determine the exact extent of perforation or laceration, after which a variety of repair techniques can be applied, including primary suturing and reinforcement with tissue flaps.

Small, Contained Perforations

Contained perforations—those where there is a limited leak of esophageal contents into a confined area without free contamination—are among the most suitable cases for laparoscopic intervention. In these scenarios, the esophageal injury is often localized, with minimal contamination of the surrounding structures, allowing for a focused, minimally invasive approach. Laparoscopic inspection enables the surgeon to assess the extent of the injury accurately and to perform a primary repair, reinforced, if necessary, with surrounding tissue or biologic sealants.

Contained perforations are particularly amenable to laparoscopic repair because they involve a relatively well-defined defect with minimal risk of widespread contamination. By intervening laparoscopically, surgeons can effectively drain localized abscesses, close small perforations, and prevent the development of more severe complications, such as mediastinitis or sepsis. Laparoscopy also allows for immediate lavage of any minor contamination within the abdominal cavity, further reducing the risk of infection.

Foreign Body Removal

In cases of esophageal trauma caused by foreign body penetration, such as knife wounds or ingested sharp objects, laparoscopy offers a valuable approach for localized inspection and removal. The lower esophagus and gastroesophageal junction are common sites for impacted foreign bodies due to the narrowing of the lumen and the sharp angle at the esophagogastric junction. For penetrating injuries where foreign bodies remain embedded in or near the esophageal wall, laparoscopy provides a direct visual path to locate and extract these objects.

Laparoscopy for foreign body removal is especially beneficial because it minimizes the risk of further damage to surrounding tissues, which is particularly crucial when removing sharp objects. The ability to perform controlled, minimally invasive retrieval reduces the need for open thoracic or abdominal surgery and enables the surgeon to avoid additional trauma to the patient's respiratory or cardiovascular systems. For stable patients, laparoscopic foreign body removal is both safe and effective, offering reduced recovery times and a lower risk of postoperative complications.

Diagnostic Exploration in Cases with Unclear Imaging

In cases where imaging is inconclusive, but an esophageal injury is suspected, laparoscopy serves as an essential diagnostic tool. Initial imaging techniques like CT scans or endoscopy may not fully reveal the extent or presence of an esophageal injury, especially in cases involving blunt trauma or indirect mechanisms of injury. A minimally invasive laparoscopic approach can offer direct visualization of the lower esophagus and surrounding structures, allowing for a definitive diagnosis without the need for a fully open surgical approach.

This diagnostic application is particularly valuable in patients with ambiguous symptoms, such as localized pain or dysphagia, where imaging does not indicate a perforation or other injury. Laparoscopy enables the surgical team to inspect the esophagus in real time and assess for subtle signs of injury, such as minor perforations or hematomas that might otherwise go undetected. By providing a direct view, laparoscopy reduces the risk of missed injuries and avoids the morbidity associated with unnecessary exploratory thoracotomies or laparotomies.

Minimal Extravasation and Low-Grade Contamination

Another indication for laparoscopic management is when minimal extravasation of esophageal contents is present, accompanied by low-grade contamination. In cases where a perforation has not led to widespread contamination of the thoracoabdominal cavity, laparoscopic repair is feasible and often preferable. Low-grade contamination typically results in confined areas of fluid collection rather than large abscesses or diffuse peritonitis. In these cases, laparoscopy allows for precise repair and drainage without the need for a full open procedure.

By containing the injury to a smaller area, the surgeon can control the leak through direct closure or reinforcement, reducing the likelihood of infection and promoting faster healing. This approach limits postoperative morbidity while effectively managing the injury with a targeted intervention. Laparoscopy is well-suited for these injuries, as it allows for selective irrigation of the contaminated area, drainage of localized collections, and primary repair of the esophageal wall.

Contraindications and Limitations of Laparoscopy in Esophageal Injuries

While laparoscopy presents an effective, minimally invasive alternative for managing certain esophageal injuries, it is not universally applicable. Due to the unique challenges posed by esophageal anatomy and the potential for rapid deterioration in esophageal trauma patients, the indications for laparoscopic intervention must be carefully weighed. This section discusses the primary contraindications and limitations associated with laparoscopy in esophageal trauma cases, focusing on hemodynamic stability, injury location, extensive contamination, technical challenges, and resource constraints.

Hemodynamic Instability

One of the most important contraindications for laparoscopy in esophageal trauma is patient hemodynamic instability. Patients with signs of shock, significant blood loss, or rapid deterioration are not suitable candidates for laparoscopy, as the procedure requires time and preparation, which may delay necessary interventions. Furthermore, laparoscopy requires pneumoperitoneum, the inflation of the abdominal cavity with carbon dioxide gas to create working space, which increases intra-abdominal pressure. This increased pressure can impair venous return, exacerbate hypotension, and worsen the patient's hemodynamic status. In such cases, open surgery via thoracotomy or laparotomy is typically favored, as it allows rapid, direct access to the injury, facilitating immediate control of bleeding and repair.

In trauma care, rapid intervention is critical, and time delays can significantly affect outcomes. Laparoscopy is therefore contraindicated in patients who are unstable or in shock, as these patients are likely to benefit more from a traditional open approach, where direct access to the esophagus and surrounding structures can be achieved quickly and without the additional physiological stress of pneumoperitoneum.

Injuries to the Upper and Mid-Esophagus

The anatomical position of the upper and mid-esophagus makes it difficult to access through the abdomen, posing a significant limitation to laparoscopic approaches. Injuries to the upper and mid-esophagus often require a thoracic approach to visualize and treat effectively, as the esophagus is surrounded by complex and dense structures in the chest, including the trachea, aorta, and large blood vessels. Laparoscopy, which accesses the esophagus from the abdominal cavity, is generally only feasible for injuries in the lower third of the esophagus near the gastroesophageal junction.

For injuries in the upper or mid-esophagus, thoracoscopy (a minimally invasive approach through the chest) or open thoracotomy is typically preferred. These approaches provide direct access to the injured area without the technical challenges and limitations posed by abdominal laparoscopy [10]. Attempting to address upper or mid-esophageal injuries laparoscopically is associated with high risk and poor visualization and is generally avoided due to the potential for complications.

Extensive or Uncontained Perforations

The extent of the esophageal injury significantly influences the choice of approach. In cases of large, uncontained perforations, where esophageal contents have freely contaminated the surrounding thoracoabdominal cavity, open surgery is often necessary. Extensive contamination requires thorough debridement, drainage, and repair to prevent severe complications such as mediastinitis, abscess formation, or sepsis. Attempting to manage extensive contamination laparoscopically can be inadequate, as laparoscopy may not allow for complete control over the contamination, and the precision needed to repair large perforations may be challenging to achieve.

In such cases, an open approach via thoracotomy or laparotomy allows for comprehensive cleaning, debridement of necrotic tissue, and effective drainage of abscesses. While laparoscopy is valuable in contained perforations with limited leakage, the high-risk nature of uncontained injuries makes open surgery the preferred method for ensuring optimal outcomes in severe esophageal trauma cases.

Limited Visualization in Active Bleeding

Active, significant bleeding within the thoracic or abdominal cavity presents another limitation to the use of laparoscopy. Blood in the operative field can obstruct the laparoscopic view, making it challenging to locate and manage the injury precisely. This limitation is particularly significant in esophageal injuries, as the dense vascular network surrounding the esophagus can lead to rapid bleeding, especially in penetrating injuries.

In scenarios with substantial bleeding, laparotomy or thoracotomy allows for quicker and more extensive exposure, facilitating direct control of bleeding sources. Attempting to manage significant hemorrhage laparoscopically is often impractical and may lead to delays in hemostasis, increasing the patient's risk of complications. Therefore, open surgery remains the standard in trauma cases with active bleeding that impairs the laparoscopic view.

Patient-Specific Factors

Patient-specific factors such as body habitus and prior abdominal or thoracic surgeries, and underlying health conditions can further limit the feasibility of laparoscopy. For instance:

- *Obesity*: Patients with significant abdominal adiposity may pose technical challenges for laparoscopy, as increased body fat can limit instrument reach and visibility. Access to the esophagus may be particularly difficult in these patients, reducing the efficacy of the laparoscopic approach [11, 12].
- *Previous surgeries*: Patients with a history of abdominal or thoracic surgeries may have extensive adhesions, which can complicate laparoscopic access and increase the risk of inadvertent injury to surrounding structures. Open surgery often allows for better control in these cases, especially when adhesions prevent adequate visualization.
- *Underlying health conditions*: Certain comorbidities, such as severe cardiovascular or pulmonary disease, may render patients unsuitable for the physiologic demands of laparoscopy, including increased intra-abdominal pressure. These patients may not tolerate pneumoperitoneum well, and open surgery is often preferred to avoid additional strain.

Resource and Expertise Constraints

Finally, the successful application of laparoscopy in esophageal trauma requires advanced skills and specific resources, which may not be available in all trauma centers, especially in low-resource settings. Trauma laparoscopy for esophageal injuries demands experience with advanced laparoscopic suturing, precise tissue handling, and complex decision-making skills that require extensive training. Centers lacking trained personnel or specialized equipment may face limitations in safely conducting laparoscopic repairs. In such settings, an open approach may be safer and more efficient, allowing surgeons to maximize patient outcomes without the risk of inadequate repair due to limited resources.

Anatomical Considerations in Laparoscopic Management of Esophageal Injuries

Laparoscopic management of esophageal injuries presents distinct challenges due to the complex anatomy of the esophagus and its proximity to critical structures. The esophagus is a long, muscular tube located within the thorax and abdomen, positioned posteriorly and surrounded by important organs, vessels, and other structures that require careful navigation and protection. Effective laparoscopic management of esophageal trauma requires a thorough understanding of these anatomical intricacies, especially as they pertain to the different regions of the esophagus and adjacent areas that may impact surgical access, visualization, and repair.

Regional Anatomy of the Esophagus

The esophagus is typically divided into three regions: the upper, middle, and lower thirds. Each region presents specific anatomical considerations that influence the approach to laparoscopic management:

- *Upper esophagus*: Located in the cervical region, this section lies close to the trachea and thyroid gland and is generally managed with open or transcervical approaches rather than laparoscopy due to its high position and proximity to dense vascular structures.
- *Middle esophagus*: The middle third of the esophagus lies within the chest cavity, positioned behind the heart and between the trachea and spine. Accessing this region requires a transthoracic approach in most cases, as it is difficult to reach from the abdominal cavity.
- *Lower esophagus*: The lower third of the esophagus, which extends through the diaphragm and meets the stomach at the gastroesophageal junction (GEJ), is the most accessible portion for laparoscopy. This section lies close to the diaphragm, liver, and gastric cardia, making it ideal for abdominal laparoscopic approaches.

For these reasons, laparoscopy is generally reserved for injuries in this lower section, where surgical access and visualization are feasible.

Gastroesophageal Junction (GEJ)

The gastroesophageal junction is a key focus in the laparoscopic management of esophageal injuries due to its anatomical accessibility from the abdominal cavity. Located just below the diaphragm, the GEJ is a natural point of transition between the esophagus and the stomach, making it an ideal entry point for laparoscopic access in trauma cases involving the lower esophagus. The GEJ is bordered by the lower esophageal sphincter (LES) and surrounded by the diaphragm's crural fibers, which form a protective barrier around this area.

To access the GEJ laparoscopically, surgeons often begin by dissecting the gastrohepatic ligament, a membranous structure connecting the stomach to the liver, which allows for improved visualization of the lower esophagus and proximal stomach. This dissection helps expose the area around the GEJ, providing better access for inspection, repair, or foreign body removal.

Hiatal Anatomy and Diaphragm

The diaphragm, specifically its hiatal opening, is a key anatomical consideration in accessing the lower esophagus laparoscopically. The esophageal hiatus is an opening in the diaphragm through which the esophagus passes before joining the stomach. It is bordered by the right and left crura of the diaphragm, which provide structural support to the lower esophagus. Understanding the diaphragmatic anatomy is crucial, as the crura can limit laparoscopic access to the esophagus and may require mobilization to achieve adequate exposure of the injury site.

In trauma cases, particularly those with blunt force or high-velocity penetrating injuries, the diaphragm may be injured alongside the esophagus. This dual injury requires careful attention during laparoscopic procedures, as repairing both structures simultaneously can be challenging. Additionally, laparoscopic manipulation of the esophagus near the diaphragm must be conducted carefully to avoid damaging the phrenic nerve, which runs along the lateral edge of the diaphragm and is responsible for diaphragmatic movement.

Proximity to Major Vascular Structures

The esophagus is closely situated to several major blood vessels, which can pose significant risks during laparoscopic intervention. In the thoracic region, the esophagus lies near the aorta, azygos vein, and inferior vena cava, making surgical dissection in this area complex and requiring precise control to avoid vascular injury. In laparoscopic management of the lower esophagus, care must be taken to avoid the celiac trunk, splenic artery, and left gastric artery, which supplies the stomach and spleen.

The left gastric artery is of particular concern in lower esophageal injuries, as it runs in proximity to the GEJ. During laparoscopy, inadvertent damage to this artery can lead to significant bleeding, complicating the procedure and increasing the risk of postoperative complications. Surgeons must remain vigilant and work carefully around these vessels to prevent unnecessary bleeding while maintaining clear visualization of the injury site.

Surrounding Organs: Liver, Stomach, and Spleen

The lower esophagus is flanked by several vital organs, including the liver, stomach, and spleen, all of which require careful handling during laparoscopic procedures. The left lobe of the liver can obstruct the view of the lower esophagus and may need to be gently retracted or mobilized to provide adequate exposure. Specialized retractors are often used laparoscopically to achieve this without causing liver injury.

The stomach, located just below the lower esophagus, is another essential consideration. In cases of perforation near the GEJ, contamination may spread into the stomach and upper abdomen, requiring inspection and cleaning to prevent infection. Laparoscopic tools and suction devices allow for thorough lavage of the area to address any contamination and ensure a clean operative field. Additionally, the spleen, positioned to the left of the stomach, must be avoided during dissection and manipulation, as it is highly vascular and prone to bleeding.

Challenges of Laparoscopic Visualization and Access

The anatomical constraints of the esophagus and its location in the posterior thorax and upper abdomen can make visualization challenging. Laparoscopy offers excellent magnification, but accessing deep structures in this confined space often requires strategic port placement and angled instruments. The need for specific instruments, such as flexible laparoscopic staplers and suction devices, is heightened when working with the esophagus due to its proximity to sensitive structures and limited maneuvering room.

Techniques and Procedural Nuances in Laparoscopic Management of Esophageal Injuries

Laparoscopic management of esophageal injuries requires a range of specialized techniques and meticulous attention to detail, as the anatomy and potential complications associated with esophageal trauma can make even minor missteps impactful. Effective laparoscopic management relies on precise port placement, careful diagnostic evaluation, adept tissue handling, and, when necessary, advanced repair techniques. Below, we explore the essential techniques and procedural nuances that enable successful laparoscopic intervention for esophageal injuries.

Access and Port Placement

Port placement is a critical factor in the success of laparoscopic procedures for esophageal injuries, as it directly affects the surgeon's ability to visualize and maneuver instruments. Standard port placement often involves a camera port near the umbilicus and additional working ports strategically located based on the location and nature of the injury [13].

For injuries in the lower esophagus and gastroesophageal junction (GEJ), a typical setup includes the primary camera port at or just below the umbilicus, along with two or three working ports in the left and right upper quadrants. This positioning allows optimal access to the distal esophagus and surrounding structures, enabling the surgeon to manipulate instruments without interference. In cases where additional exposure is needed, a fourth port may be placed to retract the liver or other nearby tissues, improving visibility and access to the GEJ. Port placement can be adjusted as needed to accommodate variations in patient anatomy, injury location, or the presence of adhesions.

Establishing Pneumoperitoneum

Creating pneumoperitoneum or insufflating the abdomen with carbon dioxide gas to create working space is an essential step in laparoscopic esophageal surgery. In trauma patients, the insufflation rate and intra-abdominal pressure require careful management, as excessive pressure can adversely affect hemodynamic stability and respiratory function. Typically, an intra-abdominal pressure of 12–15 mmHg is used, balancing sufficient space for visualization while avoiding undue physiological stress.

The pneumoperitoneum not only provides room for instrument manipulation but also helps displace abdominal organs, such as the intestines and stomach, away from the surgical field, enhancing visibility. For esophageal injuries specifically, it is important to monitor the patient's response to insufflation, as some patients with associated injuries or coexisting health conditions may experience difficulties in maintaining stable blood pressure or oxygenation under these conditions.

Diagnostic Exploration and Injury Assessment

Once the pneumoperitoneum is established, the surgeon conducts a thorough diagnostic exploration of the abdominal cavity, beginning with an inspection of the lower esophagus, stomach, and adjacent structures. This initial exploration helps identify the exact location, extent, and type of injury, which are critical factors in determining the appropriate treatment strategy. For esophageal injuries, assessing the injury site involves looking for signs of perforation, such as visible tears, bleeding, or leakage of gastric contents, and examining the extent of contamination in the surrounding areas.

In addition to visual inspection, techniques like gentle probing with atraumatic instruments can help assess tissue stability and injury depth. If contamination is localized, laparoscopy provides a minimally invasive means to manage it through irrigation and suction, effectively containing the spread of infectious material. Diagnostic laparoscopy allows the surgical team to decide whether laparoscopic repair is feasible or if conversion to open surgery is required based on the injury's complexity.

Primary Repair Techniques

For contained perforations or small tears, primary repair is often feasible laparoscopically. The repair typically involves suturing the perforation using fine, non-absorbable sutures to ensure a secure closure. In most cases, a two-layer closure technique is employed: an inner layer for the mucosa and submucosa, followed by an outer layer to reinforce the muscularis. This dual-layer approach helps create a watertight seal, reducing the risk of leaks and promoting better healing outcomes [14].

The laparoscopic suturing of the esophagus can be challenging due to the esophageal wall's thinness and proximity to surrounding structures. Surgeons use specific suturing techniques, such as intracorporeal knot tying or stapling devices, to ensure accurate closure while minimizing tissue trauma. Staplers are particularly useful in laparoscopic repairs as they allow for quick, consistent closure of the defect, especially in hard-to-reach areas. However, staplers must be used cautiously, as the tissue may be friable, especially if the injury was caused by chemical ingestion or prolonged inflammation.

Reinforcement with Tissue Flaps or Sealants

In cases where the esophageal repair site is at high risk for leakage; reinforcement with biological tissue or synthetic sealants can provide additional protection. The omentum, a fatty layer of tissue that drapes over the abdominal organs, is often mobilized and placed over the repair site to bolster it. Known as an omental patch or "omental wrap," this technique provides a vascularized tissue layer over the repair, enhancing healing and reducing the likelihood of postoperative leaks [15].

Additionally, tissue sealants such as fibrin glue can be applied over the sutured repair as an added measure to prevent leakage. These sealants create a barrier that supports the closure, particularly in cases where the tissue quality is compromised, or the defect is irregularly shaped. Using tissue reinforcements and sealants is a key step in preventing complications, especially in patients at higher risk of postoperative complications due to their injury mechanism or comorbidities.

Management of Contamination and Drainage

In esophageal trauma cases with contamination, effective management is crucial to prevent infection and further complications. Laparoscopy allows for efficient peritoneal lavage, during which sterile saline is used to irrigate the contaminated area and clear away any leaked esophageal or gastric contents. Laparoscopic suction devices are used to remove contaminated fluid, while precision instruments help minimize tissue handling to avoid spreading contaminants [16].

Once contamination has been managed, placing drains near the repair site or in areas at risk for fluid collection helps monitor for leaks and manage any residual infection. Drains provide an outlet for fluids and can be monitored in the postoperative period for early signs of leakage or abscess formation, allowing for prompt intervention if needed. Drains are typically left in place for several days, depending on the extent of the injury and the amount of contamination present.

Conversion to Open Surgery

Despite the advantages of laparoscopy, some cases may require conversion to open surgery. If the injury is more extensive than initially anticipated, if significant bleeding impairs visibility, or if laparoscopy fails to control contamination effectively, a rapid decision to convert to thoracotomy or laparotomy is made. Converting to an open approach allows the surgeon to manage complex injuries comprehensively, reducing the risk of further complications associated with prolonged laparoscopic attempts.

Conversion is not a failure but a necessary choice in many cases, prioritizing patient safety and ensuring a definitive solution to the injury.

Comparative Efficacy: Laparoscopy Versus Open Surgery for Esophageal Injuries

The management of esophageal injuries has historically relied on open surgery due to the complex anatomy and critical nature of the structures surrounding the esophagus. However, with advancements in minimally invasive techniques, laparoscopy has become a viable alternative for specific cases, offering the potential for reduced morbidity and shorter recovery times. The choice between laparoscopy and open surgery—whether thoracotomy or laparotomy—depends on various factors, including patient stability, injury location, contamination extent, and surgical expertise. This section examines the comparative efficacy of both approaches in terms of patient outcomes, recovery times, risks, and overall effectiveness in treating esophageal injuries.

Advantages of Laparoscopy

Laparoscopy offers several distinct advantages when applied to esophageal injuries, particularly in hemodynamically stable patients with injuries localized to the lower esophagus or gastroesophageal junction (GEJ). The minimally invasive nature of laparoscopy, with its small incisions and limited tissue disruption, results in reduced postoperative pain, lower infection rates, faster recovery, and shorter hospital stays compared to open surgery. Studies have shown that the smaller incisions used in laparoscopy lead to decreased inflammatory responses, which are particularly beneficial in trauma patients who may already be in a compromised state. Furthermore, the risk of wound infection and other postoperative complications is lower in laparoscopic procedures, as there is less exposure of internal tissues to external contaminants.

Laparoscopy is especially useful in cases where the esophageal injury is small, contained, or localized near the GEJ. For example, a small perforation resulting from blunt trauma or iatrogenic injury (such as from endoscopic procedures) can often be managed laparoscopically with minimal risk. In these cases, laparoscopy allows for direct visualization of the injury, immediate assessment of the surrounding area for contamination, and rapid repair without the need for large incisions. For trauma patients, the faster recovery associated with laparoscopy means that they can resume normal activities sooner, which is particularly beneficial in those who may have multiple injuries requiring longer-term rehabilitation.

The use of laparoscopy also enables a more precise diagnostic evaluation. In cases where imaging results are inconclusive, laparoscopy provides direct visualization of the esophagus and surrounding tissues, allowing the surgeon to confirm the location and extent of the injury. This diagnostic utility can reduce the incidence of unnecessary exploratory thoracotomies or laparotomies, sparing patients from the risks associated with open surgery.

Advantages of Open Surgery

Despite the benefits of laparoscopy, open surgery—thoracotomy or laparotomy—remains the gold standard for managing complex or extensive esophageal injuries. Open surgery provides superior access to the esophagus and surrounding structures, making it ideal for injuries in the upper or middle esophagus, which are difficult to reach laparoscopically. Thoracotomy, for instance, allows for direct access to the thoracic esophagus and adjacent areas, including the trachea, aorta, and major vessels, enabling comprehensive management of injuries in this challenging anatomical region. Open surgery is particularly valuable in cases of severe trauma with extensive perforations, active bleeding, or widespread contamination from esophageal contents.

Large, uncontained esophageal perforations present a high risk of mediastinitis and sepsis, which require aggressive debridement and drainage that may not be achievable laparoscopically. Open approaches allow the surgeon to thoroughly clean and debride contaminated areas, perform a secure, multi-layered closure, and place drains in appropriate locations to prevent fluid accumulation and abscess formation. This comprehensive approach reduces the likelihood of postoperative infection and improves outcomes in high-risk patients.

Additionally, open surgery provides an advantage in hemodynamically unstable patients. In situations where time is critical—such as in cases of uncontrolled bleeding or rapidly spreading infection—thoracotomy or laparotomy allows for immediate control of the injury, minimizing delays associated with laparoscopic setup and pneumoperitoneum. Open access also facilitates vascular control if there is damage to major vessels near the esophagus, reducing the risk of further hemorrhage and stabilizing the patient more effectively.

Patient Outcomes and Recovery Times

Comparative studies on laparoscopy versus open surgery in esophageal trauma show that outcomes can vary widely based on injury severity and patient condition. In cases where laparoscopy is feasible, patients often experience significantly shorter recovery times and fewer complications. Recovery benefits include reduced pain, minimized postoperative scarring, and quicker return to normal activities. Studies indicate that patients who undergo laparoscopic repair typically spend less time in the intensive care unit (ICU) and have shorter overall hospital stays, reflecting the reduced invasiveness of the procedure.

On the other hand, patients with severe or complex injuries who undergo open surgery may face longer recovery periods due to the extensive nature of the procedure. However, in these cases, the more comprehensive approach of open surgery is often necessary to ensure a complete repair and adequate management of contamination. Although open surgery is associated with higher morbidity and longer hospital stays, it provides a safer and more effective option for patients with severe esophageal trauma, improving survival rates in cases that might be challenging to manage laparoscopically.

Risk of Postoperative Complications

Postoperative complications are a major consideration in choosing between laparoscopy and open surgery for esophageal injuries. Laparoscopy's smaller incisions and reduced tissue handling lower the risk of wound infections, respiratory complications, and other common postoperative issues associated with thoracotomy or laparotomy. In patients who undergo laparoscopic management, the risk of pulmonary complications, such as pneumonia and respiratory distress, is generally lower, as the procedure avoids the rib spreading and muscle damage that can impact respiratory function in thoracic surgery.

Conversely, open surgery carries a higher risk of complications, including infection, pulmonary issues, and prolonged postoperative pain. Thoracotomy can lead to chronic pain and a range of respiratory complications due to the extensive dissection required to access the esophagus. However, despite these risks, open surgery's thorough approach provides the best option for addressing complex injuries that might otherwise result in life-threatening complications if managed laparoscopically.

Limitations of Laparoscopy and Open Surgery

While laparoscopy offers several advantages, it has limitations in complex esophageal trauma cases. Laparoscopic techniques are limited to patients with contained injuries and stable hemodynamic status, as extensive contamination and active bleeding pose challenges to the confined, indirect view provided by laparoscopy. Furthermore, laparoscopic repairs require advanced surgical skills, and not all trauma centers have the expertise or resources necessary for successful laparoscopic intervention in complex esophageal injuries.

Open surgery, while highly effective for severe injuries, is limited by its invasiveness, which can result in significant morbidity, longer recovery times, and a higher incidence of complications. In cases where a less invasive approach is feasible, the drawbacks of open surgery can outweigh its benefits, making it a less desirable option for minor or localized injuries.

Future Trends and Technological Advances in Laparoscopy for Esophageal Injuries

The management of esophageal injuries through laparoscopy is evolving rapidly, driven by technological advancements and innovative approaches that aim to improve visualization, precision, and patient outcomes. With improvements in minimally invasive surgical techniques and tools, laparoscopy is expanding beyond diagnostic uses to include therapeutic interventions for increasingly complex esophageal injuries. The future of laparoscopy in esophageal trauma management is shaped by developments in imaging, robotics, artificial intelligence (AI), augmented reality (AR), and enhanced tissue-repair materials, which collectively promise to make these procedures safer, faster, and more effective.

Enhanced Imaging and Fluorescence-Guided Surgery

Advanced imaging techniques are a significant area of development in laparoscopy, particularly for esophageal injuries where precision is crucial. Fluorescence-guided laparoscopy, using agents like indocyanine green (ICG), can illuminate blood vessels, identify tissue perfusion, and highlight areas of ischemia or injury. This approach helps surgeons better visualize subtle injuries and confirm the viability of surrounding tissues, reducing the risk of missed injuries and ensuring that the repair is performed on healthy tissue. In cases of trauma with contamination or bleeding, fluorescence-guided imaging provides valuable information on the extent of injury, making it easier to differentiate between viable and non-viable tissue.

High-definition (HD) cameras with 3D visualization capabilities are also being incorporated into laparoscopic setups, offering surgeons a more realistic and spatially accurate view of the esophagus and adjacent structures. This enhanced visualization allows for more accurate assessment and repair, which is especially beneficial when working within the complex anatomy of the esophagus.

Robotic-Assisted Laparoscopy

Robotic-assisted laparoscopic systems are gradually entering the field of esophageal surgery and bringing advanced dexterity, precision, and control to the procedure. Robotic systems, such as the da Vinci Surgical System, allow surgeons to manipulate instruments with greater accuracy, especially in confined areas or near delicate structures, such as the aorta and trachea, that are difficult to navigate with traditional laparoscopic tools. Robotic arms with wristed motion enable more complex suturing and tissue manipulation, which can improve the quality of repairs in esophageal trauma cases.

Although robotic systems remain costly and are primarily available in high-resource settings, they are becoming more accessible as technology advances and costs decrease. Future developments in robotics may allow for smaller, more portable systems that can be integrated into standard operating rooms, potentially expanding the use of robotic-assisted laparoscopy for esophageal injuries in a broader range of hospitals.

Artificial Intelligence (AI) and Decision-Support Systems

Artificial intelligence (AI) has the potential to transform the laparoscopic management of esophageal injuries by enhancing diagnostic accuracy and supporting clinical decision-making. Machine learning algorithms trained on large datasets of esophageal trauma cases can analyze real-time patient data and imaging results to provide surgeons with recommendations for treatment plans and predict the likelihood of specific complications. For instance, AI could help identify subtle signs of perforation or suggest optimal suturing patterns based on tissue thickness and elasticity, optimizing repair quality.

Furthermore, AI-powered decision-support systems could help surgeons assess the suitability of laparoscopy versus open surgery by evaluating patient factors such as hemodynamic stability, injury severity, and anticipated recovery times. These systems could provide real-time feedback, improving outcomes by guiding surgeons toward the most appropriate approach for each case.

Augmented Reality (AR) in Laparoscopy

Augmented reality (AR) is another emerging technology that could greatly benefit laparoscopic surgery for esophageal injuries. By overlaying real-time imaging data onto the surgical field, AR provides surgeons with enhanced visualization of hidden structures, such as blood vessels and nerves, reducing the risk of accidental damage. In esophageal trauma cases, where the anatomy is complex, and precision is critical, AR can help navigate around sensitive structures and optimize repair accuracy.

AR could also be integrated with preoperative imaging data, such as CT scans, to create a "roadmap" of the injury and surrounding anatomy, helping surgeons visualize the exact location of the injury before making incisions. This level of guidance could minimize the need for extensive exploration, reducing operative time and potential tissue trauma and ultimately contributing to faster recovery.

Advanced Tissue-Sealing and Repair Materials

New developments in tissue-sealing agents and biomaterials are providing additional tools for laparoscopic esophageal repair. Traditional sutures and staples are effective but can be challenging to use in fragile esophageal tissue, especially in inflamed or contaminated areas. New tissue adhesives and sealants, such as fibrin glues, are now available and can be applied laparoscopically to reinforce sutures or close small perforations. These agents provide a waterproof seal over the repaired area, reducing the risk of leaks and promoting faster healing.

Additionally, biological and synthetic graft materials, such as acellular dermal matrices, are being studied as reinforcement patches for esophageal repairs. These materials provide structural support while promoting tissue integration, making them particularly useful for large defects or areas at risk of dehiscence. In the future, advancements in bioengineered materials may enable the use of "smart" grafts that release healing-promoting agents or adapt to the surrounding tissue environment, further enhancing repair durability.

Conclusion

Laparoscopy is emerging as a valuable tool in the management of esophageal injuries, especially for cases involving the lower esophagus and gastroesophageal junction, where minimally invasive approaches offer significant benefits. Compared to traditional open surgery, laparoscopy offers advantages such as reduced postoperative pain, lower infection risk, shorter recovery times, and decreased hospital stays. These outcomes are particularly advantageous for trauma patients, who often face prolonged rehabilitation. By minimizing surgical trauma, laparoscopy also reduces the risk of respiratory complications, wound infections, and other morbidities associated with open thoracotomy or laparotomy.

Despite its benefits, the application of laparoscopy in esophageal trauma remains limited to specific cases, such as stable patients with contained injuries and minimal contamination. Open surgery continues to be essential for managing complex or extensive injuries that require comprehensive access and control, especially in hemodynamically unstable patients or those with upper and middle esophageal injuries. However, as laparoscopy technology advances—through improved imaging, robotic assistance, and new tissue-sealing materials—the scope of its application is expanding, allowing it to be safely applied in more complex cases.

The future of laparoscopy in esophageal injury management is promising, as new technologies such as augmented reality, AI, and fluorescence imaging enhance precision and reduce risks. As more trauma centers adopt these innovations, laparoscopy is likely to play an even more central role, contributing to improved patient outcomes, shorter hospital stays, and enhanced overall recovery for esophageal trauma patients.

References

1. Biffl WL, Moore EE, Feliciano DV, Albrecht RA, Croce M, Karmy-Jones R, et al. Western trauma association critical decisions in trauma: diagnosis and management of esophageal injuries. J Trauma Acute Care Surg. 2015;79(6):1089–95.
2. Petrone P, Kassimi K, Jiménez-Gómez M, Betancourt A, Axelrad A, Marini CP. Management of esophageal injuries secondary to trauma. Injury. 2017;48(8):1735–42.
3. Oderda G. Challenges in the management of acute postsurgical pain. Pharmacotherapy. 2012;32(9pt2):6S–11S.
4. Grushka J, Ginzburg E. Through the 10-mm looking glass: advances in minimally invasive surgery in trauma. Scand J Surg. 2014;103(2):143–8.
5. Goettler CE, Bard MR, Toschlog EA. Laparoscopy in trauma. Curr Surg. 2004;61(6):554–9.
6. Paspatis GA, Arvanitakis M, Dumonceau J-M, Barthet M, Saunders B, Turino SY, et al. Diagnosis and management of iatrogenic endoscopic perforations: European Society of Gastrointestinal Endoscopy (ESGE) position statement–update 2020. Endoscopy. 2020;52(09):792–810.
7. Wu JT, Mattox KL, Wall MJ Jr. Esophageal perforations: new perspectives and treatment paradigms. J Trauma Acute Care Surg. 2007;63(5):1173–84.
8. O'Malley E, Boyle E, O'Callaghan A, Coffey JC, Walsh SR. Role of laparoscopy in penetrating abdominal trauma: a systematic review. World J Surg. 2013;37:113–22.
9. Smith RS, Fry WR, Morabito DJ, Koehler RH, Organ CH Jr. Therapeutic laparoscopy in trauma. Am J Surg. 1995;170(6):632–7.
10. Fabien JJ, McCranie D, Kington D, Dougherty-Welch S. Blunt traumatic esophageal injury: decreased mortality with urgent repair. Am Surg. 2022;88(9):2212–4.
11. Hoi H, Grünbart M, Paal P, de Cillia M, Hell T, Weiss H, et al. Surgeon and patient-specific factors influencing the decision for minimally invasive or open surgery in acute bowel obstruction: a retrospective single-center analysis. Langenbeck's Arch Surg. 2022;407(8):3747–54.
12. Hayden P, Cowman S. Anaesthesia for laparoscopic surgery. Cont Educ Anaesth Crit Care Pain. 2011;11(5):177–80.

13. Martin D, Bessell J, Chew A, Watson D. Thoracoscopic and laparoscopic esophagectomy: initial experience and outcomes. Surg Endosc Other Interv Tech. 2005;19:1597–601.
14. Eroğlu A, Can Kürkçüoğlu İ, Karaoğlanoğlu N, Tekinbaş C, Yımaz Ö, Başoğlu M. Esophageal perforation: the importance of early diagnosis and primary repair. Dis Esophagus. 2004;17(1):91–4.
15. Shaqran TM, Engineer R, Abdalla EM, Alamoudi AA, Almahdi R, Aldhahri A, et al. The management of Esophageal Perforation: a systematic review. Cureus. 2024;16(7):e63651.
16. Khaitan PG, Famiglietti A, Watson TJ. The etiology, diagnosis, and management of esophageal perforation. J Gastrointest Surg. 2022;26(12):2606–15.

Diaphragmatic Injuries: Diagnosis and Treatment

18

Sebastian Eduardo Velez and Natalia Karolina Alvarez

Introduction

The diaphragm is a musculo-tendinous structure that separates the thoracic and abdominal cavities and is the primary muscle used in breathing. It is asymmetrical, and its anatomical relationships with adjacent organs influence both the type of trauma and the associated injuries. Isolated diaphragmatic injuries are rare, often asymptomatic, and may only manifest years later as complicated hernias. Traditional diagnostic methods, such as chest X-rays and computed tomography, have low sensitivity, and clinical signs are frequently nonspecific or absent, making diagnosis challenging. In stable patients, minimally invasive techniques such as laparoscopy and thoracoscopy have shown high accuracy in detecting these injuries, and, in some cases, allow for their surgical repair with an optimal safety margin—avoiding the need for laparotomy and its associated complications [1–3].

History

Since 1579, when Ambroise Paré described a strangulated diaphragmatic hernia following a gunshot wound, key valuable advances have occurred in the management of these injuries [4]. In 1886, Riolfi performed the first successful

S. E. Velez (✉)
Department of Surgery, Hospital Municipal de Urgencias, Córdoba, Argentina

Emergencies, Trauma and Critical Care Surgeon, Department of Surgery, Hospital Municipal de Urgencias, Córdoba, Argentina
e-mail: sebastianevelez@unc.edu.ar

N. K. Alvarez
Emergencies, Trauma and Critical Care Surgeon, Department of Surgery, Hospital Municipal de Urgencias, Córdoba, Argentina

© The Author(s), under exclusive license to Springer Nature Switzerland AG 2026

M. Cezillo, B. M. Pereira (eds.), *Minimally Invasive Surgery Trauma*,
https://doi.org/10.1007/978-3-032-28971-1_18

diaphragmatic repair, followed by Neuman in 1888, who reduced a strangulated stomach [5]. In the 1990s, the development of computed tomography and laparoscopy revolutionized diagnosing and treating diaphragm wounds, establishing minimally invasive methods as the standard. Technological advances and surgical improvements have made it possible to avoid laparotomy and its complications [4, 5].

Embryology, Anatomy, and Physiology

The diaphragm is a muscle-tendinous structure between the thoracic and abdominal cavities (Fig. 18.1). Embryologically, it is made up of four components: the transverse septum, the pleuroperitoneal membranes, the dorsal mesentery of the esophagus, and the muscles of the abdominal wall, which together contribute to the definitive formation of the organ. During its development, the diaphragm descends from the cervical to the lumbar region, carrying the phrenic nerves, responsible for its motor innervation [5, 6].

The diaphragm is shaped like two domes, with the right dome being slightly higher than the left and is composed of a muscular part and a central tendinous region. It is divided into three main parts:

- Lumbar (pars lumbaris): It is the strongest portion, with insertions in the lumbar spine and the lumbocostal arches.
- Costal (pars costalis): Originates from the lower ribs and connects to the central tendon.

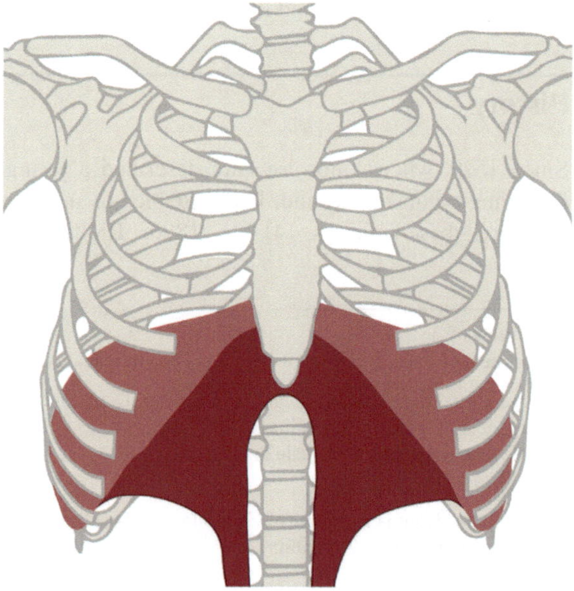

Fig. 18.1 Diaphragm location between the thorax and the abdomen

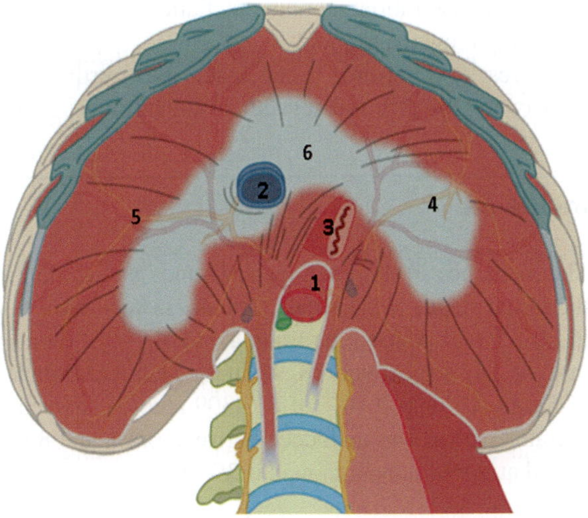

Fig. 18.2 Holes or diaphragmatic hiatus: 1. aortic hiatus (Aorta), 2. cava vein foramen (inferior vena cava), 3. esophageal hiatus (esophagus), 4. left phrenic nerve, 5. right phrenic nerve, 6. central tendon

- Sternal (pars sternalis): Is inserted into the posterior surface of the sternum.

The diaphragm has three main openings that allow the passage of vital structures [6] (Fig. 18.2):

1. Aortic hiatus: Admits the passage of the descending aorta, the thoracic duct, and occasionally, the azygos veins.
2. Foramen of the vena cava: Allows the passage of the inferior vena cava and the right phrenic nerve.
3. Esophageal hiatus: Surrounded by muscle fibers, it allows the passage of the esophagus and vagal trunks.

Anatomical Relationships

Above, the diaphragm is in contact with the lung, and with pericardium and heart in its middle region.
Below, it is related to the liver, kidneys, adrenal glands, spleen, stomach, and esophagus.

In the event of trauma, this anatomical arrangement predisposes to associated injuries and deserves special attention in the initial assessment [6].

Physiology

As the main muscle of inspiration, the diaphragm changes position depending on its state:

- During inspiration, it contracts, flattens, and moves the abdominal organs downward, below the xiphoid.
- At rest (expiration), it can reach the fourth costal cartilage on the right and between the fifth and seventh costal cartilages on the left [5, 6].

Incidence

The incidence of diaphragmatic wounds is uncertain, since many go unnoticed in the initial stages [4] (Ferrada Ordoñez). According to Feliciano et al. [7], it occurs in 10–15% of penetrating trauma and 1–7% of blunt trauma, with an approximate ratio of 2:1, respectively [8, 9]. In the National Data Bank of the American College of Surgeons, only 0.46% of 833,309 records showed diaphragm involvement. The literature reports an incidence between 0.8% and 8% [10]. In our region, it is estimated at 5.8%, mostly in men (83%) [11].

Mortality

Mortality ranges from 4% to 9% in cases of penetrating injuries and increases to between 15% and 24% for blunt diaphragm injuries [7].

Mortality may augment in cases of late presentation due to delays in diagnosis and the resulting clinical deterioration of the patient. *Murray* et al. [1] reported a mortality rate of 11% in a series of 28 patients, 50% of whom presented as emergencies requiring surgery.

Trauma Mechanism

Blunt Trauma

Under normal conditions, intrathoracic pressure is negative relative to atmospheric pressure, while intra-abdominal pressure is positive due to the presence of the viscera and the contraction of abdominal muscles [4]. When a severe abdominal trauma occurs, the pleuroperitoneal pressure gradient can reach up to +200 cm H_2O. Since the abdomen is a closed compartment, this pressure generates kinetic energy that impacts the diaphragmatic domes, causing muscle fiber rupture or detachment at fixation points [6].

On the right side, the liver absorbs much of the kinetic energy, reducing the pressure against the right hemidiaphragm and reducing the probability of ruptures. In contrast, the left hemidiaphragm is more vulnerable to injury, because it is cushioned only by the stomach and transverse colon (mobile and hollow organs) and featuring weaker embryonic fusion points [10].

Penetrating Trauma

Stab wounds in the thoracoabdominal region require exhaustive evaluation, considering the entry into the skin, dimensions, edges, and evolution. In cases of impaled elements, their extraction must be carried out in the operating room under direct control. Gunshot wounds prioritize the exclusion of vital injuries, such as heart, great vessels, or hollow viscera. In stable patients, studies should determine the trajectory of the projectile and rule out these injuries.

In our experience, penetrating wounds constitute 76% of diaphragmatic injuries (49% from firearms and the rest from stab objects), mainly associated with urban violence. The remaining 24% corresponds to blunt trauma, such as vehicle accidents or falls from a height [11].

Classification

The classification of diaphragmatic wounds, proposed by Moore et al. in 1994 [12], includes five degrees of injury. Grade 1 corresponds to a contusion, while grade 5 covers wounds that affect the entire length of the diaphragm or exceed 25 cm.

Symptoms typically appear from grade 2 onward, when lacerations smaller than 2 cm allow abdominal viscera to herniate into the thoracic cavity. These injuries, particularly on the right side, can be challenging to detect, as the liver often acts as a barrier, avoiding clear symptoms. As the lacerations enlarge (grades 3–5), clinical signs and imaging findings become increasingly evident.

Associated Injuries

Due to its location and close anatomical relationship with abdominal and thoracic organs, diaphragmatic injuries are often accompanied by trauma to other organs. At least 50% of patients with diaphragmatic injuries also present with associated injuries. In cases of penetrating trauma, such as stab or gunshot wounds, the diaphragm is rarely affected in isolation.

An analysis of the National Trauma Data Bank [10] revealed that penetrating diaphragmatic injuries are frequently associated with damage to the liver and hollow viscera. In more than half of penetrating trauma cases, the most commonly injured structures include the lungs, liver, and pleural space (resulting in hemothorax or pneumothorax). Fewer than 50% of cases involve injuries to the heart, pericardium, spleen, and small or large intestines. Less frequently, trauma affects the stomach, kidneys, and pancreas. The association between diaphragmatic injuries and injuries to the thoracic aorta—whether from blunt or penetrating trauma—occurs in 3.5–17% of cases [10].

In blunt trauma, diaphragmatic rupture reflects significant energy dissipation within the abdominopelvic cavity, often resulting in fractures of the ribs, sternum, clavicles, vertebrae, and pelvis. These fractures are associated with diaphragmatic injuries in 68.2% of cases [10].

In a study conducted at our hospital in 2021, the most commonly affected organ was the liver (49.5%), followed by the stomach (30.2%), lungs (29.3%), and spleen (27.5%). Intestinal injuries appear in 23.8% of cases [11].

Clinical Evaluation

The patient's chest and abdomen should be examined looking for superficial wounds that suggest significant injuries. While the excursion of the diaphragm depends on variables such as body composition, posture, and lung volume, any gunshot or stab wound between the fourth and twelfth intercostal spaces has the potential to injure it, particularly if penetrating wounds are present on both sides of the diaphragm. Wounds in the posterior or flank regions of the torso can also lead to diaphragmatic damage [5, 7].

A diaphragmatic rupture can result in the acute herniation of abdominal contents into the thoracic cavity. Diminished breath sounds may indicate lung collapse caused by herniation. If the stomach is herniated, air injected into a nasogastric tube may be audible in the thorax upon auscultation, though this finding is nonspecific [7].

Patients may report chest pain due to increased intrathoracic pressure or pleural compromise caused by the hernia sac. Mediastinal shift increases venous pressure and reduces venous return and cardiac output, resulting in dyspnea. If the pericardium or heart is involved, this can manifest as restrictive cardiomyopathy or cardiac tamponade [5].

In cases of delayed presentation, patients may initially show no symptoms or signs of diaphragmatic damage, many times associated injuries may be so severe that they delay definitive evaluation. Over time, the resulting diaphragmatic defect tends to enlarge, increasing the likelihood of abdominal organ herniation, particularly when the injury involves the left hemidiaphragm. In contrast, small defects on the right side may remain stable, as the liver serves as a natural barrier, preventing intestinal herniation [5].

Patients with a history of thoracoabdominal, blunt or penetrating trauma, who present with abdominal pain accompanied by nausea or vomiting should be evaluated for possible undiagnosed diaphragmatic injury, which could result in gastrointestinal obstruction secondary to herniation. Failure to diagnose and properly repair the diaphragm can result in gangrene and intestinal strangulation, with fatal outcomes [5, 13].

Diagnostic Imaging

If there is a suspicion of a diaphragm injury, specific additional imaging methods beyond those obtained during the initial trauma evaluation may be required.

Chest X-Ray Diaphragmatic injury may be evident if abdominal organs are identified in the chest. Other times, it is suggested by elusive signs such as asymmetric elevation of the hemidiaphragm, pleural effusion, basal atelectasis, mediastinal shift, irregular diaphragm contour, or lower rib fractures [5].

Specific signs include an abnormal position of the nasogastric tube projecting above the hemidiaphragm (Fig. 18.3) and the presence of gas-filled hollow viscera in the thoracic cavity (Fig. 18.4). The sensitivity of chest X-rays in the emergency room ranges from 27% to 68% for the left hemidiaphragm and 17% for the right [14].

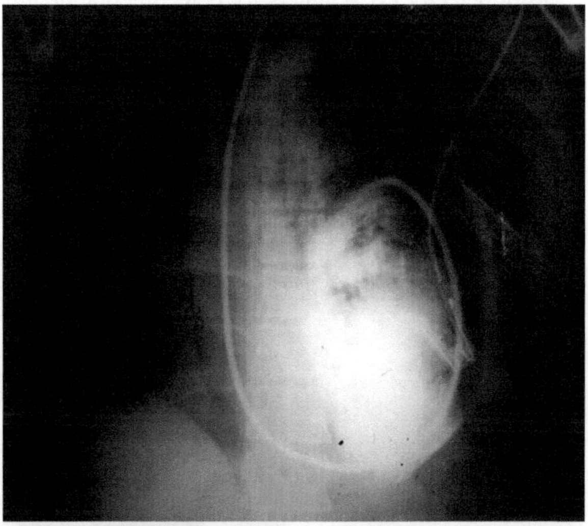

Fig. 18.3 Nasogastric tube in a chest X-ray

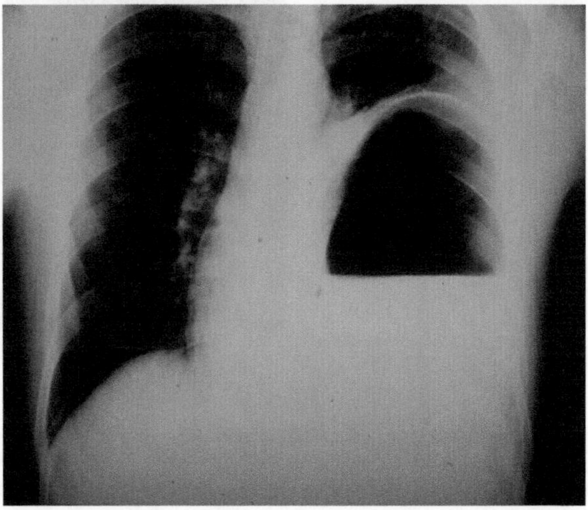

Fig. 18.4 Gastric fundus inside the thorax and air-fluid level

Ultrasound Although not standardized, ultrasound is proposed as a valuable tool during the initial assessment, particularly for patients who cannot be exposed to radiation or transported for a CT scan due to the severity of their condition or time constraints. A linear transducer with a frequency of 5.0–7.5 MHz is placed transversely on the abdomen and directed toward the diaphragm, which appears as a hyperechoic line superior to the liver. Ultrasound findings indicative of diaphragmatic injury include discontinuity of the diaphragm, herniation of the liver or hollow viscus, a floating diaphragm, and the presence of pleural effusion or subphrenic fluid [5].

Computed Tomography (CT) Scan CT scans are valuable for detecting injuries and evaluating the posterior lumbar elements of the diaphragm, such as the crural and arcuate ligaments. However, diaphragmatic injuries are often diagnosed incidentally during CT imaging, and smaller lesions may go unnoticed [7].

Multidetector CT scanners for detecting diaphragmatic injuries caused by penetrating trauma revealed moderate to high diagnostic accuracy, with a pooled sensitivity of 74% and specificity of 92% in the meta-analysis conducted by Hassankhani A. et al. [13].

Several direct and indirect CT signs can aid in diagnosing traumatic diaphragmatic injuries [13]:

- *Direct signs:*
  1. Discontinuity of the diaphragm: it means a visible gap or tear in the diaphragm muscle (Fig. 18.5).

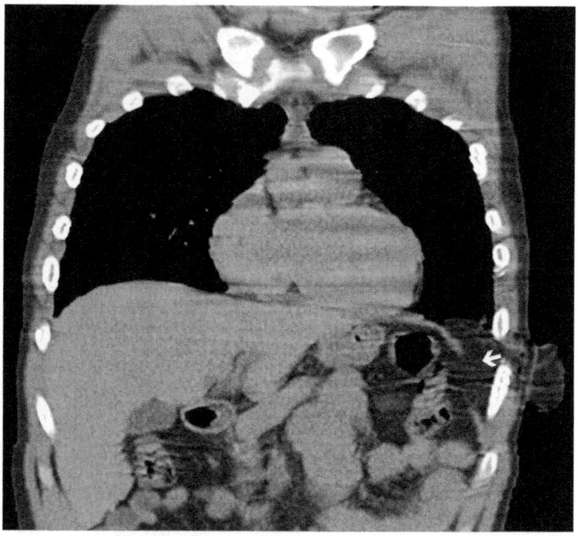

Fig. 18.5 CT scan, coronal plane. Discontinuity of the diaphragm (white arrow)

Dangling diaphragm sign: the free edge of the torn diaphragm appearing as a comma-shaped structure

- *Indirect signs:*
  1. Thickening of the diaphragm: observed close to the injury (Fig. 18.6).

Dependent viscera sign: herniated abdominal organs against the posterior chest wall (Fig. 18.7).

Collar sign: a constricted appearance of the bowel where it passes through the diaphragmatic tear (Fig. 18.8).

Hump sign: a portion of the liver herniated through the diaphragm forming a rounded mass (Fig. 18.9).

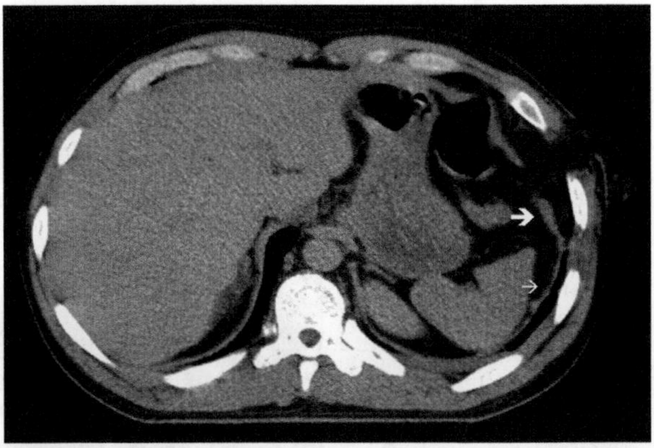

Fig. 18.6 CT scan, axial plane. Thickening of the diaphragm (large arrow), normal diaphragm thickness (small arrow)

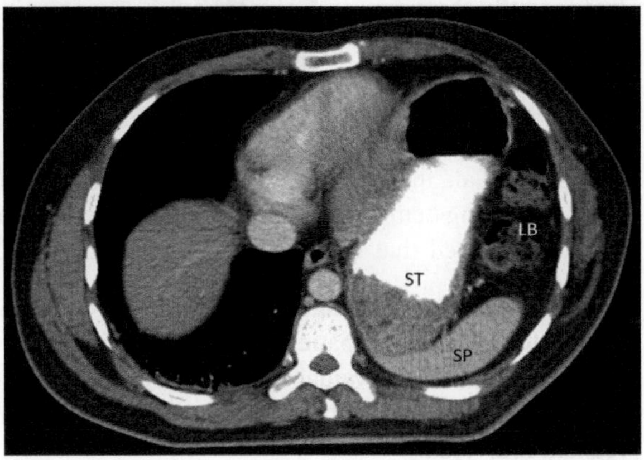

Fig. 18.7 Dependent viscera sign: herniated abdominal organs lying against the posterior chest wall. ST stomach, SP spleen, LB large bowel

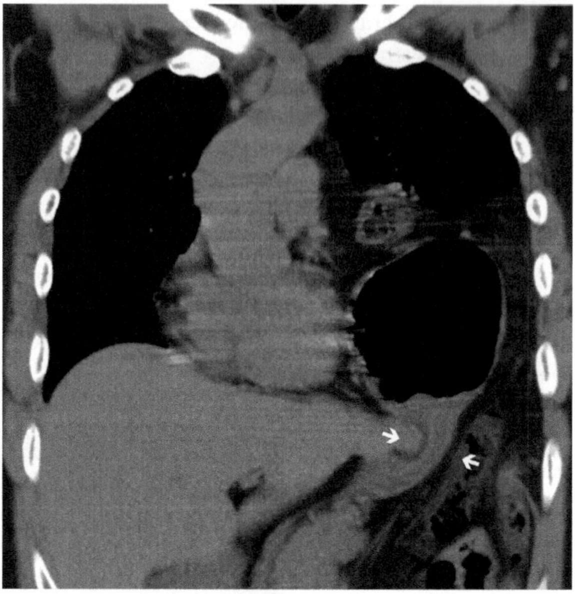

Fig. 18.8 CT scan coronal plane. The arrows show the constriction of the herniated viscera through the diaphragm

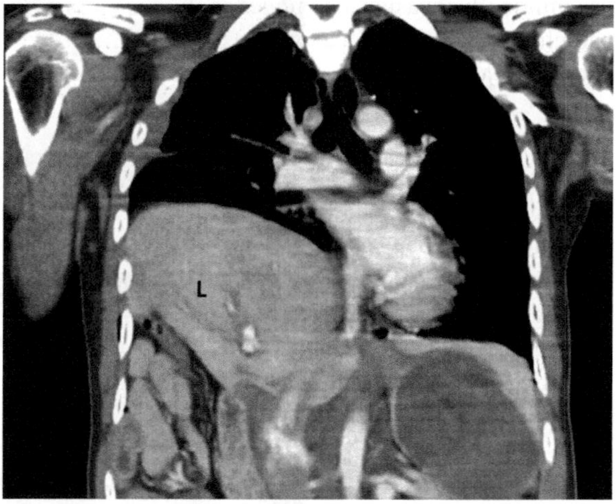

Fig. 18.9 CT-scan coronal plane. Liver located in the chest due to a diaphragmatic rupture in a blunt trauma

Magnetic Resonance Imaging (MRI) MRI studies are time-consuming and not suitable for polytrauma patients, limiting their role in the initial evaluation [13]. However, MRI can be valuable for hemodynamically stable patients who cannot undergo CT imaging, such as those allergic to iodinated intravenous contrast or pregnant individuals.

Diagnostic Laparoscopy and Thoracoscopy with a high index of suspicion for diaphragmatic injury or initial trauma images are inconclusive, and the guidelines from the Eastern Association for the Surgery of Trauma [2] and the consensus from the World Society of Emergency Surgery [14] recommend the use of diagnostic laparoscopy or thoracoscopy. Laparoscopy allows for easy visualization of both hemidiaphragms and generally carries a low risk. Furthermore, if an injury is identified, these techniques enable immediate repair. Sensitivity and specificity of laparoscopy can reach 100%, and a laparotomy can be avoided in approximately 58% of cases [15].

Minimally Invasive Treatment

When choosing a minimally invasive method to treat diaphragmatic injuries, we aim to achieve the following main objectives:

1. Perform a rapid and efficient diagnosis.
2. Perform the appropriate surgical treatment.
3. Ensure recovery with low morbidity.

The main advantages of minimally invasive surgical treatment of diaphragm wounds are rapid diagnosis, precision in surgical management, and reduction of associated complications. This approach allows for rapid identification of occult injuries, minimizing damage to surrounding tissues, and promoting faster recovery with less morbidity compared to laparotomy. It is an ideal approach when the patient is hemodynamically stable [1, 8, 15].

In patients without signs or symptoms of acute hemorrhage and shock, several authors agree that the laparoscopic, and sometimes thoracoscopic, approaches have enough arguments to be indicated [2, 14], with an average conversion rate to the conventional procedure from approximately 0.24% to 7.3% [16], mostly related to associated injuries. Laparoscopy surpasses the open procedure in terms of low rates of major complications and shorter hospital stay. On the other hand, in the review by Yue Li et al., blood loss was less compared to the open procedure and a decrease in mortality was also observed [16].

Surgical Management of Diaphragmatic Injuries

Laparoscopic Procedure

When there is suspicion of an injury to the diaphragm, either due to clinical findigs, the path of a penetrating wound or findings in imaging studies, surgery with a minimally invasive approach is indicated in stable patients.

Preoperative Preparation After performing the necessary preoperative studies, including blood type and RH factor tests, a nasogastric tube is placed to evacuate gastric contents and perform pneumatic tests to evaluate damage to the stomach. Skin antisepsis includes the chest to the neck, allowing rapid change to a thoracic approach. The exposure of the surgical area covers the abdomen from the posterior axillary lines to the pubis and, upward, above the xiphoid.

Patient Position In the operating room, the patient is positioned supine with arms extended to the sides. The table should allow adjustment of height, tilt (Trendelenburg and reverse Trendelenburg positions), and lateral tilt to provide optimal access to the surgical site. The monitor is located at the patient's head or on the shoulder ipsilateral to the affected side of the diaphragm (Fig. 18.10). Using the American technique, the surgeon is positioned on the side opposite to the injure diaphragm. The first assistant, responsible for holding the camera, is positioned on the same side as the affected diaphragm. This setup ensures optimal visualization and access to the injury site.

If there are no contraindications, pneumoperitoneum is established by umbilical puncture with a Veress needle. In patients with previous laparotomies, the open technique is used in the umbilicus, where the first 10 mm port for the camera is placed, preferably at 30°. Additionally, two 5 mm accessory ports are placed: one subcostal in the anterior axillary line and another in the midline, a few centimeters below the xiphoid. If required, a fourth 5 mm port is added for separation or aspiration (Fig. 18.11).

A CO_2 pressure is maintained between 12 and 15 mmHg, adjusting to 8 mmHg if necessary, using the tilting of the surgical table in the reverse Trendelenburg position with the feet down and lateral elevation of the affected side to improve exposure of the diaphragm. In case of increased ventilatory pressure, a chest tube is placed in the fifth intercostal space, mid-axillary line on the left side, if it has not been previously placed. We recommend starting the examination with the diaphragm: if it is

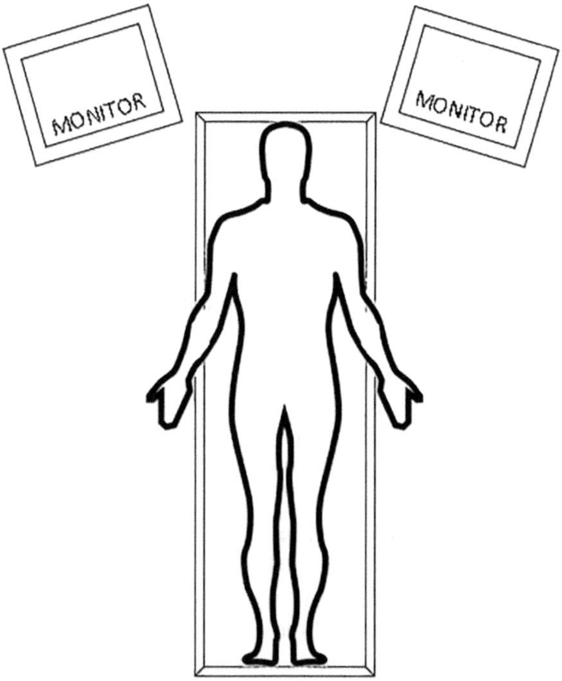

Fig. 18.10 Patient position and monitor location in the operating room

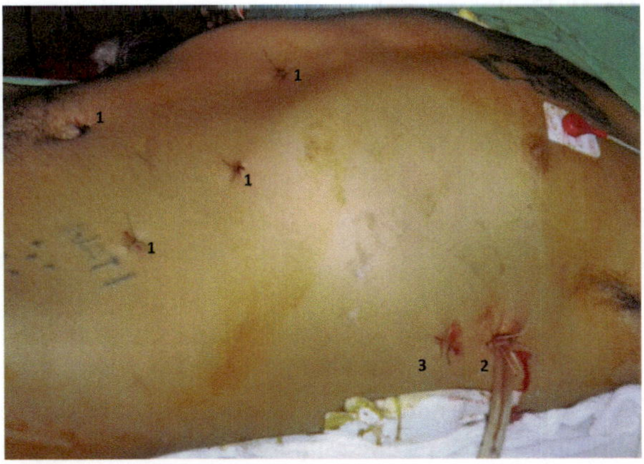

Fig. 18.11 Laparoscopy port's location [1], thoracostomy tube [2], number 3 indicates the stab entry

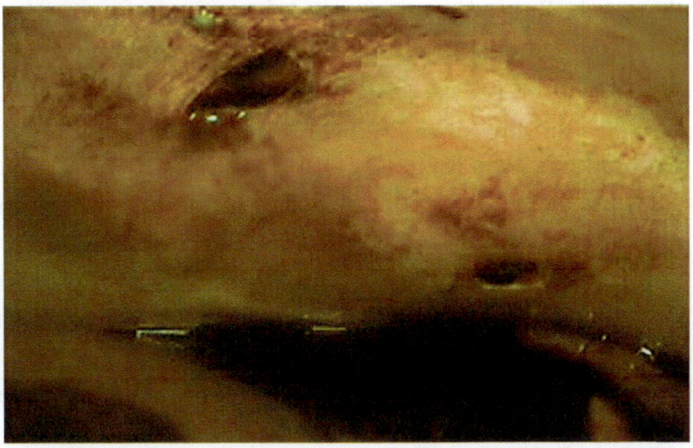

Fig. 18.12 Double perforation of the left diaphragm due to a stab wound

intact, we do not modify the carbon dioxide pressure, keeping it between 12 and 15 mmHg. In case of diaphragmatic injury, we decrease to 8–10 mmHg to avoid pressure on pulmonary ventilation (Figs. 18.12 and 18.13).

In agreement with other authors, we have not observed respiratory complications with abdominal insufflation or ventilation restrictions [9]. To mobilize the viscera, atraumatic forceps or a 5-mm aspiration cannula are used. The first maneuver consists of inspecting both sides of the diaphragm and the entire cavity, checking the surfaces of the viscera to identify blood or intestinal contents. All fluid is aspirated from the abdominal cavity, and the anterior surface of the stomach, small intestine, and colon are carefully examined. The spleen, the upper and lower surfaces of the left liver, and the diaphragm are also inspected.

When displacement of viscera into the pleural space is found, such as the greater omentum or a hollow viscera, specific measures are taken. In the case of hollow viscera, atraumatic clamps must be prepared to quickly occlude any orifice when reducing them, thereby avoiding spills. This reduction is done gently to avoid additional injuries. If reduction is difficult, the diaphragm wound can be expanded using electrocautery, cutting only what allows free descent of the contents.

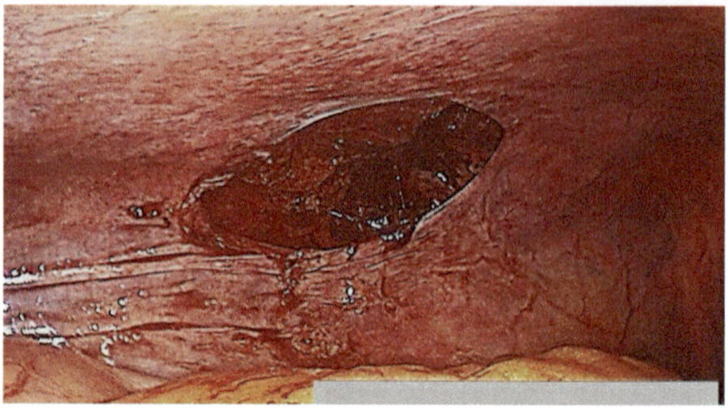

Fig. 18.13 Perforation of the left diaphragm due to a stab wound

When there is no visceral herniation and the orifices are small, it is possible to close them under pleural aspiration and assisted lung expansion with the help of the anesthetist by tracheal ventilation, without leaving a thoracostomy tube in place. If there is hollow viscus content or intestinal effusion, an exhaustive pleural lavage is performed and a chest tube is left. This lavage would reduce the possibility of pleural contamination and, consequently, the development of pleural empyema [17].

Similar maneuvers are performed on the right side, inspecting the liver surface, gallbladder, hepatic flexure of the colon, and duodenum.

All holes in the diaphragm are closed with nonabsorbable suture, such as 2-0 or 3-0 polypropylene or silk, with a 2.5 cm long 1/2 circle tapered curved needle. If only a few stitches are required (one X or two stitches), polyglactin of the same caliber can also be used. We don't recommend polyglactin for large wounds (Fig. 18.14 and 18.15).

We performed a pneumatic maneuver in case of suspected stomach injury, inflating through the nasogastric tube and filling the abdominal cavity with saline solution, verifying the absence of leaks.

Abdominal drains are only placed in case of concomitant liver injuries or hollow viscera injuries. The aponeurotic closure of the 10-mm holes is performed.

Every patient with a diaphragmatic injury requires adequate analgesia and immediate kinesiotherapy in the first 48 h to prevent atelectasis and pulmonary complications. Early mobilization and removal of pleural or abdominal drains within 48 h are encouraged.

In isolated diaphragmatic injuries, hospital discharge usually does not exceed 48 h. Before discharge, with or without chest tube, a standing chest X-ray is performed to rule out pleural effusion or unusual complications such as diaphragmatic paralysis.

Thoracoscopic Procedure The choice of abdominal or thoracic approach depends on several factors. Generally, a thoracic surgery specialist will prefer a thoracoscopy, while a general surgeon will choose the abdominal approach. We believe that both approaches can be combined if necessary, and every trauma surgeon should handle both approaches, regardless of their specialty.

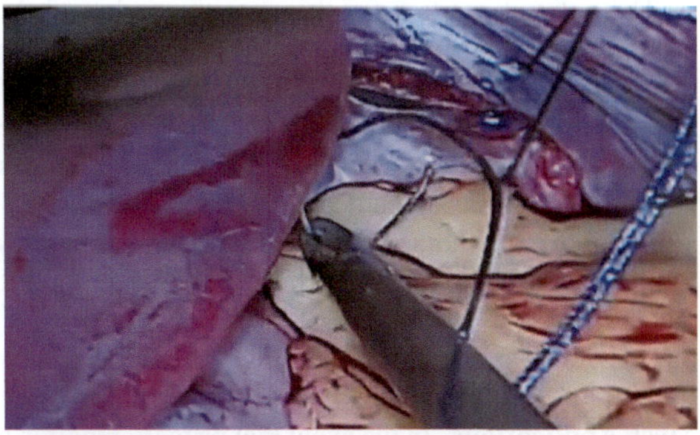

Fig. 18.14 Diaphragm wound suture with 2-0 polypropylene

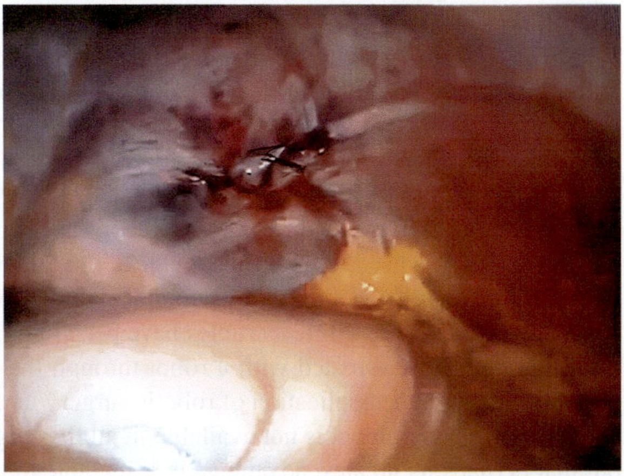

Fig. 18.15 "X" point in a wound of left diaphragm

MacDonald et al., in a 2018 review [2], explain that abdominal wounds associated with penetrating trauma require repair between 53% and 88.9%. Furthermore, 87.5% of chest injuries are hemothorax or pneumothorax and generally require only pleural drainage.

The conversion to a thoracotomy was reported in 5% of cases by Freeman, 2001 [18]. This reveals that the exclusive thoracoscopic approach could miss undetected abdominal injuries in a significant percentage in the emergency settings. MacDonald et al. [2] recommend the abdominal approach to avoid these complications.

Advantages of thoracoscopy include complete evacuation of the hemothorax, evaluation of the mediastinum, and hemostasis of intercostal injuries. Among the disadvantages, only one hemidiaphragm can be evaluated at a time, and the lateral recumbent is uncomfortable if we must convert to a laparoscopic approach.

Selective bronchial intubation is recommended, but not necessary. Some authors use single lumen orotracheal intubation for thoracoscopic procedures safely and without morbidities [9]. Correct selective intubation is verified with bronchofibroscopy or fluoroscopy in our patients.

The optimal position for thoracoscopy is lateral decubitus, contralateral to the affected diaphragm, which aids in the evaluation of the posterior diaphragm near the mediastinum. Ochsner et al. [19] propose a modified lateral position, using the movements of the operating table to transition to supine if the abdomen needs to be addressed. The ports are located in the fifth intercostal space, mid-axillary line, and additional ports are added depending on the location of the wound.

We prefer the thoracic approach in lateral decubitus, using a single port with a retractor and wound protector device (Fig. 18.16) to introduce the camera and special thoracoscopy instruments (Fig. 18.17). The diaphragmatic wound is repaired in the same way as in laparoscopy (Fig. 18.18).

Mesh Applications In the event that primary repair is not possible due to excessive loss of diaphragmatic tissue or chronic expansion of the defect (grade IV or V injury), nonabsorbable prosthetic materials can be used (e.g., polytetrafluoroethylene, polyethylene), when there is no contamination of intestinal fluids. When contamination is present, the abdomen is copiously irrigated and an autologous tissue flap (e.g., omentum, latissimus dorsi flap) or a bioprosthesis should be used [5, 20].

Robotic Surgery in Diaphragm Trauma In 2021, the World Society of Emergency Surgery published a paper showing a review of abdominal emergency pathologies where a robot was used to treat them [21]. In this review, 10 studies were selected in which the majority of surgery was completed with robots. None of them were of traumatic origin. Since 2021, 2 articles have been published describing a late-onset diaphragmatic hernia treated with a robot through the thorax with optimal results [22, 23], although the application of robotic surgery in trauma is still under analysis and clearly the equipment is not available in all the surgical centers, we must point out that perhaps its greatest advantage is being able to perform a remote operation, or telementoring, in lower volume hospitals and far from the most experienced centers, or in special environments [21].

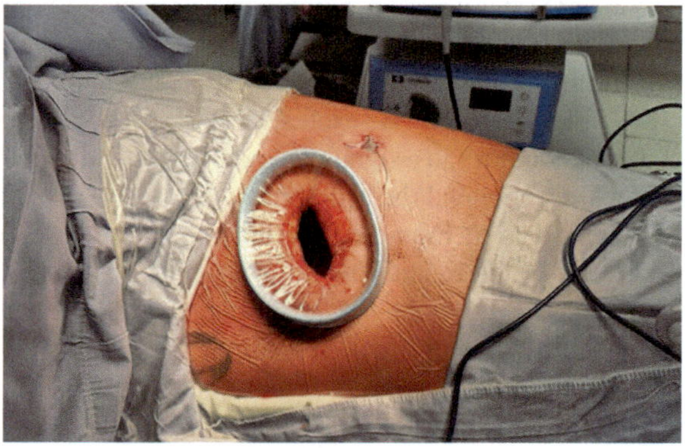

Fig. 18.16 Single-port thoracoscopy with protection and retraction accessory

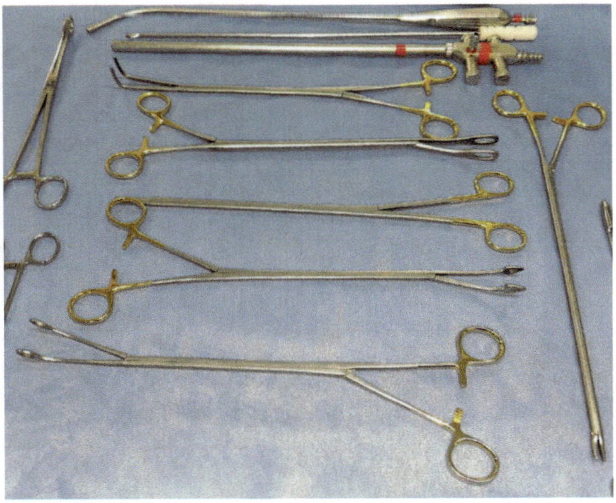

Fig. 18.17 Single-port thoracoscopy instrumentation

Chronic Diaphragmatic Hernia

Diaphragmatic hernia can be recognized late. It may appear as a finding on a chest X-ray, accompanied by nonspecific symptoms, such as an alteration in intestinal transit, or as an acute form of incarceration and strangulation, being an emergency associated with high morbidity and mortality. These symptoms may appear months or years after the initial trauma [2, 6, 20].

The approach to chronic diaphragmatic hernia can be performed through the abdominal or thoracic route, depending on the preference and experience of the surgeon. In certain cases, a combined approach may be beneficial, but is essential to anticipate this situation before starting surgery. We prefer to position the patient that allows both accesses or facilitates a change of position if necessary [7].

In uncomplicated situations, thoracic access may be preferable, as it allows better visualization and release of pleuro-pulmonary adhesions (Fig. 18.18). However, in emergency cases, the abdominal approach is recommended, which allows the status of the herniated viscera to be evaluated in a more comprehensive way [20].

Despite the benefits of the minimally invasive approach, we believe that in critically ill patients, laparotomy should be performed, with the possibility of applying a damage control protocol if metabolic acidosis is severely compromised [20].

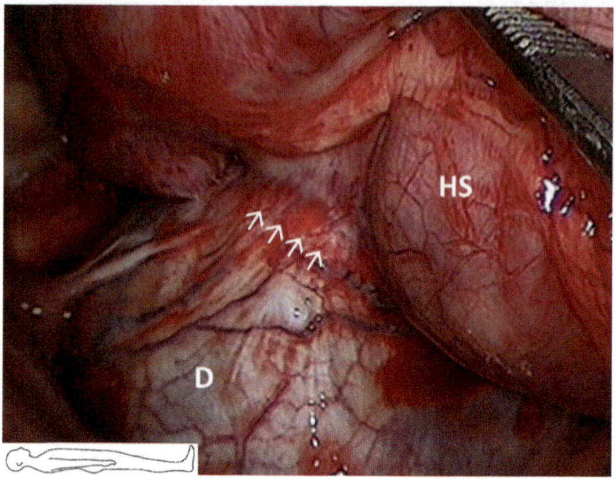

Fig. 18.18 Thoracoscopic procedure, uncomplicated left diaphragmatic hernia: D diaphragm, HS hernia sac. The arrows point to the diaphragmatic ring

Conclusions

Diaphragmatic injuries represent a challenge to the trauma surgeon, and the number of unnoticed injuries that subsequently lead to complicated hernias that must be resolved urgently is not negligible. The combination of clinical suspicion, CT scan, and minimally invasive approach are the main tools for diagnosis and treatment in hemodynamically stable patients. Our choice is laparoscopy for diagnosis and treatment of most diaphragm injuries. The thoracoscopic approach is also feasible, especially in trained surgeons or chest surgeons.

References

1. Murray JA, Demetriades D, Asensio JA, Cornwell EE 3rd, Velmahos GC, Belzberg H, Berne TV. Occult injuries to the diaphragm: prospective evaluation of laparoscopy in penetrating injuries to the left lower chest. J Am Coll Surg. 1998;187(6):626–30. https://doi.org/10.1016/s1072-7515(98)00246-4. PMID: 9849737.
2. McDonald AA, Robinson BRH, Alarcon L, Bosarge PL, Dorion H, Haut ER, et al. Evaluation and management of traumatic diaphragmatic injuries: a practice management guideline from the Eastern Association for the Surgery of trauma. J Trauma Acute Care Surg. 2018;85(1):198–207. https://doi.org/10.1097/TA.0000000000001924. PMID: 29613959.
3. Dreizin D, Borja MJ, Danton GH, Kadakia K, Caban K, Rivas LA, Munera F. Penetrating diaphragmatic injury: accuracy of 64-section multidetector CT with trajectography. Radiology. 2013;268(3):729–37. https://doi.org/10.1148/radiol.13121260. Epub 2013 May 14. PMID: 23674790.
4. Hanna W, Tata P, Ferri L, Razek T, Ortega Checa D, Herrera LR. Chapter 27: Trauma de Diafragma. In: Ferrada R, Rodriguez A, editors. Trauma. 2nd ed. Distribuna ed; 2009. p. 331–6.
5. Petrone P, Asensio JA, Marini CP. Diaphragmatic injuries and post-traumatic diaphragmatic hernias. Curr Probl Surg. 2017;54(1):11–32. https://doi.org/10.1067/j.cpsurg.2016.11.001. Epub 2016 Nov 29. PMID: 28212818.

6. Schumpelick V, Steinau G, Schluper I, Prescher A. Surgical embryology and anatomy of the diaphragm with surgical applications. Surg Clin North Am. 2000;80(1):213–39, xi. https://doi.org/10.1016/s0039-6109(05)70403-5. PMID: 10685150.
7. Feliciano DV, Cruse PA, Mattox KL, Bitondo CG, Burch JM, Noon GP, Beall AC Jr. Delayed diagnosis of injuries to the diaphragm after penetrating wounds. J Trauma. 1988;28(8):1135–44. https://doi.org/10.1097/00005373-198808000-00005. PMID: 3411640.
8. Biffl WL, Cioff WG. Chapter 32: Diaphragm. In: Felciano DV, Mattox KL, Moore EE, editors. TRAUMA. 9th ed. EEUU MacGraw HillIn ed; 2021. p. 645–56.
9. Koto MZ, Matsevych OY, Nsakala L. Evaluation of Thoracoscopy with single-lumen endotracheal tube intubation and laparoscopy in the diagnosis of occult diaphragmatic injuries in penetrating thoracoabdominal trauma. J Laparoendosc Adv Surg Tech A. 2019;29(6):785–9. https://doi.org/10.1089/lap.2018.0733. Epub 2019 Jan 10. PMID: 30628853.
10. Fair KA, Gordon NT, Barbosa RR, Rowell SE, Watters JM, Schreiber MA. Traumatic diaphragmatic injury in the American College of Surgeons National Trauma Data Bank: a new examination of a rare diagnosis. Am J Surg. 2015;209(5):864–8; discussion 868–9. https://doi.org/10.1016/j.amjsurg.2014.12.023. Epub 2015 Feb 21. PMID: 25952278.
11. González Felis L, Barrionuevo M, Obelar M, Moreno LB, González G, Garay MB, et al. Lesiones de diafragma agudas, diagnóstico y tratamiento. Rev HUcba. 2021;IV(4):32–7. ISSN 1851-3042, access 11/12/2025
12. Moore EE, Malangoni MA, Cogbill TH, Shackford SR, Champion HR, Jurkovich GJ, McAninch JW, Trafton PG. Organ injury scaling. IV: thoracic vascular, lung, cardiac, and diaphragm. J Trauma. 1994;36(3):299–300. PMID: 8145307.
13. Hassankhani A, Amoukhteh M, Valizadeh P, Jannatdoust P, Eibschutz LS, Myers LA, et al. Diagnostic utility of multidetector CT scan in penetrating diaphragmatic injuries: a systematic review and meta-analysis. Emerg Radiol. 2023;30(6):765–76. https://doi.org/10.1007/s10140-023-02174-1. Epub 2023 Oct 4. PMID: 37792116; PMCID: PMC10695863
14. Sermonesi G, Tian BWCA, Vallicelli C, Abu-Zidan FM, Damaskos D, Kelly MD, Leppäniemi A, et al. Cesena guidelines: WSES consensus statement on laparoscopic-first approach to general surgery emergencies and abdominal trauma. World J Emerg Surg. 2023;18(1):57. https://doi.org/10.1186/s13017-023-00520-9. PMID: 38066631; PMCID: PMC10704840.
15. Di Saverio S, Birindelli A, Podda M, Segalini E, Piccinini A, Coniglio C, Frattini C, Tugnoli G. Trauma laparoscopy and the six w's: why, where, who, when, what, and how? J Trauma Acute Care Surg. 2019;86(2):344–67. https://doi.org/10.1097/TA.0000000000002130. PMID: 30489508.
16. Li Y, Xiang Y, Wu N, Wu L, Yu Z, Zhang M, Wang M, Jiang J, Li Y. A comparison of laparoscopy and laparotomy for the management of abdominal trauma: a systematic review and meta-analysis. World J Surg. 2015;39(12):2862–71. https://doi.org/10.1007/s00268-015-3212-4. PMID: 26316111.
17. Zellweger R, Navsaria PH, Hess F, Omoshoro-Jones J, Kahn D, Nicol A. Transdiaphragmatic pleural lavage in penetrating thoracoabdominal trauma. Br J Surg. 2004;91(12):1619–23. https://doi.org/10.1002/bjs.4598. PMID: 15505872.
18. Freeman RK, Al-Dossari G, Hutcheson KA, Huber L, Jessen ME, Meyer DM, Wait MA, DiMaio JM. Indications for using video-assisted thoracoscopic surgery to diagnose diaphragmatic injuries after penetrating chest trauma. Ann Thorac Surg. 2001;72(2):342–7. https://doi.org/10.1016/s0003-4975(01)02803-x. PMID: 11515863.
19. Ochsner MG, Rozycki GS, Lucente F, Wherry DC, Champion HR. Prospective evaluation of thoracoscopy for diagnosing diaphragmatic injury in thoracoabdominal trauma: a preliminary report. J Trauma. 1993;34(5):704–9; discussion 709–10. https://doi.org/10.1097/00005373-199305000-00013. PMID: 8497005.
20. Giuffrida M, Perrone G, Abu-Zidan F, Agnoletti V, Ansaloni L, Baiocchi GL, et al. Management of complicated diaphragmatic hernia in the acute setting: a WSES position paper. World J Emerg Surg. 2023;18(1):43. https://doi.org/10.1186/s13017-023-00510-x. PMID: 37496073; PMCID: PMC10373334.

21. de'Angelis N, Khan J, Marchegiani F, Bianchi G, Aisoni F, Alberti D, et al. Robotic surgery in emergency setting: 2021 WSES position paper. World J Emerg Surg. 2022;17(1):4. https://doi.org/10.1186/s13017-022-00410-6. PMID: 35057836; PMCID: PMC8781145
22. Holder P, Bakeer MA. Robot-assisted repair of delayed traumatic diaphragmatic hernia: a case report. J Surg Case Rep. 2024;2024(4):rjae197. https://doi.org/10.1093/jscr/rjae197. PMID: 38572281; PMCID: PMC10987203.
23. Sideris AC, Molena D. Robotic transthoracic diaphragmatic hernia repair. JTCVS Tech. 2021;10:578–80. https://doi.org/10.1016/j.xjtc.2021.08.026. PMID: 34977813; PMCID: PMC8691652.

Role of Laparoscopy on Liver Injuries

19

Federico Castillo Suescun, Adolfo Cuendis Velázquez, Juan García Cardo, José Roberto Ramírez Nava, and Roberto Fernández Santiago

Introduction

Advances in prehospital care for trauma patients have altered fatality patterns. While most deaths still occur within the first few hours of the initial cause, survival rates have improved, and late fatalities have become less common [1, 2]. Over the years, advancements in resuscitation, imaging technologies and techniques, surgical equipment, development of the technique, and innovative devices—such as resuscitative endovascular balloon occlusion of the aorta—have significantly improved the care of injured patients, increasing their chances of surviving the initial impact [1, 2].

Liver trauma is one of the most common abdominal injuries in severely injured trauma patients [3]. The diagnosis and management of hepatic trauma have advanced with modern diagnostic and therapeutic tools. As a result, we continue to address new challenges and adapt to emerging technologies [4].

The liver is a vascularized solid organ, making hemorrhage a leading cause of mortality in severe trauma. In hemodynamically unstable patients or those experiencing rapid deterioration, immediate assessment and intervention are essential to prevent further complications. Timely surgical intervention for hemorrhage control is crucial in these cases.

Hepatobiliary injuries resulting from blunt and penetrating trauma encompass a wide range of injury patterns, including deep parenchymal disruptions, portal veins and arterial hemorrhage, hepatic and suprahepatic venous injuries, and both intrahepatic and extrahepatic biliary injuries. This chapter outlines the current approach to

F. C. Suescun (✉) · J. G. Cardo · R. F. Santiago
Servicio de cirugia general, Unidad cirugia HBP y trasplantes, Hospital universitario Marques de valdecilla, Santander España, Spain
e-mail: federicojose.castillo@scsalud.es

A. C. Velázquez · J. R. R. Nava
Adscrito a la división de cirugía general y endoscopica, Hospital General Dr. Manuel Gea González, Mexico City, Distrito Federal, Mexico

© The Author(s), under exclusive license to Springer Nature Switzerland AG 2026

M. Cezillo, B. M. Pereira (eds.), *Minimally Invasive Surgery Trauma*,
https://doi.org/10.1007/978-3-032-28971-1_19

managing hepatic injuries, emphasizing the necessity of a multidisciplinary approach for complex cases.

We must always remember that trauma does not adhere to anatomical boundaries. In this chapter, we discuss liver injuries, while injuries to the biliary tract are covered in a separate chapter.

We must also consider that not all hospitals have a complex trauma unit or access to radiodiagnostic and therapeutic services for managing severe injuries. It is crucial to identify which cases can be treated with nonoperative management, minimally invasive surgery, a combined approach, or, when necessary, conventional open surgery including damage control surgery.

Evolution of Minimally Invasive Management of Liver Trauma

The evolution of liver trauma management over the past century reflects the overall advancement of trauma surgery. In the early 1900s, the approach to hepatic trauma was primarily expectant management, which was invariably fatal for severe liver injuries [5, 6]. In 1908, Dr. James Hogarth Pringle first described controlling hepatic inflow by manually compressing the hepatoduodenal ligament to manage hepatic hemorrhage [7]. This technique later became known as the Pringle maneuver.

Decades later, experiences from World War II and post-war civilian trauma prompted the development and adoption of more aggressive surgical strategies, including formal resection, debridement of devitalized liver tissue, selective hepatic artery ligation, and perihepatic drainage [5] though these approaches were often associated with significant complications, such as infection.

Much of the difficulty in surgical management of the liver is due to its anatomy. It is suspended by superior and anterior attachments, including the coronary, triangular, and falciform ligaments, and is connected to the lesser curvature of the stomach [8]. Deceleration injuries often cause tears at these fixation points, commonly fracturing the right lobe between its anterior and posterior segments. Additionally, blunt trauma to the right upper quadrant can drive the ribs into the liver, leading to stellate-type lacerations on the dome and anterior surface [9].

Perihepatic packing regained popularity in the 1990s with the growing recognition of damage control principles and resuscitative surgical techniques, this approach allowed for resuscitation and the postponement of definitive reconstruction until physiological stabilization was achieved [10] Collectively, it became evident that major liver resection in trauma cases is inadvisable, as severe trauma combined with extensive surgery can cause irreversible physiological damage due to the lethal triad: hypothermia, coagulopathy, and acidosis [11] Another major shift in hepatic trauma management occurred with the introduction of CT and alternative hemorrhage control techniques, such as angiography and endovascular embolization.

These changes led to the adoption of a nonoperative management (NOM) approach, with selective surgical interventions when necessary. The success of NOM for solid organ injuries in hemodynamically stable children in 25 served as a catalyst for applying a similar strategy to adults. In 1990, Knudson and colleagues published a study on 52 patients with major hepatic injuries, all of whom were successfully managed nonoperatively with close monitoring. 26 Subsequent studies further confirmed the safety and effectiveness of NOM for hepatic injuries in adults, regardless of whether the injuries were caused by blunt or penetrating trauma.

These shifts facilitated the adoption of NOM with selective surgical interventions when necessary. The success of NOM for solid organ injuries in hemodynamically stable children helped pave the way for a similar approach in adults. Since 1990, several studies further confirmed the safety and efficacy of NOM for hepatic injuries in adults, regardless of whether the trauma was blunt or penetrating [4, 12].

The success of NOM for hepatic trauma depends heavily on careful patient selection, as well as the use of interventional techniques to manage the sequelae of major hepatic injuries. These techniques include angiographic embolization for hepatic arterial bleeding, endoscopic biliary decompression, acute laparoscopic management, along with the option for delayed laparoscopic drainage and percutaneous debridement and drainage of liver necrosis and abscesses.

Diagnosis

The diagnosis of liver trauma has advanced with the development of modern diagnostic and therapeutic tools. Until the 1980s, most cases of blunt abdominal trauma with suspected solid organ injury were managed through exploratory laparotomy, with many diagnoses relying on peritoneal lavage, leaving the extent of injury uncertain. The increased availability and development of multiphase computed tomography angiography (CT) have since enabled more accurate assessment, with multiple studies demonstrating the safety of nonoperative management (NOM) [13]. Furthermore, innovative multimodal approaches, such as endovascular trauma and bleeding management (EVTM), have significantly enhanced the success of selective NOM [4].

In patients with blunt trauma, clear clinical signs such as rigidity, distension, or unstable vital signs may be absent. Up to 40% of patients with significant hemoperitoneum exhibit no obvious signs. The diagnostic methods on admission are determined by the hemodynamic status.

Extended-focused abdominal sonography for trauma (E-FAST) has become a routine diagnostic tool in the trauma bay and is particularly valuable in cases of blunt injury with hemodynamic instability, as detecting intra-abdominal free fluid can prompt urgent surgical intervention in a hypotensive patient. Conversely, in hemodynamically stable patients, computed tomography (CT) scan with intravenous contrast is the gold standard in hemodynamically stable trauma patients, guiding decisions on the need for embolization or operative management [4].

The primary goal of diagnostic evaluation in stable patients is to identify those who can be safely managed nonoperatively, support decision-making in nonoperative management, and establish a baseline for future imaging comparisons. In contrast, penetrating liver injuries rarely pose a diagnostic challenge, as most surgeons advocate for immediate exploration in unstable patients [9].

Classification

Understanding the various classification schemes for liver injury is crucial for determining appropriate treatment strategies. Four major classification systems are commonly used to stratify traumatic liver injuries by severity: the Abbreviated Injury Score (AIS) [14], the American Association for the Surgery of Trauma (AAST) grading system, the Injury Severity Score (ISS) [15, 16], and the World Society of Emergency Surgery (WSES) grading system [4, 17, 18]. These systems provide a structured approach to assessing injury severity and guiding clinical decision-making [19].

For the hemodynamically stable patient with AAST grade I–IV, NOM is the most evidence-based treatment [20]. Currently, the AAST and WSES classification systems are the primary frameworks used for classifying liver trauma in clinical practice.

AAST Liver Injury Scale

The grading criteria are based on imaging findings, particularly CT scans with dual-phase imaging in the arterial and portal venous phases, as well as operative and pathological findings [21]. Although the AAST criteria is universally used to express severity of injury, it is typically used in combination with the hemodynamic status to determine operative or NOM [22] Treatment options include NOM, angiographic embolization, and operative management. Grade I and II injuries with stable hemodynamic status typically undergo NOM in the intensive care unit, whereas hemodynamically unstable and/or high-grade grade V injuries require urgent operative management. Stable grade III to IV injuries usually requires angiographic evaluation.

The WSES Classification

Categorizes liver injuries into four grades, integrating the AAST-OIS classification with the patient's hemodynamic status:

Minor (WSES Grade I): AAST I-II injuries in hemodynamically stable patients.
Moderate (WSES Grade II): AAST III injuries in hemodynamically stable patients.

Severe (WSES Grade III or IV):

AAST IV-V injuries in hemodynamically stable patients.
AAST I-IV injuries in hemodynamically unstable patients.

Table 19.1 American Association for the Surgery of Trauma (AAST) grading system for hepatic injury compared to World Society of Emergency Surgery (WSES) grading system

	Injury type	Injury description	WSES grade
I[a]	Hematoma	Subcapsular <10% of surface	Grade I Minor if hemodynamically stable—includes blunt and penetrating lesions
	Laceration	Capsular tear <1 cm depth	
II[a]	Hematoma	Subcapsular 10–50% of surface area, intraparenchymal hematoma, <10 cm in diameter	
	Laceration	1–3 cm parenchymal depth, <10 cm length	
III	Hematoma	Subcapsular >50% of the study's area or expanding, ruptured subcapsular or parenchymal hematoma, intraparenchymal hematoma >10 cm	Grade II If hemodynamically stable in blunt or penetrating lesion
	Laceration	>3 cm parenchymal depth	
IV	Laceration	Parenchymal disruption 25–75% of hepatic lobe	Severe Grade III—hemodynamically stable Grade IV[a]—AAST grades I–VI *If hemodynamically unstable*
	Vascular	Hepatic injury near major hepatic vein or near the hepatic IVC	
VI	Vascular	Hepatic avulsion	

From: Gilyard et al. [19]
Abbreviations: *IVC* inferior vena cava, *WSES* World Society of Emergency Surgery
[a]Advance grade I for multiple injuries up to grade III

This classification system helps guide clinical decision-making by considering both anatomical injury severity and the patient's physiological response (Table 19.1).

Nonoperative Management (NOM) of Liver Trauma

The current approach to liver trauma has shifted toward NOM in more than 80% of cases [23]. Several key factors have contributed to this evolution:

- Recognition that over 50% of liver injuries achieve spontaneous hemostasis.
- The precedent set by the successful implementation of NOM in pediatric patients.
- Understanding that the liver possesses a remarkable capacity for self-healing after injury.
- Advancements in liver imaging, particularly with computed tomography (CT) [9].

NOM involves close patient monitoring, ensuring rapid access to radiological evaluation, and relying on an adequate hospital infrastructure to facilitate urgent surgical intervention if needed.

To be a candidate for NOM, a patient must be hemodynamically stable, demonstrate an adequate response to initial resuscitation, and show no signs of an acute abdomen. In these cases, a multiphase CT scan should be performed to assess the extent of injury and guide further management.

NOM should be the treatment of choice for all hemodynamically stable minor (WSES I) (AAST I–II), moderate (WSES II) (AAST III), and severe (WSES III) (AAST IV–V) injuries in the absence of other internal injuries requiring surgery [4].

For penetrating trauma, patient selection must be carefully considered to ensure the safety and feasibility of NOM, in the case of a gunshot wound and even more so if thoraco-abdominal. They should be considered for NOM only in centers with experience in dealing with penetrating trauma. Even in patients presenting with stable conditions and with no evidence of other intra-abdominal/internal injuries, interval laparoscopy should always be considered to confirm the absence of other injuries requiring surgical repair.

Bile leaks are a common complication in the NOM of liver injuries, occurring in 6–20% of cases. Biliary complications can vary in their time of presentation and may require multiple treatment strategies. Management options include endoscopic retrograde cholangiopancreatography (ERCP) with stent placement, ultrasound-guided or laparoscopic drainage for persistent biliary leaks.

A less common complication is hemobilia, caused by an abnormal communication between an intrahepatic blood vessel, usually an artery, and the biliary tree. The incidence after trauma is less than 3% and is more often associated with blunt trauma than with penetrating injuries. Hemobilia presents as gastrointestinal bleeding with or without abdominal pain and jaundice caused by bile ducts occluded by blood clots. It has been reported immediately after the initial trauma or up to 4 months later [24].

Multiple studies have demonstrated that NOM is a safe and highly effective approach for hepatic trauma, with reported success rates ranging from 80% to 100% in patients with blunt abdominal trauma.

Failure of NOM in blunt trauma cases is uncommon and is typically due to:

- Hemorrhage (the most common cause)
- Peritonitis
- Abdominal compartment syndrome

Hemorrhage can often be managed through surgery, angioembolization, or a combination of both. Other potential complications of NOM include:

- Delayed bleeding diagnosis
- Undiagnosed intestinal injuries
- Bile leaks and biliary peritonitis
- Hemobilia
- Liver necrosis or abscess formation

Notably, 75% of NOM failures are linked to hemodynamic instability. However, this does not necessarily indicate an immediate need for surgery, as angiographic

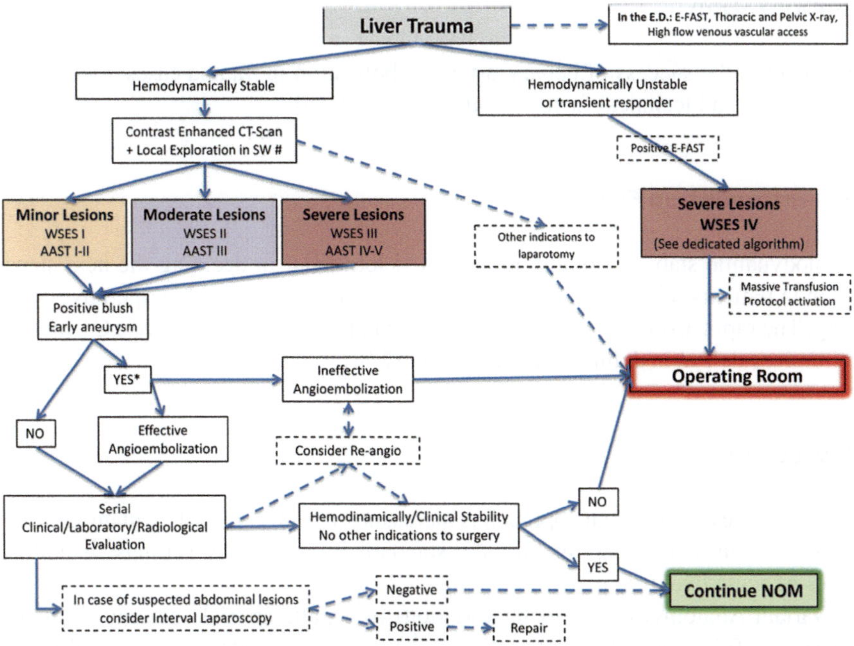

Fig. 19.1 Liver trauma management algorithm (SW stab wound. Number sign indicates wound exploration near the inferior costal margin should be avoided if not strictly necessary. Asterisk indicates angioembolization that should always be considered for adults, only in selected patients and in selected centers for pediatrics). (From: Coccolini et al. [4])

therapy may be a successful alternative in select cases [19, 25]. Figure 19.1 presents the management algorithm suggested by the World Society of Emergency Surgery (WSES).

Interventional Radiology in Liver Trauma

In the past 20 years, transcatheter arterial embolization for traumatic injury has played a pivotal role in improving survival, reducing morbidity, and decreasing operative blood loss. Its effectiveness has been demonstrated in multiple regions, including the liver, spleen, kidneys, and pelvis.

Additionally, embolization and vascular reconstruction with covered stents have proven effective in many vascular beds that are relatively inaccessible to surgical intervention. These approaches should be considered on a case-by-case basis in such scenarios [26].

Embolization

To increase the success of hepatic artery embolization in trauma cases, the following clinical and technical factors should be considered:

Pre-intervention Evaluation

Hemodynamic stability should be the key determinant in deciding the next steps. Even in patients scheduled for open surgery, CT imaging can aid in operative planning. The rapid acquisition of multiphase vascular, abdominal and pelvic CT images minimizes delays in definitive management [27].

Procedure

Arterial Access: The radial approach is increasingly being adopted by many centers. However, femoral access remains the standard in emergency settings, including cases of acute liver trauma.

Variant Anatomy: Recognizing variations in hepatic arterial anatomy is crucial for successful angioembolization. Given the high prevalence of anatomical variations, a thorough understanding of these differences can help minimize the risk of unintended nontarget embolization.

Expected Angiographic Findings

- No active extravasation. In case of traumatic injury, with CT of perihepatic hemorrhage, with or without hemodynamic instability, empiric Gelfoam embolization of the branch supplying the area of bleeding should be considered [19].
- Pseudoaneurysm: Traumatic pseudoaneurysms occur in up to 15% of patients with liver trauma [28]. Delayed rupture of a pseudoaneurysm can have devastating consequences. Pseudoaneurysms may develop in a delayed manner, making it essential to perform post-injury CT 5–7 days after the initial CT scan.
- Arteriovenous shunts occur seldom in patients with traumatic liver injury. Both arteriovenous and arterioportal shunting can be assessed using CT; however, the diagnosis is accurate with angiography [28]. Treatment typically involves coil embolization of the feeding artery. Failure to treat may result in portal hypertension.
- Late bleeding: Treatment is based on hemodynamic stability. If stable, consider slowing down the arterial pressure head. If unstable, surgical treatment is justified. Trauma patients are hypothermic, hypotensive/hypovolemic, and

coagulopathic. Once patients are warmed and volume resuscitated, bleeding may increase.

Embolic Choice

The choice of embolic agent should be guided by the presence of active arterial extravasation seen on CT or angiography.

- Coil embolization: Coil embolization is best for targeted therapy.
- Glue embolization: Cyanoacrylate “glue” is fluoroscopically visible when mixed with ethiodized oil or tantalum powder and used as a flow-directed embolic therapy [29].
- Ethylene vinyl alcohol copolymer (ONYX): This liquid embolic is like Cyanoacrylate glue, and it produces a permanent embolic effect. ONYX is intrinsically radiopaque [30].
- Gelfoam is a gelatin sponge, which initiates the clotting cascade and provides scaffolding for clot formation. The Gelfoam is, in theory, temporary, with vessel occlusion lasting 3–6 weeks [31].

Gelfoam may be used in combination with coils in cases where an injury is visualized but the catheter cannot be positioned beyond a pseudoaneurysm or arterioportal fistula.

Robotic Surgery in Liver Trauma

Robotic surgery represents the most technologically advanced approach in minimally invasive surgery. Its application has steadily gained acceptance across various surgical fields and is now routinely used in urology, gynecology, digestive, and hepato-bilio-pancreatic surgery [32] in this filed the robotic system can be used in almost all types of liver resection, including minor hepatectomy, major hepatectomy, liver donor hepatectomy, and complex liver resection.

Robotic surgery after bile duct injury is feasible and can be safely performed, with acceptable short-term results in a high-volume center, in bile duct injury repair providing the advantages of minimally invasive surgery [33].

Robotic surgery demands a higher level of technical expertise compared to open or even laparoscopic surgery. To achieve proficiency in performing standardized surgical procedures with acceptable operative and postoperative outcomes, surgeons must undergo comprehensive specialized training [34].

However, the role of robotic surgery in the emergency setting remains largely unexplored, with only limited early experiences reported in the literature. As a result, its potential applications for emergency procedures remain an open question.

Nevertheless, ongoing research and emerging evidence warrant continuous monitoring and future updates [32].

Advantages and Limitations of the Laparoscopic Approach

Difficulty Assessment, Concerns, and Controversies

The management of liver trauma is primarily guided by the patient's hemodynamic status and the presence of associated injuries, rather than solely by the radiological severity of the injury. In hemodynamically stable patients, as well as in borderline or transient responders who have no other indications for laparotomy, nonoperative management (NOM) is considered the standard of care for both blunt and penetrating liver trauma [4, 35].

Along with percutaneous drainage and angioembolization, the laparoscopic approach plays a role in the overall management of nonoperative treatment and should not be regarded as a failure of it [36]. Among its advantages, laparoscopy enables the drainage of undrained intra-abdominal fluid accumulations, including hemorrhage and biloperitoneum, facilitates the application of hemostatic agents to control liver lacerations or tears, and allows for the exclusion of concomitant hollow viscus or diaphragmatic injuries. Additionally, minimally invasive techniques offer benefits such as shorter hospital stays, reduced pain, faster recovery, and lower morbidity and mortality rates [37].

Indications

The indication and timing of laparoscopic intervention depend on the clinical scenario. In patients without an immediate indication for laparotomy but with a potential need for surgical exploration (e.g., suspected associated bowel injury), exploration should be performed after initial resuscitation is complete. Interval laparoscopy may also be required for the prevention or management of complications following NOM [38].

1. Hemorrhage drainage in blunt liver trauma when it is abundant, decreasing infection rate.
2. Diagnose the nature of abdominal or perihepatic collections, differentiating hematomas from bilomas in the early stages after trauma.
3. Bile peritonitis drainage and lavage.
4. In penetrating liver trauma, it allows to exclude associated diaphragmatic or hollow viscera injuries.

Laparoscopy in Penetrating Liver Injuries

Diagnostic laparoscopy can be valued as an option in the context of nonoperative management if, in close follow-up, there are reasonable doubts about the existence of possible associated visceral injuries [35].

The laparoscopic approach allows a clear vision of the whole abdominal cavity, and interval laparoscopy is an effective strategy to evaluate the injury and its progression while minimizing the damage and invasiveness of the surgical procedure. It could be used as a bridge to other procedures. In addition, laparoscopy should be considered an alternative to percutaneous radiological drainage and ERCP in stable patients with blunt liver trauma and hemorrhagic-bilious ascites, while avoiding the morbidity of open surgery [35].

Besides, in penetrating wounds to the upper abdomen and lower precordium, a laparoscopic transdiaphragmatic pericardial window can be used as a safe and effective modality to evaluate hemodynamically stable patients who are at risk for both cardiac and abdominal injuries [39] and to evaluate and control intercostal artery bleeding.

In the case of a penetrating and transfixing liver wound, achieving hemostasis remains the primary concern. For this rare injury, intrahepatic balloon tamponade offers a solution. A device can be improvised using a Foley catheter with a Penrose drain [40, 41] or a Sengstaken-Blakemore tube, which can be fixed as a drain or through a port hole.

Laparoscopy in Blunt Liver Injuries

Nonoperative management is considered the standard of care for blunt liver injuries in hemodynamically stable patients. However, avoiding primary surgery may lead to complications, particularly intra-abdominal collections and liver necrosis, especially when angioembolization is used.

Undrained collections may lead to complications such as hemorrhage, biliperitoneum, peritonitis, abdominal compartment syndrome, systemic inflammatory response, and/or respiratory distress. Chemical peritonitis from bile or blood causes significant pain and a physiologic ileus, delaying enteral nutrition and physical rehabilitation. Additionally, abdominal hematoma is at risk for secondary infection, particularly in the pro-inflammatory trauma state which promotes intestinal bacterial translocation [37].

Besides, laparoscopy could be used as a bridge strategy to plan an immediate or subsequent laparoscopic/laparotomy intervention. It should be considered in cases of delayed surgery, to minimize the invasiveness of surgical intervention and to tailor the procedure to the lesion [42].

Contraindications

Nonoperative management (NOM) is contraindicated in the presence of CT findings suggestive of hollow viscus injury, including free intraperitoneal or retroperitoneal air, free intraperitoneal fluid without evidence of solid organ injury, localized bowel wall thickening, or a bullet tract adjacent to a hollow viscus with surrounding hematoma. NOM should also be avoided in cases of high-energy penetrating trauma [4].

Contraindications to laparoscopy include the presence of coagulopathy, cardiopulmonary compromise, evisceration, and intra-abdominal inability to access the cavity such as when associated with burns, and the presence of multiple adhesions. However, the main contraindication to performing a laparoscopic approach is the presence of hemodynamically unstable patients.

The presence of shock, the presence of obvious lesions, or multiple organs or regions affected is another contraindication to the laparoscopic approach. In case of severe head trauma, CO_2 can raise intracranial pressure causing further deterioration of the patient [4, 43].

Patient Is Positioned: Trocars and Ports

The patient is positioned in dorsal hyperextension with legs apart and placed in a slight left or right lateral decubitus, depending on the injury site, using an inflatable bag on the back for better liver exposure. Pneumoperitoneum is established along the midline near the navel, with the Hasson trocar preferred in emergency cases. The remaining trocars are placed along the right subcostal line, maintaining a 7 cm separation between them. As for the number of trocars to carry out a laparoscopic examination of a hepatic trauma, the minimum should be three.

One of them is for the camera, in a supraumbilical position, to be able to explore the entire abdominal cavity. The other two working ports, one of 5 mm and another of 10 mm, are on both sides at the level of the midclavicular line although the left one is a little more medial. The latter would be of this diameter since it would allow us to introduce any type of topical hemostatic agent, any type of energy, endoscopic staplers, and any type of suture.

Depending on the lesions that are observed and the solution they require, the placement of more working ports will be necessary.

Inflow Control (Pringle's Maneuver)

Undoubtedly, a fundamental skill for any surgeon aiming to employ minimally invasive techniques in hepatic trauma management is the ability to perform a laparoscopic Pringle maneuver. This technique for transiently occluding hepatic inflow to control bleeding, as we previously discussed, was first described by Dr. James Hogarth Pringle in 1908; he described controlling hepatic inflow by manually

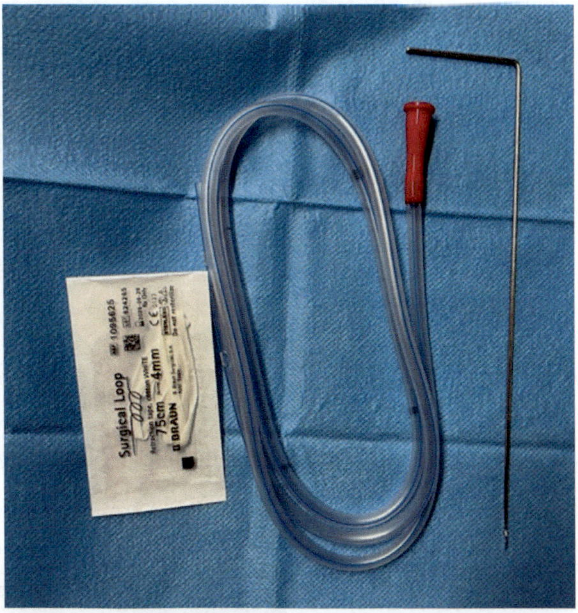

Fig. 19.2 Elements necessary to perform a laparoscopic Pringle maneuver, nasogastric tube, cotton tape, and passing threads

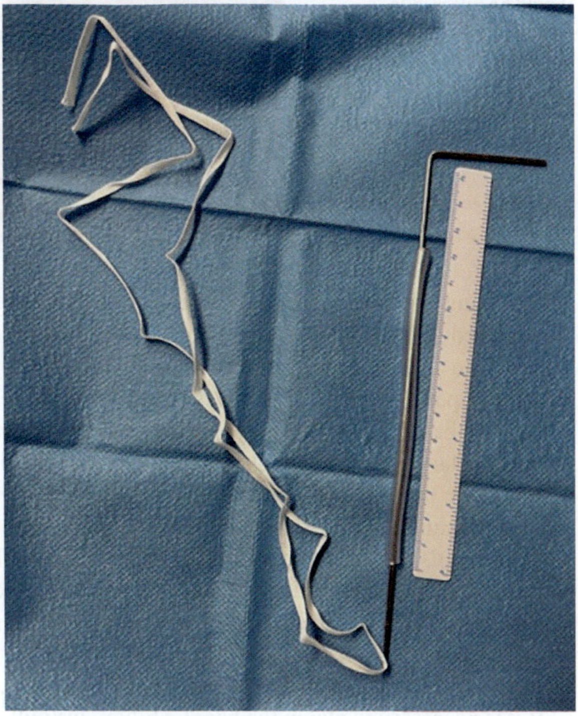

Fig. 19.3 We cut a 10–12 cm segment of the nasogastric tube and use the thread guide (once the cotton tape passes through the trocar hole and the nasogastric tube segment is introduced into the cavity)

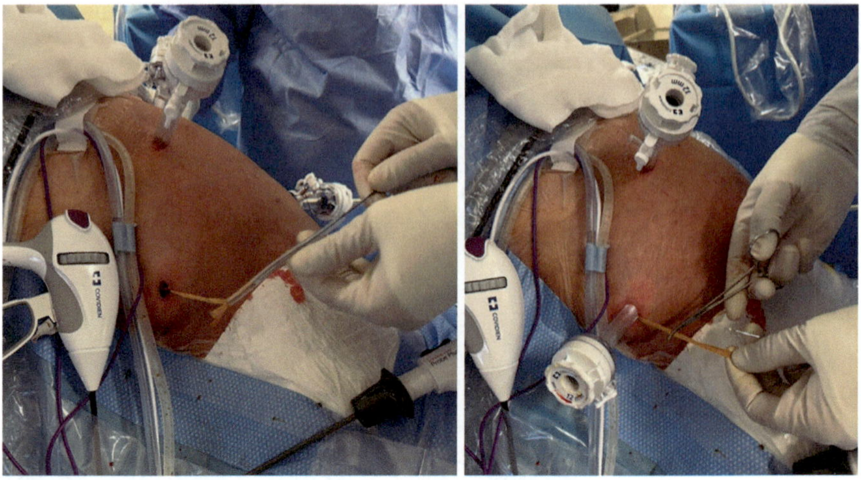

Fig. 19.4 A mosquito clamp is used for external tension control

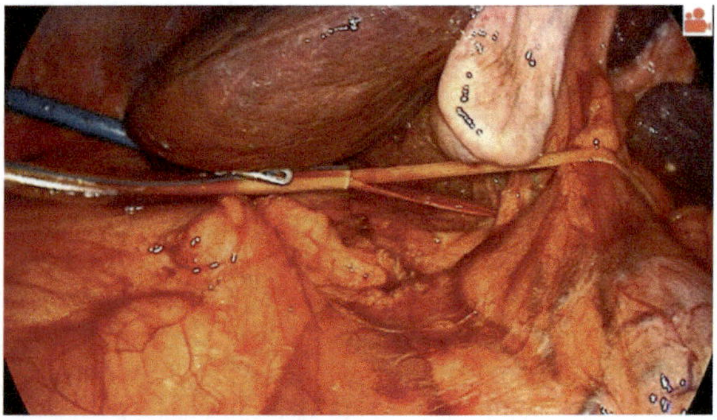

Fig. 19.5 Once the tension has been relieved, the Pringle maneuver should be released to restore hepatic inflow and minimize ischemic injury

compressing the hepatoduodenal ligament to manage hepatic hemorrhage and is widely used in liver surgery to minimize blood loss. In the case of the laparoscopic approach to liver trauma, we must also control the hepatic hilum to help control possible hepatic bleeding of portal or arterial origin.

To do this, we will place a 5- or 10-mm working port below the last right rib at the midaxillary line level, to introduce a laparoscopic clamp through there and pass it behind the hepatic hilum toward the pars flaccida of the gastrohepatic ligament. After sectioning it, we will introduce a cotton tape through another trocar and take one of its ends with the clamp that we have passed behind the hepatic hilum. We will pass the other end in front of the hilum and remove the two ends of the cotton tape through the trocar. We will temporarily remove this and introduce a 10–12 cm tube cut from a nasogastric tube into the abdominal cavity through the cotton tape. After this, we can replace the working port (Figs. 19.2, 19.3, and 19.4).

If it is necessary to clamp the hepatic hilum, we will pull on both ends of the cotton tape and the tube will tighten the tape around the hepatic hilum (Fig. 19.5), occluding the entry of hepatic blood flow with extracorporeal control of the tape [44]. Using the same entry point of the trocar into the cavity.

Techniques for Liver Hemostasis

Topical Hemostatic Agents

Topical hemostatic agents are often used in conjunction with perihepatic packing and electrocautery to control bleeding from the surface of the raw liver. There are various types depending on whether they are physical agents, biologically active agents, or combined preparations. Physical agents may be dry matrix (absorbable gelatin, oxidized regenerated cellulose, microfibrillar collagen, or microporous polysaccharide spheres) or external agents (chitosene, kaolin, or hemofiber).

Biologically active agents may be topical thrombin, fibrinogen plus human thrombin, dry fibrin sealant dressing, or albumin-glutaldehyde tissue adhesives.

Combined agents may be thrombin and gelatin or thrombin and collagen.

Virtually all of them can also be used laparoscopically, although almost all require a 10 mm port for introduction into the abdominal cavity.

Electrocautery

Conventional electrocautery or argon beam coagulation can be used to control minor bleeding from the surface of the raw liver. Cautery is probably only effective for vessels smaller than 0.5 mm in diameter; any larger vessels should be clipped or sutured.

Argon beam coagulation does not require actual contact with the liver surface to provide hemostasis, which is an advantage over conventional electrocautery, especially on more rugged surfaces.

Parenchymal Vessel Ligation

Deeper injuries to the liver parenchyma may require ligation or clamping of the vessels and bile ducts directly across the traumatic laceration.

This can be accomplished with selective clips or, occasionally, with endo staplers although the use of vascular endo staplers for hepatic vessel transection is well established, their application in hepatic parenchymal dissection is reserved for elective surgery. However, these instruments can also be utilized to achieve hemostasis in contused areas, the stapling devices and clear understanding of hepatic anatomy facilitate operative management.

Once the visible vessels and bile ducts have been controlled, residual bleeding from the liver surface can be controlled with topical hemostatic agents or electrocautery.

Direct Liver Suturing

Direct hepatic suture should not be used in case of severe bleeding, but should be used only in case of continuous staining of the hepatic parenchyma.

A topical hemostatic can be used in the middle of the sutured area to help achieve hemostasis of the area.

Suturing should be performed using monofilament 00/000 material with the largest needle that can be introduced through the trocar. The maximum amount of parenchyma should be included while tying as gently as possible to prevent tearing of the hepatic capsule. Based on experience in liver surgery, a knotless barbed suture can also be used.

Conversion to Open Surgery

Conversion to open surgery is mandatory in cases of hemodynamic instability of the patient, when perihepatic packing is required to control bleeding, when there are other complex injuries that require a laparotomy for control or if there is difficulty in visualizing structures.

Conversion rates range from 9.7% to 29.3% [43]. The reasons for converting from laparoscopy in trauma cases vary and include hemorrhage that cannot be controlled, hemodynamic instability, detection of multiple injuries, severe peritonitis, equipment failure, visualization difficulties, and complex injuries [45].

Complications

The use of laparoscopy in liver trauma treatment carries the risk of serious complications. In the event of a severe venous injury, the risk of air embolism increases significantly. Additionally, the pressure and flow of the pneumoperitoneum can reduce venous return and contribute to air embolism, potentially causing hemodynamic instability in a previously stable patient.

It should be noted that pneumoperitoneum can increase intracranial pressure in patients with pre-existing brain injuries. Tension pneumothorax may also occur in cases of thoraco-abdominal diaphragmatic injuries [46].

As with any laparoscopic procedure, other complications may occur, including incisional post hernias, iatrogenic injuries, and wound infections.

Additional complications for the trauma, NOM, and laparoscopy management include sepsis, hepatic necrosis and abscess, sterile biloma and bile leak, and gallbladder complications like infarction and perforation [47].

Future Directions

The management of hepatic injuries has evolved into a multidisciplinary approach while adhering to core trauma principles. Patient stability guides diagnostic and therapeutic decisions, with stable patients eligible for nonoperative management when resources allow. Experienced trauma and liver surgeons and interventional and therapeutic radiology play crucial roles in preventing and treating complications. Successful outcomes in complex liver trauma depend on the prompt correction of hypothermia, coagulopathy, and acidosis, along with rapid decision-making and expert judgment.

The role of laparoscopic surgery in trauma care is constantly evolving. On the one hand, diagnostic techniques and nonoperative management of trauma have developed significantly in recent years, and this could lead to a lower use of laparoscopic techniques.

However, surgeons who treat patients with severe trauma are increasingly better trained in minimally invasive surgical techniques and are more experienced in applying them to this type of patient, so it will continue to have its place in the surgical treatment of patients with severe trauma, including hepatic trauma.

References

1. Gunst M, Ghaemmaghami V, Gruszecki A, et al. Changing epidemiology of trauma deaths leads to a bimodal distribution. Baylor Univ Med Cent Proc. 2010;23(4):349–54.
2. Jastaniah A, Grushka. The role of minimally invasive surgeries in trauma. J Surg Clin North Am. 2024;104(2):437–49. https://doi.org/10.1016/j.suc.2023.10.003.
3. Brillantino A, Iacobellis F, Festa P, Mottola A, Acampora C, Corvino F, Del Giudice S, Lanza M, Armellino M, Niola R, Romano L, Castriconi M, De Palma M, Noschese G. Non-operative management of blunt liver trauma: safety, efficacy and complications of a standardized treatment protocol. Bull Emerg Trauma. 2019;7(1):49–54.
4. Coccolini F, Coimbra R, Ordonez C, et al. Liver trauma: WSES 2020 guidelines. World J Emerg Surg. 2020;15:24.
5. Richardson JD. Changes in the management of injuries to the liver and spleen. J Am Coll Surg. 2005;200(5):648–69. https://doi.org/10.1016/j.jamcollsurg.2004.11.005.
6. Peitzman AB, Richardson JD. Surgical treatment of injuries to the solid abdominal organs: a 50-year perspective from the journal of trauma. J Trauma. 2010;69(5):1011–21. https://doi.org/10.1097/TA.0b013e3181f9c216.
7. Pringle JH. V: notes on the arrest of hepatic hemorrhage due to trauma. Ann Surg. 1908;48(4):541–9. https://doi.org/10.1097/00000658-190810000-00005.
8. Skandalakis JE, Skandalakis LJ, Skandalakis PN, et al. Hepatic surgical anatomy. Surg Clin North Am. 2004;84:413–35.
9. Piper GL, Peitzman AB. Current management of hepatic trauma. Surg Clin North Am. 2010;90(4):775–85.

10. Rotondo MF, Schwab CW, McGonigal MD, et al. 'Damage control': an approach for improved survival in exsanguinating penetrating abdominal injury. J Trauma. 1993;35(3):375–82. discussion 382–3
11. Lin BC, Fang JF, Chen RJ, Wong YC, Hsu YP. Surgical management and outcome of blunt major liver injuries: experience of damage control laparotomy with perihepatic packing in one trauma centre. Injury. 2014;45:122–7.
12. Boese CK, Hackl M, Müller LP, Ruchholtz S, Frink M, Lechler P. Nonoperative management of blunt hepatic trauma: a systematic review. J Trauma Acute Care Surg. 2015;79:654–60.
13. Morrison JJ, Bramley KE, Rizzo AG. Liver trauma--operative management. J R Army Med Corps. 2011;157(2):136–44. https://doi.org/10.1136/jramc-157-02-03.
14. Linnaus ME, Langlais CS, Garcia NM, et al. Failure of nonoperative management of pediatric blunt liver and spleen injuries: a prospective Arizona-Texas-Oklahoma-Memphis-Arkansas consortium study. J Trauma Acute Care Surg. 2017;82(04):672–9.
15. Letoublon C, Amariutei A, Taton N, et al. Management of blunt hepatic trauma. J Visc Surg. 2016;153(4, Suppl):33–43.
16. Cook A, Weddle J, Baker S, et al. A comparison of the injury severity score and the trauma mortality prediction model. J Trauma Acute Care Surg. 2014;76(01):47–52, discussion 52–53
17. Coccolini F, Catena F, Moore EE, et al. WSES classification and guidelines for liver trauma. World J Emerg Surg. 2016;11(01):50.
18. Carver D, Kirkpatrick AW, D'Amours S, Hameed SM, Beveridge J, Ball CG. A prospective evaluation of the utility of a hybrid operating suite for severely injured patients: overstated or underutilized? Ann Surg. 2018; https://doi.org/10.1097/SLA.0000000000003175.
19. Gilyard S, Shinn K, Nezami N, et al. Contemporary management of hepatic trauma: what IRs need to know. Semin Intervent Radiol. 2020;37(1):35–43.
20. Fodor M, Primavesi F, Morell-Hofert D, et al. Non-operative management of blunt hepatic and splenic injuries-practical aspects and value of radiological scoring systems. Eur Surg. 2018;50(06):285–98.
21. Kozar RA, Crandall M, Shanmuganathan K, AAST Patient Assessment Committee, et al. Organ injury scaling 2018 update: spleen, liver, and kidney. J Trauma Acute Care Surg. 2018;85(06):1119–22.
22. Ruscelli P, Gemini A, Rimini M, et al. The role of grade of injury in non-operative management of blunt hepatic and splenic trauma: case series from a multicenter experience. Medicine (Baltimore). 2019;98(35):e16746.
23. Polanco P, Leon S, Pineda J, et al. Hepatic resection in the management of complex injury to the liver. J Trauma. 2008;65(6):1264–9. [discussion: 1269–70]
24. Forlee MV, Krige JE, Welman CJ, et al. Haemobilia after penetrating and blunt liver injury: treatment with selective hepatic artery embolisation. Injury. 2004;35(1):23–8.
25. Koganti D, et al. The role of diagnostic laparoscopy for trauma at a high-volume level one center. Surg Endosc. 2021;35:2667–70.
26. Padia SA, Ingraham CR, Moriarty JM, Wilkins LR, Bream PR Jr, Tam AL, et al. Society of interventional radiology position statement on endovascular intervention for trauma. J Vasc Interv Radiol. 2020;31(3):363–369.e2. https://doi.org/10.1016/j.jvir.2019.11.012.
27. Jeavons C, Hacking C, Beenen LF, Gunn ML. A review of split-bolus single-pass CT in the assessment of trauma patients. Emerg Radiol. 2018;25(04):367–74.
28. Durkin N, Deganello A, Sellars ME, Sidhu PS, Davenport M, Makin E. Post-traumatic liver and splenic pseudoaneurysms in children: diagnosis, management and follow-up screening using contrast- enhanced ultrasound (CEUS). J Pediatr Surg. 2016;51(02):289–92.
29. Darcy M. Acute gastrointestinal hemorrhage. In: Kandarpa K, Machan L, Durham J, editors. Handbook of interventional radiologic procedures. Wolters Kluwer Health; 2019. p. 232.
30. Vanninen RL, Manninen I. Onyx, a new liquid embolic material for peripheral interventions: preliminary experience in aneurysm, pseudoaneurysm, and pulmonary arteriovenous malformation embolization. Cardiovasc Intervent Radiol. 2007;30(02):196–200.

31. Medsinge A, Zajko A, Orons P, Amesur N, Santos E. A case-based approach to common embolization agents used in vascular interventional radiology. AJR Am J Roentgenol. 2014;203(04):699–708.
32. de'Angelis N, Khan J, Marchegiani F, Bianchi G, Aisoni F, Alberti D, et al. Robotic surgery in emergency setting: 2021 WSES position paper. World J Emerg Surg. 2022;17(1):4. https://doi.org/10.1186/s13017-022-00410-6.
33. Cuendis-Velázquez A, Bada-Yllán O, Trejo-Ávila M, et al. Robotic-assisted Roux-en-Y hepaticojejunostomy after bile duct injury. Langenbeck's Arch Surg. 2018;403:53–9.
34. Panteleimonitis S, Popeskou S, Aradaib M, Harper M, Ahmed J, Ahmad M, et al. Implementation of robotic rectal surgery training programme: importance of standardisation and structured training. Langenbeck's Arch Surg. 2018;403:749–60. https://doi.org/10.1007/s00423-018-1690-1.
35. Sermonesi G, Tian BWCA, Vallicelli C, "et al". Cesena guidelines: WSES consensus statement on laparoscopic-first approach to general surgery emergencies and abdominal trauma. World J Emerg Surg 2023;18(1):57. doi:https://doi.org/10.1186/s13017-023-00520-9. PMID: 38066631; PMCID: PMC10704840.
36. García IC, Villalba JS, Iovino D, "et al". Liver trauma: until when we have to delay surgery? A review Life (Basel) 2022;12(5):694. doi:https://doi.org/10.3390/life12050694.
37. Ki YJ, Jo YG, Park YC, Kang WS. The efficacy and safety of laparoscopy for blunt abdominal trauma: a systematic review and meta-analysis. J Clin Med. 2021;10(9):1853. https://doi.org/10.3390/jcm10091853.
38. Justin V, Fingerhut A, Uranues S. Laparoscopy in blunt abdominal trauma: for whom? When? and why? Curr Trauma Rep. 2017;3:43–50. https://doi.org/10.1007/s40719-017-0076-0.
39. Anderson JE, Salcedo ES, Rounds KM, Galante JM. Getting a better look: outcomes of laparoscopic versus transdiaphragmatic pericardial window for penetrating thoracoabdominal trauma at a level I trauma center. J Trauma Acute Care Surg. 2016;81(6):1035–8. https://doi.org/10.1097/TA.0000000000001173.
40. Morimoto RY, Birolini D, Rodrigues Júnior AJ, Pogget R, Horita LT. Ballon tamponade for transfixing lesions of the liver. Surg Gynecol Obstetrics. 1987;164:87–8.
41. Poggetti RS, Moore EE. Balloon tamponade for bilobar transfixing hepatic gunshot wounds. J Trauma. 1992;33:694.
42. Brooks A, Reilly JJ, Hope C, Navarro A, Naess PA, Gaarder C. Evolution of non-operative management of liver trauma. Trauma Surg Acute Care Open. 2020;5(1):e000551. https://doi.org/10.1136/tsaco-2020-000551.
43. Iordache FM, Giumba T, Bărăian C, Ghioldiş A, Făgărăşan V, Copăescu C, et al. Laparoscopy in Abdominal Emergencies. Chirurgia. 2024;119(6)
44. Piardi T, Lhuaire M, Memeo R, et al. Laparoscopic Pringle maneuver: how we do it? HepatoBiliary Surg Nutr. 2016;5(4):345–9. https://doi.org/10.21037/hbsn.2015.11.01.
45. Letoublon C, Chen Y, Arvieux C, et al. Delayed celiotomy or laparoscopy as part of the nonoperative management of blunt hepatic trauma. World J Surg. 2008;32(6):1189–93. https://doi.org/10.1007/s00268-007-9439-y.
46. Zantut LF, Ivatury RR, Smith RS, et al. Diagnostic and therapeutic laparoscopy for penetrating abdominal trauma: a multicenter experience. J Trauma 1997;42(5):825–829. discussion 829–31.
47. Green CS, Bulger EM, Kwan SW. Outcomes and complications of angioembolization for hepatic trauma: a systematic review of the literature. J Trauma Acute Care Surg. 2016;80(03):529–37.

Biliary Tract Injuries: When Laparoscopy Is Useful After Trauma

20

Marcelo A. F. Ribeiro Jr, Shailvi Gupta, David T. Efron, Steven B. Holsten, and Thomas M. Scalea

Introduction

Biliary tract injuries, regardless of etiology, present a significant challenge in both their management and treatment outcomes. The primary cause of biliary tract injuries is associated with laparoscopic surgery for the treatment of gallstones, with an estimated incidence ranging from 0.4% to 1.5%. In comparison, the incidence in open surgery is reported to be between 0.2% and 0.3% [1]. Traumatic bile duct injuries are exceedingly rare, accounting for approximately 0.1% of trauma admissions [2]. These injuries typically occur alongside other abdominal trauma, such as blunt liver injuries. Extrahepatic bile duct injuries are often associated with pancreatic, duodenal, or major vascular injuries, but these are far less common than injuries involving the intrahepatic segments of the bile ducts. Gallbladder injuries are more frequently observed in cases of penetrating trauma, and ischemic involvement of the gallbladder may occur as a result of hepatic injury in rare instances. In blunt abdominal trauma, gallbladder involvement is typically associated with high-kinetic-energy mechanisms [3, 4]. The treatment of choice for such injuries is cholecystectomy [3–6].

Diagnosis

The method used in the diagnosis of biliary tract injuries depends on the patient's hemodynamic status. Liver function tests in this scenario are unreliable, should not be used as a tool for decision-making, and are therefore unnecessary.

M. A. F. Ribeiro Jr (✉) · S. Gupta · D. T. Efron · S. B. Holsten · T. M. Scalea
Department of Surgery – R Adams Cowley Shock Trauma. Center, University of Maryland School of Medicine, Baltimore, MD, USA

© The Author(s), under exclusive license to Springer Nature Switzerland AG 2026
M. Cezillo, B. M. Pereira (eds.), *Minimally Invasive Surgery Trauma*,
https://doi.org/10.1007/978-3-032-28971-1_20

Hemodynamically stable patients should first undergo a detailed physical examination. After considering the mechanism of injury, patients at risk for significant intra-abdominal injury should have abdominal computed tomography to assess the extent of the injuries and guide the therapeutic approach. In contrast, unstable patients sustaining pelvic fractures, a positive FAST exam or signs of peritonitis should proceed directly to exploratory laparotomy, where signs such as bile leakage from the liver parenchyma, extrahepatic bile ducts, or the pancreatic region should raise high suspicion of biliary tract injury. It is important to highlight that the absence of bile leakage coming from the liver does not rule out a biliary injury. The presence of large hematomas can hide a biliary fistula, and consideration of placing a drain and follow-up imaging may be necessary in the postoperative period. Any identified intraparenchymal biliary leaks at the time of surgery are well managed by direct ductal ligation or clipping. Intraoperatively identified gallbladder injuries are best treated with cholecystectomy. Damage control surgery principles for unstable patients are crucial to controlling contamination and hemorrhage. Once the patient is stabilized, the surgeon must determine the optimal approach for drainage, repair, or referral to a specialized hepatopancreatobiliary (HPB) surgery service [7].

The Role of Laparoscopy in the Treatment of Traumatic Bile Duct Injuries

It is essential to remember that laparoscopic surgery currently has no role in the management of unstable trauma patients. Its use is reserved for stable patients who have undergone appropriate imaging that suggests biliary tract injury. The success of treating complex liver injuries nonoperatively has been associated with an increase in complications secondary to liver injuries, where some patients will likely require some type of interventional procedure. Historically, such complications were treated with laparotomy. Laparoscopy has become a valuable tool in managing both traumatic biliary injuries and later complications, offering both diagnostic and therapeutic benefits due to its minimally invasive nature and diagnostic precision. Current guidelines from the World Society of Emergency Surgery and the American Association for the Surgery of Trauma emphasize the utility of diagnostic laparoscopy in evaluating and managing biliary injuries, especially in delayed settings [8]. According to Ribeiro Jr et al. [9] the laparoscopic technique must follow a well-established systematization that can be summarized as follows:

Technical Aspects of Diagnostic and/or Therapeutic Laparoscopy in Trauma Patients.

1. *Initial Access*

   The first access should be achieved using a 10/12 mm trocar, avoiding the use of a Veress needle.

   Pneumoperitoneum should be established progressively, targeting intra-abdominal pressure levels of 12–14 mmHg. Insufflation must be discontinued immediately in cases of increased respiratory pressure, hypotension, or tachycardia.

2. *Visualization and Optics*

   Both 0° and 30° laparoscopes can be utilized, but the 30° optic is more versatile.

3. *Trocar Placement*

   If the initial survey does not mandate conversion to laparotomy, additional 5 mm or 12 mm trocars should be inserted under direct vision, without blades, and strategically positioned based on the suspected area of injury.

4. *Patient Positioning for Regional Assessment*

   Supramesocolic Region: Position the patient in reverse Trendelenburg to facilitate evaluation of the liver, gallbladder, spleen, diaphragm, pancreas, stomach, and duodenum.

   Mesocolic and Inframesocolic Regions: Adjust the position to Trendelenburg for assessment of the rectum, the pouch of Douglas, pelvic organs, cecum, and right colon.

5. *Examination of the Small Intestine*

   After moving the omentum cranially, examine the entire small intestine from the ileocecal valve to the ligament of Treitz using two atraumatic intestinal clamps. Both sides of the bowel must be systematically inspected to avoid missing injuries.

6. *Assessment of the Bladder*

   The urinary bladder should be thoroughly inspected. Methylene blue may be administered through a Foley catheter or intravenously to assist in detecting leaks.

7. *Systematic Assessment Protocol*

   Injuries may be overlooked without a systematic approach. Sequential evaluation should be performed as follows:

   1. *Diaphragm*: The first region to inspect after controlling bleeding, as injuries may cause pleural communication and hemodynamic instability.
   2. *Liver and Gallbladder*: Look for hematomas, lesions, and presence of bile in the cavity. In cases where there a high index of suspicion of extrahepatic bile duct injuries, a cholecystectomy with intraoperative cholangiography can be done to study the biliary tree.
   3. *Spleen*
   4. *Anterior Wall of the Stomach*
   5. *Division of the Gastrocolic Ligament*
   6. *Posterior Wall of the Stomach*: Elevate with forceps to inspect the retroperitoneum beneath.
   7. *Pancreas and Retroperitoneal Area*
   8. *Duodenum*: Both above and below the mesocolon.
   9. *Small Intestine*: Perform a meticulous inspection, confirming bowel integrity. Reevaluate twice if peritoneal violation or abnormal contents are noted. Spread approximately 10 cm of bowel between two atraumatic forceps,

rotate, and inspect systematically. Remove clots or fibrinous exudates to expose the bowel wall for thorough examination. Areas of contusion or hematoma should be further probed using atraumatic forceps and dry gauze.

10. *Right Colon and Retroperitoneum*: Include the cecum, ascending colon, hepatic flexure, right kidney, hilum, and ureter. Mobilize the colon to evaluate retroperitoneal structures.
11. *Transverse Colon*
12. *Left Colon and Retroperitoneum*: Include the splenic flexure, descending and sigmoid colon, left kidney, hilum, and ureter.
13. *Pelvic Cavity*: Assess the rectum and bladder.

8. *Additional Critical Areas*

    1. Pay particular attention to the inferior vena cava, aorta, and other regions requiring detailed examination. In case any hematoma is identified in zones I, II, or III it is NOT recommended to explore using laparoscopy.

By adhering to this systematic approach, surgeons can ensure comprehensive assessment and management of intra-abdominal injuries in trauma patients while minimizing the risk of missed injuries.

Injury to the Biliary Tree

Intraoperatively, laparoscopy can aid in diagnosing and managing bile duct injuries through techniques such as intraoperative cholangiography, which allows for visualization of biliary anatomy and injury identification [10]. In cases of bile peritonitis following trauma, laparoscopy facilitates abdominal washout and drainage, assisting in the control of sepsis and bile leakage [11, 12]. The primary benefits of laparoscopy can be summarized as follows:

- Diagnostic Accuracy: Laparoscopy allows for a thorough examination of the peritoneal cavity, identifying biliary tract injuries that may not be detected through other imaging modalities [13].
- Therapeutic Applications: Laparoscopy can be used to conservatively treat minor bile duct injuries (BDIs) or stabilize patients for subsequent definitive repair [14]. This includes procedures such as bile duct suturing, drainage, and complex reconstructions in select cases [15]. Currently, the complexity of the procedures that can safely be performed by minimally invasive surgery is a function of the surgical team's expertise in these types of procedures.
- Robotic surgery: In the near future, the use of robotic surgery for emergency surgery and selective trauma cases may enhance the therapeutic options to manage liver, bile ducts, and pancreatic injuries, increasing the capabilities of procedures done using minimally invasive surgery.

- Postoperative outcomes: The use of laparoscopy in managing these injuries has been associated with favorable postoperative outcomes, including reduced complications and faster recovery [16].
- Multidisciplinary approach: Optimal management often requires collaboration among surgeons, interventional gastroenterologists, and radiologists to ensure comprehensive care [1, 17].

Laparoscopy has been utilized for drainage of large, retained fluid collections, often a mixture of bile and blood, some with bacterial fluid. Drains can be placed easily using the laparoscope after a proper washout has been performed.

For definitive repair, laparoscopic techniques can be employed to suture small duct leaks, insert drains, and perform hepaticojejunostomy in selected cases [17, 18]. However, the injury's complexity, the intervention's timing, and the surgeon's expertise are critical factors in determining the feasibility of laparoscopic repair. Open surgery remains the most appropriate approach for most trauma surgeons for managing more complex injuries or when laparoscopic expertise is limited [12].

Another valuable tool associated most recently with laparoscopic procedures is represented by the use of Indocyanine green (ICG) fluorescence imaging intraoperatively. It has become an invaluable tool enhancing the visualization of biliary structures and thereby improving surgical safety and efficacy. ICG binds to plasma proteins and is excreted exclusively via bile, allowing the biliary anatomy to be clearly delineated under near-infrared light. This technique enhances the visualization of bile ducts, reducing the risk of iatrogenic injuries, which are among the most feared complications in biliary surgery. Additionally, ICG fluorescence facilitates the identification of bile leaks and ensures accurate anastomotic reconstruction during procedures such as laparoscopic hepaticojejunostomy. A 2024 systematic review by Manasseh et al. evaluated the role of ICG fluorescence imaging during laparoscopic cholecystectomy. The study found that ICG significantly enhanced the visualization of key biliary structures, such as the cystic duct and common bile duct, particularly in anatomically challenging cases. Additionally, the use of ICG was associated with a reduction in operative times in complex cases, with an average decrease of approximately 20 min compared to conventional white light imaging [19]. While the overall incidence of bile duct injuries (BDI) was low, the use of ICG showed a trend toward lower BDI rates compared to white light though the difference was not statistically significant. These findings suggest that ICG fluorescence imaging offers notable advantages in improving visualization of biliary anatomy and reducing operative time in complex cases, thereby enhancing patient safety during laparoscopic cholecystectomy.

Conclusion

Laparoscopy is increasingly recognized for its role in the management of traumatic biliary tract injuries, particularly for diagnostic purposes and, in select cases, for therapeutic interventions.

References

1. de'Angelis N, Catena F, Memeo R, et al. WSES guidelines for the detection and management of bile duct injury during cholecystectomy. World J Emerg Surg. 2020;16:30. https://doi.org/10.1186/s13017-021-00369-w.
2. Buell JF, Cronin DC, Funaki B, et al. Devastating and fatal complications associated with combined vascular and bile duct injuries during cholecystectomy. Arch Surg. 2002;137:703Y708; discussion 708Y710.
3. Ball CG, Dixon E, Kirkpatrick AW, et al. A decade of experience with injuries to the gallbladder. J Trauma Manag Outcomes. 2010;4:3.
4. Bade PG, Thomson SR, Hirshberg A, et al. Surgical options in traumatic injury to the extrahepatic biliary tract. Br J Surg. 1989;76:256Y258.
5. Epstein MG, Silva DL, Elias NC, Sica GT, Fávaro Mde L, Ribeiro Junior MAF. Isolated rupture of the gallbladder following blunt abdominal trauma: case report. Einstein (Sao Paulo). 2013;11(2):227–8. https://doi.org/10.1590/s1679-45082013000200016.
6. Reitz MM, Araújo JM, de Souza GHN, Gagliardi DP, de Toledo FVT, Ribeiro Júnior MAF. Choleperitoneum secondary to isolated subserosal gallbladder injury due to blunt abdominal trauma – a case report. Trauma Case Rep. 2022;41:100674. https://doi.org/10.1016/j.tcr.2022.100674.
7. Thomson BN, Nardino B, Gumm K, Robertson AJ, Knowles BP, Collier NA, Judson R. Management of blunt and penetrating biliary tract trauma. J Trauma Acute Care Surg. 2012;72(6):1620–5. https://doi.org/10.1097/TA.0b013e318248ed65.
8. Coccolini F, Kobayashi L, Kluger Y, et al. Duodeno-pancreatic and extrahepatic biliary tree trauma: WSES-AAST guidelines. World J Emerg Surg. 2019;14:56. https://doi.org/10.1186/s13017-019-0278-6.
9. Ribeiro MAF Jr, Tebar GK, Salgueiro J, Galindo G, Hughes JD, Sayari A, et al. Role and limitations of laparoscopy in abdominal trauma. Med Res Arch. 2023;11(8) https://doi.org/10.18103/mra.v11i8.4333.
10. Gupta V, Jayaraman S. Role for laparoscopy in the management of bile duct injuries. Can J Surg. 2017;60(5):300–4. https://doi.org/10.1503/cjs.003317.
11. Carrillo EH, Reed DN Jr, Gordon L, Spain DA, Richardson JD. Delayed laparoscopy facilitates the management of biliary peritonitis in patients with complex liver injuries. Surg Endosc. 2001;15(3):319–22. https://doi.org/10.1007/s004640000300.
12. Stassen NA, Bhullar I, Cheng JD, Crandall M, Friese R, Guillamondegui O, Jawa R, Maung A, Rohs TJ Jr, Sangosanya A, Schuster K, Seamon M, Tchorz KM, Zarzuar BL, Kerwin A, Eastern Association for the Surgery of Trauma. Nonoperative management of blunt hepatic injury: an Eastern Association for the Surgery of Trauma practice management guideline. J Trauma Acute Care Surg. 2012;73(5 Suppl 4):S288–93. https://doi.org/10.1097/TA.0b013e318270160d.
13. Zelic M, Lekic V, Bazdulj E, Hauser G. Biliary tract injuries. In: Abdeldayem H, editor. Topics in the surgery of the biliary tree. IntechOpen; 2018. https://doi.org/10.5772/intechopen.76328.
14. Coccolini F, Coimbra R, Ordonez C, et al. Liver trauma: WSES 2020 guidelines. World J Emerg Surg. 2020;15:24. https://doi.org/10.1186/s13017-020-00302-7.
15. Di Saverio S, Birindelli A, Podda M, Segalini E, Piccinini A, Coniglio C, Frattini C, Tugnoli G. Trauma laparoscopy and the six w's: why, where, who, when, what, and how? J Trauma Acute Care Surg. 2019;86(2):344–67. https://doi.org/10.1097/TA.0000000000002130.
16. Chaudhary P, Kumar R, Arora MP. Biliary tract injuries. Hellenic J Surg. 2015;87:149–55. https://doi.org/10.1007/s13126-015-0200-y.
17. Cuendis-Velázquez A, Morales-Chávez C, Aguirre-Olmedo I, Torres-Ruiz F, Rojano-Rodríguez M, Fernández-Álvarez L, Cárdenas-Lailson E, Moreno-Portillo M. Laparoscopic hepaticojejunostomy after bile duct injury. Surg Endosc. 2016;30(3):876–82. https://doi.org/10.1007/s00464-015-4282-y.

18. Dokmak S, Amharar N, Aussilhou B, Cauchy F, Sauvanet A, Belghiti J, Soubrane O. Laparoscopic repair of post-cholecystectomy bile duct injury: a advance in surgical management. J Gastrointest Surg. 2017;21(8):1368–72. https://doi.org/10.1007/s11605-017-3400-7.
19. Manasseh M, Davis H, Bowling K. Evaluating the role of Indocyanine green fluorescence imaging in enhancing safety and efficacy during laparoscopic cholecystectomy: a systematic review. Cureus. 2024;16(11):e73388. https://doi.org/10.7759/cureus.73388.

21 Gastrointestinal Injuries: When and How?

Sariya Khan, Husna Irfan Thalib, Agata Grochowska, Mable Pereira, and Marcelo Augusto Fontenelle Ribeiro Jr

Introduction

A significant number of trauma victims will sustain gastrointestinal (GI) injuries in both blunt and penetrating injuries. With the advancement of minimally invasive techniques, laparoscopy has increasingly emerged as a viable alternative to traditional laparotomy in selected trauma cases. While historically underutilized due to concerns regarding missed injuries, improved instrumentation and surgical expertise have significantly reduced the rate of missed lesions from 13% to 0.12% in experienced hands [1].

Laparoscopy is now recognized for its diagnostic accuracy, capacity to avoid unnecessary laparotomies, and potential therapeutic application in hemodynamically stable patients [2, 3]. Negative or non-therapeutic laparotomies, once common in trauma surgery, have been associated with substantial morbidity, including surgical site infections, adhesions, hernias, and even mortality [3]. Consequently, incorporating laparoscopy into trauma protocols has led to fewer complications and improved patient outcomes.

This chapter discusses the precise indications for laparoscopy in GI trauma, outlines absolute and relative contraindications, and provides a structured framework for safe and effective application of laparoscopy in abdominal trauma scenarios.

S. Khan · H. I. Thalib
General Medicine Practice Program, Batterjee Medical College, Jeddah, Saudi Arabia

A. Grochowska
Faculty of Medicine, Medical University of Lodz, Lodz, Poland

M. Pereira
Lincoln American University, School of Medicine, Georgetown, Guyana

M. A. F. Ribeiro Jr (✉)
University of Maryland, R Adams Cowley Shock Trauma Center, Baltimore, MY, USA
e-mail: mfribeiro@som.umaryland.edu

© The Author(s), under exclusive license to Springer Nature Switzerland AG 2026

M. Cezillo, B. M. Pereira (eds.), *Minimally Invasive Surgery Trauma*,
https://doi.org/10.1007/978-3-032-28971-1_21

Patient Selection: When Is Laparoscopy Appropriate in GI Trauma?

Hemodynamic Stability: A Prerequisite

Laparoscopy in trauma is only appropriate in hemodynamically stable patients or those who respond promptly to fluid resuscitation (i.e., Grade I or II hemorrhagic shock). Hemodynamic instability (SBP <90 mmHg, unresponsive to resuscitation) remains a formal contraindication [2, 4]. Patients must be appropriately screened using vital signs and metabolic indices such as pH, base excess, and serum lactate to ensure physiologic suitability [1, 2].

Injury Mechanism and Indications

Laparoscopy is most appropriate for:

- *Penetrating trauma* with uncertain peritoneal penetration (e.g., low-velocity stab wounds, tangential gunshot wounds) [2, 5].
- *Suspected diaphragmatic injuries*, especially after left thoracoabdominal injuries, which are frequently missed on CT (sensitivity ~26%) [2, 6–8].
- *Unclear abdomen* (i.e., discrepancy between physical findings and imaging) [2].
- *Suspected GI or bladder injury* based on CT or clinical findings [2, 5].
- *Presence of free intraperitoneal fluid* in blunt trauma without solid organ injury [2].
- *Intraperitoneal bladder injuries*, visualized on cystography or inferred from free fluid [2].

These indications are summarized in Table 21.1.

These situations allow laparoscopy to function diagnostically and therapeutically, with sensitivity and specificity approaching 100% in expert hands [4].

Exclusion Criteria and Contraindications

Absolute contraindications include:

- Hemodynamic instability (non-responder to fluids)
- Septic shock
- Severe cardiopulmonary dysfunction
- Severe traumatic brain injury
- Inability to establish pneumoperitoneum [2, 5].

Relative contraindications, which depend on surgeon's expertise, include:

Table 21.1 Indications for diagnostic and therapeutic laparoscopy in GI trauma

Indication	Clinical context	Supporting reference
Hemodynamically stable or stabilized after fluids	Grades I–II hemorrhagic shock; SBP ≥90 mmHg	Ribeiro et al. (2023) [2]
Penetrating abdominal trauma with unclear peritoneal breach	Tangential GSWs, anterior stab wounds	Di Saverio et al. (2019) [5]
Suspected diaphragmatic injury	Especially left thoracoabdominal wounds; CT sensitivity only ~26%	Uranues et al. (2015) [4]; Ribeiro et al. [2]
Unexplained free fluid in abdomen on CT	Especially in blunt trauma without solid organ injury	Ribeiro et al. (2023) [2]
Suspected GI, bladder, or mesenteric injury	CT findings suggestive of hollow viscus or retroperitoneal injury	Ribeiro et al. (2023) [2]
Discrepancy between physical exam and imaging	"Unclear abdomen"; avoids unnecessary laparotomy	Birindelli et al. (2020) [2]
Intraperitoneal bladder injury	Free fluid on CT or cystography leakage	Ribeiro et al. (2023) [2]
Evisceration after penetrating trauma	In selected stable cases	Matsevych et al. (2016) [9]
Failure of non-operative management (e.g., splenic trauma)	Laparoscopic splenectomy or drainage for complications	Ribeiro et al. (2023) [2]
Suspected or confirmed pancreatic injury	Hemostasis, drainage, or fluid evacuation via laparoscopy	Ribeiro et al. (2023) [2]

Table 21.2 Contraindications for laparoscopy in trauma

Absolute contraindications	Relative contraindications
Hemodynamic instability (SBP <90 mmHg, unresponsive)	COPD with CO_2 retention
Septic shock	Previous laparotomy with dense adhesions
Severe cardiopulmonary dysfunction	Obesity or large intra-abdominal mass
Severe traumatic brain injury	Umbilical or diaphragmatic hernia
Inability to achieve pneumoperitoneum	Peritoneal tuberculosis
	Obvious evisceration (in select cases)

- Extensive prior abdominal surgery (adhesions)
- Severe COPD with CO_2 retention
- Obesity or large intra-abdominal mass
- Obvious evisceration
- Umbilical or diaphragmatic hernia [2, 5]

These relative factors do not necessarily preclude laparoscopy but require experienced laparoscopic trauma surgeons to proceed safely. A summarized list of contraindications is provided in Table 21.2.

Technical Considerations: How to Perform Trauma Laparoscopy

Early Access and Trocar Placement

The placement of trocar should be customized for the zone of potential injury. A 10–12 mm Hasson or optical access is typically done at the umbilicus or supraumbilical site. Direct vision access must be used so that distended loops of bowel or adhesions, if any, are avoided, particularly in the situation where there was prior surgery. Working ports (5–10 mm) are created under direct vision along the axillary and midclavicular anterior lines, angling laterally for retroperitoneal or flank trauma. The fourth port can be inserted for retraction or suction if needed [5, 8].

Intra-abdominal Pressure Precautions

Pneumoperitoneum should be maintained at the best 10–12 mmHg to obtain the best visibility and hemodynamic tolerance. In trauma, especially in borderline cardiopulmonary patients, increased intra-abdominal pressure reduces venous return and exacerbates hypotension. Pressures above 15 mmHg should be avoided. End-tidal CO_2 monitoring and blood pressure monitoring during insufflation should be carried out closely [2, 4].

Systematic Exploration of the GI Tract to Prevent Missed Injuries

Missed injuries are a serious concern in laparoscopy for trauma and can be minimized by maintaining an algorithm of systematic inspection.

Stomach Inspection begins with the anterior wall. Inspection is facilitated by retraction of the liver, visualizing the lesser curvature and gastroesophageal junction better. Inspection of the posterior wall can include incision of the gastrocolic ligament and superior retraction of the greater curvature [1].

Small Bowel Perform a gentle bowel sweep from the ligament of Treitz to the junction of the ileum and cecum. Use atraumatic clamps to lift, roll, and inspect one loop at a time in an organized sequence. Mesenteric and antimesenteric borders have to be visualized. Skipped loops or rush sweeps are heinous culprits in perforations being overlooked [4, 9].

Colon Anterior wall is inspected directly. Posterior wall and zones in mesocolon require mobilization. In right-sided trauma, an incision is performed in the lateral peritoneal reflection crossing the white line of Toldt. Left colon and sigmoid are mobilized by coming down lateral attachments and bringing the colon medially [2, 5].

Patient Positioning for Optimal Visualization

Position is adjusted to facilitate gravitational retraction of viscera and field exposure optimization:

Trendelenburg (15–20°) Provides access to the pelvis, especially useful for examination of the bladder, sigmoid colon, and rectum.

Reverse Trendelenburg Aids in examination of the stomach, diaphragm, and upper quadrants by moving the bowel away from top abdomen.

Other tilts of the table (lateral right or left) can also further improve access to individual quadrants depending on the injured area [1, 8].

Laparoscopic Management of GI Injuries: Organ-Specific Strategies

Recently, minimally invasive surgery has become the preferred option for managing gastrointestinal injuries in trauma cases, particularly in stable patients. As surgeons gain more experience with trauma laparoscopy, they are familiar with the nuances of organ-specific strategies. This means understanding when laparoscopy is the right choice and, equally important, when timely conversion to open surgery is warranted. This section has been compiled as a practical guide for the laparoscopic management of injuries to the stomach, small bowel, colon, and duodenum. Each section below is aligned to address some of the technical tips and decision-making strategies based on the current practice.

Stomach

Stomach injuries are common, particularly in cases of anterior penetrating trauma. If the patient is stable and in the absence of significant contamination, laparoscopic repair can often be performed safely and effectively. Anterior injuries are usually straightforward, whereas posterior injuries are more complex. They may require more advanced mobilization and are associated with a higher risk [2, 5].

For linear injuries with healthy edges, a stapled repair using a laparoscopic linear stapler is often effective and safe. However, if irregular, jagged, or larger perforations are encountered, a two-layer hand-sewn closure is usually the preferred approach. An absorbable inner layer and an interrupted seromuscular outer layer can be used for this purpose. A leak test should be routinely performed to confirm repair integrity; air insufflation via an orogastric or nasogastric tube with saline irrigation should be performed prior to completing the procedure [10].

Tip Use of a 30° laparoscope and liver retractor may significantly enhance visualization, particularly for posterior wall injuries [11].

Small Bowel

Not all small bowel injuries require resection. Clean, small perforations without devascularization can generally be managed with primary repair. In the presence of devitalized bowel, crush injury, or closely grouped perforations, resection and anastomosis are recommended [12].

Anastomosis: What to Keep in Mind

- The bowel should be handled with care, and everything should be aligned properly.
- The choice between intracorporeal and extracorporeal techniques may be selected based on the location of the injury and the surgeons' experience.
- Always check perfusion before the anastomosis. Indocyanine green (ICG) can be a useful tool [13, 14].

Tip A methodical bowel run should be performed from the ligament of Treitz to the ileocecal junction. Atraumatic graspers should be used to examine both the mesenteric and antimesenteric borders [14].

Colon

Colon injury requires careful evaluation, particularly in the context of hemodynamic stability and contamination. In stable patients with isolated, clean injuries and good blood supply, laparoscopic primary repair or resection with anastomosis is often a good option. However, in cases of gross contamination, delayed presentation, or multiple systemic injuries, loop colostomy is a safer diversion method [14].

Tip The affected segment should be fully mobilized prior to definitive repair. The mesentery and other nearby structures should also be checked for hidden injuries [15].

Duodenum and Mesentery

Duodenal and mesenteric injuries require particular caution due to their complex retroperitoneal location, which can be challenging. Many duodenal injuries are retroperitoneal, and the only clues may be subtle, such as bile staining or retroperitoneal crepitus [16].

When to Convert

Be ready to convert to open surgery if the following is suspected:

- The second or third portion of duodenal injuries
- An expanding retroperitoneal hematoma
- Involvement of the pancreas or biliary tree
- Inadequate visualization even after Kocherization
- In these situations, early conversion to open surgery is not a failure, but rather a reflection of sound intraoperative judgment [16].

Safe Techniques

- A Kocher maneuver should be performed to mobilize the duodenum, allowing inspection of both the anterior and posterior surfaces.
- For mesenteric injuries, signs such as creeping fat, dusky coloration, or sluggish peristalsis, which can indicate compromised perfusion, should be assessed [17].

Tip If intraoperative visualization is suboptimal or doubt remains regarding the extent of injury, early conversion to open surgery is advised [18].

Advantages and Limitations of Laparoscopy in GI Trauma

Advantages of Laparoscopy in GI Trauma

Trauma surgery has evolved over the years, driven by technical improvements and a new concept of minimally invasive surgery. Among these, laparoscopy has been evolving into a crucial diagnostic and therapeutic tool in hemodynamically stable patients, especially in GI trauma patients [19]. The advantages of laparoscopy in GI trauma include reduced risk of postoperative infections, reduced postoperative pain, shorter hospital stay and enhanced recovery, precision, and maneuverability.

Reduced Risk of Postoperative Infections

Laparoscopy implementation in emergency surgery settings offers at least a few key advantages when applied in GI trauma. First, due to small incisions in the abdominal cavity for the camera and working trocars, there is a lower risk of surgical site occurrence (SSO), including surgical site infection (SSI) [20]. Also, laparoscopy offers a lower risk of intra-abdominal abscess. This is especially important in GI trauma patients due to damage to the digestive tract; they are primarily at risk of leakage of digestive contents and digestive enzymes, leading to chemical or bacterial peritonitis and sepsis. The trauma patients are at risk of contamination, open wounds, or delayed presentation. When the extent of tissue exposure and tool manipulation is diminished in laparoscopy, the outcomes concerning inflammatory response and wound healing are far more favorable.

Reduced Postoperative Pain

Laparoscopic approach with fewer and smaller incisions allows patients to be less burdened by pain, which translates into less opioid use. Considering the global opioid crisis, the exposure to opioids should be as low as possible to treat pain. Less pain is associated with earlier mobilization and standing after surgery. In addition, the use of opioids exposes trauma patients to impaired respiratory function, limited mobility, and overall recovery. Opioids also affect gastrointestinal motility. The gastrointestinal tract is very sensitive in critically ill, trauma patients, and many factors can affect its functioning, from the gastrointestinal barrier and absorption to motility [21].

Shorter Length of Stay and Enhanced Recovery

Laparoscopic surgery is associated with a shorter length of hospital stay and faster return to everyday activities. The length of stay of patients with abdominal trauma is significantly shorter than those who underwent laparotomy [22]. In trauma care, bed availability and resource utilization are very important parts that make the system work efficiently. It is beneficial for patients, but also for the hospital, to allow for early hospital discharge. In cases of more severe trauma, accompanying comorbidities or additional injuries significantly increase the risk of prolonged hospitalization and additional antibiotic-resistant microbial infections caused by exposure to the hospital environment.

Precision and Maneuverability

Laparoscopic surgery has evolved over many years towards better visualization of gastrointestinal injuries and improved maneuverability within the abdominal cavity to treat intestinal perforations, bleeding, or bile leakage. In addition, magnification with a high-quality view allows for accurate assessment of damage to the gastrointestinal tract and incorporates proper intervention. Laparoscopy fulfills two substantial roles: diagnosing GI tract injury and treating GI injury. This is particularly important because it allows laparotomy to be avoided if the patient's GI injury can be managed via laparoscopy. The detection of minor traumatic injuries within the GI tract allows for their early treatment before the patient's condition begins to deteriorate and, due to hemodynamic instability, requires laparotomy.

Limitations of Laparoscopy in GI

As laparoscopy is a very valuable diagnostic and therapeutic tool, it has its limitations. Those include the risk of missed injuries, difficult visualization in certain regions, technical demands, a long learning curve, and patient-related factors.

Risk of Missed Injuries

While magnification and high-quality imaging are very valuable benefits of laparoscopy, the risk of missed injuries still exists. Incomplete exploration, due to operators' lack of experience, poor visualization, intra-abdominal adhesions, no operation progress, and technical constraints, can result in false negatives with undetected injuries that may be fatal [23]. A recent study revealed that missed injuries were associated with a 23.5-fold increased risk of death and a 41.8-fold increased risk of major complications in laparotomy [24]. For laparoscopies, the rates are significantly lower as the laparoscopy has evolved for the better. However, in the past, laparoscopy had missed injury rates of nearly 20–40% in the early stages [25, 26]. However, the advances in surgical methods and modification of positioning (Trendelenburg or reverse Trendelenburg) have helped with enhancing visualization, and nowadays, missed injury rates are closer to zero [27].

Difficult Visualization in Certain Anatomical Regions

Trauma can also disrupt normal anatomy, cause hematomas, and bring contamination. Injuries in certain areas, such as the mesentery and small bowel, can be subtle and remain undetected. Considering ideal conditions, those regions are still difficult to reach by laparoscopy. Small perforations and mesenteric tears may be unnoticed unless the examination is carried out methodically and comprehensively.

Technical Demands and Long Learning Curve

Laparoscopy requires a high level of technical skill, and when performed under emergency conditions, it can be stressful. The learning curve is steep, in particular when time ticks and action is needed, and trauma has altered the patient's normal anatomy. Unfortunately, the training program for emergency surgeons performing minimally invasive surgery remains a subject of research. It appears to be poorly standardized and insufficiently studied concerning serious surgical emergencies involving GI trauma [28].

Patient-Related Factors

Laparoscopy is safe and feasible in many cases, but some special groups of patients need to be noted when considering laparoscopic intervention in GI trauma:

- Hemodynamic instability is a major contradiction; in such cases, the golden standard remains the same, and it is laparotomy when every second counts. A similar situation is for septic shock, severe cardiopulmonary dysfunction, accompanying head trauma, or inability to perform pneumoperitoneum [2].

- Obesity is associated with a high risk of postoperative complications. Additionally, laparoscopy may not be feasible due to the placement of trocars and surgical instruments. Patients with obesity are more likely to suffer from comorbidities, postoperative complications, and higher mortality during their first hospitalization [29].
- Significant intra-abdominal extensive adhesions may influence the laparoscopic approach and may contribute to a higher risk of missed injuries. Thus, conversion to an open approach is reasonable.

Most contraindications for laparoscopy remain relative and depend on the surgeon's expertise and experience.

Conversion to Open Surgery: When and Why

Despite the numerous advantages of laparoscopic surgery, in certain clinical situations it is necessary to switch to classic laparotomy. Conversion to open surgery from a laparoscopic approach is always a difficult decision. However, this should not be considered a surgical failure, but more of a sign of proper assessment of the situation, an expression of a reasonable approach, and concern for the patient's well-being.

When to Convert?

Conversion can be forced by several intraoperative factors:

- Excessive bleeding that cannot be controlled laparoscopically—when the source of the hemorrhage cannot be located or controlled in any way during laparoscopy.
- Limited visibility of the surgical field or difficulty accessing the site of gastrointestinal injury, often caused by intra-abdominal adhesions, severe inflammatory response, or obesity of the patient.
- Multiple injuries to the digestive tract; severe, complex injuries requiring rapid access to multiple sites in the abdominal cavity.
- No progress in the surgery and worsening state of the patient, inability to achieve the therapeutic goal, difficulty in creating an anastomosis, and inability to control the course of the operation.

Why to Convert?

Early recognition of situations in which continuing a laparoscopic procedure becomes ineffective, or even dangerous, is crucial. Prolonging attempts to perform a minimally invasive procedure in difficult conditions may increase the risk of complications, prolong the duration of the operation, and worsen treatment outcomes. In such cases, a quick decision to convert is a sign of good surgical practice. It is important to note that early conversion, performed at the right time, is associated with a lower risk of complications and better treatment outcomes compared to late conversion.

Advanced Techniques and Adjuncts

Indocyanine Green (ICG) for Bowel Perfusion

ICG fluorescence angiography enables real-time assessment of bowel perfusion. After intravenous injection (0.1–0.5 mg/kg), near-infrared imaging confirms adequate blood supply to resections or sites of concern, reducing the risk for anastomotic failure. It is increasingly used in trauma laparoscopy for evaluation of mesenteric and small bowel injury [30, 31].

Robotic Platforms in Trauma Surgery

Robotic laparoscopy enhances vision and accuracy of the instruments' control. Despite not being implemented on a broad scale, individual high-volume centers have used it for hemodynamically stable trauma patients predominantly for diaphragm, bladder, and some bowel injuries. Robotic systems ensure greater accuracy of suturing, especially in the deep crevices [32].

Laparoscopy for Re-look and Washout

For post-initial damage control trauma patients or non-operatively managed trauma patients, laparoscopy may be safely done for re-look procedures or peritoneal lavage. It is very useful in providing minimally invasive evaluation of bowel viability, treatment of remaining contamination, and confirmation of source control [5, 8].

References

1. Koto MZ, Matsevych OY, Aldous C. Diagnostic laparoscopy for trauma: how not to miss injuries. J Laparoendosc Adv Surg Tech A. 2018;28(5):506–13. https://doi.org/10.1089/lap.2017.0562.
2. Ribeiro MAF Jr, Tebar GK, Salgueiro JLR, et al. Role and limitations of laparoscopy in abdominal trauma. Med Res Arch. 2023;11(8) https://doi.org/10.18103/mra.v11i8.4333.
3. Renz BM, Feliciano DV. Unnecessary laparotomies for trauma: a prospective study of morbidity. J Trauma. 1995;38(3):350–6.
4. Uranues S, Popa DE, Diaconescu B, Schrittwieser R. Laparoscopy in penetrating abdominal trauma. World J Surg. 2015;39(6):1381–8. https://doi.org/10.1007/s00268-014-2904-5.
5. Di Saverio S, Birindelli A, Podda M, et al. Trauma laparoscopy and the six w's: why, where, who, when, what, and how? J Trauma Acute Care Surg. 2019;86(2):344–67. https://doi.org/10.1097/TA.0000000000002130.
6. Loffer FD, Pent D. Indications, contraindications and complications of laparoscopy. Obstet Gynecol Surv. 1975;30(7):407–27.

7. Clarke DL, Brysiewicz P, Sartorius B, et al. Hypotension of <110 mmHg is associated with increased mortality in South African patients after trauma. Scand J Surg. 2017;106(3):261–8. https://doi.org/10.1177/1457496916680129.
8. Matsevych O, Koto M, Balabyeki M, Aldous C. Trauma laparoscopy: when to start and when to convert? Surg Endosc. 2018;32(3):1344–52. https://doi.org/10.1007/s00464-017-5812-6.
9. Matsevych OY, Koto MZ, Motilall SR, Kumar N. The role of laparoscopy in management of stable patients with penetrating abdominal trauma and organ evisceration. J Trauma Acute Care Surg. 2016;81(2):307–11. https://doi.org/10.1097/TA.0000000000001064.
10. Munawar F, AlKhalifa S, AlTraiki Z, Fadul A, Abdalla M, Mamdooh H, Shanavas S, Mahamood A, Pillai R, Arif M. Meta analysis of stapled vs hand-sewn anastomosis in gastrointestinal surgery. J Surg Res. 2025:230–3. https://doi.org/10.26502/jsr.10020442.
11. Lee C, Park S. Laparoscopic techniques and strategies for gastrointestinal GISTs. J Vis Surg. 2017;3:62. https://doi.org/10.21037/jovs.2017.03.09.
12. Tantardini C, Godiris-Petit G, Noullet S, Raux M, Menegaux F, Chereau N. Management of the injured bowel: preserving bowel continuity as a gold standard. BMC Surg. 2021;21:339. https://doi.org/10.1186/s12893-021-01332-x.
13. Liao B, Xue X, Zeng H, Ye W, Xie T, Wang X, Lin S. Comparison of different surgical techniques and anastomosis methods in short-term outcomes of right colon cancer: a network meta-analysis of open surgery, laparoscopic, and robot-assisted techniques with extracorporeal and intracorporeal anastomosis. Updat Surg. 2025;77(2):309–25. https://doi.org/10.1007/s13304-025-02096-2.
14. Tang M, Wong J, Chia C, Lee D. Meta-analysis on surgical management of colonic injuries in trauma: to divert or to anastomose? Eur J Trauma Emerg Surg. 2021;47(5):1381–8. https://doi.org/10.1007/s00068-020-01555-2.
15. De Araújo Molteni R, Omar W, Traya R, Moscardi M, Kanda Y, Rattan R. Colon injuries. The Trauma Golden Hour. 2019:155–7. https://doi.org/10.1007/978-3-030-26443-7_29.
16. Bolaji T, Ratnasekera A, Ferrada P. Management of the complex duodenal injury. Am J Surg. 2022;225(4):639–44. https://doi.org/10.1016/j.amjsurg.2022.12.016.
17. Ratnasekera A, Ferrada P. Traumatic duodenal injury: current management update. Curr Surg Rep. 2020;8:1–6. https://doi.org/10.1007/s40137-020-00251-9.
18. Gao J, Li H, Yang J, Wang J, Ai T, He P, Wei G, Xiang Z, Zhao S. Surgical management of duodenal injury: experience from 92 cases. Eur J Trauma Emerg Surg. 2023;49:1367–74. https://doi.org/10.1007/s00068-023-02238-4.
19. Mandrioli M, Inaba K, Piccinini A, Biscardi A, Sartelli M, Agresta F, Catena F, Cirocchi R, Jovine E, Tugnoli G, Di Saverio S. Advances in laparoscopy for acute care surgery and trauma. World J Gastroenterol. 2016;22(2):668–80. https://doi.org/10.3748/wjg.v22.i2.668. PMID: 26811616; PMCID: PMC4716068.
20. Alkaaki A, Al-Radi OO, Khoja A, Alnawawi A, Alnawawi A, Maghrabi A, Altaf A, Aljiffry M. Surgical site infection following abdominal surgery: a prospective cohort study. Can J Surg. 2019;62(2):111–7. https://doi.org/10.1503/cjs.004818. PMID: 30907567; PMCID: PMC6440888.
21. Yan Y, Chen Y, Zhang X. The effect of opioids on gastrointestinal function in the ICU. Crit Care. 2021;25(1):370. https://doi.org/10.1186/s13054-021-03793-1. PMID: 34689805; PMCID: PMC8543814.
22. Wang J, Cheng L, Liu J, Zhang B, Wang W, Zhu W, Guo Y, Bao C, Hu Y, Qi S, Wang K, Zhao S, Laparoscopy vs. Laparotomy for the management of abdominal trauma: a systematic review and meta-analysis. Front Surg. 2022;8(9):817134. https://doi.org/10.3389/fsurg.2022.817134. PMID: 35350141; PMCID: PMC8957831.
23. Atkins K, Schneider A, Charles A. Negative laparotomy rates and outcomes following blunt traumatic injury in the United States. Injury. 2023;54(8):110894. https://doi.org/10.1016/j.injury.2023.110894. Epub 2023 Jun 14. PMID: 37330406; PMCID: PMC10526723.
24. Rodiguero G, Uequed MM, Dias LS, Baldissera N, Dalcin RR, Fonseca MK. Missed injuries in trauma laparotomy: a single-center 8-year experience. Panam J Trauma Crit Care Emerg Surg. 2025;14(1):32–7.

25. Mynster T, Wille-Jørgensen P. Single incision laparoscopic surgery: new 'toys for boys'? Color Dis. 2011;13(4):351. https://doi.org/10.1111/j.1463-1318.2011.02572.x.
26. Guth AA, Pachter HL. Laparoscopy for penetrating thoracoabdominal trauma: pitfalls and promises. JSLS. 1998;2(2):123–7. PMID: 9876725; PMCID: PMC3015287.
27. Shamim AA, Zeineddin S, Zeineddin A, Olufajo OA, Mathelier GO, Cornwell Iii EE, Fullum T, Tran D. Are we doing too many non-therapeutic laparotomies in trauma? An analysis of the National Trauma Data Bank. Surg Endosc. 2020;34(9):4072–8. https://doi.org/10.1007/s00464-019-07169-z. Epub 2019 Oct 11.
28. de'Angelis N, Marchegiani F, Schena CA, Khan J, Agnoletti V, Ansaloni L, Barría Rodríguez AG, Bianchi PP, Biffl W, Bravi F, Ceccarelli G, Ceresoli M, Chiara O, Chirica M, Cobianchi L, Coccolini F, Coimbra R, Cotsoglou C, D'Hondt M, Damaskos D, De Simone B, Di Saverio S, Diana M, Espin-Basany E, Fichtner-Feigl S, Fugazzola P, Gavriilidis P, Gronnier C, Kashuk J, Kirkpatrick AW, Ammendola M, Kouwenhoven EA, Laurent A, Leppaniemi A, Lesurtel M, Memeo R, Milone M, Moore E, Pararas N, Peitzmann A, Pessaux P, Picetti E, Pikoulis M, Pisano M, Ris F, Robison T, Sartelli M, Shelat VG, Spinoglio G, Sugrue M, Tan E, Van Eetvelde E, Kluger Y, Weber D, Catena F. Training curriculum in minimally invasive emergency digestive surgery: 2022 WSES position paper. World J Emerg Surg. 2023;18(1):11. https://doi.org/10.1186/s13017-023-00476-w. PMID: 36707879; PMCID: PMC9883976.
29. Kassahun WT, Mehdorn M, Babel J. The impact of obesity on surgical outcomes in patients undergoing emergency laparotomy for high-risk abdominal emergencies. BMC Surg. 2022;22(1):15. https://doi.org/10.1186/s12893-022-01466-6. PMID: 35033036; PMCID: PMC8761337.
30. Kudszus S, Roesel C, Schachtrupp A, Höer JJ. Intraoperative laser fluorescence angiography in colorectal surgery: a noninvasive analysis to reduce the rate of anastomotic leakage. Langenbeck's Arch Surg. 2010;395(8):1025–30.
31. Boni L, David G, Mangano A, Dionigi G, Rausei S, Spampatti S, Cassinotti E, Fingerhut A. Clinical applications of indocyanine green (ICG) enhanced fluorescence in laparoscopic surgery. Surg Endosc. 2015;29(7):2046–55.
32. Anastasiya S, Swenson G, Vasyluk A. Robotic evaluation and repair of penetrating injury of the abdominal wall. Cureus. 2024;16(7):e63685.

Laparoscopy Treatment for Splenic Injuries

22

William Sanchez, Juliana Ordoñez, and Andres Aponte

Introduction

Splenic trauma represents one of the most frequent abdominal injuries, with a global incidence of approximately 2% of all trauma admissions. The spleen is the most commonly affected intra-abdominal solid organ, involved in approximately 50–60% of abdominal injuries, predominantly in the setting of blunt trauma and, to a lesser extent, in penetrating trauma [1, 2].

Due to its high frequency and the functional importance of the spleen, the management of these injuries remains a constant challenge for trauma and emergency surgeons, who aim to develop strategies that allow organ preservation.

The spleen performs essential immunological and hematological functions, which has driven the evolution toward therapeutic approaches focused on its preservation. In recent decades, the management of splenic trauma has shifted from radical splenectomy toward more conservative strategies, including non-operative management (NOM), angioembolization, and, more recently, laparoscopy in selected patients [3].

W. Sanchez
Head of the Medical-Surgical Unit, Central Military Hospital, Bogotá, Colombia

Department of General Surgery, Central Military Hospital, Bogotá, Colombia

J. Ordoñez (✉)
Trauma and Critical Care Surgeon, Head of the Vascular Surgery Service – Central Military Hospital, Bogotá, Colombia

Department of General Surgery, Central Military Hospital, Bogotá, Colombia

A. Aponte
Department of General Surgery, Central Military Hospital, Bogotá, Colombia

© The Author(s), under exclusive license to Springer Nature Switzerland AG 2026

M. Cezillo, B. M. Pereira (eds.), *Minimally Invasive Surgery Trauma*,
https://doi.org/10.1007/978-3-032-28971-1_22

Currently, therapeutic options range from non-surgical management to minimally invasive interventions. Multicenter studies, such as those reported by Velmahos et al., have demonstrated that although non-operative management (NOM) is effective in selected patients, it presents failure rates ranging between 11% and 38% in adults, thereby creating an important space for considering laparoscopy as a therapeutic alternative [4].

Additionally, open surgery is associated with significant morbidity, including increased postoperative pain, prolonged hospital stay, pulmonary complications, surgical site infection, incisional hernias, and adhesion formation. In contrast, minimally invasive approaches have emerged as safe and effective alternatives in selected patients [5, 6].

Technological advancements, improvements in diagnostic methods, and the growing experience of trauma surgeons, as well as the availability of greater resources in specialized centers, have allowed laparoscopy to be consolidated as a key tool in the evolution of splenic trauma management.

Initial Assessment and Diagnosis

The initial evaluation of patients with blunt abdominal trauma should follow the principles of Advanced Trauma Life Support (ATLS), prioritizing hemodynamic stabilization under the XABCDE approach [2].

Hemodynamic status is the main determinant in therapeutic decision-making. Patients are considered unstable when presenting:

- Systolic blood pressure <90 mmHg
- Signs of peripheral hypoperfusion
- Altered mental status
- Respiratory compromise
- Requirement for resuscitation with fluid, transfusion, or vasopressors

Other indicators include base excess <−5 mmol/L, shock index >1, or the need for transfusion of 4–6 units of red blood cells within the first 24 h [2, 5, 6].

In these cases, immediate surgical intervention is indicated.

In hemodynamically stable patients, defined as the absence of the above-mentioned criteria, contrast-enhanced computed tomography (CT) is the diagnostic gold standard, allowing adequate characterization and classification of splenic injuries, which guides the therapeutic strategy.

Splenic Injury Classification Systems

Multiple classification systems exist based on tomographic and intraoperative findings. The most widely used is that of the American Association for the Surgery of Trauma (AAST).

Additionally, the World Society of Emergency Surgery (WSES) classification integrates clinical and radiological variables, facilitating therapeutic decision-making. [Tables 22.1 and 22.2] [7].

It is important to consider that CT may underestimate the degree of injury in some cases [7].

Table 22.1 AAST splenic injury trauma classification

Grade	Injury description	
I	Hematoma	Subcapsular, <10% surface area
	Laceration	Capsular tear, <1 cm parenchymal depth
II	Hematoma	Subcapsular, 10–50% surface area
		Intraparenchymal, <5 cm diameter
	Laceration	1–3 cm parenchymal depth not involving a parenchymal vessel
III	Hematoma	Subcapsular, >50% surface area or expanding
		Ruptured subcapsular or parenchymal hematoma
		Intraparenchymal hematoma >5 cm
	Laceration	>3 cm parenchymal depth or involving trabecular vessels
IV	Laceration	Laceration of segmental or hilar vessels producing major devascularization (>25% of spleen)
V	Laceration	Completely shatters spleen
	Vascular	Hilar vascular injury which devascularized spleen

Adapted and reproduced: Coccolini et al. [7] splenic injury trauma classification. Licencia Creative Commons Atribucion 4.0 International (CC BY 4.0)

Table 22.2 WSES splenic injury trauma classification

	WSES class	Mechanism of injury	AAST	Hemodynamic status[a, b]	CT scan	First-line treatment in adults
Minor	WSES I	Blunt/penetrating	I–II	Stable	Yes + local exploration in SW[d]	NOM[c] + serial clinical/laboratory/radiological evaluation
						Consider angiography/angioembolization
Moderate	WSES II	Blunt/penetrating	III	Stable		
	WSES III	Blunt/penetrating	IV–V	Stable		NOM[c]
						All angiography/angioembolization + serial clinical/laboratory/radiological evaluation
Severe	WSES IV	Blunt/penetrating	I–V	Unstable	No	OM

Adapted and reproduced: Coccolini et al. [7] splenic injury trauma classification. Licencia Creative Commons Atribucion 4.0 International (CC BY 4.0)

Management Strategies

The therapeutic strategy depends on hemodynamic status and the degree of splenic injury. Options include:

- Non-operative management (NOM)
- Angioembolization
- Laparoscopy

The fundamental principle for considering laparoscopy is the patient's hemodynamic stability.

Indications for Laparoscopy

Equivocal tomographic findings.
Free fluid without a clear source of bleeding.
Suspicion of unidentified intra-abdominal injuries.
Low-grade splenic injuries (AAST I–III) amenable to hemostatic control.
Failure of non-operative management [8].

Recent studies, such as that of Lin et al. (2024), in an 11-year case series of patients with severe blunt splenic trauma and hemodynamic stability, compared the role of laparoscopy versus angioembolization and other strategies, demonstrating that laparoscopy is a safe and feasible alternative in experienced centers, with no significant differences in complications or hospital stay compared to other strategies ($p > 0.05$ in all cases) [9].

Failure of Non-operative Management

Among the main factors associated with NOM failure are:

- Age >55 years
- High ISS (>25)
- Significant hemoperitoneum
- Contrast extravasation
- Pseudoaneurysms
- Subcapsular hematoma rupture
- Transfusion requirement
- Comorbidities

Other factors include pre-resuscitation hypotension, decreased level of consciousness (GCS <12), low hematocrit on admission, associated abdominal injuries, active contrast extravasation on imaging, use of anticoagulation therapy, and comorbidities such as cirrhosis, HIV infection, or substance abuse, which further increase the risk of conservative management failure [10].

Chen CY et al. [11] described the risk of rebleeding in patients undergoing non-operative management after blunt splenic trauma, finding that age >50 years, ISS >16, and a history of cardiac disease increase the risk of rebleeding at 180 days and failure of non-operative management.

Failure may manifest clinically as persistent pain, a drop in hemoglobin, or complications such as abscess formation or delayed bleeding, which may present with an increased systemic inflammatory response, fever, and elevated acute-phase reactants.

In these cases, laparoscopy offers an effective therapeutic alternative, allowing interventions ranging from drainage to hemostatic control or splenectomy.

All these prior analysis and recommendations are expressed in Fig. 22.1:

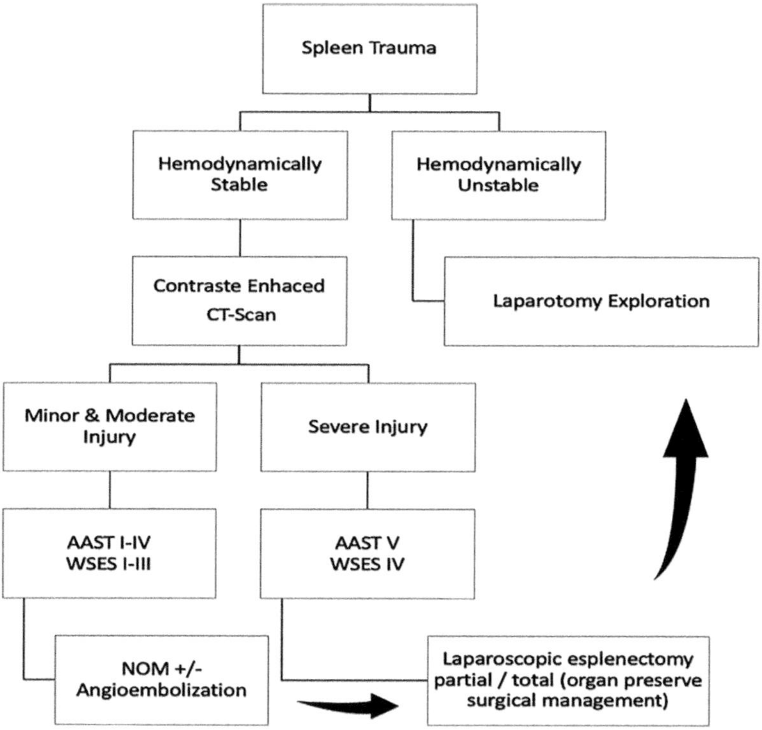

Fig. 22.1 Spleen trauma management algorithm

Laparoscopic Technique

Preoperative Preparation

Appropriate patient selection is essential for the success of the laparoscopic approach in splenic trauma. A contrast-enhanced CT scan is required to characterize the injury, along with continuous patient monitoring and complete laboratory evaluation, including complete blood count, coagulation profile, and acid–base status.

Additionally, the availability of blood products must be ensured, and the surgical team must be prepared for potential conversion to open surgery.

Patient Positioning

The patient is placed in the supine position. The surgical team stands on the patient's right side.

The operating table may be tilted to the right, achieving a right lateral decubitus position of approximately 30–45°, combined with a slight Trendelenburg position. This configuration facilitates exposure of the left upper quadrant through gravitational displacement of abdominal viscera. (Fig. 22.2).

Placement of a roll or cushion under the left thoracic region or scapula is recommended to improve opening of the subphrenic space and optimize visualization of the operative field, provided there are no contraindications.

This position also facilitates conversion to laparotomy if necessary.

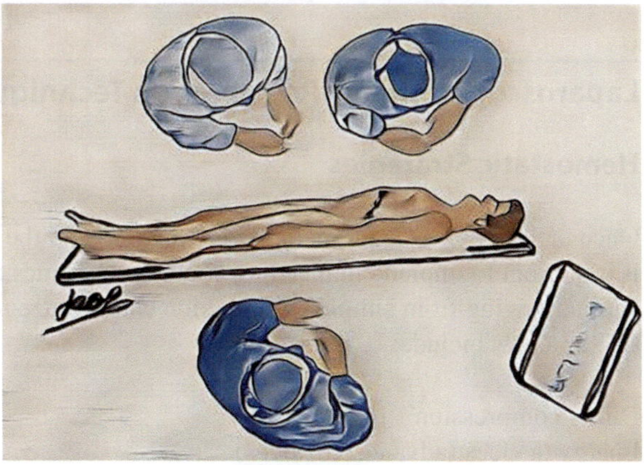

Fig. 22.2 Patient positioning and the trocar placement

Trocar Placement

Trocar placement should allow adequate triangulation directed toward the left upper quadrant, facilitating instrument manipulation.

Suggested configuration:

- 12-mm umbilical trocar (camera)
- 5-mm epigastric trocar
- 12-mm trocar in the left midaxillary line, lateral to the umbilical port
- Additional 12-mm trocar in the left flank (optional, depending on need)

Systematic Exploration

Once the trocars are placed and pneumoperitoneum is established, a systematic exploration of the abdominal cavity should be performed.

The first step is aspiration of the hemoperitoneum, which improves visualization of the surgical field.

Subsequently, the bleeding site should be identified, which may correspond to capsular lacerations or rupture of subcapsular hematomas. An intraoperative classification of the splenic injury is then performed.

It is essential to assess whether the bleeding is low-flow and potentially controllable using laparoscopic techniques.

After evacuation of the hemoperitoneum and initial assessment, the next step is to define the type of technique to be performed, whether splenic preservation or definitive splenectomy is required.

Laparoscopic Splenic Preservation Techniques

Hemostatic Strategies

Once the left upper quadrant has been assessed and the hemoperitoneum drained, it is important to implement bleeding control techniques that also allow organ preservation, ranging from simple compression using gauze to the use of meshes [12].

Strategies include:

Direct compression
Energy devices (advanced devices)
Hemostatic agents
Compression meshes

Ochsner et al., in a case series, demonstrated the effectiveness of biological sealants in achieving hemostasis as a useful intraoperative adjunct; subsequently, Kram et al. documented that in patients with splenic trauma, the use of fibrin sealants achieved splenic preservation in 86% [13].

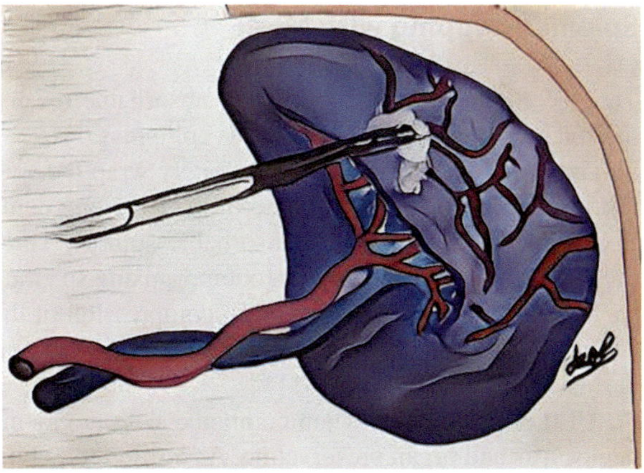

Fig. 22.3 Use of fibrin glue. (Direct focal application)

Fibrin Sealants

The technique for applying fibrin sealant involves the use of a long laparoscopic applicator (spray or cannula). Once the hemoperitoneum has been drained and hemostasis achieved with electrocautery, the field should be kept dry. (Fig. 22.3).

Techniques can be performed in two ways:

Direct focal application
Spray technique (2–5 cm distance)

Post-application irrigation should be avoided, and a waiting time of 2–3 min is recommended to allow the sealant to act.

The use of fibrin sealants has gained relevance as an adjunct in the laparoscopic management of splenic trauma, particularly in spleen-preserving strategies. Early reports, such as those by Olmi et al. [14], demonstrated effective hemostasis without the need for conversion or added morbidity. In parallel, studies on laparoscopic trauma have highlighted the role of topical hemostatic agents in achieving adequate bleeding control while minimizing surgical invasiveness. In this context, fibrin-based sealants may enhance the feasibility of minimally invasive approaches by improving local hemostasis and supporting organ preservation. However, current evidence is largely limited to small case series, and further studies are required to better define their role.

In conclusion, fibrin sealants appear to be a safe and effective adjunct when combined with conventional hemostatic techniques, such as energy devices or compression, in the laparoscopic conservative management of splenic trauma, particularly in cases of low- to moderate-grade bleeding.

Splenic Wrapping with Mesh

This technique consists of using an absorbable mesh (polyglactin) placed around the spleen to generate homogeneous compression.

The mesh should be cut to adequately wrap the spleen and placed in a bag-like fashion both anteriorly and posteriorly, achieving complete coverage of the organ. Fixation is performed using absorbable sutures. The key is to provide sufficient pressure for hemostasis without compromising splenic perfusion. (Fig. 22.4).

This technique provides uniform compression of the parenchyma, enhances the effect of topical hemostatic agents, and promotes splenic preservation, provided perfusion is not compromised [12].

All these strategies, when combined with angioembolization, further reinforce hemostasis and organ preservation. According to Schimmer et al. [15], angioembolization is an effective method for achieving hemostasis while preserving splenic function, reducing the need for post-splenectomy interventions. Although long-term outcomes remain uncertain, it is increasingly recognized, alongside laparoscopy, as a key strategy in splenic trauma management.

Laparoscopic Splenectomy

In the context of penetrating trauma, the presence of active contrast extravasation (contrast blush) on imaging in patients with similar injury grades reinforces the indication for surgery—splenectomy. Likewise, surgical treatment is appropriate when non-surgical strategies, with or without adjunctive angioembolization, are not feasible. This includes patients with conditions that preclude safe monitoring or intervention, such as pregnancy, cognitive impairment, lack of reliable social support, severe hypersensitivity to iodinated contrast, or significant renal dysfunction.

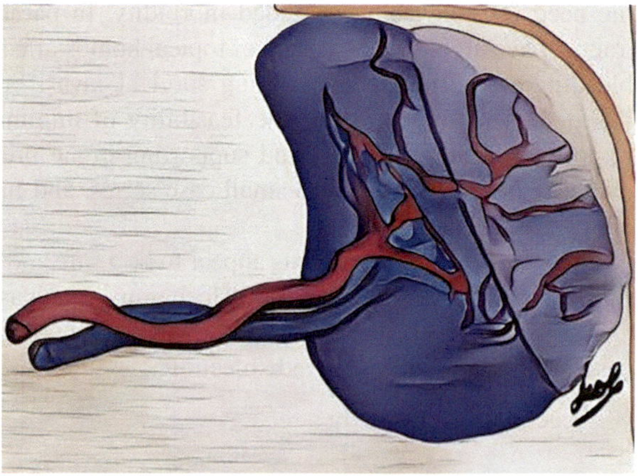

Fig. 22.4 Prosthetic mesh. (Splenic wrapping with absorbable mesh for hemostatic compression while preserving perfusion)

A percentage of patients undergoing non-operative management will fail, with global rates ranging from 8–15%; approximately 75–90% of failures occur within the first 72 h, while up to 10% may be delayed (>5–7 days) [11].

Indications

The indication for laparoscopic splenectomy is determined by the clinical characteristics and evolution of the patient. It may also be indicated when patients refuse non-surgical treatments or when technical limitations prevent effective angioembolization. These limitations may include unfavorable vascular anatomy, such as marked tortuosity of the splenic artery, celiac trunk stenosis, failure of endovascular techniques such as coil placement, or failure of laparoscopic hemostatic techniques.

Therefore, splenectomy is indicated in:

- Failure of conservative management
- High-grade injuries
- Inability to achieve hemostatic control [16]

Surgical Technique

Patient positioning in right lateral decubitus (30–45°), trocar placement using the standard configuration described above (3–5 ports) to allow triangulation toward the left upper quadrant, establishment of pneumoperitoneum, systematic evaluation of the abdominal cavity, confirmation of the bleeding source, drainage of hemoperitoneum, and assessment of the splenic injury were performed.

1. Division of the splenocolic ligament: allows mobilization of the inferior pole and facilitates exploration using monopolar energy.
2. Division of the gastrosplenic ligament: performed using advanced bipolar energy, with identification and division of the short gastric vessels.
3. Posterior mobilization (splenorenal ligament): can be performed bluntly, allowing exposure of the hilum.
4. Control of the splenic hilum: can be achieved using an endoscopic stapler with a vascular load, including both the vein and artery (Fig. 22.5). This is a critical step where care must be taken to avoid injury to the pancreatic tail.
5. Division of the splenophrenic ligament: complete release of the superior pole.
6. Complete mobilization of the spleen.
7. Verification of hemostasis.
8. Specimen extraction in a retrieval bag.

Careful verification of hemostasis is essential, and the use of hemostatic agents in the splenic bed may help prevent postoperative complications.

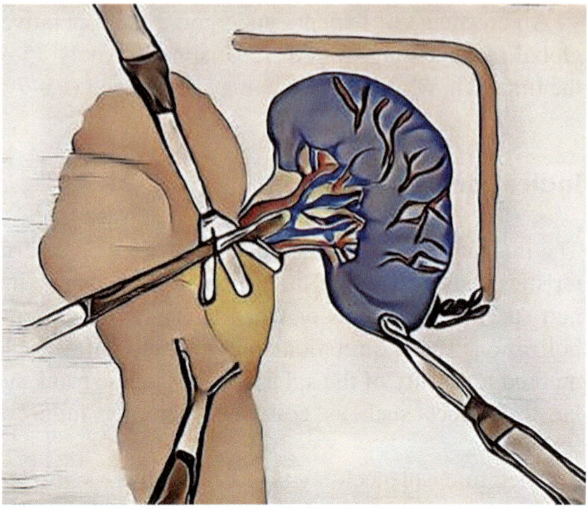

Fig. 22.5 Technique of laparoscopic splenectomy. (Control of the splenic hilum with a vascular stapler, including artery and vein, with careful preservation of the pancreatic tail)

Conclusions

The management of splenic trauma has evolved toward a conservative and minimally invasive approach, prioritizing organ preservation.

Laparoscopy has become a key diagnostic and therapeutic tool in hemodynamically stable patients, allowing both hemostatic control and splenectomy in selected cases.

The success of these strategies depends on appropriate patient selection, surgical team experience, and available resources.

Adjunctive techniques, such as fibrin sealants and mesh wrapping, play a fundamental role in splenic preservation.

In conclusion, the management of splenic trauma should be individualized, integrating patient physiology, injury severity, and institutional capabilities, with laparoscopy serving as a cornerstone in modern treatment.

Acknowledgments The authors thank Javier Adolfo Ordoñez Cortez for his contribution to the illustrations of this manuscript.

References

1. Haan JM, Bochicchio GV, Kramer N, Scalea TM. Nonoperative management of blunt splenic injury: a 5-year experience. J Trauma. 2005;58(3):492–8.
2. Feliciano DV. Abdominal trauma revisited. Am Surg. 2017;83:1193–202.
3. Pachter HL, Guth AA, Hofstetter SR, Spencer FC. Changing patterns in the management of splenic trauma: the impact of nonoperative management. Ann Surg. 1998;227(5):708–17.
4. Velmahos GC, Zacharias N, Emhoff TA, Salama A, Hirsch E, Crookes BA, et al. Management of the most severely injured spleen: a multicenter study of the Research Consortium of New England Centers for Trauma (ReCONECT). Arch Surg. 2010;145(5):456–60.

5. Fransvea P, Costa G, Serao A, Cortese F, Balducci G, Sganga G, et al. Laparoscopic splenectomy after trauma: who, when and how. A systematic review. J Minim Access Surg. 2021;17:141–6.
6. Di Saverio S, Birindelli A, Podda M, Segalini E, Piccinini A, Coniglio C, et al. Trauma laparoscopy and the six w's: why, where, who, when, what, and how? J Trauma Acute Care Surg. 2019;86(2):344–67. https://doi.org/10.1097/TA.0000000000002130. PMID: 30489508
7. Coccolini F, Montori G, Catena F, Di Saverio S, Biffl WL, Horer TM, et al. Splenic trauma: WSES classification and guidelines for adult and pediatric patients. World J Emerg Surg. 2017;12:40. https://doi.org/10.1186/s13017-017-0151-4.
8. Targarona EM, Trías M. Laparoscopic treatment of splenic injuries. Semin Laparosc Surg. 1996;3(1):44–9. https://doi.org/10.1177/155335069600300108.
9. Wu C, Lin KL, Chang YJ, Chang YR, Lin HF. Laparoscopic surgery: an effective alternative for managing severe blunt splenic injuries in patients who are ineligible for transcatheter arterial embolization. Asian J Surg. 2024;26:S1015. https://doi.org/10.1016/j.asjsur.2024.09.098.
10. Cogbill TH, Moore EE, Jurkovich GJ, et al. Nonoperative management of blunt splenic trauma: a multicenter experience. J Trauma. 1989;29(10):1312–7. https://doi.org/10.1097/00005373-198910000-00002.
11. Chen CY, Lin HY, Hsieh PW, et al. Risk factors of 180-day rebleeding after management of blunt splenic injury without surgery and embolization: a national database study. World J Emerg Surg. 2025;20:11. https://doi.org/10.1186/s13017-025-00586-7.
12. Uranüs S, Mischinger HJ, Pfeifer J, et al. Hemostatic methods for the management of spleen and liver injuries. World J Surg. 1996;20(8):1107–12. https://doi.org/10.1007/s002689900169.
13. Ochsner MG, Maniscalco-Theberge ME, Champion HR. Fibrin glue as a hemostatic agent in hepatic and splenic trauma. J Trauma. 1990;30(7):884–7. https://doi.org/10.1097/00005373-199007000-00020.
14. Olmi S, Scaini A, Erba L, et al. Use of fibrin glue (Tissucol) as a hemostatic in laparoscopic conservative treatment of spleen trauma. Surg Endosc. 2007;21:2051–4. https://doi.org/10.1007/s00464-007-9288-7.
15. Schimmer JA, van der Steeg AF, Zuidema WP. Splenic function after angioembolization for splenic trauma in children and adults: a systematic review. Injury. 2016;47:525–30.
16. Birindelli A, Martin M, Khan M, Gallo G, Segalini E, Gori A, et al. Laparoscopic splenectomy as a definitive management option for high-grade traumatic splenic injury when nonoperative management is not feasible or failed: a 5-year experience from a level one trauma center with minimally invasive surgery expertise. Updat Surg. 2021;73(4):1515–31. https://doi.org/10.1007/s13304-021-01045-z. PMID: 33837949; PMCID: PMC8397689.

Laparoscopic Approach for Pancreatic Injuries

23

Marcus Cezillo, Jorge Roberto Marcante Carlotto, and Marcos Dal Vesco Neto

Introduction

The pancreas is a retroperitoneal organ, located posteriorly in the abdominal cavity, protected by adjacent visceral and bony structures. This anatomical position provides relative protection against external injuries, so pancreatic trauma accounts for less than 2% of lesions in polytrauma patients [1–4].

The most frequent injury mechanism is blunt trauma, classically associated with abdominal impact against the steering wheel in car accidents. Penetrating injuries, although less prevalent, usually cause greater parenchymal destruction and are generally related to stab or gunshot wounds [1–4].

The retroperitoneal location of the pancreas poses significant diagnostic challenges. The clinical presentation is often nonspecific, which contributes to delayed diagnosis and, consequently, higher morbidity and mortality. Moreover, associated injuries are common, mainly involving the large intestine, stomach, and duodenum [4].

The first report of laparoscopy in a trauma patient dates back to 1925, when the method was used to investigate the presence of free blood in the pelvic cavity and visceral ruptures [5]. Since then, laparoscopy has become established in trauma primarily as a diagnostic tool, allowing avoidance of non-therapeutic laparotomies. In selected cases, it also plays a therapeutic role, with reports of its application in procedures such as repair and drainage of hollow and solid organ injuries, splenectomy, nephrectomy, and repair of diaphragmatic lesions [6–8].

In the specific context of pancreatic trauma, however, laparoscopy has not yet become routine practice. Most injuries are still managed through exploratory laparotomy, with laparoscopic treatment reports being scarce in the literature. Between

M. Cezillo
Trauma Surgery Department, Hospital de Base do Distrito Federal (HBDF), Brasília, DF, Brazil

J. R. M. Carlotto (✉) · M. D. V. Neto
Hospital de Clínicas de Passo Fundo, Passo Fundo, Brazil

© The Author(s), under exclusive license to Springer Nature Switzerland AG 2026

M. Cezillo, B. M. Pereira (eds.), *Minimally Invasive Surgery Trauma*,
https://doi.org/10.1007/978-3-032-28971-1_23

2000 and 2020, approximately 40 cases of pancreatic management via laparoscopy in trauma patients were described, highlighting the rarity of this practice [9, 10].

Indications

The main requirement for performing laparoscopy in trauma patients is hemodynamic stability. Candidates are those who are stable upon hospital admission or who demonstrate a satisfactory response to initial fluid resuscitation.

In critically ill patients or in those with tissue hypoperfusion, the adverse physiological effects of pneumoperitoneum are not well tolerated and may pose significant risks [6–8, 11].

Another indispensable prerequisite is the availability of a trained and experienced surgical team in laparoscopy, as well as adequate material and human resources, ensuring that the procedure can be performed rapidly, safely, and effectively, regardless of the time of surgery.

Contraindications

Laparoscopy in trauma is contraindicated in certain clinical situations, with hemodynamic instability being the most important. Patients in shock already present established organ dysfunction, and the creation of pneumoperitoneum—by reducing venous return, decreasing cardiac preload, impairing splanchnic flow, and increasing peripheral vascular resistance—tends to aggravate the clinical condition [6–8, 11].

Severe traumatic brain injury associated with abdominal trauma is also an absolute contraindication since pneumoperitoneum elevates intracranial pressure, reduces cerebral perfusion pressure, and contributes to the progression of secondary central nervous system injury.

Some conditions represent relative contraindications, in which the decision must be individualized according to team experience and available resources [6–8, 11]. These include:

- multiple prior abdominal surgeries,
- major abdominal vascular injuries,
- complex retroperitoneal lesions,
- multiple associated injuries,
- extensive duodenal injuries.

Patient Selection

The ideal scenario for laparoscopic management of pancreatic trauma is a hemodynamically stable patient, a victim of blunt trauma, with the diagnosis previously established by contrast-enhanced abdominal and pelvic computed tomography (CT) [1, 12].

Penetrating pancreatic injuries, on the other hand, are frequently associated with damage to the main pancreatic duct and multiple associated visceral lesions, which limit the indication for a minimally invasive approach [1, 4].

The main techniques employed in therapeutic laparoscopy of the pancreas include:

- distal pancreatectomy, with or without splenectomy,
- suturing and drainage of selected pancreatic injuries.

In general, injuries classified as grade II, III, and IV according to the American Association for the Surgery of Trauma (AAST) Pancreas Injury Scale can be treated laparoscopically, provided that the hospital infrastructure and a surgical team trained in advanced laparoscopy are available.

In lesions located on the right side of the pancreas, with involvement of the superior mesenteric vessels and injury to the main pancreatic duct, an associated endoscopic approach is mandatory, often requiring placement of a pancreatic stent. In such cases, concomitant duodenal injury is not uncommon, increasing the complexity of management [1, 4].

Thus, the greater the severity and extent of the pancreatic injury, the higher the demand for hospital infrastructure, multidisciplinary support, and prior surgical experience in advanced laparoscopic procedures.

Videolaparoscopy also plays a role in the treatment of post-traumatic pancreatitis. Infected pancreatic necrosis should preferably be managed through percutaneous drainage. However, in patients who do not show adequate clinical response, video-assisted retroperitoneal debridement (VARD) is a viable and effective alternative [13].

Positioning

The patient should be placed in the supine position, preferably with legs apart or comfortably supported in stirrups. The use of a thermal blanket and mechanical compression stockings is mandatory, aiming to maintain normothermia and prevent thromboembolic events.

The laparoscopic tower should be positioned at the head of the patient, while the lead surgeon stands between the patient's legs.

Positioning variations help ensure successful access:

- For access to the pancreas and manipulation of the head, neck, or body, a 30° reverse Trendelenburg position is recommended, facilitating displacement of the transverse colon.
- For manipulation of the pancreatic tail and/or splenic hilum, a 45° right lateral decubitus position provides better operative field exposure.

Trocar placement should be in a straight line or in a discrete semicircle at the level of the umbilical scar. Typically, four trocars are used, with at least one 12 mm port recommended to allow the introduction of laparoscopic staplers.

In procedures restricted to the pancreatic tail or in cases of video-assisted retroperitoneal debridement, the patient should be placed in the right lateral decubitus position, with pads positioned under the right axilla, right flank, and between the lower limbs.

In this configuration, the laparoscopic tower is placed on the patient's left side, while the surgeon positions themselves on the right side. Trocars are distributed along the left costal margin, ensuring proper ergonomics and access to retroperitoneal structures.

Equipment

Laparoscopic pancreatic surgery is considered a major procedure and therefore requires specific, high-quality equipment to ensure safety and effectiveness.

The main recommended instruments include:

- 4K laparoscopic camera, providing superior definition and anatomical detail
- Advanced bipolar forceps or ultrasonic dissection device, indispensable for precise hemostasis and safe tissue dissection.
- 12-mm trocar, necessary for introducing staplers and larger caliber instruments
- Laparoscopic stapler, with cartridges of different thicknesses, enabling adequate hemostasis and transection of pancreatic parenchyma and associated vessels.
- Self-retaining laparoscopic retractor, used to mobilize and retract the left lobe of the liver and the stomach, ensuring wide exposure of the operative field.
- Metallic clips and polymer clips with internal locking mechanism, employed for ligation of vessels and small-caliber structures.

Adequate availability of these resources is essential for the safe performance of laparoscopic pancreatectomy and for the execution of possible additional intraoperative maneuvers, given the complexity and anatomical variability of pancreatic injuries.

Pancreatic Exposure

Exposure and systematic inspection of the pancreas should be performed through three main approaches:

1. Access to the omental bursa by opening the gastrocolic ligament, which allows broad visualization of the anterior surface of the pancreas.
2. Complete Kocher maneuver combined with mobilization of the hepatic flexure of the colon, enabling inspection of the posterior surface of the pancreatic head.

3. Mobilization of the spleen and pancreatic tail toward the midline, ensuring complete access to the pancreatic tail and splenic hilum.

Adequate and complete mobilization of the pancreas is essential not only for accurate diagnosis but also to avoid overlooking injuries during laparoscopic exploration.

In addition to identifying the pancreatic injury, it is crucial to determine its parenchymal location, verify the integrity of the main pancreatic duct, investigate signs of pancreatitis or pancreatic fistula, and systematically assess for associated injuries in other intra-abdominal organs.

Distal Pancreatectomy With or Without Splenectomy

The main indication for distal pancreatectomy in the trauma setting corresponds to grade III injuries according to the American Association for the Surgery of Trauma (AAST) Pancreas Injury Scale. Preoperative diagnosis using contrast-enhanced computed tomography (CT) is essential, as it allows better planning of the approach in polytrauma patients [14–16]. In selected cases, magnetic resonance imaging with magnetic resonance cholangiopancreatography (MRCP) may be used to assess the integrity of the main pancreatic duct.

The first step in distal pancreatectomy is adequate exposure of the pancreas. The stomach can be retracted with the aid of a self-retaining retractor or alternatively sutured to the anterior abdominal wall with nonabsorbable stitches.

Pancreatic dissection can be carried out laterally to medially or medially to laterally. Our preference is to begin by mobilizing the splenic flexure of the colon, then exposing the inferior border of the pancreas, which should be mobilized to the right of the rupture site.

When the spleen is injured or when dissection between the pancreatic tail and the splenic hilum is hindered by intense inflammatory processes, distal pancreatectomy with splenectomy is a valid option. In such cases, the splenic artery and vein are ligated at the pancreatic transection site, followed by sectioning of the splenic attachments for specimen removal.

Whenever possible, however, the preferred strategy is spleen preservation, including the splenic vessels, gastrosplenic ligament, and short gastric vessels, due to the positive impact on the patient's immunological preservation.

The pancreas should be transected to the right of the laceration site, using a laparoscopic stapler with a cartridge appropriate for tissue thickness. Additional suturing of the pancreatic stump or the use of sealants has not demonstrated significant benefit in reducing biochemical leak or pancreatic fistula rates according to current literature.

For better mobilization, the pancreas may be retracted using a cardiac tape, allowing lateral exposure and control of small arterial branches and venous tributaries.

The specimen can be retrieved through an enlarged umbilical trocar site. In cases of distal pancreatectomy with splenectomy, extraction can be performed via a suprapubic transverse incision, ensuring en bloc removal.

Systematic drainage of the pancreatic stump is mandatory, given that, in trauma settings, the pancreatic parenchyma is usually soft, increasing the risk of biochemical leak and postoperative pancreatic fistula.

The feasibility of the laparoscopic approach for lesions located to the left of the superior mesenteric vessels has been established in recent reports. In a 2023 systematic review by Catellani et al., involving 30 cases of laparoscopic distal pancreatectomy for blunt pancreatic trauma, the following outcomes were observed [9]:

- Mean operative time: 160.6 min.
- Estimated blood loss: 400 mL.
- Mean hospital stay: 14.9 days.

These results suggest that laparoscopy is both feasible and safe in selected cases, provided that the procedures are conducted by teams trained in advanced laparoscopic techniques and supported by adequate infrastructure.

Suture and Drainage

In the context of isolated pancreatic injuries diagnosed through imaging, those classified as grade I and II by the American Association for the Surgery of Trauma (AAST) should preferably be managed conservatively, that is, without invasive procedures, aiming to reduce morbidity [16].

When such low-grade injuries are identified intraoperatively, suture and drainage represent viable treatment options. In small injuries or lacerations (AAST grade I), simple drainage may be sufficient, or in some cases, no drainage at all [14]. However, the latter strategy is rarely adopted due to the high rate of postoperative complications, especially the development of pancreatic fistula from unrecognized ductal injury. Therefore, the recommended approach is closed suction drainage [16].

For more extensive contusions or lacerations (AAST grade II), closed suction drainage is strongly recommended. It is crucial to confirm the absence of associated pancreatic fistula since its presence would indicate a more severe injury requiring a change in therapeutic strategy [16].

In addition to drainage, in grade II lesions pancreatic suturing (pancreatorrhaphy) may be performed, especially in cases with active bleeding, using stitches with hemostatic function. The use of an omental patch is also described as an adjunctive resource although current evidence lacks statistical significance to prove its effectiveness. Alternative methods, such as tissue sealants, have been tested but have not demonstrated superiority over conventional techniques. [17].

A study by Ho et al. showed that when comparing conservative management (pancreatorrhaphy and/or drainage) with pancreatic resection, there was a significantly higher incidence of intra-abdominal abscesses in the resection group (42.9%) compared to the non-resection group (8.7%) ($p = 0.0009$) [16].

The choice of suture material and caliber depends on surgeon preference and the extent of injury. Absorbable sutures such as polyglactin or polydioxanone 3–0 or 4–0 are valid options although nonabsorbable sutures such as silk or polypropylene of equivalent calibers are often preferred. Sutures are usually performed with separate stitches, either simple or in "X" configuration, with hemostatic purpose [18].

Regarding drain type, closed suction drains (e.g., Blake or Jackson-Pratt) are recommended. Open systems such as siliconized Penrose drains can be used but are less preferred due to increased infection risk [18].

In high-grade injuries (AAST grade III, IV, V), suturing and drainage become controversial since these lesions frequently evolve with complications such as pancreatic fistulas or pseudocyst formation, making pancreatic resection the preferred approach [8].

Pancreatic drainage may still be considered in cases of main pancreatic duct injury in the head region—to the right of the superior mesenteric vessels—provided there is no associated duodenal or distal biliary tract injury. This approach aims to avoid major surgeries, such as pancreaticoduodenectomy (Whipple procedure), in emergency settings [8].

In such cases, endoscopic retrograde cholangiopancreatography (ERCP) with sphincterotomy of the sphincter of Oddi and/or stent placement at the papilla is often performed to optimize biliopancreatic drainage and reduce fistula output [8].

In summary, suture and drainage are appropriate strategies for intraoperative management of low-grade pancreatic injuries, especially in hemodynamically stable patients. For more severe injuries, located to the right of the superior mesenteric vessels and without duodenal or biliary involvement, wide drainage may be employed as a temporary measure until definitive surgical treatment can be performed.

Video-Assisted Retroperitoneal Debridement (VARD)

The Video-Assisted Retroperitoneal Debridement (VARD) technique was originally developed as a minimally invasive approach for necrosectomy in cases of severe acute pancreatitis with necrosis. Although its main indication remains necrosectomy in post-pancreatitis settings, the method may also be applied in selected cases of pancreatic trauma [19].

Candidates for VARD are generally patients who have previously undergone surgical treatment with suturing and drainage or pancreatic resection and subsequently developed necrotic collections or retroperitoneal abscesses [19].

The procedure is performed under general anesthesia, with the patient in supine or slightly right lateral position, enabling adequate exposure of the left flank. A reverse Trendelenburg position is recommended to optimize access to the retroperitoneal space [20].

The first incision should be planned according to CT findings indicating the need for intervention, and the location of any previously placed drains should also be considered. A 3 cm transverse incision is made, guided by imaging or immediately adjacent to the drain, followed by blunt dissection to the retroperitoneal space. When available and well-positioned, the previous drain may serve as a guide. [19].

A 12 mm trocar, preferably with optical view and balloon system, is inserted into the necrotic or abscess cavity. The retroperitoneal cavity is then insufflated with CO_2 at 15 mmHg to create an adequate working space. Additional 5 mm and 12 mm trocars are inserted for working instruments. [19].

After wide debridement of necrotic tissue and hemostasis, the cavity is thoroughly irrigated with approximately 2 liters of saline solution. One or more large-bore drains are left in place, preferably closed suction drains (e.g., Blake) or, alternatively, open siliconized Penrose drains. Another option is the SUMP drain, which allows continuous drainage with irrigation, though it is not a closed system [19].

A variation of the VARD technique involves the use of a cystoscope. In this method, percutaneous puncture of the necrotic site is guided by ultrasonography. After confirmation with fluoroscopy using iodinated contrast, a 0.035″ hydrophilic guidewire is introduced, and the tract is progressively dilated to allow insertion of a 30 Fr sheath. The cystoscope is then advanced, permitting removal of necrotic material through its working channel and lavage with saline solution. At the end of the procedure, a large-bore drain is placed [21].

The main advantage of VARD is the reduced risk of peritoneal contamination, as the access route is limited to the retroperitoneal space. However, limitations include restricted access and limited visualization, which may compromise the completeness of debridement and require multiple interventions. Hollemans et al. demonstrated the superiority of minimally invasive techniques compared with open surgery, with a significant reduction in mortality (44% vs. 73%; $p = 0.005$) [20].

Although VARD is widely used in necrotizing pancreatitis, its application in traumatic pancreatic injury remains poorly supported by strong evidence. Nevertheless, it may be considered in selected cases, depending on clinical judgment and resource availability.

Postoperative Complications of Pancreatic Trauma Surgery

Complications following surgical treatment of pancreatic trauma are diverse and may occur in 26–86% of patients. Among the most frequent are infectious complications, such as abscesses, and pancreas-specific complications, such as pancreatic fistula and pseudocyst formation [17].

Due to the high complication rate, Biffl et al. conducted a study involving 1240 patients with pancreatic injury, identifying independent risk factors for the development of pancreatic complications [22]. These include:

- high-grade pancreatic injuries,
- penetrating trauma mechanism,
- treatment performed in low-volume centers.

These findings reinforce the importance of managing patients with pancreatic trauma in specialized reference centers, with trained teams and adequate infrastructure.

Tybuski et al. analyzed post-traumatic infection and observed an incidence nearly three times higher of infectious complications in patients with pancreatic trauma compared to those without pancreatic injury. Interestingly, the infection rate was similar among different treatment strategies (suture, drainage, or resection), suggesting that the type of procedure itself does not directly influence infectious risk [23].

Pancreatic fistula is the most common complication after trauma and may occur following both conservative and surgical approaches. Reported incidence ranges from 5% to 37%. This rate is comparable between open and laparoscopic approaches; however, laparoscopy is associated with shorter hospital stays, faster recovery, and reduced postoperative pain [24].

In the 2016 update by the International Study Group of Pancreatic Fistula (ISGPF), pancreatic fistula is defined as any measurable drainage with an amylase level greater than three times the upper limit of normal serum amylase in the institution. Fistulas are classified into three categories (Table 23.1): A, B, and C [23, 25, 26].

Management depends on the severity of the fistula. In addition to appropriate drainage, conservative treatment includes initial fasting and parenteral nutrition. Enteral nutrition may be initiated in patients with low-output fistulas, provided that drainage volume does not increase. Octreotide use, although not proven to accelerate closure, may be beneficial in reducing output, especially in high-output fistulas associated with hypovolemia and electrolyte disturbances [26].

Persistent fistulas may require surgical reintervention, with individualized evaluation needed to define the appropriate management strategy [17].

Table 23.1 Classification of pancreatic fistulas according to established clinical, laboratory, and therapeutic criteria

Grade	Definition	Characteristics
A	Biochemical leak, not a "true" pancreatic fistula	No clinical impact, amylase level >3 times the upper limit of normal serum amylase
B	Requiring change in management	Persistent drainage >3 weeks, percutaneous or endoscopic drainage, or peripancreatic fluid collections
C	Requires reoperation, results in organ failure or death	Severe condition requiring surgical intervention or resulting in fatal outcomes

Final Considerations

Pancreatic trauma is rare but associated with high morbidity and mortality, primarily due to delayed diagnosis and the occurrence of postoperative complications.

Minimally invasive approaches, such as laparoscopy, have been increasingly applied in the management of abdominal trauma and have shown clear advantages in selected cases. Their use in pancreatic trauma is feasible and safe in experienced hands, offering benefits such as reduced pain, shorter hospital stay, and lower morbidity.

Nonetheless, the choice of approach must always take into account the patient's hemodynamic stability, the extent of associated injuries, and the infrastructure available at the treating center.

Although evidence regarding the use of laparoscopy in pancreatic trauma is still limited to case reports and small series, accumulated experience in hepatopancreatobiliary surgery and pancreatic resections for benign and malignant disease supports its application in this context.

The future perspective lies in the expansion of minimally invasive surgery for trauma care, guided by technological advances, improved training, and centralization of complex cases in high-volume centers.

References

1. Soltani T, Jurkovich GJ. Diagnosis and management of pancreatic trauma: what you need to know. J Trauma Acute Care Surg. 2025;98(5):681–91.
2. Sayad P, Cacchione R, Ferzli G. Laparoscopic distal pancreatectomy for blunt injury to the pancreas. A case report. Surg Endosc. 2001;15(7):759.
3. Hasanovic J, Agic M, Rifatbegovic Z, Mehmedovic Z, Jakubovic-Cickusic A. Pancreatic injury in blunt abdominal trauma. Med Arch. 2015;69(2):130–2.
4. Debi U, Kaur R, Prasad KK, Sinha SK, Sinha A, Singh K. Pancreatic trauma: a concise review. World J Gastroenterol. 2013;19(47):9003–11.
5. Kim DH, Kim M, Lee DS, Hong TH, Park H, Cho H. Role of laparoscopic surgery in managing hemodynamically stable abdominal trauma patients: a single level I trauma center, propensity score matching study. Eur J Trauma Emerg Surg. 2024;50(5):2517–25.
6. Iordache FM, Giumba T, Bărăian C, Ghioldiş A, Făgărăşan V, Copăescu C, Tomulescu V, Binţinţan V, Duţă C, Popescu R, Şurlin V, Ulmeanu D, Nicolau A, Diaconescu B, Calu V, Liţescu M, Bartoş A, Totolici B, Molnar C, Zărnescu NO, Coroş M, Pantea S, Timofte DV, Tarcoveanu E. Laparoscopy in abdominal emergencies. Romanian association for endoscopic surgery consensus. Part I (trauma). Chirurgia (Bucur). 2024;119(6):701–11.
7. Sobocki J, Pędziwiatr M, Bigda J, Hołówko W, Major P, Mitura K, Myśliwiec P, Nowosad M, Obcowska-Hamerska A, Orłowski M, Proczko-Stepaniak M, Szeliga J, Wallner G, Zawadzki M, Expert Group: Prof. Tomasz Banasiewicz, Prof. Andrzej Budzyński, Prof. Adam Dziki, Prof. Michał Grąt, Prof. Marek Jackowski, Prof. Wojciech Kielan, Prof. Andrzej Matyja, Prof. Krzysztof Paśnik, Prof. Piotr Richter, Prof. Antoni Szczepanik, Prof. Mirosław Szura, Prof. Wiesław Tarnowski, Prof. Krzysztof Zieniewicz. The Association of Polish Surgeons (APS) clinical guidelines for the use of laparoscopy in the management of abdominal emergencies. Part II. Wideochir Inne Tech Maloinwazyjne. 2023;18(3):379–400.
8. Sermonesi G, Tian BWCA, Vallicelli C, Abu-Zidan FM, Damaskos D, Kelly MD, Leppäniemi A, Galante JM, Tan E, Kirkpatrick AW, Khokha V, Romeo OM, Chirica M, Pikoulis M, Litvin

A, Shelat VG, Sakakushev B, Wani I, Sall I, Fugazzola P, Cicuttin E, Toro A, Amico F, Mas FD, De Simone B, Sugrue M, Bonavina L, Campanelli G, Carcoforo P, Cobianchi L, Coccolini F, Chiarugi M, Di Carlo I, Di Saverio S, Podda M, Pisano M, Sartelli M, Testini M, Fette A, Rizoli S, Picetti E, Weber D, Latifi R, Kluger Y, Balogh ZJ, Biffl W, Jeekel H, Civil I, Hecker A, Ansaloni L, Bravi F, Agnoletti V, Beka SG, Moore EE, Catena F. Cesena guidelines: WSES consensus statement on laparoscopic-first approach to general surgery emergencies and abdominal trauma. World J Emerg Surg. 2023;18(1):57.

9. Catellani B, Caracciolo D, Magistri P, Guidetti C, Menduni N, Yu H, Odorizzi R, Guerrini GP, Ballarin R, Di Sandro S, Di Benedetto F. Laparoscopic management of blunt pancreatic trauma in adults and pediatric patients: a systematic review. Biomed Res Int. 2023;28(2023):9296570.
10. Vijay A, Abdelrahman H, El-Menyar A, Al-Thani H. Early laparoscopic approach to pancreatic injury following blunt abdominal trauma. J Surg Case Rep. 2014;2014(12):rju129.
11. Sylivris A, Liu ZF, Shakerian R, Loveday BPT, Read DJ. Paradigms in trauma laparoscopy for anterior abdominal stab wounds: a scoping review. Injury. 2024;55(2):111298.
12. Koto MZ, Matsevych OY, Mosai F, Balabyeki M, Aldous C. Laparoscopic management of retroperitoneal injuries from penetrating abdominal trauma in haemodynamically stable patients. J Minim Access Surg. 2019;15(1):25–30.
13. Fong ZV, Fagenholz PJ. Minimally invasive debridement for infected pancreatic necrosis. J Gastrointest Surg. 2019;23(1):185–91.
14. Coccolini F, Kobayashi L, Kluger Y, Moore EE, Ansaloni L, Biffl W, Leppaniemi A, Augustin G, Reva V, Wani I, Kirkpatrick A, Abu-Zidan F, Cicuttin E, Fraga GP, Ordonez C, Pikoulis E, Sibilla MG, Maier R, Matsumura Y, Masiakos PT, Khokha V, Mefire AC, Ivatury R, Favi F, Manchev V, Sartelli M, Machado F, Matsumoto J, Chiarugi M, Arvieux C, Catena F, Coimbra R. WSES-AAST expert panel. Duodeno-pancreatic and extrahepatic biliary tree trauma: WSES-AAST guidelines. World J Emerg Surg. 2019;11(14):56.
15. Moren AM, Biffl WL, Ball CG, de Moya M, Brasel KJ, Brown CVR, Hartwell JL, Inaba K, Ley EJ, Moore EE, Peck KA, Rizzo AG, Rosen NG, Sperry JL, Weinberg JA, Coimbra R, Shatz DV, Martin MJ. Blunt pancreatic trauma: a Western Trauma Association critical decisions algorithm. J Trauma Acute Care Surg. 2023;94(3):455–60.
16. Ho VP, Patel NJ, Bokhari F, Madbak FG, Hambley JE, Yon JR, Robinson BR, Nagy K, Armen SB, Kingsley S, Gupta S, Starr FL, Moore HR 3rd, Oliphant UJ, Haut ER, Como JJ. Management of adult pancreatic injuries: a practice management guideline from the eastern association for the surgery of trauma. J Trauma Acute Care Surg. 2017;82(1):185–99.
17. Subramanian A, Dente CJ, Feliciano DV. The management of pancreatic trauma in the modern era. Surg Clin N Am. 2007;87(6):1515–32. https://doi.org/10.1016/j.suc.2007.08.007.
18. Byrge N, Heilbrun M, Winkler N, Sommers D, Evans H, Cattin LM, Scalea T, Stein DM, Neideen T, Walsh P, Sims CA, Brahmbhatt TS, Galante JM, Phan HH, Malhotra A, Stovall RT, Jurkovich GJ, Coimbra R, Berndtson AE, et al. An AAST-MITC analysis of pancreatic trauma: staple or sew? Resect or drain? J Trauma Acute Care Surg. 2018;85(3):435–43. https://doi.org/10.1097/TA.0000000000001987.
19. Rey Chaves CE, Azula Uribe MC, Benavides Largo S, Becerra Sarmiento L, Gómez-Gutierrez MA, Cuevas López L. Video-assisted retroperitoneal debridement for necrotizing pancreatitis: a single-center experience in Colombia. BMC Surg. 2024;24:293. https://doi.org/10.1186/s12893-024-02586-x.
20. Hollemans RA, Bakker OJ, Boermeester MA, Bollen TL, Bosscha K, Bruno MJ, Buskens E, Dejong CH, van Duijvendijk P, van Eijck CH, Fockens P, van Goor H, van Grevenstein WM, van der Harst E, Heisterkamp J, Hesselink EJ, Hofker S, Houdijk AP, Karsten T, et al. Superiority of step-up approach vs open necrosectomy in long-term follow-up of patients with necrotizing pancreatitis. Gastroenterology. 2019;156(4):1016–26. https://doi.org/10.1053/j.gastro.2018.10.045.
21. Houghton EJ, García Vázquez AA, Zeledón ME, Andreacchio A, Ruiz G, Palermo M, Gimenez ME. Necrotizing pancreatitis: description of videoscopic assisted retroperitoneal debridement (VARD) technique with covered metallic stent. Arq Bras Cir Dig. 2018;31(2):e1379. https://doi.org/10.1590/0102-672020180001e1379.

22. Biffl WL, Ball CG, Moore EE, et al. A comparison of management and outcomes following blunt versus penetrating pancreatic trauma: a secondary analysis from the western Trauma Association multicenter trials group on pancreatic injuries. J Trauma Acute Care Surg. 2022;93(5):620–6. https://doi.org/10.1097/TA.0000000000003766.
23. Tyburski JG, Dente CJ, Wilson RF, et al. Infectious complications following duodenal and/or pancreatic trauma. Am Surg. 2001;67(3):227–31.
24. Mukherjee K, Morrow SE, Yang EY. Laparoscopic distal pancreatectomy in children: four cases and review of the literature. J Laparoendosc Adv Surg Tech A. 2010;20(4):373–7. https://doi.org/10.1089/lap.2009.0240.
25. Bassi C, Marchegiani G, Dervenis C, et al. The 2016 update of the International Study Group (ISGPS) definition and grading of postoperative pancreatic fistula: 11 years after. Surgery. 2017;161(3):584–91. https://doi.org/10.1016/j.surg.2016.11.014.
26. Vasquez JC, Coimbra R, Hoyt DB, et al. Management of penetrating pancreatic trauma: an 11-year experience of a level-1 trauma center. Injury. 2001;32(9):753–9. https://doi.org/10.1016/S0020-1383(01)00143-0.

Urinary Tract Injuries

24

Nicolas de Cesaro Schpchacki, Karine Matos de Albuquerque, Marcos Arcoverde Fortes Filho, Seth Rabinowitz, and Marcelo Augusto Fontenelle Ribeiro Jr

Introduction and Mechanisms of Injury

Urinary tract injuries (UTIs) are a significant part of trauma-related genitourinary injuries, the incidence and severity are often related with the anatomical location and trauma mechanism. Although UTIs account for a relatively small proportion of all trauma admissions, urologic organs may be involved in 10% of abdominal trauma, and their diagnosis and management require high knowledge and timely intervention to prevent complications such as infection or loss of the renal function [1]. These injuries may often involve different parts of the genitourinary tract as the kidneys, ureters, bladder, or urethra and may present different symptoms as hematuria, urinary retention, or signs of peritonitis. The management of each organ depends on the kind of trauma, hemodynamic status of the patient and the extent of injuries.

Authors Nicolas de Cesaro Schpchacki, Karine Matos de Albuquerque, Marcos Arcoverde Fortes Filho and Seth Rabinowitz have equally contributed to this chapter.

N. de Cesaro Schpchacki
Pontifícia Universidade Católica do Rio Grande do Sul (PUCRS), Porto Alegre, Brazil
e-mail: n.schpchacki@edu.pucrs.br

K. M. de Albuquerque
Faculty of Medicine, University of Porto, Porto, Portugal

M. A. F. Filho
Centro Universitário UniFacid | IDOMED, Teresina, Brazil
e-mail: 202051925256@alunos.facid.edu.br

S. Rabinowitz
School of Medicine, University of Maryland, Baltimore, MD, USA
e-mail: Sethrabinowitz@som.umaryland.edu

M. A. F. Ribeiro Jr (✉)
University of Maryland, R Adams Cowley Shock Trauma Center, Baltimore, MD, USA
e-mail: mfribeiro@som.umaryland.edu

© The Author(s), under exclusive license to Springer Nature Switzerland AG 2026

M. Cezillo, B. M. Pereira (eds.), *Minimally Invasive Surgery Trauma*,
https://doi.org/10.1007/978-3-032-28971-1_24

Renal injuries most result from blunt trauma as motor vehicle accidents or falls, leading to contusions, lacerations or hematomas caused by external forces or direct trauma. Penetrating trauma, including stab or gunshot wounds, may cause vascular disruption or deep parenchymal injury, often classified as grade III to V based on the American Association for the Surgery of Trauma (AAST) renal injury scale [2]. Ureteral trauma is rare but may occur due to deceleration or associated pelvic fractures, leading to partial or complete transections. Penetrating trauma is more likely to cause direct laceration or transection of the ureter [3].

Bladder injuries are frequently seen in the context of pelvic fractures. Probably, these may result in intraperitoneal or extraperitoneal bladder ruptures, commonly associated with the presence of urine extravasation [4].

Urethral injuries typically occur after a pelvic fracture during blunt trauma, where the distribution of the forces disrupts the membranous urethra, especially at the bulbomembranous junction. Alternatively, penetrating mechanisms such as gunshot or straddle injuries may lead to anterior or posterior urethral transections, depending on the trajectory and force [1].

Diagnostic Imaging

Imaging plays a pivotal role in guiding minimally invasive surgery (MIS) through identifying locations and severity of urinary tract injuries. For renal trauma, computed tomography (CT) with intravenous contrast is considered the gold standard, capable of detecting parenchymal lacerations, hematomas, and vascular injuries. A delayed-phase CT is particularly useful for identifying urine leakage and allows for renal injuries classifications, which help guide the decision for MIS [2, 3]. In cases of ureteral trauma, CT with delayed-phase imaging or intravenous pyelography (IVP) is used to detect urine leakage or obstruction, while intraoperative retrograde pyelography may confirm ureteral transections [3]. Bladder injuries are best assessed with CT cystography, which distinguishes between intraperitoneal and extraperitoneal ruptures. Although ultrasound can detect pelvic free fluid, it lacks specificity for bladder injury diagnosis [4]. For urethral trauma, retrograde urethrography (RUG) remains the gold standard, especially in patients presenting with pelvic fractures or blood at the meatus. RUG effectively delineates partial from complete disruptions and informs catheter placement and surgical decision-making. While CT or MRI is not routinely employed for urethral evaluation, it may be useful for identifying confounding pelvic injuries [4, 5].

Minimally Invasive Techniques for Urinary Tract Injuries

Over the past few decades, the emergence of novel minimally invasive techniques has further advanced the boundaries of trauma care. Laparoscopic and robotic-assisted approaches have enhanced the accuracy of diagnosis and the efficiency of the treatment for UTIs, particularly in hemodynamically stable patients, while reducing morbidity. Techniques are derived from Di Saverio et al. [4], Griffin et al. [10], Lee et al. [8], Tsai et al. [5], Kasperczak et al. [2], and Serafetinidis et al. [3].

Diagnostic Laparoscopy

- *Purpose*: Diagnostic Laparoscopy is proposed as a strategy to reduce unnecessary exploratory laparotomies in trauma patients with suspected intra-abdominal injuries. Negative laparotomy rates are significantly high and carry a notable procedure-related morbidity and cost. Diagnostic laparoscopy enables the direct visualization of renal hematomas, ureteral leaks, or bladder ruptures in stable patients, allowing assessment of injury extent and more selective intervention [4, 6, 7].
- *Technique*: A standard setup includes a 10–12 mm umbilical camera port and two 5 mm working ports along the midclavicular line. Systematic exploration of the peritoneum, retroperitoneum, and pelvis is performed, with suction-irrigation to clear the blood or urine. Methylene blue instillation or cystoscopy can be used to confirm ureteral or bladder injuries [7]. Surgeons must be vigilant for the risk of a tension pneumothorax caused by the pneumoperitoneum due to an undiagnosed diaphragmatic rupture [6, 7].
- *Specifics*: When completed in 20–30 min, diagnostic laparoscopy reduces non-therapeutic laparotomy rates by 50–60% in stable trauma patients [4]. Diagnostic accuracy is high, with sensitivity and specificity ranging from 75% to 100%. In selected series, a median of 57% of trauma patients undergoing DL had negative findings, sparing them an unnecessary exploratory laparotomy. Diagnostic laparoscopy has reduced non-therapeutic laparotomies by 19%, with no missed injuries in the laparoscopy group [6, 7].

General Setup for Treatment

- *Patient Positioning*: For bladder and ureteral repairs, patients are usually positioned supine with a 15–20° Trendelenburg tilt to improve pelvic exposure. Renal injuries are most effectively managed with a 45° modified flank position, elevating the operative side. This configuration uses a beanbag positioner, cross-chest straps, and table flexion to optimize the surgical field between the costal margin and iliac crest. Proper padding and secure strapping are crucial to maintain stability and avoid pressure-related complications [4, 8]. For urethral trauma, positioning varies with the injury site. Anterior urethral repairs with laparoscopic or robotic-assisted approaches are generally done in the dorsal lithotomy position. In selected posterior urethral injuries, a supine position with slight Trendelenburg tilt is preferred [1, 9].
- *Portal Placement*: A 3–4 port configuration includes a 10–12 mm umbilical camera port, two 5–10 mm working ports (midclavicular line, 2–3 cm below costal margin), and an optional 5 mm lower quadrant port. Retroperitoneal access shifts ports laterally toward the posterior axillary line to provide direct access to the retroperitoneal space and facilitate ergonomic instrument handling [8, 10].
- *Materials*: Core instruments include a 30° laparoscope, atraumatic graspers, needle drivers, and laparoscopic scissors. Energy devices such as ultrasonic

shears (e.g., Harmonic) or advanced bipolar sealing systems (e.g., LigaSure) assist in precise dissection and hemostasis. Hemostatic agents are used to control bleeding (e.g., fibrin sealants, oxidized cellulose); 3–0 or 4–0 absorbable sutures (polyglactin) are used for soft tissue approximation, and double-J stents are used for ureteral repair to ensure patency. Robotic systems provide articulated instruments and 3D visualization, improving precision in confined operative fields [8, 10].

Kidneys

- *Diagnosis*: Laparoscopy identifies renal injuries by direct inspection of perirenal hematomas or parenchymal lacerations, typically after medial mobilization of the colon and opening of Gerota's fascia; injury grades III–IV (AAST) are most suitable for minimally invasive repair [4, 8]. Therapeutic laparoscopy can be employed for lesion staging and, if needed, for repair or nephrectomy. However, this approach is not recommended in hemodynamically unstable patients and is not routinely employed for initial diagnosis of renal trauma.
- *Treatment*: Laparoscopic management of renal trauma is reserved for hemodynamically stable patients at high-expertise centers, and is typically considered in selected high-grade injuries (AAST grade III–IV). The contraindications for this intervention, as with other laparoscopic procedures, include hemodynamic instability, head injury, retinal detachment, coagulopathy, significant hemorrhage within Gerota's fascia and multiple organ involvement. Renal lacerations are managed using 3–0 absorbable sutures in a running or interrupted fashion, with optional use of omental or fat bolsters and fibrin sealants to reinforce closure. Hilar clamping with laparoscopic bulldog clamps may be necessary to control bleeding during suturing [11].

Ureters

- *Diagnosis*: Laparoscopy detects urine leakage or retroperitoneal fluid. Intraoperative confirmation can be achieved through the use of renally excreted dyes, such as methylene blue or indigo carmine, or through ureteroscopic evaluation [3]. These techniques allow direct inspection of ureteral integrity and are particularly valuable in stable trauma patients already undergoing surgical exploration. A delay in the diagnosis is related to negative outcomes [11].
- *Treatment*: Partial transections are repaired with uretero-ureterostomy using 4–0 absorbable sutures and a double-J stent, often reinforced with omentum wrap. In cases of complete transection injuries, ureteroneocystostomy or transureteroureterostomy may be required, depending on location and extent of tissue loss [10]. A closed-suction drain is recommended to monitor for urinary leakage and prevent urinoma formation [11].
- *Specifics*: In laparoscopic or robotic ureteral repair, the ureter is typically identified using anatomical landmarks such as the psoas muscle and the gonadal vessels. Proper spatulation of the ureteral ends is essential to create a wide, tension-free anastomosis and reduce the risk of stricture formation. When available, robotic assistance may enhance precision during intracorporeal suturing [10].

Bladder

- *Diagnosis*: Retrograde cystography (CT or fluoroscopic) is the gold standard for diagnosing bladder injuries in stable patients with gross hematuria and/or pelvic fracture [11, 12]. Laparoscopy reveals intraperitoneal ruptures through direct visualization or identification of free pelvic fluid, while extraperitoneal injuries are confirmed by methylene blue instillation or cystoscopy [4, 5, 11].
- *Treatment*: In hemodynamically stable patients with isolated intraperitoneal injuries, laparoscopic repair is considered safe and effective, particularly in centers with appropriate expertise [11–13]. Uncomplicated extraperitoneal injuries are usually managed conservatively with catheter drainage, while surgical repair is reserved for complex extraperitoneal injuries, such as those involving the bladder neck, concomitant rectal or vaginal injuries, or bony spicules penetrating the bladder wall [13]. Intraperitoneal ruptures are closed in two layers using 3–0 absorbable sutures—first continuous mucosal, followed by seromuscular closure; extraperitoneal ruptures may be managed laparoscopically or robotically in select cases when surgical repair is required [14].
- *Specifics*: Transperitoneal access clears clots via suction-irrigation. A Foley catheter remains for 3 weeks, with cystogram confirming no leakage. A pelvic drain is placed. Robotic repair improves extraperitoneal outcomes [5, 10].

Urethra

- *Diagnosis:* Urethral injuries are suspected in trauma patients presenting with bleeding from the meatus, urinary retention, or a high-riding prostate on digital rectal exam; while laparoscopy has limited diagnostic utility, it can aid in assessing concurrent pelvic damage or guiding suprapubic access under direct vision [1, 3, 11].
- *Treatment:* Partial anterior injuries may be treated endoscopically or laparoscopically in select cases, while complete posterior disruptions require delayed urethroplasty after suprapubic urinary diversion. Laparoscopic or robotic-assisted primary repair may be considered in stable patients with penetrating trauma and accessible injury sites [1, 10].
- *Specifics:* Retrograde urethrography is obligatory before catheterization in suspected urethral trauma. A suprapubic catheter placement may be performed under laparoscopic guidance to prevent visceral injury [3, 9].

Retroperitoneal Exploration

- *Diagnosis*: In hemodynamically stable patients, laparoscopy evaluates non-expanding retroperitoneal hematomas, urinary leaks, or suspicious collections. This approach may help prevent unnecessary open exploration. Findings such as confined fluid, contained bleeding, or urine extravasation can guide targeted intervention [4, 6, 7, 11].
- *Treatment*: Medial mobilization of the colon and opening of Gerota's fascia is essential to expose the kidney and proximal ureter, accessing the retroperitoneal space. Fluid collections are evacuated using suction, and injuries to structures such as the renal capsule or ureter are repaired with 3–0 or 4–0 absorbable sutures [15]. Methylene blue may be instilled via catheter to assist localization

if urinary extravasation is suspected. A closed-suction drain is placed in the retroperitoneal space to monitor for persistent leakage or bleeding [7, 8, 10].

- *Specifics*: Port configuration is laterally adapted to optimize retroperitoneal access to the retroperitoneum, typically using a 10–12 mm camera port and two 5–10 mm working ports along the posterior axillary line. The patient is placed in lateral decubitus or modified flank position depending on the site of the suspected injury. Instruments include suction-irrigation systems, atraumatic graspers, needle drivers, and drains [8, 16].

Indications and Contraindications

- *Indications*: Stable patients with suspected renal (grade III–IV), ureteral, or intraperitoneal bladder injuries are candidates for diagnostic and therapeutic MIS. Penetrating injuries with controlled bleeding are suitable in selective cases [2, 4, 10].
- *Contraindications*: Hemodynamic instability, grade V renal injuries, or complex bladder neck/prostate injuries require open surgery or embolization. Diffuse intraperitoneal contamination precludes MIS [2, 3, 5].
- *Selection Criteria*: Surgeon expertise, equipment availability, and injury severity guide decisions all influence surgical decision-making. High-volume centers provide more experience and resources and, in turn, better outcomes [8] (Table 24.1).

Table 24.1 Illustrates the main indications and contraindications for MIS in UTI

Lesion Type	Indications for MIS	Contraindications for MIS
Renal (Grade III–IV)	Hemodynamically stable, localized parenchymal laceration	Hemodynamic instability, uncontrolled bleeding
Ureteral (Partial)	Stable, with localized leak; suitable for uretero-ureterostomy	Extensive tissue loss, instability
Ureteral (Complete)	Stable, suitable for ureteroneocystostomy or transureteroureterostomy	Hemodynamic instability, poor visualization
Bladder (Intraperitoneal)	Stable, confirmed rupture; repair via laparoscopy/robotics	Instability, severe contamination, complex bladder neck injuries
Bladder (Extraperitoneal)	Selected stable cases with technical feasibility	Large, contaminated injuries or associated pelvic fractures
Urethral (Partial)	Stable, with minimal disruption; possibly endoscopic/laparoscopic	Complete disruption, pelvic instability, instability
Urethral (Complete)	Delayed repair after suprapubic diversion; rarely MIS in acute setting	Immediate primary repair in unstable patients
Retroperitoneal injury	Non-expanding hematoma, confined leaks or collections	Expanding hematoma, unstable patient, unclear anatomy

Advantages and Limitations

- *Advantages*: MIS reduces blood loss, postoperative pain, hospital stay (3–5 days), wound infections, adhesions and incisional hernias. Renal function is preserved in 85% of grade III–IV injuries. Furthermore, diagnostic laparoscopy demonstrated the avoidance of unnecessary laparotomy in 50% of cases [2, 4, 5].
- *Limitations*: Steep learning curve requires advanced training. Deep retroperitoneal access remains challenging, with 5–10% conversion to open surgery due to bleeding or complex injuries [8, 17].

Complications

- *Intraoperative*: Bleeding or adjacent organ injury (e.g., bowel, spleen) may occur but can be mitigated by careful dissection and imaging [4, 8].
- *Postoperative*: Urinary leakage, infections, or ureteral stenosis are potential risks. Watertight closures, stents, and antibiotics reduce complications. Fistula rates are 26% in conservative bladder rupture management, which emphasizes the importance of surgical repair [5].
- *Prevention*: Precise suturing, saline testing, and drainage (e.g., Jackson-Pratt drains) are critical. Simulation training improves skills, especially in intraoperative complications management [8].

Clinical Evidence and Outcomes

Minimally invasive surgery, particularly laparoscopy, is very used as a diagnostic approach and demonstrated to decrease the outcome of non-therapeutic laparotomies, and also the hospital stays compared to open surgeries [4]. Bladder repair through laparoscopy demonstrates benefits of 80–90% comparable to open surgery, and the use of robotic approaches may be useful to manage extraperitoneal bladder injuries [5, 10]. Additionally, in renal trauma, minimally invasive approaches conserve renal function in approximately 85% of injuries. Furthermore, embolization is required in 27.27% of severe cases, and conservative management is successful in 19.79% of these patients [2]. In addition, in the acute phase, laparoscopic-assisted placement of suprapubic catheters is considered safe and effective. The standard of care for urethral disruptions is delayed urethroplasty following urinary diversion, achieving success rates of 85% in experienced centers [1, 3]. Overall, the European Association of Urology guidelines support the use of minimally invasive techniques in hemodynamically stable trauma patients, as these approaches may reduce postoperative morbidity while maintaining favorable clinical outcomes.

Future Perspectives

- *Technological Advancements*
  The integration of indocyanine green (ICG) fluorescence with the Da Vinci Xi robotic system demonstrates substantial promise in the minimally invasive management of urinary tract trauma. This approach has been particularly impactful in procedures such as nephrectomy and pyeloplasty, where precise anatomical visualization is critical. Intravenously administered ICG enables real-time perfusion imaging, enhancing the surgeon's capacity to discriminate between pathological and healthy tissues. In reconstructive operations, ICG has proved to enhance the visualization of the renal pelvis and ureter, reducing the rate of unintentional trauma to urological or adjacent vascular structures [18].
  Robotic surgical systems have significantly expanded the scope of minimally invasive techniques in urologic procedures. The advent of single-port platforms, which allow all of the operative instruments to be inserted through a single 2.5 cm incision, represents a notable advancement in minimizing access-related morbidity. These systems utilize flexible, wristed instruments, allowing for internal triangulation, mimicking conventional laparoscopic maneuverability while reducing the number of incisions [10].
  A recent reintroduction of haptic feedback into robotic surgery enables the operator to perceive variations in tissue resistance and tension during dissection, suturing and reconstruction, enhancing tactile awareness. This sensory input, long absent from earlier robotic platforms, may improve the precision of tissue handling and reduce intraoperative complications [10, 18].
  Beyond mechanical innovations, the integration of artificial intelligence (AI) and machine learning (ML) into the realm of minimally invasive urology is emerging as a transformative frontier. These digital tools are being utilized throughout the perioperative pathway—from pre-surgical planning and intraoperative guidance to real-time data analytics and postoperative surveillance [11, 18].
  Single-port laparoscopy in trauma, though still in development, holds significant promise for expanding its role and efficacy. Despite limited clinical data, its potential for reducing access trauma and improving cosmesis supports further refinement of the technique and accumulation of evidence-based outcomes [19].
- *Training*
  Low-cost simulation platforms (approximately $800 USD for initial setup and $7 per session) aimed at renal and ureteral trauma have demonstrated effectiveness in enhancing surgical skills, thereby facilitating wider implementation of minimally invasive techniques. This specific training model replicates both arterial and venous renal injuries within the context of laparoscopic radical and partial nephrectomies, offering a novel and economically accessible solution for practicing laparoscopic management of renal hilar vascular injuries. It is particularly well-suited for surgical education among urology residents and trainees [8].
  Simulation-based education has become a fundamental element in surgical training, enabling residents to acquire and refine operative skills in a risk-free setting prior to clinical application. The traditional model of the "teaching hospital" has

progressively evolved into specialized centers of excellence in minimally invasive urology, where large surgical volumes, concentrated expertise, and purpose-built training infrastructure foster optimal environments for surgical education. As these training modalities advance, they are set to play a key role in enhancing surgeon proficiency, speeding up skill acquisition, and supporting the safe implementation of advanced minimally invasive techniques in urologic trauma.

Acknowledgments The authors used artificial intelligence tools (e.g., ChatGPT) to assist with language and grammar editing. All content was written and reviewed by the authors, who remain fully responsible for the accuracy and originality of the final text.

Competing Interests The author declares no conflicts of interest.

References

1. Morey AF, Brandes SB, Dugi DD 3rd, Armstrong JH, Breyer BN, Broghammer JA, et al. Urotrauma: AUA guideline. J Urol. 2014;192(2):327–35. https://doi.org/10.1016/j.juro.2014.05.004.
2. Kasperczak M, Zaręba A, Pawłowski-Kasperczak K, Kasperczak F, Antczak A. Renal trauma: a 4-year retrospective review of injury severity, treatment approaches, and outcomes from a polish trauma center. Clin Pract. 2025;15:67. https://doi.org/10.3390/clinpract15040067.
3. Serafetinidis E, Campos-Juanatey F, Hallscheidt P, et al. Summary paper of the updated 2023 European Association of Urology guidelines on urological trauma. Eur Urol Focus. 2023;10:475–85. https://doi.org/10.1016/j.euf.2023.08.011.
4. Di Saverio S, Birindelli A, Podda M, et al. Trauma laparoscopy and the six w's: why, when, who, where, what, and how? J Trauma Acute Care Surg. 2020;88(2):344–52. https://doi.org/10.1097/TA.0000000000002130.
5. Tsai CH, Wang YC, Wu SC, Hsieh CH. Laparoscopic repair of extraperitoneal urinary bladder rupture after blunt abdominal trauma. Am Surg. 2012;78(9):E386–7.
6. Jeon S, Choi K-K. Single-incision laparoscopy in abdominal trauma: current evidence, clinical applications, and evolving role—a narrative review. J Clin Med. 2025;14(10):3610. https://doi.org/10.3390/jcm14103610.
7. SAGES. Guidelines for diagnostic laparoscopy. Society of American Gastrointestinal and Endoscopic Surgeons (SAGES). 2010; Available from: https://www.sages.org/publications/guidelines/guidelines-for-diagnostic-laparoscopy/
8. Lee JY, Mucksavage P, McDougall EM. Simulating laparoscopic renal hilar vessel injuries: preliminary evaluation of a novel surgical training model for residents. J Endourol. 2012;26(4):393–7. https://doi.org/10.1089/end.2011.0432.
9. Urological Trauma Panel, EAU Guidelines. EAU guidelines on urological trauma. Arnhem: European Association of Urology; 2023. Available from: https://d56bochluxqnz.cloudfront.net/documents/full-guideline/EAU-Guidelines-on-Urological-Trauma-2023_2023-03-20-083114_kgdg.pdf
10. Griffin C, Crute W, White W. Robotic-assisted laparoscopic repair of a penetrating extraperitoneal bladder injury. Urology. 2023; https://doi.org/10.1016/j.urology.2023.08.009.
11. WSES Working Group. 2023 WSES guidelines for the prevention, detection, and management of urinary tract injuries in emergency surgery. World J Emerg Surg. 2023;18:45. https://doi.org/10.1186/s13017-023-00513-8.
12. Jaiswal Y, Agarwal A, Yadav P, Khandelwal M, Kumar R. Laparoscopic management of intraperitoneal bladder rupture due to blunt abdominal trauma: a rare case report. Int J Res Med Sci. 2023;11(4):1610–3. https://doi.org/10.18203/2320-6012.ijrms20231662.

13. Reddy D, Laher AE, Moeng M, Adam A. Bladder trauma: a guideline of the guidelines. BJU Int. 2023;133(4):365–74. https://doi.org/10.1111/bju.16236.
14. Kapoor R. Two-layer laparoscopic repair of intraperitoneal bladder rupture in blunt abdominal trauma: a case report with literature review. Surg Laparosc Endosc Percutan Tech. 2012;22(4):e204–5. https://doi.org/10.1097/SLE.0b013e31824ea67e.
15. Engelsgjerd JS, LaGrange CA. Ureteral Injury. [Updated 2023 Jul 4]. In: StatPearls [Internet]. Treasure Island (FL): StatPearls Publishing; 2025. Available from: https://www.ncbi.nlm.nih.gov/books/NBK507817/.
16. Koto MZ, Matsevych OY, Mewa Kinoo S, Singh B. Laparoscopic management of retroperitoneal injuries from penetrating abdominal trauma in haemodynamically stable patients. S Afr J Surg. 2018;56(1):37–40. Available from: https://www.researchgate.net/publication/323262194
17. Yamamoto R, Cestero RF, Kameyama N, Sasaki J. Characteristics of laparoscopic surgery for trauma patients and risks of conversion to open laparotomy. World J Surg. 2022;46(11):2616–24. https://doi.org/10.1007/s00268-022-06714-7.
18. Becker B, Rosenbaum CM. Current milestones and future horizons in minimally invasive urologic surgery. J Clin Med. 2024;13(21):6573. https://doi.org/10.3390/jcm13216573. PMID: 39518714. PMCID: PMC11546464
19. SCARLESS Study Group, Ahmed I, Cook JA, et al. Single port/incision laparoscopic surgery compared with standard three-port laparoscopic surgery for appendicectomy: a randomized controlled trial. Surg Endosc. 2014;29(1):77–85. https://doi.org/10.1007/s00464-014-3416-y.

Part III

Specific Conditions and Populations

Civil-Military Partnership to Develop Minimally Invasive Surgery

25

Kenneth Stransky, Christopher Dyke, Gordon G. Wisbach, and Tamara J. Worlton

Introduction

Minimally invasive surgery was conspicuously absent during the recent wars in Iraq and Afghanistan. This led some authors to conclude that laparoscopic surgery was irrelevant in combat trauma. This may have been due to laparoscopy only becoming widespread shortly before the war broke out. Senior surgeons may not have been comfortable with the technical skills to do diagnostic laparoscopy and felt that it was "simpler" to do an exploratory laparotomy. In fact, the non-therapeutic laparotomy rate between 2002 and 2011 in Iraq and Afghanistan was a whopping 32.2% [1]. Additionally, a review of 15 years of data from these wars demonstrated an incisional hernia rate of 19% [2]. Both of these numbers are significantly higher than reported rates for civilian trauma literature [3]. These statistics alone argue for increased availability and utilization of minimally invasive techniques even in war-related trauma.

One argument against the availability of laparoscopic equipment was that it was too cumbersome, particularly canisters of CO_2, for the mobility of forward surgical teams [4, 5]. This highlights the necessity of an integrated civilian and military approach to laparoscopic surgery. Civilian minimally invasive surgeons, particularly ones in low-resource and humanitarian settings, have been working on low-cost, mobile solutions for laparoscopy. Some surgeons have worked with gasless

K. Stransky · C. Dyke
Department of Surgery, Walter Reed National Military Medical Center, Bethesda, MD, USA

G. G. Wisbach
Department of Surgery, Navy Medicine Readiness & Training Command, San Diego, CA, USA

T. J. Worlton (✉)
Department of Surgery, Uniformed Services University of the Health Sciences, Bethesda, MD, USA
e-mail: tamara.worlton@usuhs.edu

© The Author(s), under exclusive license to Springer Nature Switzerland AG 2026

M. Cezillo, B. M. Pereira (eds.), *Minimally Invasive Surgery Trauma*,
https://doi.org/10.1007/978-3-032-28971-1_25

laparoscopy to completely eliminate the need for gas [6–8]. Companies are developing low-cost laparoscopes that plug directly into a laptop computer, thus forgoing the need for a heavy monitor and light box [9]. These are all potential areas of military and civilian development of technology to benefit all. This chapter will discuss the intersection of military and civilian minimally invasive surgery from the US perspective.

Minimally Invasive Surgery to Strengthen Global Relationships

The US Department of War (DoW) is strongly invested in strengthening ties with partner nations, improving interoperability with our partners and allies, and building capacity and capability within global healthcare systems [10]. The global COVID-19 pandemic highlighted the importance of military and civilian integration in research and development as well as bolstering overburdened healthcare systems around the world [11–13].

Minimally invasive surgery (MIS) has been shown to improve patients' ability to return to work faster, less postoperative pain, shorter hospital stays, and reduce the risk of incisional hernia. However, many countries struggle with the initial investment into the needed equipment and with the required learning curve for laparoscopy [14, 15]. Global outreach through high-income country (HIC) academic institutions, non-governmental organizations (NGOs) and surgical societies has heavily focused on this over the last decade [16–18].

The DoW also uses MIS GHE for building capability and capacity globally [19]. The US Navy hospital ships have multiple operating rooms with laparoscopic capability and, more impressively, had robotic surgery capability in 2018 during a medical mission in the Indo-Pacific region [20]. Having robust mobile assets for laparoscopy and robotic surgery can aid countries that are still developing MIS capability and exchange best practices about complex MIS cases in countries with well-established programs [21]. These exchanges can build professional relationships and aid joint research. Additionally, these missions can introduce technology that is not yet available in a country to local surgeons who may not be able to access it otherwise.

Training Military Surgeons in MIS

As a specialty, MIS is broad covering areas that include bariatric surgery, foregut, abdominal wall reconstruction, solid organ, hepatobiliary, and advanced endoscopy. The decision to pursue subspecialty training leads to a great reduction in the learning curve for not only operative technique but also the preoperative evaluation, postoperative progression, and management of complications for potential patients. While none of the specific domains of MIS currently require subspecialty training, in both the military and civilian practices in the US, domains like bariatric and foregut surgery are increasingly performed solely by surgeons who have completed an MIS fellowship.

Operative exposure in general surgery residencies across the US is variable and may not produce a practice-ready surgeon for these complex procedures. For example, while foregut caseload has steadily increased in recent years, residents graduating in 2024 only performed an average of 4.8 laparoscopic anti-reflux procedures and 6.3 gastric reduction cases for obesity during their final year of training [22, 23].

Given the transient nature of military medicine with deployments, frequent changes of duty station, and terminal separation from the service, this accelerated pathway toward expertise is especially important in the military. There likely will be a singular MIS-trained surgeon at a military treatment facility, and it is more common for young military surgeons to be placed in positions of leadership, like medical director of a metabolic and bariatric surgery program, sooner after training than a civilian counterpart. The need for minimally invasive subspecialty surgical training through nonmilitary-civilian hospitals is crucial to meet the current surgical procedural and educational needs of the active-duty military surgeon as well as to bring current and cutting-edge MIS techniques to military hospitals and surgical training programs.

Application Process

The application process for the active-duty US military surgeons has additional steps when compared to civilian counterparts. Each service (Army, Navy, and Air Force) generally funds one or two MIS fellowship spots per service per year. The selected applicants for each service are then allowed to apply for a training position in an accredited MIS fellowship program through the Fellowship Council. Fellowship programs are a minimum of 1 year and provide in-depth experience in the pre- and postoperative management of patients who have complex gastrointestinal abdominal pathology while focusing on the acquisition of technical skills in these areas [24].

Mutual Benefit of Military-Civilian Partnership

Subspecialty training of military surgeons in civilian centers creates a partnership that is mutually beneficial to both parties. Owing to a service-specific selection process prior to an application through The Fellowship Council, the military generally produces competitive applicants as they have already been chosen from a pool of surgeons interested in MIS fellowship. Additionally, military surgeons are associated with a sense of professionalism, dependability, and a strong work ethic, which lead to more predictable and teachable trainees. Military applicants likely know their future duty station and general makeup of their expected surgical practice which leads to more focused training during fellowship and no need for a job search during fellowship training. Finally, military funding of a surgeon's salary and healthcare benefits during civilian MIS fellowship is a huge benefit to these programs as salaries for fellows are easily greater than $70,000 for 1 year.

The benefits to the DoW are, perhaps, greater than that gained by a civilian partner in MIS fellowship training. The most significant is that they receive a practice ready surgeon who is capable of taking on complex laparoscopic, robotic, and endoscopic cases while serving in educational and leadership roles needed to continue to provide services like bariatric surgery and train future military surgeons. Advanced skills, like laparoscopic suturing and intracorporeal intestinal anastomosis, are mastered through exposure to a large case volume and complex procedure selection. Currently, case log minimums for an Advanced GI MIS program are 150 surgical cases (20 foregut, 25 bariatric, 10 inguinal hernia, 10 ventral hernia, 85 complex cases) and 50 flexible endoscopy cases, though most fellows perform more than 400 total procedures (3). This case volume, as well as case variety is unlikely to be to be met consistently at a single military treatment facility in a single year, and the addition of a fellow would detract from the training experience of a general surgery resident. This operative and clinical experience provided at a civilian training center also makes it possible to obtain the clinical designator of a Fellow of the Association of Metabolic and Bariatric Surgery and greatly reduces the case volume needed to be able to serve as the medical director of an MBSAQIP comprehensive bariatric surgery center. This is well worth the one-year investment for the Department of Defense. The translation of technology from civilian institutions to the military is a major benefit of all civilian training, however as explored in the next section, the military has contributed to technological advancements in MIS.

Military Development of Robotic Surgery for the Battlefield

The US military played a substantial role in the development of robotic surgery as it exists today. Interests in "telesurgery" led to the integration of virtual reality and surgical instrument manipulation. The collaboration of the NASA Ames research center and the Stanford Research Institute (SRI) led to the development of the Green Telepresence Surgery System. Dr. Richard Satava, a general surgeon at Silas B. Hayes Army Hospital, was assigned to the Defense Advanced Research Projects Agency (DARPA) in 1992 and continued to work on this platform with the intention of bringing telesurgery to the battlefield [25]. The concept of this system was to provide a forward surgical presence by mounting a surgical robot on a vehicle which could be controlled remotely by a surgeon. Military testing in 1996 demonstrated that a microwave telecommunication link between the forward surgical hospital and the mounted surgical unit could be used successfully to perform remote surgery over a 5-km distance [26]. Despite the promising applications, latency in communication was a limiting factor. DARPA continued research throughout the 1990s in collaboration with civilian laboratories, investigating parameters such as latency and haptics. The SRI Green Telepresence system, developed by DoW-funded research and tested by military surgeons, ultimately became the Intuitive da Vinci system that dominates the market today [27].

The da Vinci platform was used for additional research and development of a comprehensive critical care and surgical suite that could be used in a deployed setting. The "trauma pod" includes the robotic patient cart which could be docked to a custom gurney with attached vitals monitors. A surgical nurse subsystem and automatic supply dispenser work in tandem to allow for a completely automated experience without the need for a bedside nurse or scrub technician. The system also included portable X-ray and console that are used to operate the components remotely. The platform was used to successfully perform a bowel anastomosis and place a vascular shunt. Limitations discussed by these authors included sterility concerns and a lack of capability to obtain intravenous access and administer anesthesia [28].

Size is a significant limiting factor for deployment in the acute trauma setting. Both the trauma pod and the da Vinci system alone are not devices which can be carried by a combat medic in the field. Reichenbach et al. created a miniature surgical robot that packs to about the size of a briefcase [29]. Their prototype had two robotic arms which could have various surgical tools attached, including cautery, suction, and graspers. Radiofrequency transceivers were used to allow a surgeon to control the robot from a remote computer with haptic controls. Latency response times were recorded with an average of 80 ms compared to a wired remote connection which approximated 20 ms. In addition to portability, another difference from existing systems is that the robot is designed to perform open procedures and surgeries. This is a major departure from the da Vinci, which can be used for minimally invasive surgery only.

The prevalence of robotic surgery has increased annually within military treatment facilities (MTF) just as it has for the entire healthcare system. Global robotic cases reported by Intuitive Surgical® in 2017 were 877,000, an increase from 136,000 in 2008 [30]. In the USA, over 600,000 robotic surgery cases were reported in 2017, which was a threefold increase [31]. Procedures within the DoW increased from 3712 in 2018 to 4117 in 2019 [32]. Surgical training and simulation have also incorporated robotic curricula for trainees, which have been adopted at all MTFs with residency programs.

Robotic surgery has been widely adopted by the military healthcare system. Much of the modern robotic surgery technology was developed by teams attempting to develop telesurgery systems in partnership with the military. Currently, there is no active telesurgery being conducted by the US military; however, as technology improves, research continues so that remote surgery may become feasible in the near future. One exciting arena for telesurgery research is explored in the next section.

Military and Civilian Integration for the Development of Surgery in Space

The development of surgical capabilities in space is a burgeoning area of research for both military and civilian applications, as humanity ventures further into space exploration and considers long-term missions to the moon, Mars, and beyond. The unique challenges of microgravity, limited resources, and isolation necessitate innovative solutions for medical care, including surgery.

The military, especially in the context of space exploration and operations, focuses on developing advanced medical technologies for situations that could arise during long-term missions beyond Earth's orbit. Main areas of focus are exploring surgical capabilities in space, often with a focus on combat scenarios, rapid response, and resource efficiency. Preparing astronauts, including military personnel, to address medical emergencies while underway involves highly advanced technology and training. These remote capabilities incorporate telemedicine, multi-use medical kits and robotic-assisted and autonomous surgery supported by immersive medical simulation training [33, 34]. Military organizations collaborate with civilian space agencies to share knowledge and resources, leveraging advancements in civilian space medicine for military applications.

The civilian sector focuses largely on supporting space missions from a scientific and healthcare perspective, ensuring the well-being of astronauts on long-duration missions. Civilian space agencies and private space companies are heavily involved in these developments. Main related areas of focus are space surgery research, medical care for long-duration missions and implementing space-based surgical laboratories [35].

As space exploration moves toward longer missions into deep space, collaboration between military and civilian sectors will be critical to develop robust, scalable solutions for surgery in space. These solutions will require a combination of advanced technology, highly trained astronauts with specialized medical skills, and continual research into the impacts of space on human health [36]. Military-civilian partnerships are paving the way for more advanced medical interventions during long-duration space missions and improving healthcare access in remote areas on Earth.

Conclusion

Integration of military and civilian investment into MIS pushes forward innovation and access to technology in both sectors in the US and abroad. More widespread application of MIS in combat situations could be cost-effective and mobile and would potentially save non-therapeutic laparotomies. Future directions of military-civilian integration in MIS trauma is exploring telesurgery both earthbound and in space.

Disclaimer The opinions or assertions contained herein are the private ones of the author/speaker and are not to be construed as official or reflecting the views of the Department of War, the Uniformed Services University of the Health Sciences or any other agency of the US Government.

The authors have no conflict of interest.

References

1. Mitchell TA, Hutchison T, Becker TE, Aden JK, Blackbourne L, White CE. Nontherapeutic laparotomy in American combat casualties: a 10-year review. J Trauma Acute Care Surg. 2014;77(3):S171–5.
2. Moas V, Eskridge S, Clouser M, Kurapaty S, Dyke C, Souza J. Incisional hernia incidence following laparotomy for combat trauma: investigating 15 years of US war surgery. J Trauma Acute Care Surg. 2020;89(2S Suppl 2):S200–6.
3. Rios-Diaz AJ, Cunning J, Hsu JY, Elfanagely O, Marks JA, Grenda TR, et al. Incidence, burden on the health care system, and factors associated with incisional hernia after trauma laparotomy. JAMA Surg. 2021;156(9):e213104.
4. Stockinger ZT, Turner CA, Gurney JM. Abdominal trauma surgery during recent US combat operations from 2002 to 2016. J Trauma Acute Care Surg. 2018;85(1S Suppl 2):S122–8.
5. Stockinger ZT, Turner CA, Gurney JM. Re: laparoscopy in a combat theater of operations. J Trauma Acute Care Surg. 2018;85(6):1132–3.
6. Mishra A, Bains L, Jesudin G, Aruparayil N, Singh R, Shashi. Evaluation of gasless laparoscopy as a tool for minimal access surgery in low-to middle-income countries: a phase II noninferiority randomized controlled study. J Am Coll Surg. 2019;231(5):511–9.
7. Hwang JH, Kim SR, Kim JH, Kim BW. Gasless single-port access laparoscopy using a J-shaped retractor in patients undergoing adnexal surgery. Surg Endosc. 2021;35(6):2457–64.
8. Dawkins B, Aruparayil N, Ensor T, Gnanaraj J, Brown J, Jayne D, Shinkins B. Cost-effectiveness of gasless laparoscopy as a means to increase provision of minimally invasive surgery for abdominal conditions in rural north-East India. PLoS One. 2022;17(8):e0271559.
9. Lukish JR, Ellis-Davy J. A novel low cost minimally invasive surgical system allows for the translation of modern pediatric surgical technology to low- and middle-income nations. J Pediatr Surg. 2022;57(6):1099–103.
10. Moten A, Schafer D, Burkett EK. Global Health Engagement and the Department of Defense as a vehicle for security and sustainable global health. Mil Med. 2018;183(1-2):14–7.
11. Koehlmoos TP, Korona-Bailey J, Janvrin ML, Madsen C, Schneider E. The collaborative research and service delivery partnership between the United States healthcare system and the U.S. Military Health System during the COVID-19 pandemic. Health Res Policy Syst. 2022;20(1):81.
12. Pasquier P, Luft A, Gillard J, Boutonnet M, Vallet C, Pontier JM, et al. How do we fight COVID-19? Military medical actions in the war against the COVID-19 pandemic in France. BMJ Mil Health. 2021;167(4):269–74.
13. Ayemoba O, Adekanye U, Iroezindu M, Onoh I, Lawal I, Suleiman A, et al. The Nigerian military public health response to COVID-19: a 14-month appraisal. Health Secur. 2022;20(3):203–11.
14. Tanoli O, Ahmad H, Khan H, Khan A, Aftab Z, Khan MI, et al. Laparoscopy in low- and middle-income countries: a survey study. Cureus. 2023;15(6):e40761.
15. Djote SM, Muhie DA, Alemayehu GD. Advancing laparoscopy in resource-limited settings. BMC Surg. 2024;24(1):98.
16. Vargas G, Price RR, Sergelen O, Lkhagvabayar B, Batcholuun P, Enkhamagalan T. A successful model for laparoscopic training in Mongolia. Int Surg. 2012;97(4):363–71.
17. Asfaw ZK, Todd R, Abasi U, Marcela Bailez M, Narvaez J, Carrasquilla A, et al. Use of virtual platform for delivery of simulation-based laparoscopic training curriculum in LMICs. Surg Endosc. 2023;37(2):1528–36.
18. Henao Ó, Escallón J, Green J, Farcas M, Sierra JM, Sánchez W, Okrainec A. Fundamentos de cirugía laparoscópica en Colombia con telesimulación: una herramienta adicional para la formación integral de cirujanos [Fundamentals of laparoscopic surgery in Colombia

using telesimulation: an effective educational tool for distance learning]. Biomedica. 2013;33(1):107–14. Spanish.

19. Lim RB, Ahnfeldt E, Wisbach G, Worlton T. Why the military committee is important to SAGES? Surg Endosc. 2023;37(1):774–9.
20. Worlton TJ, Braden J, Gadbois K, Lefringhouse J, Lockrow E. The impact of robotic-assisted technology on attitudes of host nation individuals participating in Pacific partnership 2018: improving partnerships through technology. Mil Med. 2020;185(5-6):368–70.
21. Aryankalayil J, Atwood R, Johnson M, Fitch J, Ayvar A, Natuzzi E, et al. Beyond the expected: evaluating preoperative predictors of a difficult cholecystectomy aboard the USNS comfort. Ann Surg Open. 2024;5(2):e411.
22. Sohail AH, Martinez KA, Flesner SL, Martinez C, Nguyen H, Jreisat BH, et al. Operative experience of esophageal surgery among general surgery residents in the United States: an analysis of ACGME operative case logs. J Surg Educ. 2024;81(5):639–46.
23. Case Log National Report. https://apps.acgme.org/ads/Public/Reports/CaselogNationalReportDownload?specialtyId=99&academicYearId=30. Accessed 5 Jan 2025.
24. Fellowship Council – Directory of Fellowships. https://www.fellowshipcouncil.org/directory-of-fellowships/. Accessed 5 Jan 2025.
25. Wahlstedt ER, Kronstedt SM, Saffati G, Hinojosa-Gonzalez DE, Mucher ZR. Overview of robotic surgery in the U.S. military: from conception to utilization, and future applications. Mil Med. 2024;190:usae222.
26. Satava RMMD, FACS. Surgical robotics: the early chronicles: a personal historical perspective. Surg Laparosc Endosc Percuta Tech. 2002;12(1):6–16.
27. Lane T. A short history of robotic surgery. Ann R Coll Surg Engl. 2018;100(6):5–7.
28. Garcia P, Rosen J, Kapoor C, Noakes M, Elbert G, Treat M, et al. Trauma pod: a semi-automated telerobotic surgical system. Int J Med Robotics Comput Assist Surg. 2009;5:136–46.
29. Reichenbach M, Frederick T, Cubrich L, Bircher W, Bills N, Morien M, et al. Telesurgery with miniature robots to leverage surgical expertise in distributed expeditionary environments. Mil Med. 2017;182(S1):316–21.
30. Childers CP, Maggard-Gibbons M. Estimation of the acquisition and operating costs for robotic surgery. JAMA. 2018;320:835–6.
31. Lunardi N, Abou-Zamzam A, Florecki KL, Chidambaram S, Shih I, Kent AJ, et al. Robotic technology in emergency general surgery cases in the era of minimally invasive surgery. JAMA Surg. 2024;159(5):493–9.
32. Wahlstedt ER, Kronstedt SM, Saffati G, Hinojosa-Gonzalez DE, Mucher ZR. Overview of robotic surgery in the U.S. military: from conception to utilization, and future applications. Mil Med. 2024;17:usae222.
33. USSPACECOM Deputy Commander Discusses Deep Space Exploration. US Space Command. Updated Oct 25, 2022. https://www.spacecom.mil/Newsroom/News/Article-Display/Article/3198458/usspacecomdeputy-commander-discusses-deep-space-exploration/ Accessed Feb 14 2025.
34. NASA-STD-3001. NASA Space Flight Human System Standard, Volume 2, Revision D: Human Factors, Habitability, and Environmental Health. Approved: 09-15-2023.
35. Schmidt MA, Marge M, The human research program for civilian spaceflight. In: Schmidt MA, Legato MJ, editors. Building a space-faring civilization. Academic, 2025. pp. 319–333. ISBN 9780443138508.
36. Ad Hoc Committee of Members of the Space Medicine Association and the Society of NASA Flight Surgeons. Human health and performance for long-duration spaceflight. Aviat Space Environ Med. 2008;79:629–37.

Is There a Role for Minimally Invasive Surgery in the Military Setting?

26

Olivia Parry, Justin Sleeter, Donald Jenkins, Jennifer Gurney, and John Holcomb

Introduction

> Good surgery must be done as far forward as possible. If it is too good, in the sense of too elaborately equipped, it will not be far enough forward and if it is too far forward it will not be good enough. —William H Ogilvie, 1887–1971

Historically, laparoscopic surgery has had limited use in the deployed military setting. The reasons are multifactorial. These include limited resources, logistical limitations on resupply and sterilization, and the current trend in the U S Military to emphasize smaller, more mobile surgical teams pushed as far forward as possible into austere locations [1–3]. Further, the primary mission of these surgical assets is to provide damage control surgery and resuscitation to traumatically injured casualties, which rarely allows for the use of minimally invasive techniques. In an evaluation of US combat operations from 2002 to 2016 using the Department of Defense Trauma Registry, the most comprehensive military trauma registry currently in existence, 26,548 abdominal surgery procedures were identified in the deployed environment. Of these, only 18 laparoscopic procedures were documented, the majority of which were performed at mature long-standing Level 3 fixed military treatment facilities in Iraq and Afghanistan with substantially more resources than farther forward locations. Further, laparoscopic surgery was not introduced until 2006 [4]. While this registry does not capture non-trauma surgery, open procedures vastly

O. Parry (✉) · J. Sleeter · J. Gurney
Brooke Army Medical Center San Antonio, San Antonio, TX, USA
e-mail: jennifer.m.gurney.mil@health.mil

D. Jenkins
University of Texas Health Sciences Center San Antonio, San Antonio, TX, USA
e-mail: jenkinsd4@uthscsa.edu

J. Holcomb
University of Alabama at Birmingham, Birmingham, AL, USA
e-mail: jbholcomb@uabmc.edu

© The Author(s), under exclusive license to Springer Nature Switzerland AG 2026

M. Cezillo, B. M. Pereira (eds.), *Minimally Invasive Surgery Trauma*,
https://doi.org/10.1007/978-3-032-28971-1_26

outnumber laparoscopy. Other examples are limited to case reports with small patient numbers and limited data on outcomes [5–8]. Given the paucity of experience, resource demand, and potentially limited utility, should laparoscopic surgery even be considered in the deployed environment?

While the deployed historic precedent is limited, there is no arguing that minimally invasive surgery (MIS) can reduce morbidity, decrease recovery time, postoperative pain, and hospital length of stay [9]. This can result in a quicker return to duty for active military members, which is the ultimate goal of the military surgeon [10]. Further, while previous conflicts have been primarily low intensity expeditionary warfare with a focus on expedited casualty evacuation to higher levels of care in the setting of US Air superiority, this may not always be the case. Future wars with peer or near-peer adversaries is a real possibility. In these large-scale combat operations with potentially restricted air evacuation capability, the dwell time of patients may be much higher [11]. In such scenarios, there might be a larger role for minimally invasive surgery in austere locations, as has been demonstrated in the recent Russo-Ukrainian war [5].

In this chapter, we discuss the differences encountered in a deployed austere environment, logistical considerations, patient selection, and potential uses of laparoscopic surgery in trauma and emergency general surgery patients.

Levels of Care in the Deployed Environment

In the deployed environment, military doctrine describes an integrated medical support system designed to triage, treat, evacuate, and then ultimately return a Soldier, Sailor, Marine, or Airmen back to duty. This system is organized into different levels of care that patients transition through from point of injury on the battlefield to hospitals within the United States or safe havens in other countries, as historically done in World War II. These levels are organized based on distribution of medical resources and progressive capabilities. They are referred to as the Four Roles of Care [10].

Role 1

Role 1 or unit-level medical care starts at the point of injury and consists of immediate lifesaving measures. All military members are trained in basic first aid. The first care rendered is usually self-aid and buddy-aid following Tactical Combat Casualty Care (TCCC) principles, such as controlling exsanguinating hemorrhage with tourniquets [12]. Medical personnel at this level are usually limited to embedded medics, corpsman, or sometimes a physician assistant or physician, who can provide more advanced procedures and initial resuscitation. There are no surgeons present and there is limited holding capacity, so casualties are rapidly evacuated to the next level of care.

Role 2

Role 2 surgical team constructs have evolved over time and are meant to fill the large gap between on-scene and specialized definitive level care. This has been driven by a recognition that most trauma patients who die, die prior to arrival at definitive care facilities [13, 14]. They altogether provide lifesaving resuscitation and surgical care, but the different iterations have aimed at becoming more maneuverable and therefore less robust the farther forward they go into austere, resource limited environments. The structure implemented can be an opportunistic empty building the team outfits into a triage area and operating room tent or even a helicopter. The operating room staffing at minimum includes an anesthesia provider, medic, nurse, and surgeon. Diagnostic capabilities may be limited to Ultrasound or portable X-ray, holding capacity can be as little as 4 or as much as 10 casualties, with limited selected pharmacologic resources. Blood products are limited by processing and storage capacity, and are usually reliant on replenishment via medical evacuation, but can be extended with use of a walking blood blank if the mission permits. Further, given the austere operating environment sterility is very difficult. Thus, the primary objective is for patient stabilization, usually in the form of damage control surgery and resuscitation [15, 16].

Role 3 and Role 4

Role 3 s, the highest level of care on the battlefield, are military treatment facilities utilizing tents or fixed buildings on a larger forward operating base, function as an aeromedical hub, and most resemble a level 2 trauma hospital in the civilian sector. Capabilities include emergency medicine, intensive care, specialty surgeons, dental care, extended holding capacity with robust ancillary support including laboratory, radiology, and pharmacy. Definitive surgeries are performed here, and then coordination for evacuation can be arranged if the patient is unable to return to duty. Role 4 s exist outside of the theater of operations; most well-known, for example, is Landstuhl Regional Medical Center in Germany.

Resources Required for Laparoscopic Surgery

The footprint and resources for laparoscopy are large compared to open surgery and therefore must be considered when the team is expected to be mobile. Table 26.1 shows a comprehensive list of equipment and instruments needed, some of which are also used in open cases. A surgical table that articulates and changes position to optimize visualization would be the largest physical concern, followed by a laparoscopic tower complete with light source, carbon dioxide (CO_2) insufflation, and screens. Additionally, ancillary requirements must be considered with storage for larger and longer specialized instrument sets that aren't translatable to open surgery (rigid laparoscope camera, fiberoptic light cord, laparoscopic stapler, CO_2 gas tanks,

Table 26.1 Devices and instruments in laparoscopic surgery

Powered Operating Room Table
Bean Bag mattress
Tables accessories (foot board/leg supports/padding)
Sequential Compression device
Power Supply
Imaging Systems
Laparoscope
Light Source and Light Cable
Video Camera
Video Monitor
Insufflator
CO2 Tank
Backup cylinder and accessories (wrench and key)
Filter for CO2 unit or tubing
Access Instruments and Trocars
Veress needle
Balloon, straight or Hasson Trocars (5 mm, 11 mm, 12 mm, often disposable)
Suture passing instrument for trocar sites (i.e. Carter-Thomason or Karl Storz suture-passer)
Laparoscopic Retractors
Liver Retractor and external holding device
Hand Instruments
Atraumatic Graspers, 5 mm
Crocodile grasper, 5 mm
Laparoscopic Bowel Clamp, 10 mm
Laparoscopic Babcock
Laparoscopic scissors, 5 mm
Laparoscopic Clip Appliers and Staplers
Multiload disposable clip applier, 5 and 10 mm
Endo-GIA Stapler, 12 mm (Disposable) cartridges of various lengths (30, 45, 60 mm) and staple heights (2.0, 2.5, 3.5, 4.8 mm)
Endoscopic EEA Stapler (varying diameters)
Suction Instruments
Endoscopic suction/irrigation, 5 mm and 10 mm
External suction tubing
Suction canister and either portable or wall suction
Laparoscopic Suturing Instruments
Laparoscopic needle drivers
Endostitch, 10 mm (requires double pointed shuttle needle and thread)
Energy Devices
Standard monopolar and bipolar device with laparoscopic hook extender, 5 mm
Patient grounding pad
Endoscopic Ligasure device, 5 mm (straight and Maryland available)
Ultrasonic Device (i.e. Ultrasonic Shears and Harmonic Scalpel)
Accessory Equipment
Flexible Endoscope
Heating blankets
Portable Xray/C-arm

and laparoscopic graspers) and their repeated sterilization. Other important adjuncts include fluoroscopic capability either with a C-arm or flat plate, which may be needed for contrasted studies such as cholangiograms. Finally, a large and sustainable power source is required to successfully and safely run the above equipment [17].

Of these requirements, CO_2 cylinders seem to be the most limiting factor. This is due to the multiple logistical challenges of obtaining them in the field. These include their heavy weight (83 Kg when full), inability to be refilled, and difficulty in transportation due to their designation as a class 3 hazardous material [18, 19]. This classification immensely increases the required regulations that must be followed for air and ground transport [20]. Thus when considering these hurdles in the setting of limited transport space, CO_2 has not been a priority for the military in austere deployed locations. To overcome these challenges, some military surgeons have found innovative workarounds. In one deployed location, a surgical team utilized beverage grade CO_2 canisters retrofitted to laparoscopic insufflators. They were able to achieve approximately three to four surgeries per canister. Interestingly, compared to commercially available CO_2 cylinders, beverage CO_2 has higher purity standards (99.5% vs 99.9%) [21, 22].

Thus, given the robust resources required, the most feasible level of care in the current deployed environment that could support laparoscopic surgery would be at either a role 3 or 4, and historically has been vastly outnumbered by open procedures in the trauma patients at these locations [4, 7]. There have been small case series reported of laparoscopic and thoracoscopic procedures done at lower levels of care, but these consist of small numbers of patients with limited data on long-term outcomes if any at all [5, 7, 8, 18]. Further, such levels of fixed and well-staffed care are not immediately in place and only arise after prolonged theater operations.

Evolution of the Minimally Invasive Skillset

Over the past 20 years, there has been a drastic paradigm shift towards minimally invasive procedures in surgical residencies. Multiple studies have analyzed national Accreditation Council for Graduate Medical Education (ACGME) operative logs of general surgeons in training and have shown a steady decline in open surgeries and a rise in laparoscopic, endovascular, and percutaneous procedures [23–27]. One of the more recent studies comparing graduating residents from 2005 to those completing training in 2011 showed an increase in the median complex laparoscopic operations by 82% with a decrease in open thoracic and abdominal surgeries by 5% [28]. In the 2017–2018 academic year, the ACGME general surgery-defined category minimums were updated to reflect this change, with slightly over 20% of the overall case volume of 850 cases required to be laparoscopic [29]. During this time, there have also been advancements in laparoscopic equipment. This has primarily been focused on imaging systems with increased resolutions up to 4 K and recent use of 3D displays, which drastically improve the visualization [30]. Finally, the past decade has seen an increase in the use of robotic minimally invasive surgery in training programs, with one survey finding that over 73% of the respondent programs had a formal robotics curriculum, and more than half of the programs felt more time dedicated to robotic training was needed [31]. With this paradigm shift, the skillset of young surgeons is changing compared to their predecessors, which may make minimally invasive surgery more relevant and approachable in the deployed setting in the future. This trend, however, raises concerns about the preparedness of young military surgeons to deploy, as most cases will be open abdominal surgeries. This was exemplified in a 2012 survey of 246 active-duty surgeons with recent deployments, where less than half felt their residency training prepared them adequately. Specifically, citing a lack of open abdominal vascular and extremity vascular experience [32]. This lack has since been recognized, and simulation training to address this gap was first implemented in September of 2010 with the Advanced Surgical Skills for Exposure in Trauma Course (ASSET). [33] The outcomes of this case-based hands-on fresh cadaver course were recently evaluated showing that over the past decade, military surgeons who took the course had improved self-confidence and scored higher on post-test competency [34]. Thus, while the MIS skillset and equipment continue to improve, it is still important to maintain a balance that includes exposure to open cases, and simulation might be one avenue to achieve this goal.

Patient Selection

Similar to stateside standard operations, implications and application of laparoscopy for both trauma and emergency general surgery in the deployed environment hinges on correct patient selection. A trauma patient in hemorrhagic shock will not tolerate the hemodynamic changes incumbent upon insufflation, the decreased visualization and most importantly the delay in time to hemorrhage control that is inherent to laparoscopy. Further, selected patients should not have other indications necessitating immediate laparotomy such as evisceration or peritonitis [35]. Other potential contraindications in polytrauma patients include severe traumatic brain injury with increased intracranial pressure, or eye injuries such as retinal detachment and severe myopia [36]. Thus, injured trauma patients selected for laparoscopic surgery must be hemodynamically stable and have no other indications for laparotomy. Commonly accepted mechanisms for consideration of diagnostic laparoscopy in trauma include low-energy penetrating injuries, such as tangential low-velocity gunshot wounds, or stabbings [37]. In blunt trauma patients, the potential for multiple injuries has been considered a contraindication for laparoscopy as more advanced skills may be necessary. However, it has been shown to be safe by experienced surgeons [38, 39]. Unique to combat theaters, many contemporary combat casualties experience combined penetrating and blunt polytrauma mechanisms in the form of blast injuries, which must be considered. For emergency general surgery pathologies, such as appendicitis or acute cholecystitis, the same principles apply in terms of stability of the patient to tolerate peritoneal insufflation [40].

Other considerations that are unique to the deployed surgeon include complex tactical/mission-specific parameters, such as how to treat non-coalition patients (local nationals, partner nation forces, foreign citizens), diagnostic capability, supplies, holding capacity, transport times/capability, and, importantly, mission readiness of the operative team to perform their primary mission. Thus, even if an appropriate patient for laparoscopic surgery is identified, other factors may limit the ability of a deployed operative team to successfully perform it [41].

Potential Uses in Trauma

In trauma, laparoscopy can be both diagnostic and therapeutic, and when used in the correct patient population has been shown to reduce morbidity by avoiding non-therapeutic laparotomies, postoperative pain, wound infection rate, hospital length of stay, and potentially cost [42–45]. In the deployed environment, as previously mentioned, there is limited experience with laparoscopic surgery given the unique challenges in a resource-limited and austere location.

In hemodynamically stable trauma patients with low-velocity tangential ballistic wounds, fragment injuries, or stab wounds to the abdomen, diagnostic laparoscopy could be utilized to evaluate for peritoneal penetration without the morbidity of a large laparotomy or wound exploration. In patients with low force fragmentation injuries, Computed Tomography (CT) has already been shown to be safe and effective at predicting non-operative management at a combat support hospital [46]. In a resource-limited environment, where there might be no access to Computed Tomography, diagnostic laparoscopy could alleviate the need to evacuate and potentially result in a quicker return to duty for the patient. Depending on the skills of the surgeon, if specific injury patterns are diagnosed that are amenable to laparoscopic repair, such as traumatic diaphragm hernias, laparotomy could be avoided [6, 47, 48]. If limited small bowel injuries are discovered and full exploration was appropriately completed laparoscopically, the laparotomy incision can potentially be minimized for ex-vivo repair.

In blunt trauma, laparoscopy is even more controversial. A theoretical application would be in a stable blunt trauma patient with a positive Focused Assessment with Sonography in Trauma (FAST) showing only minimal free peritoneal fluid and lack of three-dimensional imaging to help differentiate hollow viscus from solid organ injury. In a resource-limited environment, however, Diagnostic Peritoneal Aspiration may be a better option [49].

Minimally invasive surgery can also be considered in thoracic trauma. In stable patients with blunt or penetrating thoracic injuries, early video-assisted thoracoscopic surgery (VATS) has been proven to reduce morbidity, length of stay, and cost for retained hemothorax [50–52]. While normally, this is not a pathology encountered or treated at lower role deployed environments given the emphasis on early evacuation, future conflicts with possibly longer dwell times and reduced transportation capacity may make this more relevant.

Ultimately, as previously emphasized, the use of laparoscopy or thoracoscopy for trauma patients in the deployed environment is mostly dependent on the resources available and the tactical/clinical context.

Emergency General Surgery

While the mission of the deployed surgeon is primarily to treat trauma casualties, urgent emergency general surgical issues often arise [41, 53]. Common etiologies include kidney stones, appendicitis, hernia, testicular torsion, acute cholecystitis, ectopic pregnancy, ovarian torsion, diverticulitis, perforated ulcers, anorectal disorders, and soft tissue infections. For most emergency general surgery cases (EGS), laparoscopy has become standard of care in the non-deployed setting in patients who are clinically stable. In an austere environment, as alluded to previously, the decision whether to perform surgery versus transporting to a higher level of care or out of theater is multifactorial. Most EGS patients will tolerate a delay of intervention with appropriate antibiotics without significantly increased morbidity or mortality and can be considered for evacuation, even though delay may not be ideal [54–61]. Resource utilization is another important consideration, as efforts should be made to avoid compromising the primary mission of taking care of trauma casualties, especially if non-operative treatments are available and safe.

For patients requiring surgery for an emergency general surgery (EGS) condition, as well as selected nonemergent patients whose treatment falls within the capabilities of the deployed facility, minimally invasive surgery (MIS) should be considered when available. Potential benefits include reduced postoperative pain and an earlier return to duty [62]. Future operational environments involving prolonged field care and delayed evacuation timelines may further increase the need for this capability.

Conclusion

Given the complex tactical, resource, and logistical restraints in a deployed location, open surgery vastly outnumbers minimally invasive techniques, and it remains critical for military surgeons to be efficacious and experienced with open procedures. However, if laparoscopic options are available and safe in the clinical context, their use can be beneficial for the patient and ultimately serve the primary goal of returning a military member to active duty sooner. In this chapter we have considered possible applications, which may have increased relevance in future wars with limited evacuation capability. Thus, laparoscopic surgery in the right setting, with the right patient, and at the right time is both feasible and potentially beneficial, albeit rare in the deployed environment.

References

1. Nessen SC, Cronk DR, Edens J, Eastridge BJ, Little TR, Windsor J, Blackbourne LH, Holcomb JB. US Army two-surgeon teams operating in remote Afghanistan--an evaluation of split-based Forward Surgical Team operations. J Trauma. 2009; https://doi.org/10.1097/TA.0B013E31819CE302.
2. Remick KN. The Surgical Resuscitation Team: surgical trauma support for U.S. Army Special Operations Forces. J Spec Oper Med. 2009;9:20–5.
3. Nessen SC, Cronk DR, Edens J, Eastridge BJ, Blackbourne LH. US Army split forward surgical team management of mass casualty events in Afghanistan: surgeon performed triage results in excellent outcomes. Am J Disaster Med. 2009; https://doi.org/10.5055/ajdm.2009.0045.
4. Stockinger ZT, Turner CA, Gurney JM. Abdominal trauma surgery during recent US combat operations from 2002 to 2016. J Trauma Acute Care Surg. 2018;85:S122–8. https://doi.org/10.1097/TA.0000000000001804.
5. Lurin I, Vorovskiy O, Makarov V, Khoroshun E, Nehoduiko V, Ryzhenko A, Chobey S, Gorobeiko M, Dinets A. Management of thoracoabdominal gunshot injuries by using minimally invasive surgery at role 2 deployed field hospitals in Ukraine. BMC Surg. 2024;24:1–8.
6. Israelit SH, Krausz MM. Laparoscopic management of a combat military injury during the Lebanon War in August 2006. J Trauma. 2009; https://doi.org/10.1097/TA.0B013E31802E7489.
7. Bradley MJ, Rodriguez CJ, Ritter EM, Bailey JA. Laparoscopy in a combat theater of operations. J Trauma Acute Care Surg. 2018;85:648–9.
8. Paul MG, Kim MD, Tylka MBL, Crabtree MTG, Drost MT, Newcomb LEW, Mc Guire CAM. Laparoscopic surgery in a mobile army surgical hospital deployed to the former Yugoslavia. Surg Laparosc Endosc. 1994;4:441–7.
9. Di Saverio S. Emergency laparoscopy: a new emerging discipline for treating abdominal emergencies attempting to minimize costs and invasiveness and maximize outcomes and patients' comfort. J Trauma Acute Care Surg. 2014;77:338–50.
10. Heaton LD. Emergency war surgery. Am J Surg. 1965; https://doi.org/10.1016/0002-9610(65)90072-3.
11. Remondelli MH, Remick KN, Shackelford SA, Gurney JM, Pamplin JC, Polk TM, Potter BK, Holt DB. Casualty care implications of large-scale combat operations. J Trauma Acute Care Surg. 2023;95:S180.
12. Tactical combat casualty care handbook, Version 5: Army, U.S.: 9781678198312: Amazon.com: Books. https://www.amazon.com/Tactical-Combat-Casualty-Handbook-Version/dp/1678198315/ref=sr_1_1?dib=eyJ2IjoiMSJ9.R65_WZ-QB9Bq4iwXltQJ0A.OJcJNGhVpwdFrN5D_iTNdaiB2uaUHLiYKVULSgPi_O4&dib_tag=se&keywords=9781678198312&linkCode=qs&qid=1732055123&s=books&sr=1-1. Accessed 18 Nov 2024.
13. Eastridge BJ, Mabry RL, Seguin P, et al. Death on the battlefield (2001-2011): implications for the future of combat casualty care. J Trauma Acute Care Surg. 2012; https://doi.org/10.1097/TA.0b013e3182755dcc.
14. Kotwal RS, Montgomery HR, Kotwal BM, Champion HR, Butler FK, Mabry RL, Cain JS, Blackbourne LH, Mechler KK, Holcomb JB. Eliminating preventable death on the battlefield. Arch Surg. 2011; https://doi.org/10.1001/archsurg.2011.213.
15. Shackelford SA, Del Junco DJ, Mazuchowski EL, Kotwal RS, Remley MA, Keenan S, Gurney JM. The golden hour of casualty care: rapid handoff to surgical team is associated with improved survival in war-injured US Service members. Ann Surg. 2024; https://doi.org/10.1097/SLA.0000000000005787.
16. Kotwal RS, Howard JT, Orman JA, Tarpey BW, Bailey JA, Champion HR, Mabry RL, Holcomb JB, Gross KR. The effect of a golden hour policy on the morbidity and mortality of combat casualties. JAMA Surg. 2016; https://doi.org/10.1001/jamasurg.2015.3104.

17. Instruments and devices used in laparoscopic surgery - UpToDate. https://www.uptodate.com/contents/instruments-and-devices-used-in-laparoscopic-surgery/print. Accessed 18 Nov 2024.
18. Stockinger ZT, Turner CA, Gurney JM. Re: Laparoscopy in a combat theater of operations. J Trauma Acute Care Surg. 2018; https://doi.org/10.1097/TA.0000000000002109.
19. Department of the Air Force Office of the Chief of Safety Washington, DC 20330. 2024.
20. Hazardous Material, Part II, Chapter 204.
21. Carbon Dioxide Grade Specifications. https://www.mathesongas.com/wp-content/uploads/2022/05/Grade-Specifications-Liquid-Carbon-Dioxide.pdf. Accessed 4 Feb 2025.
22. International Society of Beverage Technologists Carbon Dioxide Guidelines | Food Safety. https://www.food-safety.com/articles/4422-international-society-of-beverage-technologists-carbon-dioxide-guidelines. Accessed 4 Feb 2025.
23. Unawane A, Kamyab A, Patel M, Flynn JC, Mittal VK. Changing paradigms in minimally invasive surgery training. Am J Surg. 2013;205:284–8.
24. Richards MK, McAteer JP, Drake FT, Goldin AB, Khandelwal S, Gow KW. A national review of the frequency of minimally invasive surgery among general surgery residents: assessment of ACGME case logs during 2 decades of general surgery resident training. JAMA Surg. 2015;150:169–72.
25. McCoy AC, Gasevic E, Szlabick RE, Sahmoun AE, Sticca RP. Are open abdominal procedures a thing of the past? An analysis of graduating general surgery residents' case logs from 2000 to 2011. J Surg Educ. 2013;70:683–9.
26. Carson JS, Smith L, Are M, Edney J, Azarow K, Mercer DW, Thompson JS, Are C. National trends in minimally invasive and open operative experience of graduating general surgery residents: implications for surgical skills curricula development? Am J Surg. 2011;202:720–6.
27. Eckert M, Cuadrado D, Steele S, Brown T, Beekley A, Martin M. The changing face of the general surgeon: national and local trends in resident operative experience. Am J Surg. 2010;199:652–6.
28. Malangoni MA, Biester TW, Jones AT, Klingensmith ME, Lewis FR. Operative experience of surgery residents: trends and challenges. J Surg Educ. 2013;70:783–8.
29. Defined Category Minimum Numbers: General Surgery Effective for Program Graduates Beginning Academic Year 2017–2018 Review Committee for Surgery.
30. Subido EDC, Pacis DMM, Bugtai NT. Recent technological advancements in laparoscopic surgical instruments. AIP Conf Proc. 2018;10(1063/1):5023977.
31. George LC, O'Neill R, Merchant AM. Residency training in robotic general surgery: a survey of program directors. Minim Invasive Surg. 2018;2018:8464298.
32. Tyler JA, Ritchie JD, Leas ML, Edwards KD, Eastridge BE, White CE, Margaret Knudson M, Rasmussen TE, Russell Martin R, Blackbourne LH. Combat readiness for the modern military surgeon: data from a decade of combat operations. J Trauma Acute Care Surg. 2012; https://doi.org/10.1097/TA.0B013E3182625EBB.
33. Bowyer MW, Kuhls DA, Haskin D, Sallee RA, Henry SM, Garcia GD, Luchette FA. Advanced Surgical Skills for Exposure in Trauma (ASSET): the first 25 courses. J Surg Res. 2013;183:553–8.
34. Saberi RA, Parker GB, Mohsin N, Gilna GP, Cioci AC, Urrechaga EM, Buzzelli CMD, Schulman CI, Proctor KG, Garcia LRGD. Advanced surgical skills for exposure in trauma (ASSET) course improves military surgeon confidence. Am J Disaster Med. 2024;19:45–51.
35. Zantut LF, Ivatury RR, Smith RS, Kawahara NT, Porter JM, Fry WR, Poggetti R, Birolini D, Organ CH. Diagnostic and therapeutic laparoscopy for penetrating abdominal trauma: a multicenter experience. J Trauma. 1997;42:825–31.
36. Kindel T, Latchana N, Swaroop M, et al. Laparoscopy in trauma: an overview of complications and related topics. Int J Crit Illn Inj Sci. 2015;5:196.
37. Salim A, Velmahos GC. When to operate on abdominal gunshot wounds. Scand J Surg. 2002;91:62–6.
38. Koto MZ, Matsevych OY, Mosai F, Patel S, Aldous C, Balabyeki M. Laparoscopy for blunt abdominal trauma: a challenging endeavor. Scand J Surg. 2019;108:273–9.

39. Marcus Cezillo M, Robson Uwagoya M, Paola Panadés M, Samanta Bueno M, Hugo Gregoris M. Laparoscopy in the context of trauma: Too slow or too fast? | ACS. https://www.facs.org/for-medical-professionals/news-publications/news-and-articles/acs-brief/reviews/laparoscopy-in-context-of-trauma/. Accessed 15 Dec 2024.
40. Orlando R, Crowell KL. Laparoscopy in the critically ill. Surg Endosc. 1997;11:1072–4.
41. Maj Andrew Hall U. CDR Jacob Glaser U, Maj D. Marc Northern U, et al. Emergency General Surgery in Deployed Locations. 2018. https://jts.health.mil/assets/docs/cpgs/Emergency_General_Surgery_in_Deployed_Locations_01_Aug_2018_ID71.pdf. Accessed 15 Dec 2024.
42. Zafar SN, Onwugbufor MT, Hughes K, Greene WR, Cornwell EE, Fullum TM, Tran DD. Laparoscopic surgery for trauma: the realm of therapeutic management. Am J Surg. 2015;209:627–32.
43. Ki YJ, Jo YG, Park YC, Kang WS. The efficacy and safety of laparoscopy for blunt abdominal trauma: a systematic review and meta-analysis. J Clin Med. 2021; https://doi.org/10.3390/JCM10091853.
44. Li Y, Xiang Y, Wu N, Wu L, Yu Z, Zhang M, Wang M, Jiang J, Li Y. A comparison of laparoscopy and laparotomy for the management of abdominal trauma: a systematic review and meta-analysis. World J Surg. 2015;39:2862–71.
45. Hajibandeh S, Hajibandeh S, Gumber AO, Wong CS. Laparoscopy versus laparotomy for the management of penetrating abdominal trauma: a systematic review and meta-analysis. Int J Surg. 2016;34:127–36.
46. Beekley AC, Blackbourne LH, Sebesta JA, McMullin N, Mullenix PS, Holcomb JB. Selective nonoperative management of penetrating torso injury from combat fragmentation wounds. J Trauma. 2008; https://doi.org/10.1097/ta.0b013e31816093d0.
47. Ertekin C, Onaran Y, Güloglǔ R, Günay K, Taviloğlu K. The use of laparoscopy as a primary diagnostic and therapeutic method in penetrating wounds of lower thoracal region. Surg Laparosc Endosc Percutan Tech. 1998; https://doi.org/10.1097/00019509-199802000-00007.
48. Saribeyoglu K, Pekmezci S, Baca B, et al. Laparoscopy offers diagnosis and treatment in abdominal stab injuries. Surg Laparosc Endosc Percutan Tech. 2007;17:396–401.
49. Feliciano DV. Diagnostic modalities in abdominal trauma. Peritoneal lavage, ultrasonography, computed tomography scanning, and arteriography. Surg Clin North Am. 1991;71:241–56.
50. Meyer DM, Jessen ME, Wait MA, Estrera AS. Early evacuation of traumatic retained hemothoraces using thoracoscopy: a prospective, randomized trial. Ann Thorac Surg. 1997;64:1396–401.
51. Chou YP, Lin HL, Wu TC. Video-assisted thoracoscopic surgery for retained hemothorax in blunt chest trauma. Curr Opin Pulm Med. 2015;21:393.
52. Smith JW, Franklin GA, Harbrecht BG, Richardson JD. Early VATS for blunt chest trauma: a management technique underutilized by acute care surgeons. J Trauma. 2011;71:102–7.
53. Pannell D, Nathens AB, Ricard J, Savage E, Tien H. Acute nontraumatic general surgical conditions on a combat deployment. Can J Surg. 2015;58:S135–40.
54. Sippola S, Grönroos J, Tuominen R, Paajanen H, Rautio T, Nordström P, Aarnio M, Rantanen T, Hurme S, Salminen P. Economic evaluation of antibiotic therapy versus appendicectomy for the treatment of uncomplicated acute appendicitis from the APPAC randomized clinical trial. Br J Surg. 2017;104:1355–61.
55. Polo M, Duclos A, Polazzi S, Payet C, Lifante JC, Cotte E, Barth X, Glehen O, Passot G. Acute cholecystitis-optimal timing for early cholecystectomy: a French Nationwide Study. J Gastrointest Surg. 2015;19:2003–10.
56. Meier CM, Latz H, Kraemer J, Wagenpfeil S, Graeber S, Glanemann M, Simon A. Acute appendicitis in children: can surgery be postponed? Short-term results in a cohort of 225 children. Langenbeck's Arch Surg. 2017;402:977–86.
57. Wang CH, Chou HC, Liu KL, Lien WC, Wang HP, Wu YM. Long-term outcome of patients with acute cholecystitis receiving antibiotic treatment: a retrospective cohort study. World J Surg. 2014;38:347–54.
58. Yadao S, Lamture Y, Huse S. Uses of antibiotics alone in case of uncomplicated appendicitis. Cureus. 2022;14:e28488.

59. Wojciechowicz KH, Hoffkamp HJ, van Hulst RA. Conservative treatment of acute appendicitis: an overview. Int Marit Health. 2010;62:265–72.
60. Daniels L, Ünlü Ç, De Korte N, et al. Randomized clinical trial of observational versus antibiotic treatment for a first episode of CT-proven uncomplicated acute diverticulitis. Br J Surg. 2017;104:52–61.
61. Edwards CR, Dolan JP, Fang R, Standaert RE. Treatment of gallbladder disease during operations Iraqi Freedom and Enduring Freedom. Surg Endosc. 2009;23:2702–7.
62. O'reilly MJ, Mooney MJ, Modesto V, Byrne M. Laparoscopic cholecystectomy: use and preparation for operation desert shield. Surg Laparosc Endosc. 1991;1:50–1.

Actual Experience Using Minimally Invasive Surgery in Battlefield from Ukraine

27

Kostiantyn Gumeniuk, Oleksandr Usenko, Igor Lurin, Igor Kryvoruchko, and Andrii Dinets

Video-Assisted Thoracoscopy (VATS)

Terminology

Video-thoracoscopy (derived from the Latin "video", meaning "to look", and the Greek "θώραξ", meaning "thorax", referring to the chest, and "σκοπέω", meaning "scope", meaning "to look", "to observe") is a diagnostic and therapeutic method aiming to examine the pleural cavity and chest organs by using a special endoscopic video camera. In this technique, the video camera and surgical instruments are typically inserted separately through the 5–12 mm thoracoports. Also, video-thoracoscopy might be performed by using multi-port video-thoracoscopy.

In contrast to video-thoracoscopy, thoracoscopy is a method of visualising the surgical space performed not through the video camera-monitor system but with the help of an optical direct visualisation device, namely a thoracoscope. At present, this method is not employed due to the indisputable benefit of video-thoracoscopy.

K. Gumeniuk
National Military Medical Clinical Center - Head Military Clinical Hospital, Kyiv, Ukraine

O. Usenko
Shalimov National Institute of Surgery and Transplantology, Kyiv, Ukraine

I. Lurin
National Academy of Medical Sciences of Ukraine, Kyiv, Ukraine

State Institution of Science "Research and Practical Center of Preventive and Clinical Medicine", State Administrative Department, Kyiv, Ukraine

I. Kryvoruchko
Kharkiv National Medical University, Kharkiv, Ukraine

A. Dinets (✉)
National Academy of Medicla Sciences of Ukraine and Verum Expert Clinic, Kyiv, Ukraine

© The Author(s), under exclusive license to Springer Nature Switzerland AG 2026

M. Cezillo, B. M. Pereira (eds.), *Minimally Invasive Surgery Trauma*,
https://doi.org/10.1007/978-3-032-28971-1_27

Video-assisted thoracoscopic surgery (VATS) is a minimally invasive surgical technique in which access to the pleural cavity and chest organs is achieved through an incision of up to 5.0 cm in length made in one of the intercostal spaces. The video camera is inserted either through the same incision or through an additional thoracoport. A fundamental aspect of VATS is the absence of wound dilators, which are employed in other techniques to reduce the risk of injury to the intercostal vascular and nerve bundles. In instances where a wound dilator is positioned within the surgical incision, even when performing mini-accesses (incisions up to 5.0 cm), such surgical procedures are designated as video-assisted thoracotomy (mini-thoracotomy) or video-assisted thoracotomy (mini-thoracotomy).

General Principles for Video-Thoracoscopy Application for the Management of the Wounded Patients

Video-thoracoscopic surgery places more rigorous demands on the preoperative examination and the precision of the preoperative diagnosis in wounded patients. This is because, during video-thoracoscopy, the operating team has a restricted view of the surgical field within a two-dimensional confined space, limited ability to manipulate intrathoracic organs, and the inability to perform manual palpation of organs. Consequently, in the preoperative period, the surgeon must have a comprehensive understanding of the patient's condition in order to evaluate the feasibility of performing minimally invasive surgery and anticipate the surgical trajectory, considering individual anatomical characteristics.

Prior to the surgical procedure, the anaesthesiologist and the surgeon should plan specific features of anaesthetic support during the surgical operation. In the event of the discovery of concomitant pathology, it is incumbent upon the surgeon to engage in discourse with the relevant specialists in order to circumvent any potential risks that may arise during the course of surgery and in the postoperative period.

It is incumbent upon the surgeon to undertake a critical assessment of clinic's capabilities, correlating them with the potential danger to the patient and the risk of possible complications. This is particularly crucial when acquiring new techniques. It is of the utmost importance that the surgeon's ambitions are never placed above the life and health of the patient, which is an important ethical and professional aspect.

It is unethical to perform video-thoracoscopy without the requisite technical equipment to perform the full scope of the operation.

For the optimal execution of video-thoracoscopy, it is imperative to address key considerations such as the selection of anaesthesia, the patient's position on the operating table, the number and placement of trocars, the precise revision of the pleural cavity, and the intricacies of technical manoeuvres during the procedure.

Indications and Contraindications for Video-Thoracoscopy in War Settings

The timing and purpose of video-thoracoscopy for chest wounds and traumas allow for the distinction of the following indications and contraindications:

1. A video-thoracoscopy is an emergency procedure that should be performed within 1–2 h of admission to a deployed field hospital or other medical military facility. This is done to exclude or eliminate the consequences of life-threatening gunshot wounds.
2. An urgent procedure is indicated within 48 h after injury occurs. This is performed for the management of haemothorax or haemopneumothorax in cases where the drainage of the pleural cavity is ineffective.
3. A delayed procedure is undertaken to eliminate early and late pleural complications or to remove foreign bodies that do not threaten the life of the wounded.

Indications for video-thoracoscopy in the context of gunshot wounds and chest trauma.

1. Emergency video-thoracoscopy is indicated in the following circumstances:
   (a) Penetrating chest wound in the "heart zone"
   (b) Small and moderate haemothorax or haemopneumothorax
2. Urgent video-thoracoscopy is indicated in the following circumstances:
   (a) Intrapleural bleeding that persists at a rate of 300 ml or more for a minimum of 1 h
   (b) Emphysema of the soft tissues of the chest, which improves with adequate drainage within 1 day
   (c) Diaphragmatic injury with a predominant clinical picture of thoracic injury
   (d) The presence of a "rib valve" for video-assisted fixation of floating ribs
3. Postponed video-thoracoscopy is indicated for the following:
   (a) Preservation of leakage in the pleural cavity with adequate drainage for 3 days
   (b) The presence of foreign bodies in the chest wall, lung and mediastinum, which may lead to complications
   (c) Control and correction in case of dysfunction of drainage tubes
   (d) Pleural complications (coagulated haemothorax, infected haemothorax, pleural effusion, pleural empyema, etc.) that occurred within 14 days of the injury

It is important to note that all video thoracoscopies must be conducted under optimal combat and medical conditions.

The following conditions preclude the use of video-thoracoscopy in the management of gunshot wounds and chest trauma:

A. Absolute contraindications include
   1. The presence of the agonal state in the wounded
   2. Coagulopathy of various genesis that cannot be corrected
   3. Gunshot wounds with significant haemodynamic disorders
   4. Unstable haemodynamics with ineffective anti-shock therapy
   5. Acute myocardial infarction
   6. Acute cerebrovascular accident
   7. Advanced haemothorax

8. Haemomediastinum with compression of the airways and central vessels
9. Reliable signs of damage to the trachea and large bronchi
10. Reliable signs of oesophageal injury
11. Large chest defects and penetrating gunshot wounds with open pneumothorax or haemopneumothorax
12. Insufficient material and technical support for minimally invasive surgical interventions
13. Insufficient level of surgeons' training skills in video-thoracoscopic operations

B. Relative contraindications
1. Intolerance to single-lung ventilation
2. Obliteration of the pleural cavity on the side of the gunshot wound
3. Previous thoracotomy on the side of the gunshot wound
4. Thoracoabdominal injuries with a predominant pattern of damage to the abdominal cavity

Conversion During Video-Thoracoscopy

While video-thoracoscopy offers significant diagnostic and therapeutic capabilities, several conditions require conversion to open surgery at the stage of pleural cavity revision or during the main stage of surgery. The term "conversion" means a transition from video-assisted mini-thoracotomy to traditional thoracotomy, or vice versa. It is recommended that video-assisted mini-thoracotomy be employed whenever feasible, as it offers the benefits of minimal trauma, optimal visualisation, and the potential for open surgery, which is particularly advantageous in patients with injuries.

Indications for Conversion in Chest Wounds and Traumas

1. Ineffectiveness of single-lung ventilation and low-volume ventilation.
2. Emergence of unstable haemodynamics that cannot be corrected with medication.
3. Inability to perform a complete revision of the pleural cavity and its organs by video-thoracoscopy.
4. Infeasibility of the operation in the presence of haemopericardium or heart injury.
5. Detection of injuries to the main vessels.
6. Detection of a tense mediastinal haematoma.
7. Persistent haemorrhage in the event of vascular damage to the pleural cavity, where video-thoracoscopy is unable to promptly halt the bleeding.
8. Identification of gunshot wounds to the lung apex.
9. Detection of a significant gunshot wound to the lung.
10. Detection of tracheal, large bronchial or oesophageal wounds.

11. The risk of inadequate suturing of the lung wound (especially in the area of its root).
12. The surgeon's decision to perform conversion due to intraoperative findings will increase the duration of the intervention compared to open surgery.

The Positioning of the Wounded on the Operating Table

The positioning of the wounded on the operating table is contingent upon the type of gunshot wound, the functional status of the casualty and the purpose of the surgical intervention. If the casualty is placed in the supine position, a roller is positioned beneath the chest on the side of the surgical incision. This serves to partially enlarge the intercostal spaces and facilitate access to the chest organs. It is preferable to position the upper limb of the injured individual in a manner that differs from the conventional approach, which involves extending the arm over the head and resting it on an armrest. Instead, the limb should be positioned and secured below the body in a posterior abduction position at the shoulder joint, with flexion at the elbow joint and pronation at the wrist joint. This position of the limb helps to prevent injury to the brachial plexus branches due to incorrect positioning and ischaemia of the limb tissues and does not interfere with the manipulation of surgical instruments and a video camera during surgery. The advantages of supine positioning are its simplicity and speed, as well as the ability to perform the majority of surgical techniques on the anterior, upper and lower mediastinum, lung root, anterior and lateral lung, and anterior and lateral chest walls. Additionally, it provides the anaesthetist with free access to the main veins. The anaesthetist can gain free access and control of the intubation tube, manipulate it with ease, and perform sanitary fibrobronchoscopy with greater technical proficiency during surgery. Furthermore, there is less respiratory distress during single-lung ventilation and less cardiac distress. However, the most significant disadvantages of placing the patient in the supine position are the considerable limitations it imposes on the surgeon's view and ability to manipulate the posterior chest wall, the posterior surface of the lung, and the near-total absence of the possibility of accessing the posterior mediastinum.

To facilitate lateral positioning of the patient on the operating table, a roller is placed beneath the table to widen the intercostal spaces on the side of the surgery. The patient is positioned on the uninjured side, lying prone. The upper limb on the surgical side is positioned and secured on the armrest situated in front of and above the head, with the shoulder and elbow joints in a flexed position. The upper limb on the uninjured side is positioned in a straight manner on the armrest with flexion of the shoulder joint. The lower limb on the "healthy" side is flexed at the hip and knee joints, while the non-surgical side is extended. The advantages of positioning a patient on their side include the ability to comprehensively examine the majority of the chest and mediastinum structures on the surgical side, as well as the capacity to utilise surgical techniques in these areas. From a technical perspective, the position of the patient on their side is universally applicable to the operating surgeon, as it allows for the completion of a range of tasks. However, this position also has notable disadvantages. In the event of surgical intervention with separate lung ventilation, the lung on the side of the intervention is excluded from ventilation, while the lung on the uninjured side in the lateral position experiences reduced ventilation rates. This results in a notable decline in the oxygenation of tissues. In the absence of separate lung ventilation, the potential for pathological secretions (blood or pus) to enter the lung on the uninjured side via the bronchial tree during surgery represents a further risk of impaired ventilation and reduced oxygenation of human tissues. The utilisation of carbon dioxide insufflation into the pleural cavity, resulting from the displacement of mediastinal organs, has the potential to cause a significant deterioration in lung ventilation, blood oxygenation and cardiovascular activity. Furthermore, the lateral position of the patient presents certain challenges with regard to the performance of rehabilitation fibrobronchoscopy during surgery. While the lateral position of the patient on the operating table offers certain advantages, it should only be employed in cases of wounded patients with a high functional reserve of the lungs and cardiovascular system.

The abdominal position on the operating table is indicated only when wide access to the posterior mediastinum or posterior chest wall is necessary and the requisite surgical procedures cannot be performed in the supine or lateral position. Furthermore, the abdominal position presents challenges for anaesthetic practitioners in monitoring the intubation tube and performing sanitary fibrobronchoscopy during surgery. In cases where surgery is performed for an extended period (3–6 h) in the abdominal position, various positional manifestations may occur, including pressure ulcers, plexitis, and brachial plexus neuritis.

It can be concluded that there is no definitive optimal position for gunshot wounds and chest injuries on the operating table. The decision regarding the position of the wounded on the operating table is dependent on several factors, including the type of wound, the trajectory of the wound canal, the extent of damage to the internal organs of the chest, the functional reserves of the vital organs of the wounded, the intended outcome of the surgical intervention, and the technical capabilities of anaesthetic and surgical support. Consequently, this decision is made on a case-by-case basis.

Principles of Pleural Cavity Revision in Patients with Combat Trauma

The insertion of thoracoports through existing post-traumatic gunshot wounds is not a recommended procedure in the majority of cases. This is because the location of such wounds does not always meet the requirements for a comprehensive examination of the pleural cavity. Furthermore, the insertion of a thoracoport through a gunshot wound limits the ability to examine and manipulate the wound itself from the pleural cavity. Additionally, the procedure does not comply with the rules of asepsis, as all penetrating gunshot wounds are primarily contaminated. Nevertheless, if the surgical intervention allows for the introduction of a video thoracoscope or one of the "working" instruments to provide the optimal location for the main stage of the operation, then it is permissible to install a thoracoport through the wound gunshot canal. Nevertheless, such manipulations should only be performed after the gunshot wound canal has undergone thorough surgical treatment.

The most logical sequence for examining the pleural cavity is based on the principle of priority. The pericardium is initially examined, followed by the mediastinum and lung root. If the revision reveals evidence of damage to the heart or major vessels, it is recommended that the operation be continued using the traditional open method. Subsequently, the diaphragm is examined. In the event of damage being identified, a decision must be made as to whether further video-thoracoscopy, video-laparoscopy or laparotomy is required. Subsequently, the lung and chest wall are subjected to a final examination. This sequence of revision circumvents the potential for missteps that may arise when a surgeon promptly identifies a wound channel opening on the parietal pleura with a lung injury and commences suturing while failing to consider the possibility of more significant injuries.

In the event of bilateral pneumothorax, the examination of the pleural cavities is conducted in an alternating sequence. In this case, the full functioning of one lung is first established by draining the pleural cavity and eliminating pneumothorax, which is confirmed by X-ray examination. In cases of bilateral pneumothorax, the initial priority should be the elimination of pneumothorax on the right side, given that a more rapid and pronounced disruption to haemodynamic function occurs due to the superior ease with which the superior and inferior vena cava can be compressed by air compared to the aorta. It can be reasonably deduced that decompression of the right pleural cavity will result in a more rapid stabilisation of haemodynamic parameters than decompression of the left pleural cavity.

Each video-thoracoscopy must be followed by a comprehensive chest revision to guarantee the reliability of haemostasis, lung aerostasis, and the integrity of adjacent organs.

The Principles of Video-Thoracoscopic Removal of Foreign Bodies (Bullets and Fragments)

The indications for the removal of bullets and fragments using video-thoracoscopic techniques are the presence of a foreign body in the peripheral zone of the lung, in the tissues of the chest wall, or of freely located bodies in the pleural cavity. The use of video-thoracoscopic techniques for the removal of foreign bodies located in the root of the lung is contraindicated due to the high probability of damage to the large vessels of the lung and the occurrence of massive bleeding.

In the majority of cases, the video-thoracoscopic removal of bullets and fragments located in the middle zones of the lung is an ineffective procedure due to the substantial mass of lung tissue, which precludes the accurate determination of the foreign body's precise location. Furthermore, the attempted removal of such foreign bodies carries a significant risk of injury to the intrapulmonary vessels of the lung, which can be challenging to access and treat using minimally invasive techniques.

Furthermore, the creation of a substantial wound channel following the removal of a foreign body makes complete suturing a challenging endeavour. In light of the aforementioned considerations, the lung may exhibit a violation of its tightness in the early postoperative period, as well as the formation of an intrapulmonary haematoma.

The removal of bullets and fragments located in the mediastinum using video-thoracoscopy is only feasible if no damage has been sustained to the mediastinal organs and large vessels. In the event of damage to the mediastinal organs and large vessels (pericardium, heart, trachea, large bronchi, oesophagus, etc.) during the removal of mediastinal foreign bodies, it is not advisable to prolong the operation through a minimally invasive method. Instead, a transition to thoracotomy is required. In certain cases, however, it may be possible to complete the operation video-thoracoscopically through an individualised approach.

In the event of technical difficulties during the removal of a bullet or fragment by the video-thoracoscopic method, which could result in a significant prolongation of the surgical intervention or potentially lead to damage to organs and major vessels, a transition to an open intervention should be considered. It is therefore evident that conventional X-rays are insufficient for the assessment of the feasibility of a video-thoracoscopic removal of foreign bodies in the preoperative period. It is imperative to utilise spiral computed tomography of the chest organs with three-dimensional reconstruction and to conduct a comprehensive analysis of the obtained images, with a clear representation of the topographical and anatomical features of the area of the intended surgical intervention, and an assessment of the actual technical possibilities of video-thoracoscopy. As a consequence of the unavailability of SCT of the OGK at the II level of medical care in military mobile hospitals and advanced surgical groups, the removal of bullets and fragments should be postponed until the provision of care at a higher III and IV level. The removal of foreign bodies via video-thoracoscopy at the second level of care is feasible only when performing operations for urgent indications, provided that there are no technical challenges in detecting and removing a bullet or fragment.

A notable limitation of video-thoracoscopy is the inability to perform direct palpation of anatomical structures, as well as palpatory detection and clarification of the location of foreign bodies within the chest organs. Consequently, a variety of techniques and instruments have been employed in clinical settings to ascertain the precise location of foreign bodies. Such modern devices include endoscopic ultrasound devices and devices for endoscopic tactile mechanoreception. In routine clinical practice, intraoperative fluoroscopy is employed for the detection of foreign bodies during surgical procedures.

Additionally, intraoperative utilisation of a magnet is a potential avenue for exploration. This necessitates the utilisation of endosurgical instruments that are responsive to the magnetic field. Before the utilisation of such instruments, it is imperative to ascertain that upon connection of the magnet to the component of the instrument that will be situated extracorporeally, magnetic contact will be established between the tip of the instrument and the metallic object. Nevertheless, this approach can only be employed in the presence of magnetically sensitive projectiles and fragments.

In instances where the precise location of the foreign body remains uncertain following a video-thoracoscopic examination of the pleural cavity and instrumental palpation of the lung, the method of direct lung palpation may be employed. In this manner, the operating surgeon's finger is inserted through the thoracoportal passage in closest proximity to the foreign body within the chest. The lung is then fixed using an endoscopic atraumatic clamp to prevent its displacement during palpation. This method allows for the detection of foreign bodies in the peripheral zones of the lung, which would otherwise remain undetected during visual inspection through a video camera.

Following the removal of a foreign body from the lung parenchyma, it is essential to monitor the haemostasis and aerostasis of the lung. Any bleeding vessels are then treated with electrocoagulation or ligation. Any areas of the lung that are leaking are then sutured.

It should be noted that in the case of gunshot wounds to the peripheral parts of the lung, due to the high kinetic energy and the presence of residual burning gunpowder on the surface of the wounding shells, thermal cauterisation of the lung tissue occurs along the wound channel. This often results in the preservation of the tightness of the lung. Consequently, the suturing of lung tissue following the removal of a bullet or fragment is not always feasible.

Video-Thoracoscopy for Cardiac Gunshot Wounds (Haemopericardium, Tamponade)

A gunshot wound to the heart is life-threatening and associated with high mortality. Fast evacuation of these patients to the stage of qualified surgical care (Role 3 and 4 hospitals) and timely and high-quality diagnosis of such wounds are the basis for successful surgical treatment. In the presence of haemopericardium and tamponade, left-sided thoracotomy is the basic approach to resuscitation. The use of video-thoracoscopy is an additional possible approach in the presence of highly qualified specialists and equipment, with mandatory consideration of the condition of the wound.

N.B! In the presence of a haemothorax, it is necessary to drain the pleural cavity of the affected side before video-thoracoscopy, with possible subsequent autohaemotransfusion.

N.B.! The surgical team must be ready for rapid repositioning if necessary!

Position of the patient on the operating table is supine; the right side can be used if there are no contraindications.

Access: The trocar insertion points and their number do not differ from those used in typical surgical accesses for visualisation and access to the heart.

Technique: Surgical intervention in the presence of haemopericardium (Fig. 27.1) and cardiac tamponade should be performed rapidly.

1. Complete high-quality visualisation of the heart and selection of a safe area of the pericardium for dissection (Figs. 27.2 and 27.3).
2. The pericardial wall is then grasped with a thoracoscopic clamp with soft branches and dissected with scissors.

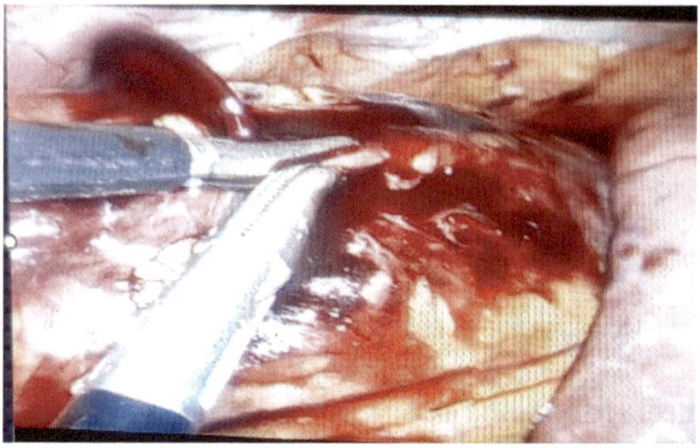

Fig. 27.1 Illustration of video-thoracoscopic pericardial dissection

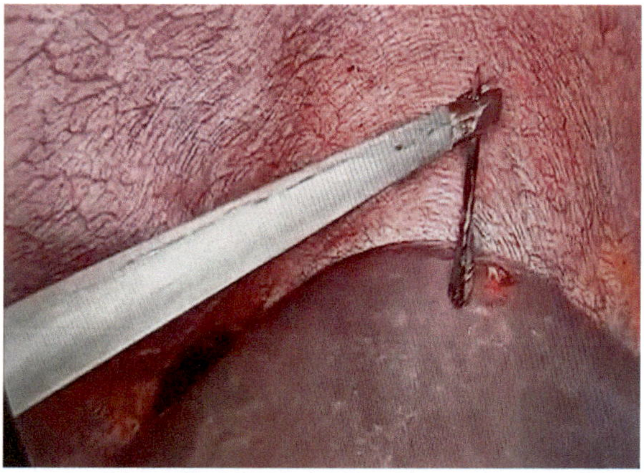

Fig. 27.2 Video-laparoscopy: removal of a foreign body "flash" in a gunshot wound to the right liver lobe

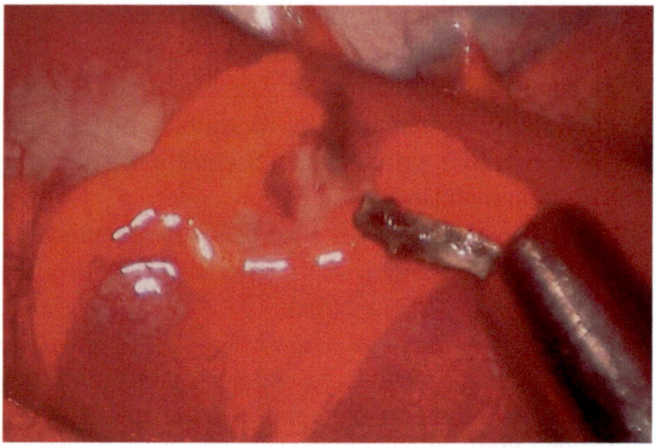

Fig. 27.3 Video-laparoscopy view of the gunshot shrapnel wound of the small intestine segment, followed by removal of metal fragments with a magnet tool

3. The release of a large amount of blood under pressure should not cause panic in the surgeon and the operating team! The most important person in this situation is the anaesthetist—his clear instructions will be the basis for further action.
4. Once the condition has been stabilised and the haemopericardium has been eliminated, the anaesthesiologist will notify the attending physician of all vital signs. At this point, it is necessary to remove blood from the pleural cavity using an electric suction device.
5. It is essential to monitor for active bleeding from the site of the heart injury!

   N.B.! In most cases, the right part of the heart is accompanied by active bleeding, which requires prompt and effective surgical intervention. The decision regarding the choice and method of suturing is at the discretion of the surgeon. Video-thoracoscopic suturing of a heart wound on a working heart is a technically challenging procedure.
6. In the absence of active bleeding, the surgical intervention is concluded with the cleansing of the pleural cavity and the establishment of drainage.

   N.B.! A patient who has sustained a gunshot wound to the heart, following the removal of haemopericardium and tamponade, requires prompt transfer to a highly specialised cardiac surgical centre. If bullets or fragments are present in the heart, subsequent fatal complications may ensue.

Video-Laparoscopy

Terminology: The term "video-laparoscopy" is derived from the Latin "video", meaning "to watch", "to see", and the Greek "lapara", meaning "groin" or "abdomen". The term "σκοπεο" (scope), which translates to "I look, I observe", is a contemporary diagnostic and therapeutic approach that employs a specialised endoscopic video camera for the examination of the abdominal cavity. In this technique, the video camera and surgical instruments are most often installed through separate incisions, with 5–12 mm special ports being used. An example of the video-laparoscopic image is shown on Fig. 27.4, an Illustration of video-laparoscopy with a gunshot wound to the abdomen.

General Principles of Video-Laparoscopy for Gunshot Wounds

Indications and Contraindications for Video-Laparoscopy

Video-laparoscopy can be performed for diagnostic or therapeutic purposes.

1. Emergency video-laparoscopy (within the first 1–2 h after the injury) is performed upon admission to a mobile hospital or other medical institution to prevent or treat the consequences of gunshot wounds that threaten life.
2. Urgent video-laparoscopy must be performed within 3 h.

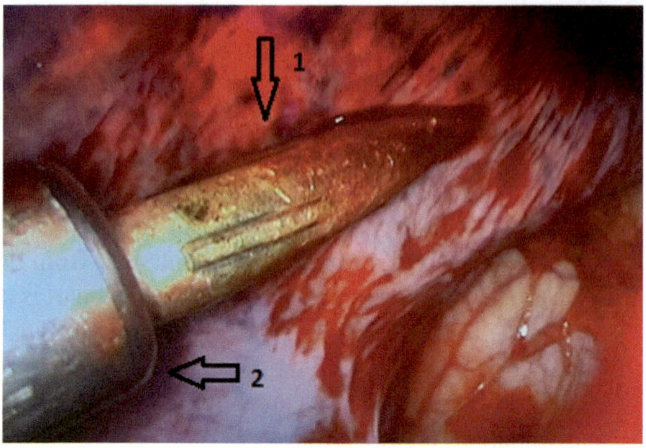

Fig. 27.4 Video-laparoscopy showing the step of bullet (marked as 1) removal by using a surgical magnet (marked as 2)

Indications for video-laparoscopy for gunshot wounds and life-threatening injuries:

1. Emergency video-laparoscopy (within the first 1–2 h after the injury) is performed upon admission to a deployed field hospital or other medical facility to prevent or treat the consequences of gunshot wounds that threaten life.
2. Urgent video-laparoscopy must be performed within 3 h.

Indications for video-laparoscopy for gunshot wounds and life-threatening injuries:

1. To verify the diagnostic service of the penetration of the nature of the damage
2. In the presence of penetration of gunshot damage to the abdominal cavity with stable haemodynamics
3. In the presence of haemoperitoneum and free fluid in the abdominal cavity

Contraindications to video-laparoscopy for gunshot wounds

1. Agonal state of the wounded
2. Severe condition—shock of the III and IV stages
3. Multiple penetrating gunshot wounds of the abdomen
4. Combined severe wounds of the skull, chest organs, torso, and limbs
5. Presence of defects of the abdominal wall
6. Presence of eventration of internal organs
7. Gunshot wounds with significant haemodynamic disorders
8. Unstable haemodynamics with the ineffectiveness of anti-shock therapy
9. Acute myocardial infarction
10. Acute cerebral circulation disorders
11. Reliable clinical signs of heart injury

A. Relative contraindications

1. Severe thoracoabdominal injuries with a predominant pattern of damage to the abdominal organs
2. History of acute myocardial infarction
3. Heart failure class 3–4 according to the NYHA classification
4. Presence of heart failure
5. History of heart and aortic surgery
6. Coagulopathy
7. Portal hypertension
8. Diffuse peritonitis
9. Previous abdominal surgery
10. Obesity stage II or higher (BMI >35 kg/m^2)
11. Severe obstructive pulmonary disease
12. Lack of experience in surgery
13. Technically complex and time-consuming

Video-Laparoscopy for Gunshot Injuries to the Diaphragm

In the context of contemporary gunshot wounds to the diaphragm, it is essential to recognise that these injuries have a direct impact on the thoracoabdominal area. To a lesser extent, there is also involvement of the abdomen and thorax. Such injuries are considered as severe, with damage to the internal organs of the chest and abdominal cavities. Timely and accurate diagnosis is fundamental to the success of surgical treatment.

N.B.! Once a thoracoabdominal wound has been identified, and there are no contraindications to video-laparoscopy. The next step is to drain the pleural cavity as appropriate for the affected side.

The patient is positioned supine on the operating table. It is also possible to utilise the lateral position.

Access: The site of trocar introduction and the number of trocars used do not differ from those employed during surgical procedures on the upper abdomen. The primary objective is to ensure the convenience of the surgical procedure and to facilitate a comprehensive video examination of the damaged portion of the diaphragm.

Technique: At revision, the presence of air is noted, which serves as a sign of gunshot damage to the diaphragm. The abdominal cavity is usually seen with haemoperitoneum, which may also be present in the event of damage to other porous organs. In the event of a gunshot wound to the diaphragm, damage is sustained to the diaphragmatic surface.

1. In the context of video-laparoscopy, it is of paramount importance to rapidly ascertain the nature of the gunshot wound to the diaphragm by the AAST classification (American Association for the Surgery of Trauma). The AAST comprises five grades, from I to V, which are used to assess the severity of

diaphragmatic injuries [1, 2]. In addition to this, the possibility of operating video-laparoscopically must be assessed. In the event of significant diaphragmatic defects accompanied by the presence of internal organ eversion into the thoracic cavity and persistent active bleeding, a conversion to open surgery is indicated. Time must not be wasted! The primary objective is to save the life of the wounded individual!

N.B.! In the event of a damaged diaphragm during video-laparoscopy, it is possible to perform a pleural cavity sanitation procedure with blood removal and the quick removal of existing foreign bodies (such as bullets and/or fragments of projectiles) using a surgical magnet tool.

2. It is recommended to suture the damaged diaphragm with non-absorbable suture material, with sufficient tissue grip in the suture maintained to prevent the suture eruption and failure of the suture site.
3. In such cases, the optimal choice is a continuous type of suture, with knotted sutures proving particularly efficacious.
4. Following the end of the surgical procedure, it is imperative to observe any signs of tightness or haemorrhage. It is also possible that other injuries may have been sustained. The subdiaphragmatic space should be drained.

Video-Laparoscopy for Gunshot Injuries to the Liver and Gallbladder

A gunshot injury to the liver and gallbladder might be diagnosed as thoracoabdominal injury, which necessitates a meticulous and comprehensive examination of both the chest and abdominal cavities.

The Procedure Protocol

The patient is positioned supine on the operating table.

Access: The number and location of trocars inserted during the procedure are consistent with those typically used for surgical interventions on the liver and gallbladder.

Technique: In the course of a video-laparoscopy for gunshot wounds to the liver and gallbladder, the presence of haemoperitoneum of varying sizes is discerned through the observation of signs indicative of intra-abdominal bleeding and the detection of bile impurities.

1. The assessment of gunshot injury to the liver should follow the AAST (American Association for the Surgery of Trauma, 1994) classification [2, 3]. The subsequent step of the procedure entails the evacuation of blood, clots, and bile through the utilisation of an electric suction apparatus. A comprehensive and accurate revision of the injured area is essential for a successful operation (Fig. 27.2).

   N.B! Should the necessity arise, the Pringle manoeuvre must be performed.

   It should be noted that according to the Advanced Trauma Life Support (ATLS) definitions set forth by the American College of Surgeons Trauma Committee, a casualty is considered an "unstable" patient if they exhibit any of the following: systolic blood pressure below 90 mmHg with a heart rate above

120 beats per minute, signs of vasoconstriction of the skin (cool, clammy, decreased capillary refill), altered level of consciousness, and/or shortness of breath [4].
2. If a comprehensive revision of the region of the gunshot injury to the liver, particularly the diaphragmatic surface, is necessary, the liver should be mobilised along its ligaments (the falciform ligament and the ligamentum teres hepatis).
3. If the liver sustains a minor tangential or marginal gunshot injury according to the AAST I–II degree classification, it is possible to perform suturing of the damaged area with intracorporeal P-shaped Vicryl sutures. It is recommended that argon plasma coagulation, other forms of coagulation and the utilisation of contemporary local haemostatic agents (Floseal, Hemopatch, Surgicel) be employed.
4. In cases where foreign bodies (such as bullets or other projectile fragments) are present within the liver parenchyma, it is essential to exercise caution when considering their removal via endovideosurgical methods. This is due to the potential for significant bleeding to occur.

   In all other cases where liver injuries have been diagnosed according to the AAST classification grades III, IV, or VI, conversion is indicated. It is recommended that, where feasible, liver packing be performed following the principles of damage control surgery (DCS).
5. Following the endovideosurgical treatment of a gunshot liver injury, the subhepatic space is drained.

   In the event of a diagnosed gunshot wound to the gallbladder, the surgical tactics include endovideosurgical cholecystectomy. The assessment of the nature of the gunshot injury to the gallbladder is conducted by the AAST (American Association for the Surgery of Trauma) classification system [2].

   In the event of technical difficulties, it is important to consider the potential options for cholecystectomy, including approaches from the neck, the bottom, or a combination of both. It is crucial to emphasise the importance of preserving the gallbladder in cases of gunshot wounds.

   N.B.! It is also essential to have a comprehensive understanding of the anatomy of the liver, gallbladder, and extrahepatic bile ducts. This knowledge enables the rapid identification of critical anatomical structures and the accurate assessment of the nature of the gunshot wound, which in turn informs the subsequent surgical approach.

Video-Laparoscopy for Gunshot Wounds to the Stomach

The patient is positioned supine on the operating table.

Access: The insertion places of trocars and their number do not differ from the typical accesses for gastric surgery.

Technique: Video-laparoscopy starts with the revision of the abdominal cavity concerning the presence of wounds to the stomach, or in case of haemoperitoneum of various sizes with signs of intra-abdominal bleeding and into the gastric lumen, the presence of content in the stomach and bile impurities.

1. A rapid assessment of the nature of the gunshot wound to the stomach is essential during video-laparoscopy by the AAST (American Association for the Surgery of Trauma) classification [2].

   N.B.! In contemporary gunshot wounds of the stomach, it is essential to consider the potential for damage to the posterior wall of the stomach. If a revision of the posterior wall of the stomach is required, this should be performed by dissection using electrocoagulation of the gastric ligament (lig. gastrocolicum).
2. In case of a minor tangential or marginal gunshot wound to the stomach (AAST I or II grades), it is possible to proceed with intracorporeal two-row Vicryl sutures. A variety of contemporary staplers may be employed for marginal stapling resection of the affected regions of the stomach. It is important to note that the appropriate cassettes should be utilised for gastric surgery.
3. Intraoperative fibro-gastroscopy is indicated to check for foreign bodies (bullets, projectile fragments, etc.) within the stomach followed by their removal in case of identification. This procedure is also undertaken to prevent gastric bleeding.
4. Conversion is indicated for all other cases with a significant gunshot wound to the stomach and according to the AAST classification (III, IV, VI grades). If feasible, gastric resection should be considered by the principles of damage control surgery (DCS). In the presence of peritonitis, surgery with anastomosis is contraindicated.
5. Following laparoscopic gastric surgery, a leak test should be conducted by introducing air into the gastric tube.
6. Following laparoscopic gastric surgery, the abdominal cavity is drained and a nasogastric tube is placed.

   N.B.! An understanding of the anatomy is beneficial in rapidly identifying crucial structures within the stomach, evaluating the characteristics of the gunshot wound, and determining the most appropriate subsequent surgical approach.

Video-Laparoscopy in the Context of Gunshot Wounds to the Small Intestine

In contemporary gunshot wounds of the small intestine, it is important to note that isolated injuries to a single segment of the intestine are uncommon. In most cases, multiple injuries to different segments at varying levels are caused by a single projectile. To achieve complete visualisation and to avoid all areas of potential gunshot injury, it is essential to perform an audit from the duodenojejunal junction to the ileocecal angle (Fig. 27.3).

The patient is positioned supine on the operation table.

Access: The locations of trocar insertion and the number of trocars should not differ from those typically employed for surgical procedures on abdominal hollow organs. Additional trocars may be inserted if necessary.

Technique: In the context of video-laparoscopy in cases of gunshot wounds to the small intestine, the presence of varying degrees of haemoperitoneum is usually expected, accompanied by the presence of bile and small intestinal contents.

1. A rapid assessment of the nature of the gunshot wound to the small intestine according to the AAST classification is essential during video-laparoscopy [2]. This should include the removal of blood, clots, bile, and small intestinal contents using an electric suction device. A comprehensive and accurate examination of the small intestine is essential for a successful surgical outcome.

   N.B.! To conduct a qualitative revision of all segments of the small intestine, it is essential to utilise special atraumatic laparoscopic instruments. Additionally, it is necessary to move the strand of the large forceps into the epigastrium, extending to the liver. Furthermore, changing the position of the operating table from the lateral position to the Trendelenburg position will facilitate the visualisation of all segments of the small intestine.
2. In the presence of a minor, tangential, marginal gunshot wound of the small intestine according to the AAST classification of grade I or II, it is possible to suture the area of the gunshot wound with intracorporeal nodal Vicryl sutures.

   Subserous haematomas and non-penetrating wounds should be subject to a minimum of treatment and closed with separate nodal sutures. Furthermore, intramural haemorrhage into the small bowel wall should be considered as a sign of perforation. In case of a gunshot wound measuring up to half the diameter of the intestine lumen, resection with a three-quarter anastomosis is recommended. Resection of the small intestine may be indicated for cases with multiple perforations in the following conditions: short area of the intestine loop, complete obstruction of the intestine, wall rupture, large size and irregular configuration of the gunshot defect, longitudinal tears of the intestine, a wound or large haematoma in the mesenteric margin of the intestine, as well as detachments from the mesentery. Additionally, resection may be necessary in cases of transverse mesenteric tear with ischaemia or necrosis of the intestinal wall. In case of a gunshot wound to the mesentery of the small intestine, it is of the utmost importance to ascertain the viability of the affected intestinal segment and, if necessary, to perform an obstructive resection. The damaged intestine segment may be resected with application of the surgical stapler. It is crucial to utilise the appropriate cassettes for small bowel surgery, as this is a vital aspect of the procedure.
3. The decision to perform a video-laparoscopic obstructive resection of the damaged segment of the small intestine by damage control surgery (DCS) tactics must be justified. In the event of diagnosed significant gunshot injuries to the small intestine (AAST III, IV, V grades), it is not feasible to perform a comprehensive qualitative revision of all its segments. In such cases, conversion is the recommended course of action.

   In the absence of contraindications, the intestine resection may be performed with anastomosis using a linear stapler apparatus of the "side-to-side" type. An alternative approach is a mini-laparotomy with extracorporeal anastomosis, which may be performed by using a stapler or manually. In the context of these surgical procedures, a case-by-case approach is essential, taking into account the condition of the patient, the duration of the surgical intervention, the existing caseload of patients requiring surgery in combat settings, and the surgeon's skills. In the event of peritonitis, the performance of surgery with anastomosis is contraindicated.

4. The application of special surgical magnets may facilitate the removal of foreign bodies (such as bullets or projectile fragments) from the intestinal lumen or mesentery. It is important to note that haemorrhage may occur following their removal.
5. The surgery must be finished with the installation of the drainage tubes to the abdominal cavity, and a nasogastric tube is inserted for decompression purposes.

   N.B.! Awareness of the anatomical structures involved is beneficial in rapidly identifying the essential anatomical features of the small intestine, evaluating the characteristics of the gunshot wound, and selecting the optimal surgical approach. In these surgical interventions, the surgeon's skills are of paramount importance.

Video-Laparoscopy for Gunshot Wounds to the Colon

In patients with gunshot wounds to the colon, it is important to note that mesoperitoneal injuries present with varying clinical signs, and diagnosis might be challenging to diagnose such an injury in the first place. This increases the likelihood of undiagnosed wounds to the colon, which might subsequently lead to complications and increase mortality. Gunshot wounds to the abdomen with injury to the colon and the subsequent development of faecal peritonitis represent a significant and potentially fatal complication.

The patient is positioned supine on the operation table.

Access to the surgical site is achieved by the following approach: the insertion sites for the trocars and the number of trocars used do not differ from those typically employed in colon surgery.

The technique employed for patients with gunshot injury to the colon is described below.

1. It is imperative to rapidly ascertain the nature of the gunshot wound of the colon by the AAST classification [2], which necessitates the removal of blood and colon contents through the utilisation of an electric suction device. In the event of faecal contamination of the abdominal cavity, the area must be thoroughly cleaned with antiseptic solutions in a sterile environment. A comprehensive and meticulous revision and mobilisation of the colon, particularly the mesoperitoneal sections, is pivotal to the success of the surgical procedure.

   N.B.! To achieve a high-quality revision of all parts of the colon, it is essential to utilise special atraumatic laparoscopic instruments, relocate the large cecum to the epigastrium in proximity to the liver, reposition the loops of the small intestine, and alter the orientation of the operating table from the lateral and the Trendelenburg positions.

   N.B.! It should be noted that further visualisation of the gunshot wounds of the colon be required, intraoperative fibro-colonoscopy represents a valuable diagnostic option.

2. In the presence of a minor, tangential, marginal gunshot wound to the colon, classified as AAST grade I or II, it is possible to suture the area with intracorporeal two-row nodal Vicryl sutures. The wound must be less than 1.0 cm in diameter. The articulating suturing and cutting device Echelon Flex EC 60 and its analogues may be employed to perform marginal stapling resection of the gunshot wound. We have previously conducted such surgical procedures and have achieved favourable clinical outcomes.

   The indications for obstructive resection of the colon include the following injuries, according to the AAST classification: grades III, IV, and V multiple gunshot defects in a limited area of the intestine, as well as complete interruption of the intestine. In addition, the following conditions require surgical intervention: a large size and irregular configuration of the gunshot defect, longitudinal tears of the intestine, a wound or large haematoma in the mesenteric margin of the intestine, as well as detachments from the mesentery. Furthermore, transverse tear of the mesentery with ischaemia or necrosis of the intestinal wall necessitates surgical intervention. In such cases, the principles of DCS must be adhered to. In the event of a modern gunshot wound to the colon with faecal contamination, it is contraindicated to perform a primary anastomosis.
3. Video-laparoscopy allows for the performance of a range of colostomies for colon wounds caused by gunshot injuries, including Hartmann-type operations, which involve creating a stoma at the site of the gunshot wound. It is important to note that the mobilisation of the colon must be performed correctly during such operations to avoid any tension or deterioration of the blood supply.
4. Following the completion of video-laparoscopic surgery on the colon, the abdominal cavity, pelvis and nasogastric tube are duly drained, and the nasogastric tube is placed.
5. An application of surgical magnet tools should be considered in the case-based approach to remove projectiles, bullets, or shells with the ferromagnetic properties (Fig. 27.4).

   N.B.! A comprehensive understanding of the anatomy is essential for rapidly identifying the crucial structures within the colon, and its associated vasculature, and accurately assessing the severity of the gunshot wound and the extent of contamination. This information is crucial for determining the appropriate surgical approach and tactics. In these surgical procedures, the surgeon's experience and professional skills are of paramount importance. Given the time-consuming nature of surgical interventions, it is essential to consider the condition of the wounded, the flow of other wounded, and the combat and tactical situation. The tactics of DCS are of particular significance for such wounded individuals.

Video-Laparoscopy in Case of Gunshot Wounds of the Spleen

In the case of existing entrance or exit gunshot wounds, primary surgical treatment is required. During endovideosurgery, it is necessary to perform tamponade on these wounds with a napkin and antiseptics, as well as temporary skin sealing (using a skin clamp or suture) to facilitate a full-fledged carboxyperitoneum. Following

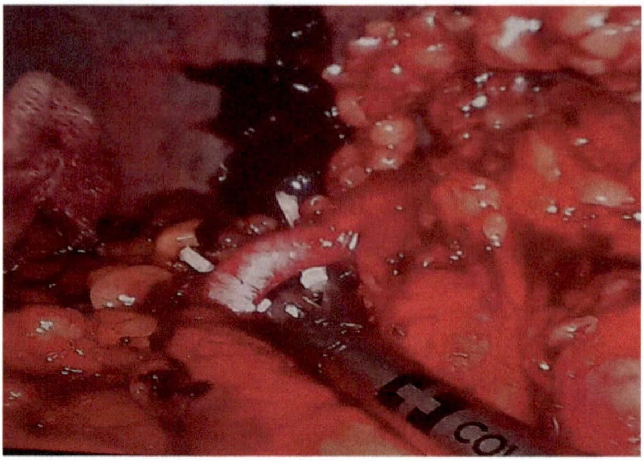

Fig. 27.5 Photograph of video-laparoscopy view showing mobilisation of the splenic artery in the patient with a gunshot wound to the spleen

video-laparoscopy, these gunshot wounds should be evaluated and the decision should be made whether or not to close the gunshot entry wounds by suturing.

It worth mentioning, that in cases of gunshot wounds to the spleen, splenectomy is the preferred surgical option. This is due to the high risk of rebleeding during video-laparoscopic organ-preserving surgery, considering the high-damage ballistics properties of modern wounding projectiles. An illustration of laparoscopic removal of the spleen is showed in Fig. 27.5.

The patient may be positioned in one of two ways: (1) lying on their back, or (2) lying on their right side (right lateral position).

Access: The number and placement of trocars remain consistent with a typical splenectomy for various injuries.

Technique: In the event of a gunshot injury to the spleen, the presence of varying degrees of haemoperitoneum with indications of intra-abdominal bleeding is identified during video-laparoscopy.

1. During video-laparoscopy, it is essential to rapidly ascertain the nature of the gunshot spleen injury by the AAST classification [2], with the removal of blood and clots via an electric suction device. A comprehensive and meticulous revision of the spleen is paramount to the success of the procedure.
2. In the presence of minor tangential or marginal gunshot damage to different splenic poles, organ-preserving surgery is a viable option according to the AAST grade I classification. It is recommended that argon plasma coagulation, coagulation and the use of modern local haemostatic agents (Floseal, Hemopatch, Surgicel) be employed. In all other cases, splenectomy is the recommended course of action.
3. To mitigate the bleeding from the damaged splenic parenchyma, it is recommended to tamponade the area with a napkin, which will reduce blood leakage and enhance visualisation.

   N.B.! An understanding of the relevant anatomy is beneficial in facilitating rapid identification of crucial structures, such as the splenic artery and its branches, as well as the splenic vein. It is essential to recall the necessity of dissecting the splenic ligaments and mobilising them. This entails the initial dissection of the medial ligament, which should commence immediately from the splenic gate.

4. The mobilisation of the splenic gate should be performed expeditiously and meticulously, with the arteries and veins clipped utilising splenic traction and constant electrocautery. Following the completion of the splenectomy, it is imperative to conduct meticulous monitoring of the haemostatic process.
5. The excised spleen is placed in a reservoir bag. It is possible to destroy the spleen in the reservoir, which will facilitate the removal of its remains from the abdominal cavity. Alternatively, the entire macrophage can be removed through a separate incision in a specific location.
6. In the event of the presence of foreign bodies (such as bullets or fragments), the latter should be extracted using dedicated magnetic instruments if they are situated near the damaged spleen.
7. The bed of the removed spleen is drained through a separate trocar puncture, or one of the access points for laparoscopic instruments in the left hypochondrium may be utilised.

   N.B! The removal of foreign bodies is not a priority in the context of the treatment of wounded individuals. It is necessary to take into account the condition of the wounded person, the time required for their search and removal, which should not be lengthy, and their size and location.

   N.B! The efficacy of a video-laparoscopic splenectomy for gunshot wounds is contingent upon the expertise of the surgeon, the proficiency of the operating team, and the presence of clear indications for this surgical intervention.

Video-Laparoscopy for Management of Gunshot Wounds to the Kidney

Before performing video-laparoscopy, it is essential to diagnose the presence of the contralateral kidney and confirm its integrity using supplementary instrumental techniques, such as ultrasonography.

If an entrance or exit gunshot wound is present, primary surgical treatment must be conducted at the time of endovideosurgical intervention. This may entail the packing of the wound area with surgical pads followed by washing the cavity with antiseptic solutions, as well as the temporary sealing of the skin (using a skin clamp or suture). Following the performance of video-laparoscopy, it is imperative to conduct an evaluation of the entrance and exit (if applicable) gunshot wounds and to decide whether or not to suture the gunshot holes.

Position of the wounded on the operating table.

The wounded are positioned on the operating table in one of two ways: (1) supine or (2) lateral (right or left).

Access: The trocars and their number are the same as in a typical nephrectomy for various diseases.

Technique: It should be noted that in the case of a gunshot wound to the kidney, a retroperitoneal haematoma of varying sizes is usually expected. The presence of the haematoma is the indicator of the damage to the kidney and a sign of retroperitoneal bleeding.

1. In the event of a wide retroperitoneal haematoma, it is necessary to open it to conduct a comprehensive revision of the gunshot wound area of the kidney.
2. It is of the utmost importance to remove any blood clots and identify the source of bleeding using an electric suction device.
3. To reduce the signs of bleeding from the renal parenchyma, it is possible to tamponade this area with a napkin.
4. The extent of the gunshot wound should be evaluated according to the AAST classification system [2].
5. It is recommended that organ-preserving surgery be performed whenever feasible. This procedure involves the use of electrocautery to seal the injury and suturing of the gunshot wound to the kidney in cases where the injury is classified as AAST I, II, or III grades.
6. In the event of the presence of foreign bodies (bullets, fragments), it is imperative that these are removed with the assistance of specialised magnetic tools from the kidney parenchyma, perinephric tissue, or other pertinent anatomical regions.

   It should be noted that the removal of foreign bodies is not a priority. Instead, the condition of the wounded, the time required for their search and removal (which should be limited), and their size and location must be taken into account.
7. In the event of a substantial gunshot injury to the kidney (AAST IV or V grades), the patient should undergo a nephrectomy.

   N.B.! Knowledge of anatomy is beneficial in rapidly identifying crucial anatomical structures, such as the renal artery, vena cava (which may be present in multiple locations), and ureter. It is important to be aware of the anatomy and location of the inferior vena cava, aorta, duodenum, and spleen, as these structures may be of significance in the context of the injury.
8. The procedure should be carried out as rapidly as possible, with the injured kidney being mobilised medio-laterally. It is then necessary to visualise the relevant anatomical structures, namely the renal artery, renal vein, and ureter, and to perform the appropriate clips: artery → vein → ureter → nephrectomy.
9. It is imperative to maintain control of the haemostatic process.
10. The excised kidney is placed in a bag, which serves as a reservoir. A further incision is made in a specific location to facilitate the removal of the macro drug. The bed of the excised kidney is drained through a separate trocar puncture.

    N.B.! The success of video-laparoscopic nephrectomy in gunshot wounds is contingent upon the professionalism of the surgeon, the operating team, and the presence of clear indications for this surgical intervention.

Suggested references of the combat trauma from the Russo-Ukrainian war are listed below [5–10].

References

1. Moore EE, Malangoni MA, Cogbill TH, Shackford SR, Champion HR, Jurkovich GJ, McAninch JW, Trafton PG. Organ Injury scaling IV: thoracic vascular, lung, cardiac, and diaphragm. J Trauma Inj Infect Crit Care. 1994;36(3):299–300.
2. Injury Scoring Scale. A resource for Trauma Care Professionals. https://www.aast.org/resources-detail/injury-scoring-scale.
3. Coccolini F, Catena F, Moore EE, Ivatury R, Biffl W, Peitzman A, et al. WSES classification and guidelines for liver trauma. World J Emerg Surg. 2016;11:50. https://doi.org/10.1186/s13017-016-0105-2.
4. Xu J, Murphy SL, Kochanek KD, Arias E. Mortality in the United States, 2021. NCHS Data Brief. 2022;456:1–8.
5. Lurin I, Khoroshun E, Makarov V, Nehoduiko V, Cherniavskyi Y, Gorobeiko M, Marchenko O, Dinets A. A rare case of endoscopic removal of the metal fragment from the segmental bronchus after gunshot injury to the chest in combat patient injured in the war in Ukraine. Int J Surg Case Rep. 2024;123:110288. https://doi.org/10.1016/j.ijscr.2024.110288. Epub 2024 Sep 14. PMID: 39277908; PMCID: PMC11417572.
6. Lurin I, Khoroshun E, Makarov V, Negoduiko V, Shypilov S, Bunin Y, Gorobeiko M, Dinets A. Management of gunshot injury to the abdominal aorta and inferior vena cava: a case report of a combat patient wounded in the Russo-Ukrainian war. Int J Emerg Med. 2024;17(1):113. https://doi.org/10.1186/s12245-024-00690-6. PMID: 39237874; PMCID: PMC11375833.
7. Lurin I, Vorovskiy O, Makarov V, Khoroshun E, Nehoduiko V, Ryzhenko A, Chobey S, Gorobeiko M, Dinets A. Management of thoracoabdominal gunshot injuries by using minimally invasive surgery at role 2 deployed field hospitals in Ukraine. BMC Surg. 2024;24(1):183. https://doi.org/10.1186/s12893-024-02475-3. PMID: 38877409; PMCID: PMC11177506.
8. Lurin I, Khoroshun E, Negoduiko V, Makarov V, Shypilov S, Boroday V, Gorobeiko M, Dinets A. Retrieval of ferromagnetic fragments from the lung using video-assisted thoracoscopic surgery and magnetic tool: a case report of combat patient injured in the war in Ukraine. Int J Emerg Med. 2023;16(1):51. https://doi.org/10.1186/s12245-023-00527-8. PMID: 37620806; PMCID: PMC10464422.
9. Gumeniuk K, Lurin I, Savytskyi O, Nehoduiko V, Makarov V, Smolianyk K. Surgical tactics in fire kidney injury and the first experience in performing laparoscopic nephrectomy at the II level of medical support (role II) in combat conditions: case report. Int J Surg Case Rep. 2023;106:108046. https://doi.org/10.1016/j.ijscr.2023.108046. Epub 2023 Apr 15. PMID: 37068453; PMCID: PMC10130198.
10. Kazmirchuk A, Yarmoliuk Y, Lurin I, Gybalo R, Burianov O, Derkach S, Karpenko K. Ukraine's experience with management of combat casualties using NATO's four-tier "changing as needed" healthcare system. World J Surg. 2022;46(12):2858–62. https://doi.org/10.1007/s00268-022-06718-3. Epub 2022 Sep 7.

Pediatric Patient

28

Robson Uwagoya, Diana Delgado Lindeman, Rodrigo Chaves Ribeiro, and Simone de Campos Vieira

Introduction

Children are Not Just Small Adults!

Management for pediatric trauma patients should follow the same systematic approach used for adults, including steps such as initial assessment and resuscitation. Caring for children with multiple trauma can be challenging for teams not accustomed to managing trauma in pediatric age groups. It is of the essence that pediatric advanced support materials are available everywhere to ensure best quality treatment from the resuscitation phase [1].

Pediatric patients face more significant challenges in interaction and communication, especially in environments with unfamiliar people. Also, they tend to display behaviors withdrawn during the emotional instability associated with shock. These factors contribute to difficulties in achieving effective communication of health status. Healthcare providers should be able to adapt their communication while treating pediatric trauma patients [1, 2, 15].

What distinguishes pediatric trauma are the significant anatomical, physiological, and metabolic differences compared to adults. These distinctions necessitate a tailored approach, even though the fundamental principles of trauma care remain

R. Uwagoya
Department of Pediatric Surgery, Grupo de Pesquisa e Extensão em Cirurgia (GPEC), Antonio Giglio Municipal Hospital, Osasco, SP, Brazil

D. D. Lindeman (✉)
Department of Pediatric Surgery, Antonio Giglio Municipal Hospital, Osasco, SP, Brazil

R. C. Ribeiro
Department of Pediatric Surgery, Children's Cancer Hospital, Barretos Cancer Hospital, Barretos School of Health Sciences Dr. Paulo Prata, São Paulo, SP, Brazil

S. de Campos Vieira
Department of Pediatric Surgery, Federal University of São Paulo, São Paulo, SP, Brazil

© The Author(s), under exclusive license to Springer Nature Switzerland AG 2026

M. Cezillo, B. M. Pereira (eds.), *Minimally Invasive Surgery Trauma*,
https://doi.org/10.1007/978-3-032-28971-1_28

consistent. Pediatric patients exhibit unique injury patterns, and their physiological responses to trauma differ markedly. For instance, the smaller body size and developing musculoskeletal system in children influence how injuries manifest, while their elevated metabolic rate accelerates the progression of shock or hypoxia [2, 15].

In order to provide effective pediatric trauma care, it is critical to have an understanding of these variations in anatomical, physiological, and metabolic disorders. Besides, recognizing the specific clinical presentations and pathophysiology of common pediatric trauma conditions is equally critical. Conditions such as head injuries, abdominal trauma, and fractures have distinct presentations in children, often requiring different therapeutic approaches than those used in adults. Familiarity with these nuances is essential to avoid mismanagement and improve patient outcomes [3].

Ultimately, although foundational skills for treating trauma in adults and children overlap, a more profound understanding of pediatric-specific factors is essential to ensure optimal care. Pediatric trauma centers are specifically equipped to address these unique challenges, and targeted training can significantly enhance the confidence and competence of healthcare providers managing pediatric trauma cases. Those principles should be disseminated to environments and people that care for traumatized pediatric patients everywhere [1, 3].

In addition to the considerations above, hypothermia poses a specific concern in pediatric patients. Although hypothermia is a recognized issue in adult trauma care, it is far more pronounced in pediatric patients due to their larger surface-area-to-volume ratio [2, 3, 15].

Depending on the age of the child, numerous frames of biopsychosocial significance can be your wait. These milestones can be adversely affected by the physical and psychological after-effects of trauma. In addition, trauma often affects the entire family unit, resulting in parental divorce, losing jobs and psychological distress for siblings [3].

Children have different trauma mechanisms than adults, and we cannot forget that this also changes, according to the child's age, as shown in Table 28.1.

Table 28.1 Common mechanisms of pediatric trauma by age group

Age group	Common mechanisms of trauma
Infants (<1 year)	Falls from heights (e.g., changing tables, cribs), non-accidental trauma (child abuse), suffocation
Toddlers (1–4 years)	Falls (stairs, playground equipment), burns (scald injuries), drowning, motor vehicle accidents (as pedestrians), poisoning, accidents with animals
School-aged (5–9 years)	Pedestrian injuries (hit by vehicle), bicycle accidents, falls, sports injuries
Adolescents (10–18 years)	Motor vehicle collisions (drivers/passengers), sports-related trauma, violence (e.g., assaults, gunshot wounds)

Pediatric Trauma by Topography

Trauma in children should always be considered as multisystemic due to the proximity of organs, and healthcare givers should rule out those possible injuries accordingly [1].

Blunt abdominal trauma is often treated nonoperatively, more frequently when compared to adult trauma. The guiding parameter is hemodynamic stability [4].

Pediatric surgery manages its patients in a conservative manner until the need for surgical intervention is proven. That is, the goal is to avoid as many complications and unnecessary procedures as possible in order to reduce childhood morbidity and mortality, as well as complications that can lead to future difficulties in the child's life [4].

Liver and Spleen Trauma

The liver and spleen are the most affected organs in pediatric trauma. As described in Table 28.2, most pediatric abdominal trauma is blunt, leading to injuries in these two organs. Typically, liver and spleen injuries result from automobile accidents, falls from heights, and sports activities [4].

There is already evidence suggesting that liver and spleen trauma can be approached conservatively in children, provided the child does not show signs of hemodynamic instability, that there are no other concomitant injuries indicating surgery (hollow viscus, for instance), and that the hospital has permanent capacity to provide monitoring, imaging, exams, operating rooms, and surgeons [4, 5].

To make that occur of form safe and effective, the child must remain in an intensive care unit (ICU), with constant monitoring and hemodynamic support. There exists evidence that shows success rates of up to 95% for conservative treatment of liver and spleen trauma in pediatric patients [5].

The main factors of failure of conservative treatment are described in Table 28.3.

Table 28.2 Organs most affected in trauma, by age group

Age group	Most commonly affected organs
Infants (0–1 year)	Cranial injuries and bone fractures due to skeletal fragility and falls
Preschoolers (1–5 years)	Abdominal injuries, particularly liver and spleen, often resulting from falls and household accidents
School-aged (6–12 years)	Splenic and hepatic injuries, frequently associated with sports activities and bicycle accidents
Adolescents (13–18 years)	Complex abdominal injuries, including renal and pancreatic trauma, typically caused by motor vehicle accidents and high-energy trauma

Table 28.3 Main reasons for conservative treatment failure

Organ	Reasons for conservative treatment failure
Liver	Uncontrolled hemorrhage, hepatic abscess formation, hepatic necrosis
Spleen	Continuous bleeding, pseudoaneurysm development, delayed splenic rupture
Pancreas	Pancreatic fistulas, pseudocyst formation, retroperitoneal infection and associated injuries
Kidneys	Persistent hemodynamic instability, hematoma expansion, signs of renal ischemia
Hollow viscera	Undiagnosed intestinal perforation, peritonitis, sepsis

Kidney

High-grade renal injuries are also frequently treated conservatively in children. Studies indicate that, unlike adults, children have a greater ability to spontaneously heal the kidney after trauma [6, 7].

Patients with grade IV and V renal injuries were analyzed and treated conservatively, achieving success rates between 40% and 84% [4, 7].

Pancreas

Pancreatic injuries are rarer but can occur in up to 10% of cases in children, due to the height of bicycle handlebars. The impact of the handlebars on the upper abdomen can cause pancreatic trauma, which is the most common mechanism, followed by trauma from automobile accidents [4, 8].

Conservative treatment of pancreatic injury also occurs, following the principle of patient hemodynamic stability. The child must also remain properly monitored and provided with intensive support [8, 9].

The most common reason for failure in the conservative treatment of pancreatic injuries is the formation of pseudocysts. Surgery should be indicated when a pancreatic fracture with compromise of the principal pancreatic duct is identified. In such cases, pancreatectomy with preservation of the spleen, if possible, is indicated [9].

Hollow Viscera

As discussed previously, penetrating trauma is rarer in pediatric patients, so trauma to the hollow viscera typically occurs due to rapid deceleration, which can cause avulsions and injuries. However, they can also result from high-energy impacts directly to the abdomen or from fewer penetrating traumas [4, 10].

Conservative treatment is limited in these cases, as most hollow viscera injuries require surgical intervention due to the risk of peritonitis and sepsis. However, in selected cases of intramural hematomas without perforation, intensive and close care with all available resources can be successfully performed [10].

As observed, pediatric trauma presents not only physical injuries but also the unique challenges posed by each child's behavior and emotional response. Children may exhibit a range of symptoms, with some being more cooperative and others more resistant or fearful. This requires healthcare professionals to be sensitive to both the child's physical and emotional needs [10].

Recognizing the injuries is essential, but equally important is understanding how to manage the child's fears and stress. A thoughtful approach helps prevent psychological trauma and long-term emotional effects. Additionally, addressing the child's needs can reduce the psychological and financial strain on the family, fostering a more supportive environment for both the child and their parents [10].

Minimally Invasive Surgery (MIS) in Pediatric Trauma

The videolaparoscopic technique has consistently demonstrated its superiority in the management of polytrauma patients. It is well-established in the medical community that minimally invasive methods lead to better postoperative outcomes, significantly reducing recovery time, pain levels, and the overall use of healthcare resources in the post-surgical period. This approach minimizes tissue trauma and enhances the body's ability to heal more quickly, leading to shorter hospital stays and fewer complications [11].

In pediatric trauma patients, where performing a thorough physical examination is often more difficult due to the child's age and cooperation, videolaparoscopy plays a crucial role as a diagnostic tool. It offers a less invasive alternative to traditional diagnostic methods, helping to identify internal injuries while avoiding the need for larger, more invasive procedures like laparotomy. This is particularly important, as laparotomies in pediatric patients are associated with a significantly higher risk of morbidity, mortality, and postoperative complications [11].

Although there is still a limited amount of data specifically supporting the superiority of videolaparoscopy in pediatric trauma cases, emerging research is increasingly showing positive outcomes. Studies suggest that the use of laparoscopy in this population not only helps reduce mortality rates but also lowers the number of unnecessary exploratory laparotomies, commonly referred to as "negative laparotomies" or "unnecessary laparotomies." As more data becomes available, it is likely that videolaparoscopy will continue to gain recognition as an effective and safer option in the management of pediatric trauma patients [11, 12].

Indications for Laparoscopy in Pediatric Trauma

Laparoscopy in pediatric Trauma follows similar principles to those used in adults, offering minimally invasive surgery, reduced morbidity, and faster recovery. It is contraindicated in cases of hemodynamic instability. Due to the need for stable conditions for adequate visualization and management of lesions, videolaparoscopy can be used for both diagnoses in hemodynamically stable patients [13].

Main indication for MIS in pediatric trauma:

- *To explain free fluid in the cavity:* When free fluid is detected in the abdominal cavity, videolaparoscopy allows direct visualization to determine its source and guide further management.
- *To investigate causes of severe abdominal pain:* In cases where the cause of significant abdominal pain is unclear, videolaparoscopy provides real-time assessment of potential injuries, offering a more accurate diagnosis.
- *To investigate injuries when the belt sign is positive:* The presence of the "belt sign," often indicative of abdominal trauma in children involved in motor vehicle accidents, can be further investigated using videolaparoscopy to detect underlying injuries.

The videolaparoscopy is essential to diagnose and treat pediatric patients who do not present clinical signs on exams and who have inconclusive imaging findings. Children with blunt trauma may have vague symptoms, and the extent of the injury may not be immediately apparent on routine imaging tests such as X-rays, CT scans, or ultrasounds. In these cases, laparoscopy provides direct visualization of the abdominal cavity, allowing surgeons to identify and treat hidden injuries that may not be detected by traditional imaging methods [11, 13].

By providing an accurate, minimally invasive approach to diagnosing and treating injuries like liver or splenic ruptures, laparoscopy reduces the need for more invasive procedures, such as exploratory laparotomies, and promotes quicker recovery times with fewer complications [11–13].

In cases of penetrating injuries in the abdomen or thoracoabdominal region, videolaparoscopy can be used to assess the presence of peritoneal penetration and determine the extent of abdominal injuries in cases of stab or low-velocity gunshot wounds. This technique offers real-time visualization of the peritoneal cavity, abdominal organs, and any potential injuries. Furthermore, videolaparoscopy facilitates minimally invasive treatment, allowing for suturing, hemostasis, and even organ repair during the procedure [13].

The ability to directly view the injury site and manage it laparoscopically can reduce unnecessary exploratory laparotomies by up to 52%. This approach not only enhances diagnostic accuracy, but also reduces the risks and complications associated with open surgery [11, 13].

In summary, videolaparoscopy offers a highly effective and minimally invasive approach for managing pediatric trauma, particularly in cases of blunt and penetrating abdominal trauma, thoracoabdominal injuries, and diaphragmatic and cardiac trauma. By enabling precise diagnosis, direct visualization, and therapeutic intervention, laparoscopy improves clinical outcomes while minimizing the risks and complications associated with traditional open surgery. However, its use must be carefully considered based on the patient's hemodynamic stability, the nature of the trauma, and the availability of appropriate surgical expertise. As pediatric trauma care continues to evolve, laparoscopy will undoubtedly remain a critical tool in improving patient outcomes and minimizing the need for more invasive interventions [11–13].

However, the effectiveness of these benefits is intrinsically linked to the surgeon's skill. Technical proficiency, both in trauma and in minimally invasive surgery, is crucial for performing the procedure safely and successfully, minimizing risks and promoting optimal recovery. Studies indicate that the surgeon's experience in laparoscopic surgery is directly related to a reduction in complications and improved clinical outcomes in pediatric trauma patients. Therefore, the surgeon's technical competence is a key factor for the success of laparoscopic surgery in pediatric trauma victims [11–13].

To facilitate the understanding of the indications and contraindications of pediatric laparoscopy, we can use the criteria already described in this chapter and also follow the flowchart of care, as shown in Figs. 28.1 and 28.2.

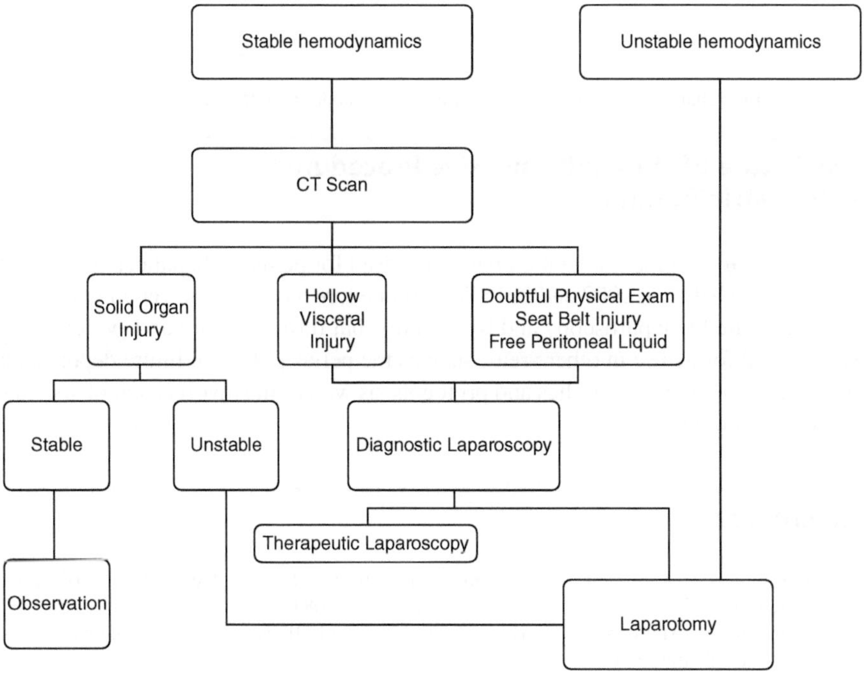

Fig. 28.1 Flowchart of videolaparoscopy in blunt abdominal trauma

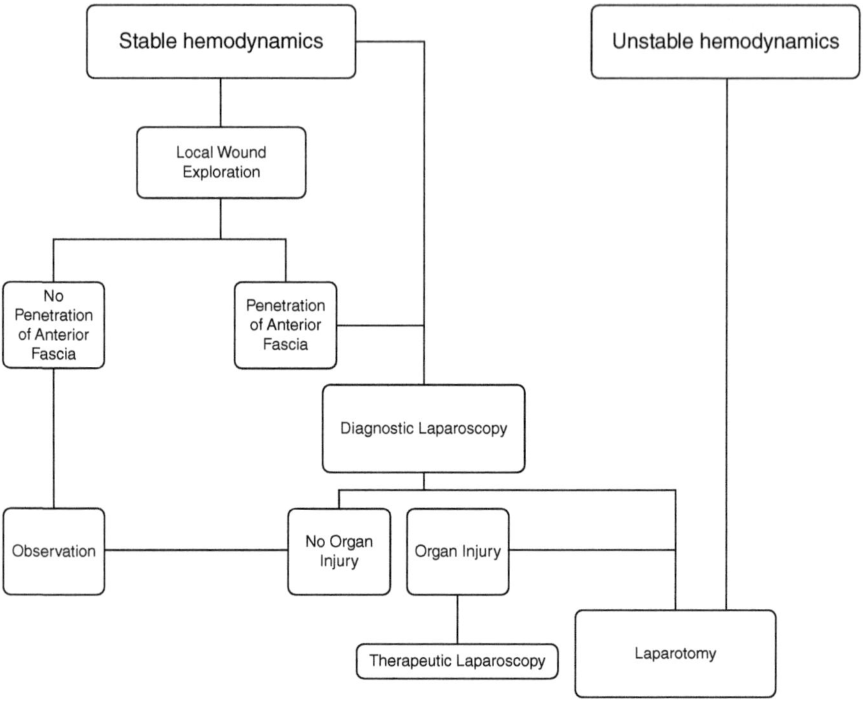

Fig. 28.2 Flowchart of videolaparoscopy in penetrating abdominal trauma

The Future of Minimally Invasive Procedures in Pediatric Trauma

Indications for angioembolization have increased for pediatric hepatic, splenic, and renal trauma between 2007 and 2015. This procedure has shown lower complication rates compared to laparoscopy and laparotomy, but further studies and evidence are still needed for its use in other areas, such as the pelvis [14]. The future depends on the development of new studies and protocols, as well as the involvement of specialists in the field [14].

References

1. Mikrogianakis A, Grant V. The kids are alright. Emerg Med Clin North Am. 2018;36(1):237–57. https://doi.org/10.1016/j.emc.2017.08.015.
2. Pereira JR GA, Andreghetto AC, Basile-Filho A, Andrade JI. Trauma no paciente pediátrico. Medicina, Ribeirão Preto. 1999;32:262–81.
3. Peden M, Oyegbite K, Ozanne-Smith J, et al. World report on child injury prevention. World Health Organization (WHO) and UNICEF; 2008.

4. Train AT, Naseem H-U-R, Chen Z, Wilding GE, Bass KD, Noyes K, et al. Predictors and outcomes of laparoscopy in pediatric trauma patients: a retrospective cohort study. J Laparoendoscopic Adv Surgic Tech. 2019; https://doi.org/10.1089/lap.2019.0322.
5. Holmes JH, Wiebe DJ, Tataria M, Mattix KD, Mooney DP, Scaife ER, et al. Nonoperative management of blunt liver and spleen injury in children: evaluation of practice guidelines. J Trauma Acute Care Surg. 2002;
6. Cunha SC, et al. Analysis of the efficacy and safety of conservative treatment of blunt abdominal trauma in children: retrospective study. Conservative treatment of blunt abdominal trauma in children. Rev Col Bras Cir. 2023;50 https://doi.org/10.1590/0100-6991e-20233429-en.
7. GovindarajanKK,etal.Highgraderenaltraumaduetobluntinjuryinchildren:doallrequireintervention? Brazil J Nephrol. 2019;41(2):172–5. https://doi.org/10.1590/2175-8239-jbn-2018-0186.
8. Stylianos S. Evidence-based guidelines for resource utilization in children with isolated spleen or liver injury. J Pediatr Surg. 2000;35:164.
9. Holmes, J. H., Wiebe, D. J., Tataria, M. O, Mattix, K. D., Mooney, D. P., Scaife, E. R., … Nance, M. L. (2005). The failure of nonoperative management in pediatric solid organ injury: a multi-institutional experience. J Trauma: Injury Infect Critic Care, 59(6), 1309–1313. doi:https://doi.org/10.1097/01.ta.0000197366.38404.79.
10. Motta DC, Scarpelini S. Lesões traumáticas de vísceras ocas. Medicina (Ribeirão Preto). 2007;40(4):531–7. out./dez.
11. Feliz A, Shultz B, McKenna C, Gaines BA. Diagnostic and therapeutic laparoscopy in pediatric abdominal trauma. J Pediatr Surg. 2006;41(1):72–7. https://doi.org/10.1016/j.jpedsurg.2005.10.008.
12. Gaines BA, Rutkoski JD. The role of laparoscopy in pediatric trauma. Semin Pediatr Surg. 2010;19(4):300–3. https://doi.org/10.1053/j.sempedsurg.2010.08.
13. Teixeira JF. Laparoscopic surgery in the pediatric population and its applications. Res Soc Develop. 2023;12(9):e2212943176. https://doi.org/10.33448/rsd-v12i9.43176.
14. Wise BV, Mudd SS, Wilson ME. Management of blunt abdominal trauma in children. J Trauma Nurs. 2002;9(1):6–14. https://doi.org/10.1097/00043860-200209010-00002.
15. Stringel G, Xu ML, Lopez J. Minimally invasive surgery in pediatric trauma: one institution's 20-year experience. JSLS. 2016;20(1):e2015.00111. https://doi.org/10.4293/JSLS.2015.00111.

Obese Patients

29

Renato Diniz Lins and Rodrigo Caselli Belém

Introduction

Obesity is a complex chronic disease, defined by excessive accumulation of body fat, which has reached epidemic proportions globally. This condition is associated with a myriad of comorbidities, including cardiovascular diseases, type 2 diabetes, obstructive sleep apnea, and certain types of cancer. In the context of trauma, the presence of an elevated Body Mass Index (BMI) adds an intricate layer of physiological, anatomical, and logistical considerations that can affect diagnosis, treatment, and ultimately, patient outcomes [1, 2]. One of the most debated areas is the "obesity paradox," which suggests a nonlinear and, at times, counterintuitive relationship between body weight and mortality after severe traumatic injuries. Furthermore, obesity fundamentally alters the physiological and immunological response to acute stress, influencing directly the recovery.

Epidemiology

The prevalence of obesity is alarming. In the United States, approximately 40% of adults are obese, while globally, about 13% of the adult population falls into this category [3, 4]. This increasing proportion of obese individuals means that trauma systems are increasingly caring for this population.

The link between a patient's body mass index and their chances of survival after a traumatic injury has sparked considerable discussion, often leading to findings that seem to contradict each other. A significant study by Dvorak and collaborators, analyzing over 415,000 patients, shed light on a fascinating concept: the "obesity paradox." They observed a "U"-shaped pattern in mortality, meaning that individuals who were overweight (BMI 25.0–29.9) surprisingly had a lower risk of death.

R. D. Lins (✉) · R. C. Belém
Hospital de Base do Distrito Federal (HBDF), Brasilia, DF, Brazil

© The Author(s), under exclusive license to Springer Nature Switzerland AG 2026

M. Cezillo, B. M. Pereira (eds.), *Minimally Invasive Surgery Trauma*,
https://doi.org/10.1007/978-3-032-28971-1_29

Even those with Class I Obesity (BMI 30.0–34.9) didn't show a significantly higher mortality risk when compared to people of normal weight. This unexpected resilience in patients with moderately higher BMI might be due to several factors. Some theories suggest they have greater metabolic reserves, a protective "preconditioning" from existing conditions like obstructive sleep apnea, or even a different inflammatory response influenced by their adipose tissue, as proposed by Di Giacinto and colleagues [4]. However, it's vital to understand that this potential benefit doesn't extend to more severe obesity. Patients with Class II (BMI 35.0–39.9) and Class III Obesity (BMI $\geq$ 40.0) consistently face a progressively higher mortality risk [3]. On the other end of the spectrum, and perhaps more intuitively, those who are underweight (BMI < 18.5) generally experience the worst survival outcomes after trauma.

In contrast, other studies challenge the universality of the obesity paradox in mortality. Brown and colleagues (2005), in an analysis of 1153 critically injured blunt trauma patients, concluded that obesity was an *independent risk factor for mortality* (OR 1.6) [1]. This finding directly contradicts the idea of a protective effect for survival in certain BMI categories. Similarly, Drury and team (2021) found no significant differences in mortality among different BMI groups in their cohort of trauma patients [2]. Hakam and colleagues (2021), in a study focusing on renal trauma, also observed that, after adjusting for injury severity, the obesity paradox *did not hold* for mortality, with only the BMI extremes (underweight and Class III obesity) associated with an increase in mortality [7].

The key to this apparent contradiction may lie in the specificity of the injury type or the magnitude of the "cushion" effect of fat. Patel and colleagues (2021) investigated the impact of obesity on anterior abdominal gunshot wounds (AAGSW) and found evidence of a protective effect [9]. Obese patients with AAGSW were less likely to have abdominal fascial penetration and sustained fewer visceral injuries, suggesting that extra adipose tissue can act as a protective barrier against penetration and internal damage [9]. Di Giacinto et al. (2021) also mention this "cushion effect," noting that obese individuals are relatively protected from abdominal and pelvic injuries in motor vehicle accidents due to their soft tissues although they are more prone to pelvic ring injuries or fractures of peripheral structures [4]. Patel et al. (2021) observed significantly lower NISS (New Injury Severity Score) scores, shorter hospital stays, and shorter surgical duration in these patients, with a high rate of non-therapeutic laparotomies (57.1% with no visceral injuries) [9]. These results suggest that for penetrating injuries in areas with a large volume of adipose tissue, obesity may confer an advantage.

However, even when there is a possible protective effect on mortality or a reduction in initial injury severity, the literature consistently shows a significant increase in morbidity in obese trauma patients [1–10]. Elmhiregh and colleagues (2022), in a study on polytraumatized patients with operatively treated fractures, demonstrated that obesity was associated with a significant increase in total hospital length of stay (36 vs. 27 days), ICU length of stay (13 vs. 8 days), and a higher incidence of ICU admissions and mechanical ventilation. Nelson et al. (2012) reported that obese patients showed higher organ failure scores (Marshall, Murray, SOFA) compared to normal-weight patients, indicating significant organ dysfunction. This aligns with Di Giacinto et al. (2021), who highlight that obesity is associated with a higher risk of post-traumatic morbidity, including higher incidence of ICU admission, long hospital stay, and frequent complications such as pulmonary embolism, prolonged mechanical ventilation, infections, bedsores, wound dehiscence, acute renal failure, and multi-organ failure. The underlying pathophysiology of this increased morbidity is complex and involves the interaction of mechanical, metabolic, and immunological factors. Obese individuals are in a chronic low-grade pro-inflammatory state, which can exacerbate the acute inflammatory response to trauma and contribute to a higher risk of infectious complications and organ dysfunction [4].

Systematization of Care and Diagnostic Challenges

The Advanced Trauma Life Support (ATLS) systematic approach, based on the xABCDE sequence, is universally applied to all trauma patients, including obese ones [11]. However, the application of these principles requires significant adaptations to overcome the anatomical and physiological challenges posed by obesity.

X (Exsanguinating Hemorrhage Control) Initial control of external hemorrhages is fundamental. In obese patients, the visualization of wounds and the application of direct pressure can be difficult due to folds and volume of tissue [11].

A (Airway with Cervical Spine Protection) Airway management is one of the greatest challenges. Obese patients often have shorter necks with excess soft tissue (Figs. 29.1 and 29.2), in addition to a high prevalence of obstructive sleep apnea (OSAS), which increases the risk of a difficult airway. Di Giacinto et al. (2021) emphasize that obese patients present increased complexity in airway management, often leading to difficult oxygenation and even "cannot ventilate, cannot

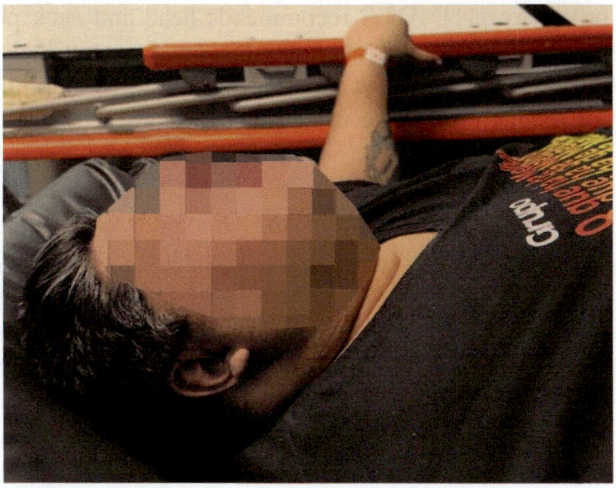

Fig. 29.1 Short necks with excess soft tissue are the greatest challenges of the airway management

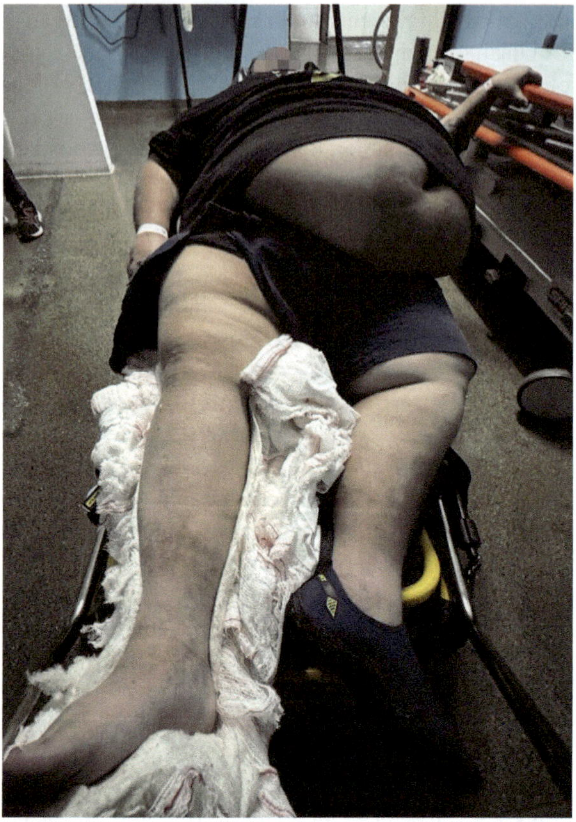

Fig. 29.2 Positioning of the patient is a challenge of the airway management

oxygenate" scenarios [4]. The accumulation of adipose tissue in the cervical region can distort airway anatomy, making laryngoscopy and intubation difficult [11]. Furthermore, reduced lung compliance and increased metabolic demand result in faster desaturation during intubation attempts, decreasing the "time reserve" for the procedure [11]. ATLS recommends head and neck positioning in a "ramped" or reverse Trendelenburg position to optimize glottic visualization, the use of larger blade laryngoscopes or videolaryngoscopy, and modifications of medication doses for intubation, based on ideal body weight to avoid overdose and hemodynamic instability [11].

B (Breathing and Ventilation) Obesity is associated with reduced lung volumes, decreased chest wall and lung compliance, and increased work of breathing [6, 11]. These physiological changes predispose the obese trauma patient to hypoventilation and respiratory failure. Mechanical ventilation is complex, and tidal volumes should be calculated based on ideal body weight, not actual weight, to prevent ventilator-induced lung injury (barotrauma and volutrauma) [6, 11]. Higher PEEP (positive end-expiratory pressure) may be beneficial to maintain oxygenation, but requires careful monitoring [11].

C (Circulation with Hemorrhage Control) Vascular access can be notoriously difficult in obese patients due to the difficulty in locating superficial veins (Fig. 29.3). Di Giacinto et al. (2021) state that ensuring venous access is a priority but can be very difficult, often requiring ultrasound guidance [4]. They also note that standard 25-mm intraosseous needles may not be long enough for patients with BMI > 43 kg/m^2, recommending a 45-mm needle [4]. ATLS emphasizes obtaining large-bore venous access, which may require techniques such as ultrasound guidance for insertion or the use of intraosseous access as a rapid alternative [11]. Nelson et al. (2012) found that obese patients received significantly lower volumes of IV fluids (crystalloid and colloid) than normal-weight or underweight counterparts when corrected for BMI, especially in the initial hours post-trauma [10]. This suggests *inadequate resuscitation* due to underestimation of volume requirements, leading to persistent shock and metabolic acidosis, despite initial blood pressure readings that might not reflect the true hypoperfusion [10]. The estimation of blood volume should be based on ideal body weight to avoid overestimation and consequent fluid over-resuscitation, which could exacerbate pulmonary and cardiac complications in patients with cardiometabolic comorbidities [6, 11].

D (Disability and Neurological Assessment) Neurological assessment can be challenging. Obesity makes complete visual inspection of the body and palpation of

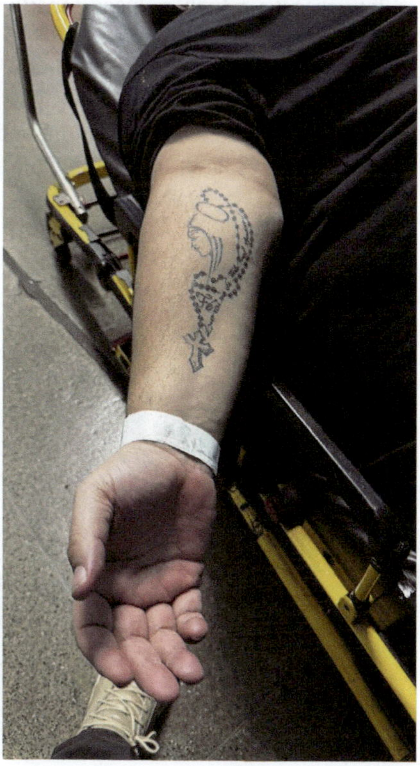

Fig. 29.3 Lack of apparent superficial veins, impairing its locating

important areas difficult, which can lead to delays in injury diagnosis [11]. Di Giacinto et al. (2021) also mention that assessing motor, sensory, and reflex functions is more challenging in morbidly obese patients due to their size, previous impaired perception of pain, and reduced joint mobility and muscle strength [4].

E (Exposure and Environmental Control) Full exposure of the patient is essential to identify all injuries, but the presence of skin folds and larger body surface area increase the risk of hypothermia, which can worsen coagulopathy and outcomes [11]. Environmental temperature control, the use of warming blankets, and fluid warming are crucial [11]. Furthermore, obesity can make it difficult to manage patient dignity and privacy during exposure (Fig. 29.4).

Adjuncts to Diagnosis Imaging methods are particularly problematic. Di Giacinto et al. (2021) highlight that ultrasonography is technically complex in obese patients due to the hypo-echogenicity of adipose tissue and the distance to target organs, recommending 2-MHz probes for greater depth [4]. X-ray, CT, and MRI equipment have size and weight restrictions (Figs. 29.5 and 29.6), often requiring multiple scans, leading to increased timing, radiation exposure, and risk of motion artifacts [4]. The weight capacity of computed tomography (CT) and magnetic resonance imaging (MRI) equipment may be exceeded, preventing crucial examinations. Even when the patient fits, image quality can be degraded due to X-ray beam attenuation or fat artifacts, which reduces sensitivity for detecting injuries and can lead to delayed or inaccurate diagnoses [6, 11]. The observation by Patel et al. (2021) that obese patients with AAGSWs had lower NISS scores and fewer visceral injuries [9] suggests that while obesity may protect against more severe injuries in certain scenarios, this can also lead to an initial underestimation of severity and a higher number of procedures "non-therapeutic" if diagnostic evaluation is not optimized.

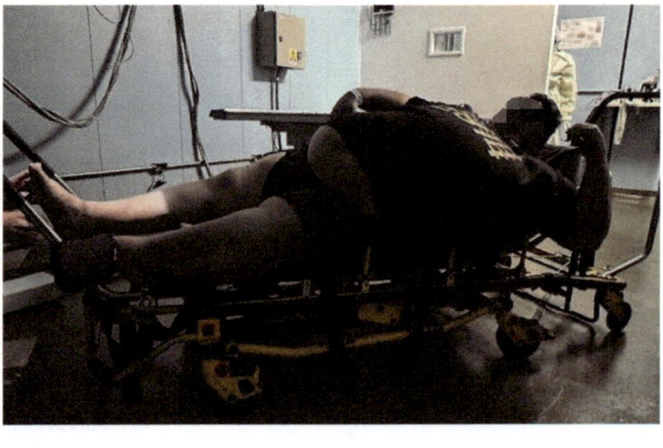

Fig. 29.4 Obesity can make it difficult to manage patient dignity and privacy during exposure

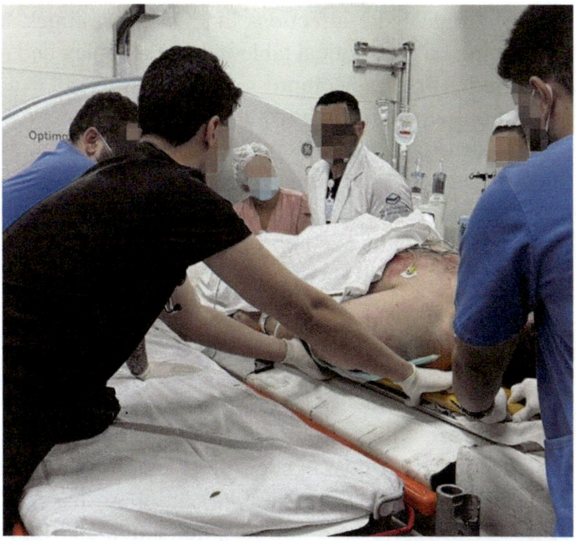

Fig. 29.5 X-ray, CT, and MRI equipment have size and weight restrictions

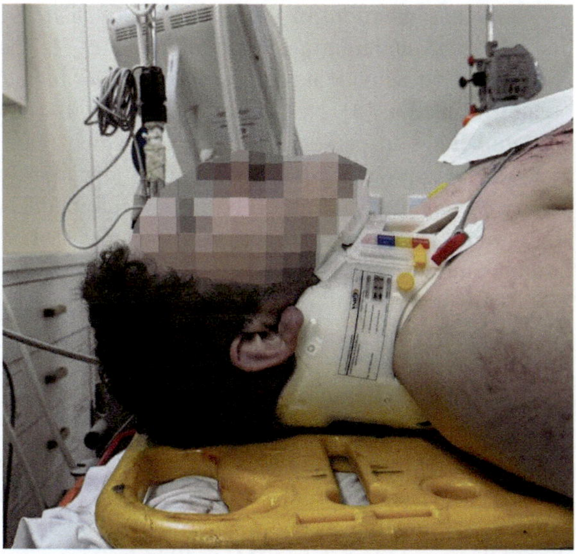

Fig. 29.6 X-ray, CT, and MRI equipment have size and weight restrictions

Treatment

The treatment of the obese trauma patient is complex and demands adaptations at various stages of care, aiming to mitigate consistently observed morbidity.

Surgical Management Obesity imposes substantial challenges during surgical procedures. Di Giacinto et al. (2021) state that in surgery, obesity results in significantly longer intervention times, higher intraoperative blood loss, and increased rates of surgical site infections [4]. Operative times are frequently longer, patient positioning on the surgical table is more complex and requires care to prevent pressure injuries or nerve compression [6, 7]. Surgical exposure is hampered by excess adipose tissue, requiring larger incisions and deeper retraction. Visualization of anatomical structures may be compromised, increasing the risk of iatrogenic injuries. Furthermore, surgical wounds in obese patients are more prone to postoperative complications such as surgical site infections, dehiscence (wound opening), and delayed healing, due to compromised adipose tissue vascularization [6, 7]. The finding by Patel et al. (2021) of a high rate of non-therapeutic laparotomies in AAGSWs in obese patients [9] suggests that for certain injuries, selective non- operative management (SNOM) may be a viable strategy, potentially reducing the risks associated with unnecessary surgeries [9].

Critical Care Obese trauma patients are more likely to be admitted to ICUs and stay for longer periods, in addition to requiring more days on mechanical ventilation [1–4, 7]. Nelson et al. (2012) reported that obese patients had higher incidences of intensive care unit hospitalization and longer hospital stays [10]. They are at higher risk of developing complications such as acute kidney injury (AKI) [5, 7], various infections [5], acute respiratory distress syndrome (ARDS), myocardial infarction, and multiple organ failure [1, 6, 7]. The dysregulated inflammatory response in obese patients can lead to a higher incidence of sepsis and persistent organ dysfunction [4]. Nutrition for critically ill obese patients must follow specific guidelines to prevent malnutrition, which often implies a hypocaloric and hypoproteic approach [6]. Early mobilization, fundamental for recovery, is hampered and requires specialized bariatric equipment (beds, lifts, walkers) and collaboration from multidisciplinary teams [6]. Prophylaxis for venous thromboembolism (VTE) is crucial, as obesity is an independent risk factor for VTE. Di Giacinto et al. (2021) highlight that mechanical devices often do not fit obese patients, and higher doses of low-molecular-weight heparins (e.g., enoxaparin 0.5 mg/kg BID) may be required to achieve therapeutic levels although universal recommendations are still lacking [4].

Specific Morbidity The impact of obesity on morbidity is widely recognized and consistent across studies [1–10]. A study by Liu and colleagues (2024) on surgical stabilization of multiple rib fractures (SSRF) in obese patients demonstrated that morbid obesity (BMI > 40 kg/m^2) was associated with a longer hospital stay, higher hospital costs, and an increase in adverse events [7]. Notably, this association with severe respiratory complications (tracheostomy, ARDS/respiratory failure, prolonged mechanical ventilation) was observed *exclusively* in patients with *flail chest* [7]. This suggests that chest wall rigidity and compromised respiratory physiology due to obesity exacerbate the dysfunctions caused by severe thoracic injuries, making the management of these cases particularly challenging and prolonged.

Laparoscopy in the Trauma Patient with Obesity

The use of laparoscopy in obese polytrauma patients is an increasingly relevant topic, as the prevalence of obesity continues to rise worldwide. Although obesity imposes significant technical and anesthetic challenges, laparoscopy offers potential advantages in terms of diagnosis, therapy, and postoperative outcomes, particularly when compared with traditional laparotomy.

Historically, obesity was considered a limiting factor for the laparoscopic approach due to longer operative times, increased risk of complications, and higher rates of conversion to laparotomy [12–16]. However, recent studies have shown that when performed by experienced teams, laparoscopy is feasible and safe even in patients with elevated BMI. In addition to reducing wound-related complications such as infection and dehiscence, the minimally invasive approach can favor faster recovery and shorter hospital stay [17].

Pneumoperitoneum Pressure

The induction and maintenance of pneumoperitoneum in obese patients require special attention. Increased abdominal wall thickness, higher baseline intra-abdominal pressure, and respiratory limitations impose risks of hypercapnia and ventilatory difficulties [16]. It is recommended to use moderate insufflation pressures (12–15 mmHg) to ensure adequate exposure without excessively compromising respiratory function, adjusting according to pulmonary compliance and hemodynamic tolerance. In some cases, association with abdominal wall elevation techniques may allow a lower insufflation pressure, thereby minimizing cardiopulmonary effects.

Exposure of the Operative Field

Laparoscopic exposure is particularly challenging in obese patients due to thickened abdominal wall, accumulation of intra-abdominal fat, and reduced ability to tolerate steep Trendelenburg positioning. Limited inclination, owing to restrictive ventilation and increased diaphragmatic pressure, reduces visceral displacement and may compromise visibility. Strategies to optimize the operative field include:

- Use of longer trocars and alternative entry sites, such as the left upper quadrant [12]
- Suspension or umbilical elevation techniques to create additional working space [13, 15]
- Careful positioning on bariatric operating tables, using straps and supports to prevent sliding in partial Trendelenburg
- Selective use of 30° optics and angle adjustments during the procedure

Management of Bowel Loops

Excess mesenteric fat and reduced mobility of the bowel loops make laparoscopic exploration more difficult in obese patients. Increased bowel content in the operative field, associated with limited retraction, may prolong operative time and increase the risk of inadvertent injury [16]. Systematic exploration—evaluating quadrant by quadrant, with atraumatic long instruments and suction devices—is essential to avoid missed injuries. The use of intracavitary gauze pads and irrigation-aspiration techniques can assist in retraction and help detect bleeding or small perforations. Additionally, the baseline low-grade inflammation in obese individuals can amplify the inflammatory response to minor injuries, increasing postoperative morbidity when intraoperative lesions are missed.

Hepatic Management in the Obese Patient

In obese trauma patients, hepatic exposure during laparoscopy represents a particular technical challenge. The enlarged liver, often associated with steatosis, restricts visualization and hinders safe manipulation of instruments in the right upper quadrant. This limitation may compromise both diagnostic accuracy and therapeutic interventions such as hemostasis or repair of capsular injuries.

Several strategies have been described to optimize hepatic exposure. Patient positioning is crucial, with reverse Trendelenburg combined with left lateral tilt improving gravitational displacement of the liver and enhancing visibility of the subhepatic region. Gastric decompression can also facilitate cephalad displacement of the liver, while partial mobilization of the falciform or round ligaments may further increase exposure when required.

The use of dedicated liver retractors plays a central role in this context. Rigid retractors provide strong lifting capacity but may be limited in maneuverability in obese patients. Conversely, flexible liver retractors (Fig. 29.7) offer a significant advantage by adapting to the contour of the enlarged fatty liver and distributing the retraction force over a broader surface [18]. This reduces the risk of capsular tears and allows for stable, prolonged exposure of the operative field without compromising visibility. When introduced through auxiliary trocars, flexible retractors create a working space in the subhepatic region while maintaining ergonomic instrument positioning.

It should be noted that excessive intra-abdominal fat and elevated intra-abdominal pressure from pneumoperitoneum may exacerbate hepatic concealment, reinforcing the importance of careful pressure modulation and ergonomic trocar placement. In experienced hands, the combination of these technical adjustments—positioning, decompression, ligament mobilization, and use of flexible retractors—allows for safer and more effective laparoscopic management of liver-related injuries in obese patients, minimizing the need for conversion to laparotomy.

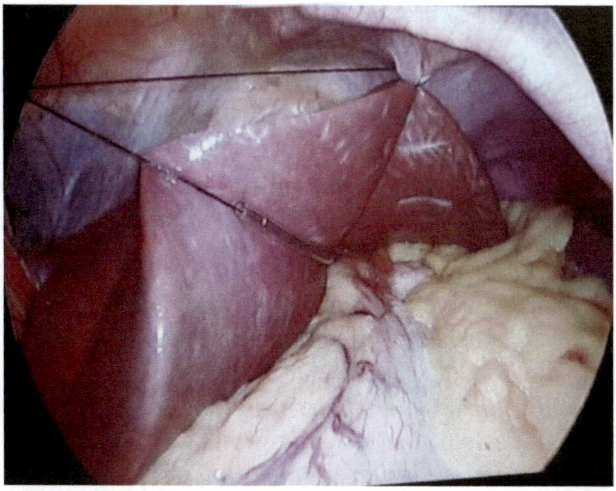

Fig. 29.7 Flexible liver retractors offer a significant advantage by adapting to the contour of the enlarged fatty liver and distributing the retraction force over a broader surface

Advantages and Limitations

In abdominal trauma, laparoscopy has a consolidated role both as a diagnostic and therapeutic tool in hemodynamically stable patients [14, 17]. It allows direct inspection of abdominal viscera, control of minor bleeding, suturing of bowel injuries, and even splenectomy or segmental resections in specialized centers. In obese patients, these benefits are particularly important since laparotomy carries additional risks related to prolonged mechanical ventilation, venous thromboembolism, and abdominal wall complications.

On the other hand, laparoscopy in obese trauma patients still faces important limitations. The anesthetic risks associated with sustained pneumoperitoneum, positioning difficulties, and the need for appropriate instruments make the procedure dependent on team experience and the availability of structural resources such as bariatric operating tables, long trocars, and high-definition imaging systems.

Conclusion

The management of trauma in obese patients is a multifaceted clinical landscape that defies simplistic notions. While the "obesity paradox" may suggest potentially better survival in certain BMI ranges for trauma patients, this apparent advantage is often overshadowed by a substantial increase in morbidity, prolonged hospital stays, and greater resource utilization. Obesity imposes significant challenges at every stage of care, from pre-hospital rescue and diagnosis to surgery and intensive care recovery. The complexity of physiological, anatomical, and logistical factors demands a highly individualized and adapted approach, following the systematized principles of ATLS care.

Challenges

The challenges in managing trauma in obese patients are diverse and require a coordinated and multifaceted response from healthcare systems:

1. *Resources and Infrastructure:* The need for bariatric equipment is a growing demand that many hospitals are still unable to fully meet. Examples include:

    - *Bariatric Stretchers and Beds:* With greater width, length, and weight capacity (often exceeding 300 kg, and potentially reaching 500 kg or more), these are crucial for safe patient transport and accommodation, preventing injuries to both the patient and the staff [6].
    - *Bariatric Wheelchairs:* With reinforced frames and wider seats, they allow for safe patient mobility within the hospital.
    - *Bariatric Lifts and Patient Hoists:* Designed to lift and transfer patients with significant weights, they minimize physical strain on staff and reduce the risk of overload injuries [6].
    - *Bariatric Surgical Tables:* With increased weight capacity and width, they allow for safe patient positioning for surgical procedures and adequate access to the operative field [6].
    - *Large-Sized Blood Pressure Cuffs:* Essential for accurate blood pressure readings, avoiding underestimation of hypotension [6].
    - *Imaging Equipment with Wider Openings and Increased Weight Capacity:* CT scanners and MRI machines with tables that support significantly higher weights and wider openings are crucial for accurate diagnosis, as the lack of such equipment can render evaluation of internal injuries impossible or severely compromised [6].
    - *Other:* Reinforced commodes, bedside chairs, grab bars, and bariatric walkers, canes, and crutches are important for patient autonomy and safety during recovery.

2. *Team Training:* Healthcare professionals, from paramedics to intensivists and surgeons, need specialized training in safe handling, clinical assessment, airway and ventilation management, and prevention of specific complications in obese patients. ATLS provides the foundation, but deeper understanding of obesity-specific considerations is crucial. Di Giacinto et al. (2021) noted that current guidelines lack specific recommendations for obese patients, emphasizing the intellectual, procedural, and technical challenges involved [4]. Nelson et al. (2012) pointed out the necessity to increase the training of health professionals specifically for these special patients to manage the most encountered critical issues [10].
3. *Accurate Diagnosis:* The limitations of diagnostic imaging are a significant obstacle. Research should focus on developing new imaging technologies or optimizing existing ones for this population. The ability to use BMI as a predictive factor for selective non-operative management in certain injuries (such as

AAGSW) [9] represents an opportunity to improve diagnosis and avoid unnecessary surgeries.
4. *Complication Management:* The higher incidence of wound infections [5], VTE, respiratory failure, and multiple organ failure demands constant vigilance and aggressive, adapted treatment protocols. The increase in specific complications like ARDS, myocardial infarction, and AKI [5, 7] in obese patients requires more robust therapeutic approaches. Understanding the chronic pro-inflammatory state in obesity and its influence on the trauma response is fundamental for modulating the immune response and preventing adverse outcomes [4].
5. *Physiopathological Understanding:* Despite the debate about the paradox, further studies are needed to delve into the biological mechanisms that could confer resilience in some obese patients, or to explain why morbidity is invariably higher. The understanding of how the "cushion effect" operates in different types of trauma and the modulation of the inflammatory response (including the role of adipokines and cytokines) are crucial areas for the development of targeted therapies [4].
6. *Optimization of Care:* It is crucial to develop and implement evidence-based guidelines that address the peculiarities of obese patients at each stage of trauma, aiming to optimize survival outcomes and, crucially, reduce morbidity and promote a complete functional recovery. This includes considering strategies like SNOM for specific cases where BMI may act as a protective factor [9].
7. *Laparoscopy:* Laparoscopy in obese trauma patients should be regarded as a valuable tool, provided that hemodynamic stability, experienced surgical teams, and adequate resources are available. Despite the inherent technical challenges—particularly those related to pneumoperitoneum, exposure of the surgical field, and bowel handling—current evidence suggests that its benefits outweigh the risks in selected cases, reducing morbidity, length of stay, and avoiding non-therapeutic laparotomies.

In summary, the obese trauma patient is not just a patient with extra weight; they represent a distinct clinical entity that demands a specialized approach and dedicated resources. Overcoming these challenges will not only improve care for this growing population but also strengthen the overall capacity of trauma systems.

References

1. Brown CV, Neville AL, Rhee P, Salim A, Velmahos GC, Demetriades D. The impact of obesity on the outcomes of 1,153 critically injured blunt trauma patients. J Trauma. 2005;59(5):1048–51.
2. Drury B, Kocharians C, Dong F, Tran L, Beroukhim S, Hajjafar R, et al. Impact of obesity on mortality in adult trauma patients. Cureus. 2021;13(2):e13352.
3. Dvorak JE, Lester ELW, Maluso PJ, Tatebe L, Schlanser V, Kaminsky M, Messer T, Dennis AJ, Starr F, Bokhari F. The obesity paradox in the trauma patient: Normal may not be better. World J Surg. 2020;44(6):1817–23.

4. Di Giacinto I, Guarnera M, Esposito C, Falcetta S, Cortese G, Pascarella G, et al. Emergencies in obese patients: a narrative review. J Anesth Analg Crit Care. 2021;1(1):13.
5. Elmhiregh A, Ahmed AF, Dabboussi AM, Ahmed GO, Abdelrahman H, Ibrahim T. The impact of obesity on polytraumatized patients with operatively treated fractures. Injury. 2022;53(9):2519–23.
6. Gray S, Dieudonne B. Optimizing care for trauma patients with obesity. Cureus. 2018;10(7):e3021.
7. Hakam N, Nabavizadeh B, Sadighian MJ, Holler J, Shibley P, Li KD, et al. The impact of obesity on renal trauma outcome: an analysis of the National Trauma Data Bank from 2013 to 2016. World J Surg. 2021;45(12):3633–42.
8. Liu YF, Chen TL, Tseng CH, Wang JY, Wang WC. Impact of obesity on outcomes after surgical stabilization of multiple rib fractures: evidence from the US nationwide inpatient sample. PLoS One. 2024;19(2):e0299256.
9. Patel BM, Samsonov AP, Patel JR, Onursal E, Jung MK, Talty N, et al. Obesity and anterior abdominal gunshot wounds: a cushion effect. Cureus. 2021;13(11):e19838.
10. Nelson J, Billeter AT, Seifert B, Neuhaus V, Trentz O, Hofer CK, et al. Obese trauma patients are at increased risk of early hypovolemic shock: a retrospective cohort analysis of 1,084 severely injured patients. Crit Care. 2012;16(3):R77.
11. American College of Surgeons. Advanced Trauma Life Support® (ATLS®) student course manual. 10th ed. Chicago: American College of Surgeons; 2018.
12. Barbaresso R, Parikh S, Pasic R. Should laparoscopy be performed in the morbidly obese? Gynecol Obstet Clin Med. 2024;4:e000049.
13. Gemici K, Tanrikulu Y, Buldu I, et al. A novel safe laparoscopic entry technique in obese patients: an umbilical elevation technique. Int J Clin Exp Med. 2016;9(5):8411–5.
14. Engin O, Sunamak O. Diagnostic laparoscopy in abdominal trauma patients. Ann Laparosc Endosc Surg. 2016;1:14.
15. Polat M, Incebiyik A, Tammo O. Abdominal access in laparoscopic surgery of obese patients: a novel abdominal access technique. Ann Saudi Med. 2023;43(3):236–42.
16. Hasson AM. Risk of pneumoperitoneum in obese: old myths and new realities. World J Laparosc Surg. 2011;4(2):97–102.
17. Jo H, Kim D. Diagnostic and therapeutic laparoscopy for abdominal trauma: a single surgeon's experience. J Trauma Inj. 2021;34(4):248–56.
18. Babadopulos RFAL, Moura-Jr LG, Fechine V, Rocha MBS, Antunes N, Costa TA, De-Moraes MO. Técnica de exposição da junção esofagogástrica obtida por meio de afastador flexível de fígado em cirurgia bariátrica: ensaio clínico randomizado. ABCD Arq Bras Cir Dig. 2021;34(4)

Part IV

Special Considerations and After Trauma Care

Laparoscopy in the Trauma Non-operative Management: General View

30

Federico Coccolini, Antonella Lopes, and Camilla Cremonini

Introduction

While laparoscopy has been commonly accepted by general surgeons, in the trauma field it is gaining ground during the last decades hand in hand with the concept of non-operative management (NOM) for both blunt and penetrating injuries to reduce the number of negative laparotomies.

The use of laparoscopy on patients with trauma was first reported in the 1970s [1]. First of all, the purpose of laparoscopy was only the diagnosis, and open laparotomy was performed only in cases that needed further procedures such as vessel ligation, bowel resection, or suturing impossible to perform by laparoscopy. Several studies have reported that diagnostic laparoscopy in patients with trauma has a high diagnostic accuracy of nearly 100% [2]. Diagnostic laparoscopy is beneficial in avoiding unnecessary nontherapeutic laparotomy, which is usually accompanied by more complications than laparoscopy [3]. With the development of the laparoscopic technique and equipment, there has recently been an increase in the number of reports on therapeutic laparoscopy in patients with trauma [4]. Recently, the laparoscopic procedure comprises both diagnostic and therapeutic purposes. First, similar to the non-trauma field, several studies showed that laparoscopy had advantages in terms of blood loss during surgery and hospital stay compared to laparotomy.

F. Coccolini (✉) · A. Lopes · C. Cremonini
Department of General, Emergency and Trauma Surgery, Pisa University Hospital, Pisa, Italy

© The Author(s), under exclusive license to Springer Nature Switzerland AG 2026

M. Cezillo, B. M. Pereira (eds.), *Minimally Invasive Surgery Trauma*,
https://doi.org/10.1007/978-3-032-28971-1_30

Non-operative Management of Abdominal Trauma

Blunt and Penetrating

Trauma surgeons have begun to embrace this philosophy in adult injuries during the past three decades. With the use of modern diagnostic and therapeutic tools, the increase of selective NOM in blunt abdominal trauma in hemodynamically stable patients has been clearly shown by several studies and by the latest guidelines [5–9].

This trend has been supported by technological advancements in both diagnostic and therapeutic areas (such as CT scans, angiography, angio-embolization, and the use of integrated or hybrid operating rooms) as well as by specialized institutional backing and appropriate infrastructure.

About injury mechanism, it's essential to discuss penetrating abdominal trauma (PAT) and blunt abdominal trauma (BAT). Few studies have been conducted on laparoscopy in patients with blunt abdominal trauma (BAT), probably because there are many ambiguous blunt regions, such as hematomas and bruised organs. Laparoscopy in BAT, compared to PAT, had a higher morbidity and conversion rate. Anyway, laparoscopy for BAT and PAT is mostly performed in hemodynamically stable patients. There is still controversy regarding the indications, safety, and efficacy of laparoscopy for BAT. It can be dangerous for patients with hemodynamic instability, and it can miss serious blunt injury [10].

In 1960, Shaftan was the first to report selective NOM of abdominal penetrating wounds, supporting "observant and expectant treatment" instead of the then-mandatory celiotomy [11].

Since then NOM of penetrating abdominal trauma in hemodynamically stable patients without signs of peritonitis or evisceration has been extensively accepted, as it has been shown to reduce morbidity due to negative laparotomy [12, 13].

The concept of conservative management for gunshot wounds has been more controversial: the higher risks of vascular and visceral injuries and the morbidity and mortality as a consequence of missed injuries are the main concerns [14, 15]. Although initially met with some resistance, selective non-operative management (NOM) of abdominal stab wounds has now become standard practice in many trauma centers.

Laparoscopy in Trauma

Currently, laparoscopic surgery is widely accepted as a treatment for non-traumatic disease, and the controversy surrounding its technical issues has reduced. There have been considerable improvements in laparoscopic skills and laparoscopic equipment over the past few decades. This evolution was possible because of the development of various useful instruments, including high-resolution cameras, suturing devices, staplers, and energy devices, that allow for effective hemostasis and resection [10].

Recent studies included laparoscopic procedures such as bowel resection, bowel repair, bladder repair, splenectomy, distal pancreatectomy, diaphragm repair, and hemostasis [10, 16–20]. In early studies, laparotomy was needed for these procedures. Large-scale randomized controlled trials have shown that, in terms of stomach and colon cancers, the outcomes of laparoscopic surgery are similar and non-inferior to the outcomes of open surgery [21, 22]. This suggests that only minimal advancements are needed to address the technical challenges related to bowel surgery. However, performing laparoscopic procedures on retroperitoneal organs like the duodenum and pancreas continues to be a subject of debate. The retroperitoneal laparoscopic approach demands a higher level of expertise and technical proficiency compared to other methods used in bowel surgery. Therefore, trauma surgeons must possess substantial experience and advanced surgical skills. The possibility of open conversion may be high in severe bleeding and retroperitoneal organ injury [10]. Computed tomography (CT) or focused assessment with sonography for trauma (FAST) may help to decide to attempt therapeutic laparoscopy [10]. If there are no specific findings on physical examination and there is no severe bleeding in CT or FAST, therapeutic laparoscopy may be attempted. Recently, interventional radiology has evolved considerably for hemostasis in patients with hemorrhagic pelvic fracture, liver laceration, spleen rupture, or major vascular trauma [23, 24].

Many of these trauma patients are managed in the ICU: here's the concept of bedside laparoscopy. It's a very quick strategy when performed by a skilled equipe and studies have demonstrated a near 100% diagnostic accuracy [25].

Bedside Laparoscopy in the Critically Ill

Critically ill patients treated in the intensive care unit (ICU) can present with many abdominal conditions [26] that need a rapid diagnosis and timely treatment because of their general frailty. Clinical evaluation is not always reliable due to sedation or analgesia. In some cases, it can be misleading, causing a delayed diagnosis, which can be detrimental to this category of patient [27]. Furthermore, the accuracy of diagnostic tests such as ultrasound or CT scans is reduced. In particular, ultrasound benefits from patient compliance and is operator-dependent [28], while a CT scan requires intra-hospital transportation with its established rates of related complications and mortality [29, 30]. These include patient-related or equipment-related adverse events such as hypotension, respiratory distress, dysrhythmias, central line disconnections, oxygen supply problems, or accidental extubation. Due to the physiological instability of ICU patients, the challenges in conducting a physical examination, the decreased reliability of diagnostic tests, and the time-sensitive nature of these conditions, exploratory laparotomy has traditionally been the preferred treatment when a definitive diagnosis has not been made. To date, there are no data regarding the rate of positive intra-abdominal findings in exploratory laparotomies in critically ill patients. Nonetheless, a negative laparotomy is a reality that surgeons encounter in their practice, and some reports on other types of patients [31, 32] suggest that this rate and the associated comorbidities are far from negligible. In a retrospective analysis of 817 patients who underwent an exploratory laparotomy after abdominal gunshot wounds, Sosa et al. found a negative laparotomy to be associated with a 22% morbidity rate and an average length of stay of 5.1 days, while Weigelt et al. in a retrospective study enrolling 248 patients, reported a 14% postoperative morbidity rate with a mean hospital stay of 5 days [32, 33]. Bedside laparoscopy (BSL) is a minimally invasive procedure that allows surgeons to assess the abdominal cavity directly in the ICU, thus avoiding unnecessary exploratory laparotomy or incidents related to intra-hospital transfer.

Since its introduction, laparoscopy has significantly improved surgical outcomes, leading to a marked reduction in postoperative morbidity, pain, and hospital stay. It facilitates a quicker and less painful recovery, while offering comparable results to traditional laparotomy in all other surgical parameters. However, when treating critically ill patients, the benefits of laparoscopy are often, in the authors' view, underestimated. Even today, when facing a suspected intra-abdominal issue, surgeons and anesthesiologists remain cautious about the potential advantages of laparoscopy, often opting for a laparotomic approach instead. This is largely due to concerns over the cardiac and respiratory risks of pneumoperitoneum, particularly in vulnerable, already compromised patients. The procedure can be conducted safely in a brief but thorough manner directly in the ICU, avoiding a superfluous transportation in those with negative findings in BSL or effectively diagnosing an intra-abdominal pathology allowing transportation and operational treatment (either radiologic, laparoscopic, or laparotomic) only for patients who require them. To our knowledge, the optimal approach after a positive finding in BSL is yet to be studied, and therefore no standardized algorithm exists. As already stated above, the safety profile of BSL is remarkable, showing very low procedure-related morbidity rates, with the most common complication being superficial wound infection. Also, mortality rates, although undoubtedly high, are not to be ascribed to BSL but instead to the poor general conditions particular to ICU patients. The low procedure-related morbidity and mortality rates should further encourage surgeons to use BSL [34].

Penetrating Trauma

In stable patients with abdominal penetrating injuries and either confirmed or suspected peritoneal involvement, laparoscopy allows for both the diagnosis and potential treatment of occult injuries, such as those involving hollow organs or the diaphragm.

During the past decades, selective non-operative management became the standard of practice in penetrating injuries; many reports documented its efficacy and safety for stab wounds and its growing role in the management of gunshot wounds too [35–37].

Many authors focused on the failure of this kind of approach finding stomach injuries and injury to the extra-hepatic biliary tract being lesions that may not manifest with evident peritonitis [37]. Lang et al. published their data demonstrating an improvement in the management of penetrating injuries with standardized protocols by the adoption of a much more aggressive approach with the use of laparoscopy: "We have selectively adopted newer modalities and applied them to specific problem areas, which we have identified from previous audits. The use of DL to assess stable patients with left thoracoabdominal penetrating injuries has reduced the incidence of delayed diagnosis of hollow visceral injury and of occult diaphragmatic injury" [35].

Diaphragmatic Injuries

Diaphragmatic injuries are frequent after both blunt and penetrating trauma with rates as high as 5% for blunt trauma and 15% for patients after penetrating injuries to the lower chest and upper abdomen [38, 39]. Adamthwaite, in 1984, was the first to suggest a minimally invasive approach for identifying a traumatic diaphragmatic injury [40];

Diagnostic laparoscopy has gained more and more consent among trauma surgeons both as a diagnostic and therapeutic tool [41]. Laparoscopy, in fact, is the most accurate and safe method to completely evaluate the entire diaphragmatic dome, allowing not only for DI diagnosis but also for definitive repair of the injury with minimal morbidity and good outcomes [42]. Hemodynamically stable patients that have sustained a penetrating trauma of the thoracoabdominal region (especially on the left side) with no signs of peritonitis or other organ injuries are the perfect candidates that may benefit from this minimally invasive option. Hence, when a DI is suspected based on the mechanism but not detected, a diagnostic laparoscopy should always be considered.

Alternatively, a thoracoscopy may be used to evaluate the diaphragm from above. This is commonly used when evacuation of retained hemothorax or empyema is needed [43, 44] although some elect this surgical strategy anyway. Repair of the diaphragm is feasible using minimally invasive techniques such as laparoscopy or thoracoscopy [45, 46].

Blunt Trauma

The role of laparoscopy in blunt trauma is not well defined yet: the lack of randomized studies and the fewness of the prospective ones have made this concept still unclear [47, 48].

Non-operative management for stable patients with blunt trauma has become the standard of care, primarily with regard to liver and spleen trauma. A CT scan can assist in identifying patients suitable for this type of management, even though its accuracy in detecting associated hollow-viscus injuries is limited. Laparoscopy has become a useful tool when it comes to those "unclear abdomen": patients who have been treated conservatively but present with nonspecific symptoms in contrast with negative imaging and clinical findings. A minimally invasive approach can lead to a rapid diagnosis and, when needed, to therapeutic options, avoiding laparotomy and all the implications that come with it. Under these circumstances, we can speak of "interval laparoscopy" as a valuable extension of the non-operative strategy, ruling out doubts in case of an unclear abdomen, detecting occult injuries or even treating complications. A limpid example of the application of interval laparoscopy is in liver trauma management, not only blunt but also penetrating injuries. Hemodynamic status and clinical examinations are the main standards used to decide on non-operative management [49, 50], in association with radiological and laboratory evaluation. The absence of standard early follow-up protocols remains a problem; however, strict clinical, laboratory, and imaging monitoring are mandatory: in case of doubtful clinical findings or in the occurrence of complications such as subcapsular hematoma or biliary leaks, laparoscopic evacuation and lavage with drain placement can be used as a bridge strategy, in the same context as ERCP or percutaneous drainage.

Pediatric Population

Various discussions regarding the use of laparoscopy in pediatric blunt trauma have been published [51, 52]; in 2017, Linnaus et al. presented the first prospective multicenter study showing that almost half of NOM failures are for reasons other than persistent hemorrhage [53]: occult isolated pancreatic injuries and hollow-viscus injuries have already been reported as a considerable percentage of failures of NOM [54].

The ongoing use of laparoscopy even in pediatric trauma patients is gaining success not only as a diagnostic tool, but also in the treatment scenario, as interval laparoscopy [55, 56].

Conclusion

Interval laparoscopy, whether in adult or pediatric trauma, and for both blunt and penetrating injuries, should not be regarded as a failure of non-operative management. Rather, it serves as a valuable adjunct in reducing morbidity and avoiding unnecessary laparotomies. It can be performed in the operating room or at the bedside in the ICU as bedside laparoscopy.

Laparoscopy is now considered a feasible approach at various stages of trauma management, particularly when viewed as part of non-operative care.

References

1. Di Saverio S, Birindelli A, Podda M, Segalini E, Piccinini A, Coniglio C, Frattini C, Tugnoli G. Trauma laparoscopy and the six w's: Why, where, who, when, what, and how? J. Trauma Acute Care Surg. 2019;86:344–67.
2. O'Malley E, Boyle E, O'Callaghan A, Coffey JC, Walsh SR. Role of laparoscopy in penetrating abdominal trauma: A systematic review. World J. Surg. 2013;37:113–22.
3. Shamim AA, Zeineddin S, Zeineddin A, Olufajo OA, Mathelier GO, Cornwell EE III, Fullum T, Tran D. Are we doing too many non-therapeutic laparotomies in trauma? An analysis of the National Trauma Data Bank. Surg. Endosc. 2019;34:1–7.
4. Cirocchi R, Birindelli A, Inaba K, Mandrioli M, Piccinini A, Tabola R, Carlini L, Tugnoli G, Di Saverio S. Laparoscopy for trauma and the changes in its use from 1990 to 2016: A current systematic review and meta-analysis. Surg Laparosc Endosc Percutaneous Tech. 2018;28:1–12.
5. Knudson MM, Maull KI. Nonoperative management of solid organ injuries. Past, present, and future. Surg Clin North Am. 1999;79:1357–71.
6. Christmas AB, Wilson AK, Manning B, Franklin GA, Miller FB, Richardson JD, et al. Selective management of blunt hepatic injuries including nonoperative management is a safe and effective strategy. Surgery. 2005;138:606–10.
7. Rutledge R, Hunt JP, Lentz CW, Fakhry SM, Meyer AA, Baker CC, et al. A statewide, population-based time-series analysis of the increasing frequency of nonoperative management of abdominal solid organ injury. Ann Surg. 1995;222:311–22.
8. Coccolini F, Montori G, Catena F, et al. Splenic trauma: WSES classification and guidelines for adult and pediatric patients. World J Emerg Surg. 2017;12:40.
9. Coccolini F, Coimbra R, Ordonez C, et al. Liver trauma: WSES 2020 guidelines. World J Emerg Surg. 2020;15:24.
10. Ki Y-J, Jo Y-G, Park Y-C, Kang W-S. The efficacy and safety of laparoscopy for blunt abdominal trauma: a systematic review and meta-analysis. J Clin Med. 2021;10(9):1853.
11. Shaftan GW. Indications for operation in abdominal trauma. Am J Surg. 1960 May;99:657–64.
12. Leppäniemi AK, Haapiainen RK. Selective nonoperative management of abdominal stab wounds: prospective, randomized study. World J Surg. 1996;20(8):1101–5. discussion 1105–6
13. Como JJ, Bokhari F, Chiu WC, Duane TM, Holevar MR, Tandoh MA, Ivatury RR, Scalea TM. Practice management guidelines for selective nonoperative management of penetrating abdominal trauma. J Trauma. 2010;68(3):721–33.
14. Navsaria PH, Berli JU, Edu S, Nicol AJ. Non-operative management of abdominal stab wounds—an analysis of 186 patients. S Afr J Surg. 2007;45(4):128–32.
15. Al Rawahi AN, Al Hinai FA, Boyd JM, Doig CJ, Ball CG, Velmahos GC, Kirkpatrick AW, Navsaria PH, Roberts DJ. Outcomes of selective nonoperative management of civilian abdominal gunshot wounds: a systematic review and meta-analysis. World J Emerg Surg. 2018;13:55.
16. Shah SM, Shah KS, Joshi PK, Somani RB, Gohil VB, Dakhda SM. To study the incidence of organ damage and postoperative care in patients of blunt abdominal trauma with haemoperitoneum managed by laparoscopy. J Minimal Access Surg. 2011;7:169–72.
17. Johnson JJ, Garwe T, Raines AR, Thurman JB, Carter S, Bender JS, Albrecht RM. The use of laparoscopy in the diagnosis and treatment of blunt and penetrating abdominal injuries: 10-year experience at a level 1 trauma center. Am J Surg. 2013;205:317–20.
18. Memon MR, Sanghi AG, Abbasi SA, Memon AA. Role of laparoscopy in blunt abdominal trauma. Rawal Med J. 2013;38:40–3.
19. Lin HF, Chen YD, Chen SC. Value of diagnostic and therapeutic laparoscopy for patients with blunt abdominal trauma: A 10-year medical center experience. PLoS One. 2018;13:e0193379.
20. Matsevych O, Koto M, Balabyeki M, Aldous C. Trauma laparoscopy: When to start and when to convert? Surg. Endosc. 2018;32:1344–52.
21. Bonjer HJ, Deijen CL, Abis GA, Cuesta MA, Van Der Pas MH, De Lange-De Klerk ES, Lacy AM, Bemelman WA, Andersson J, Angenete E. A randomized trial of laparoscopic versus open surgery for rectal cancer. N Engl J Med. 2015;372:1324–32.

22. Park YK, Yoon HM, Kim Y-W, Park JY, Ryu KW, Lee Y-J, Jeong O, Yoon KY, Lee JH, Lee SE, et al. Laparoscopyassisted versus Open D2 Distal Gastrectomy for Advanced Gastric Cancer: Results From a Randomized Phase II Multicenter Clinical Trial (COACT 1001). Ann Surg. 2018;267:638–45.
23. Fox N, Schwartz D, Salazar JH, Haut ER, Dahm P, Black JH, Brakenridge SC, Como JJ, Hendershot K, King DR, et al. Evaluation and management of blunt traumatic aortic injury: A practice management guideline from the Eastern Association for the Surgery of Trauma. J. Trauma Acute Care Surg. 2015;78:136–46.
24. Coccolini F, Coimbra R, Ordonez C, Kluger Y, Vega F, Moore EE, Biffl W, Peitzman A, Horer T, Abu-Zidan FM. Liver trauma: WSES 2020 guidelines. World J Emerg Surg. 2020;15:1–15.
25. Zemlyak A, Heniford BT, Sing RF. Diagnostic laparoscopy in the intensive care unit. J Intensive Care Med. 2015;30(5):297–302.
26. Reintam Blaser A, Starkopf J, Malbrain ML. Abdominal signs and symptoms in intensive care patients. Anaesthesiol. Intensive Ther. 2015;47:379–87.
27. Crandall M, West MA. Evaluation of the abdomen in the critically ill patient: Opening the black box. Curr Opin Crit Care. 2006;12:333–9.
28. Wang HP, Chen SC. Upper abdominal ultrasound in the critically ill. Crit. Care Med. 2007;35(Suppl. S5):S208–15.
29. Aliaga M, Forel JM, De Bourmont S, Jung B, Thomas G, Mahul M, Bisbal M, Nougaret S, Hraiech S, Roch A, et al. Diagnostic yield and safety of CT scans in ICU. Intensive Care Med. 2015;41:436–43.
30. Beckmann U, Gillies DM, Berenholtz SM, Wu AW, Pronovost P. Incidents relating to the intra-hospital transfer of critically ill patients. An analysis of the reports submitted to the Australian Incident Monitoring Study in Intensive Care. Intensive CareMed. 2004;30:1579–85.
31. Lowe RJ, Boyd DR, Folk FA, Baker RJ. The negative laparotomy for abdominal trauma. J. Trauma. 1972;12:853–61.
32. Weigelt JA, Kingman RG. Complications of negative laparotomy for trauma. Am. J. Surg. 1988;156:544–7.
33. Sosa JL, Baker M, Puente I, Sims D, Sleeman D, Ginzburg E, Martin L. Negative laparotomy in abdominal gunshot wounds: Potential impact of laparoscopy. J. Trauma. 1995;38:194–7.
34. Palladino A, Vallicelli C, Perrina D, Convertini G, Coccolini F, Ansaloni L, Sartelli M, Catena F. Bedside Laparoscopy in the Critically Ill: A Review of the Literature. J Clin Med. 2024;13(6):1530. https://doi.org/10.3390/jcm13061530. PMID: 38541756; PMCID: PMC10971438
35. Laing GL, Skinner DL, Bruce JL, Bekker W, Oosthuizen GV, Clarke DL. A multi faceted quality improvement programme results in improved outcomes for the selective non-operative management of penetrating abdominal trauma in a developing world trauma centre. Injury. 2014;45(1):327–32.
36. Muckart DJ, Abdool-Carrim AT, King B. Selective conservative management of abdominal gunshot wounds: a prospective study. Br J Surg. 1990;77(6):652–5.
37. Cirocchi R, Birindelli A, Inaba K, Mandrioli M, Piccinini A, Tabola R, Carlini L, Tugnoli G, Di Saverio S. Laparoscopy for trauma and the changes in its use from 1990 to 2016: a current systematic review and meta-analysis. Surg Laparosc Endosc Percutan Tech. 2018;28(1):1–12.
38. Brandt ML, Luks FI, Spigland NA, DiLorenzo M, Laberge JM, Ouimet A. Diaphragmatic injury in children. J Trauma. 1992;32(3):298–301. Epub 1992/03/01
39. Zantut LF, Ivatury RR, Smith RS, Kawahara NT, Porter JM, Fry WR, et al. Diagnostic and therapeutic laparoscopy for penetrating abdominal trauma: a multicenter experience. J Trauma. 1997;42(5):825–9. discussion 9–31. Epub 1997/05/01
40. Adamthwaite DN. Traumatic diaphragmatic hernia: a new indication for laparoscopy. Br J Surg. 1984;71(4):315. Epub 1984/04/01
41. Powell BS, Magnotti LJ, Schroeppel TJ, Finnell CW, Savage SA, Fischer PE, et al. Diagnostic laparoscopy for the evaluation of occult diaphragmatic injury following penetrating thoracoabdominal trauma. Injury [Internet] May [cited 2022 Jan 27]. 2008;39(5):530–4. https://pubmed.ncbi.nlm.nih.gov/18336818/

42. Mjoli M, Oosthuizen G, Clarke D, Madiba T. Laparoscopy in the diagnosis and repair of diaphragmatic injuries in left-sided penetrating thoracoabdominal trauma: Laparoscopy in trauma. Surg Endosc [Internet]. 2015 Mar 1 [cited 2022 Jan 27];29(3):747–52. https://pubmed.ncbi.nlm.nih.gov/25125096/
43. Schuster K, Davis KA. Diaphragm. In: Moore EE, Feliciano DV, Mattox KL, editors. Trauma. 8th ed. McGraw-Hill Education; 2017. p. 539–49.
44. Hanna WC, Ferri LE. Acute Traumatic Diaphragmatic Injury [Internet]. Vol. 19, Thoracic Surgery Clinics. Thorac Surg Clin; 2009 [cited 2022 Jan 23]. p. 485–9. https://pubmed.ncbi.nlm.nih.gov/20112631/
45. Hanna WC, Ferri LE, Fata P, Razek T, Mulder DS. The current status of traumatic diaphragmatic injury: lessons learned from 105 patients over 13 years. Ann Thorac Surg [Internet]. 2008 Mar [cited 2021 Mar 8];85(3):1044–8. https://pubmed.ncbi.nlm.nih.gov/18291194/
46. Matthews BD, Bui H, Harold KL, Kercher KW, Adrales G, Park A, et al. Laparoscopic repair of traumatic diaphragmatic injuries. Surg Endosc Other Interv Tech [Internet]. 2003 Feb 1 [cited 2022 Jan 29];17(2):254–8. https://pubmed.ncbi.nlm.nih.gov/12399834/
47. Johnson JJ, Garwe T, Raines AR, et al. The use of laparoscopy in the diagnosis and treatment of blunt and penetrating abdominal injuries: 10-year experience at a level 1 trauma center. Am J Surg. 2013;205(3):317–21.
48. Nicolau AE. Is laparoscopy still needed in blunt abdominal trauma? Chirurgia. 2011;106:59–66.
49. Lamb CM, Garner JP. Selective non-operative management of civilian gunshot wounds to the abdomen: a systematic review of the evidence. Injury. 2014;45(4):659–66.
50. Coccolini F, Montori G, Catena F, Di Saverio S, Biffl W, Moore EE, Peitzman AB, Rizoli S, Tugnoli G, Sartelli M, Manfredi R, Ansaloni L. Liver trauma: WSES position paper. World J Emerg Surg. 2015;10:39.
51. Linnaus ME, Langlais CS, Garcia NM, et al. Failure of nonoperative management of pediatric blunt liver and spleen injuries: A prospective Arizona-Texas-Oklahoma-Memphis-Arkansas Consortium study. J Trauma Acute Care Surg. 2017;82:672–9.
52. Tharakan SJ, Kim AG, Collins JL, Nance ML, Blinman TA. Laparoscopy in pediatric abdominal trauma: A 13-year experience. Eur J Pediatr Surg. 2016;26:443–8.
53. Goldman R, Zilkoski M, Mullins R, et al. Delayed celiotomy for the treatment of bile leak, compartment syndrome, and other hazards of nonoperative management of blunt liver injury. Am J Surg. 2003;185:492–7.
54. Holmes JH, Wiebe DJ, Tataria M, Mattix KD, Mooney DP, Scaife ER, Brown RL, Groner JI, Brundage SI, Tres Scherer LR III, et al. The failure of nonoperative management in pediatric solid organ injury: a multi-institutional experience. J Trauma. 2005;59(6):1309–13.
55. Parrado R, Notrica DM, Garcia NM, Alder AC, Eubanks JW, Maxson RT, Letton RW, Ponsky TA, St Peter SD, Leys C, Bhatia A, Tuggle DW, Lawson KA, Ostlie DJ. Use of laparoscopy in pediatric blunt and spleen injury: an unexpectedly common procedure after cessation of bleeding. J Laparoendosc Adv Surg Tech A. 2019;29(10):1281–4.
56. Alemayehu H, Clifton M, Santore M, et al. Minimally invasive surgery for pediatric trauma-a multicenter review. J Laparoendosc Adv Surg Tech A. 2015;25:243–7.

Role of Laparoscopy After Non-Operative Management (NOM) of Liver and Splenic Injuries

31

Bruno Monteiro Pereira, Pablo R. Ottolino Lavarte, and Marcelo A. F. Ribeiro Jr.

Introduction

Blunt abdominal trauma remains one of the leading causes of morbidity and mortality worldwide, particularly among young adults and individuals involved in motor vehicle accidents, falls, and assaults. The liver and spleen are the most frequently injured solid organs in blunt abdominal trauma due to their anatomical position and vascularity [1].

Over recent decades, there has been a paradigm shift in the management of these injuries. Non-operative management (NOM) has become the standard of care for hemodynamically stable patients, supported by advances in diagnostic imaging, critical care, and interventional radiology. NOM has significantly decreased the need for laparotomy, reducing morbidity, reducing hospital length of stay, and preserving splenic and hepatic function [1–3].

B. M. Pereira (✉)
University of Vassouras, Surgical Group® President, Campinas Brazil. World Society of the Abdominal Compartment Past-President, Campinas, Brazil
e-mail: adm@gruposurgical.com.br

P. R. Ottolino Lavarte
Trauma and Emergency Unit, Dr. Sótero del Río Hospital, Pontifical Catholic University of Chile, Santiago, Chile

M. A. F. Ribeiro Jr.
R Adams Cowley Shock Trauma Center, University of Maryland School of Medicine, Baltimore, MD, USA

Pontifical Catholic University of Sao Paulo, Sorocaba, Brazil
e-mail: mfribeiro@som.umaryland.edu

© The Author(s), under exclusive license to Springer Nature Switzerland AG 2026

M. Cezillo, B. M. Pereira (eds.), *Minimally Invasive Surgery Trauma*,
https://doi.org/10.1007/978-3-032-28971-1_31

However, NOM is not without limitations. Failure rates, although generally low, are present and can lead to delayed hemorrhage, missed hollow viscus injuries, bile leaks, or other complications that require surgical intervention. This has led to an interest in minimally invasive techniques as adjuncts to NOM, with laparoscopy emerging as a valuable tool bridging conservative management and open surgery [3].

Laparoscopy provides both diagnostic and therapeutic capabilities, allowing direct visualization of intra-abdominal organs, identification of missed injuries, and treatment of complications while minimizing surgical trauma.

Minimally invasive surgery (MIS) has become an important diagnostic and therapeutic tool in select trauma patients as it has been shown to improve outcomes although internationally accepted guidelines are lacking. The most accepted current indications for laparoscopy for trauma patients are unexplained peritonitis, uncertain CT findings, any discrepancy between image findings and physical exam, free fluid in the intra-abdominal/intrathoracic cavity without major organ injuries or positive contrast extravasation on CT, uncertain peritoneal violation, and penetrating trauma in the thoracoabdominal transition in hemodynamically stable patients (the most well-defined indication) [1–3].

Historical Background

Historically, trauma surgery relied heavily on exploratory laparotomy as the primary diagnostic and therapeutic tool. In the 1980s and early 1990s, the surgical community began to recognize the significant morbidity associated with negative or non-therapeutic laparotomies, especially in stable patients. With the development of focused abdominal sonography for trauma (FAST) and computed tomography (CT), it became possible to more accurately assess intra-abdominal injuries without immediate surgical exploration.

By the late 1990s, NOM became the gold standard for most blunt hepatic and splenic injuries in stable patients. During this same period, laparoscopy began to gain acceptance in elective general surgery and gradually in trauma, though its application in trauma lagged due to concerns about missed injuries and limited access in unstable patients.

The twenty-first century ushered in a new era of enhanced laparoscopic capabilities, better instrumentation, and surgeon experience. These advances, combined with the understanding that certain complications of NOM (e.g., persistent bleeding, bilomas, pseudoaneurysms, and peritoneal signs without clear source) require surgical insight, created a niche for laparoscopy as a valuable diagnostic and therapeutic tool in the post-NOM setting [1–8].

Epidemiology and Injury Patterns

Liver and splenic injuries account for approximately 50–70% of all blunt abdominal trauma cases. The spleen is the most commonly injured organ in blunt trauma, followed closely by the liver. The American Association for the Surgery of Trauma (AAST) grading scale remains the gold standard for classifying the severity of liver and splenic injuries, ranging from Grade I (minor lacerations or contusions) to Grade V (vascular avulsions or shattered organs) [2–6].

Risk factors for failure of NOM include:

- High-grade injuries (AAST Grade IV and V)
- Presence of large hemoperitoneum
- Associated vascular injuries (pseudoaneurysm, arteriovenous fistula)
- Advanced patient age and comorbidities
- Delayed presentation or inadequate monitoring

Recognition of these factors aids in the early identification of patients who may require intervention [3–8].

NOM protocols involve:

- Continuous vital signs monitoring
- Serial hemoglobin and hematocrit assessments
- Repeat imaging studies (contrast-enhanced CT) to evaluate injury evolution.
- ICU admission for high-grade injuries or unstable patients
- Ready access to OR
- Availability of angiography and embolization in case of vascular injury or bleeding

Contraindications include hemodynamic instability refractory to resuscitation, signs of peritonitis, evisceration, or suspicion of hollow viscus injury requiring surgical repair.

When NOM Fails

Failure of NOM is primarily detected by clinical deterioration, including:

- Hemodynamic instability despite resuscitation
- Increasing abdominal pain or distension
- Declining hemoglobin levels suggesting ongoing bleeding

Radiologic indicators include expanding hematomas, active contrast extravasation on CT scans, and pseudoaneurysm formation.

Decision-making algorithms recommend prompt surgical consultation when these signs appear. While immediate laparotomy has traditionally been the intervention of choice, laparoscopy is increasingly considered when the patient is stable enough and the surgical team has adequate expertise [2–8].

Rationale for Laparoscopy After NOM

While NOM has an impressive success rate—reportedly >85% for liver injuries and > 90% for splenic injuries—certain cases evolve unfavorably. The role of laparoscopy is particularly crucial in the following scenarios:

- *Unclear clinical deterioration* in a patient initially managed non-operatively.
- *Suspected missed hollow viscus or diaphragm injuries.*
- *Ongoing low-grade bleeding* or contained hematomas with risk of rupture.
- *Complications such as bile leaks, abscesses, or splenic infarction* [11].
- *Retained hemoperitoneum* causing abdominal compartment syndrome or sepsis.

By allowing a targeted, controlled exploration with minimal physiologic impact, laparoscopy can effectively address these complications while preserving the benefits of a less invasive approach [2–4, 6, 8, 9].

Current Evidence and Indications for Laparoscopy After NOM

The Evidence Base

Over the last two decades, an increasing body of literature has supported the use of laparoscopy in trauma, particularly in cases where non-operative management (NOM) of liver and splenic injuries encounters complications. Multiple retrospective series, cohort studies, and systematic reviews have highlighted the safety, feasibility, and efficacy of laparoscopy as an intermediate step between observation and open surgery.

A review published in *The Journal of Trauma and Acute Care Surgery* (2020) analyzed over 500 cases of post-NOM complications and reported that laparoscopy avoided laparotomy in 65% of patients requiring surgical re-evaluation. Similarly, a multicenter European study (Laparoscopy in Trauma Study Group, 2021) showed that diagnostic laparoscopy had a 95% sensitivity for detecting post-traumatic hemoperitoneum or missed injuries, and was therapeutic in nearly half of the cases.

While no large randomized controlled trials currently exist comparing laparoscopy versus laparotomy after failed NOM, the trend in high-volume trauma centers is toward a stepwise, minimally invasive escalation strategy, starting with laparoscopy when feasible [2–10].

Indications for Laparoscopy After NOM

Laparoscopy after NOM should be considered in specific scenarios where imaging is inconclusive or clinical deterioration suggests evolving intra-abdominal pathology. The primary indications include [2–10, 12]:

Hemodynamic Deterioration Without Clear CT Findings

- Patients who initially met criteria for NOM but develop signs of peritonitis, tachycardia, or hypotension without radiologic evidence of free fluid progression.
- Laparoscopy can rule out hollow viscus injury, diaphragm rupture, or minor ongoing bleeding.

Suspected Missed Injuries

- Hollow viscus injuries (e.g., small bowel, colon), which may not be immediately apparent on imaging.
- Diaphragmatic injuries, especially on the left side, are notoriously difficult to detect by CT or ultrasound.

Persistent or Delayed Hemoperitoneum

- Especially relevant in liver injuries with slow oozing or splenic pseudoaneurysms.
- Retained clots may lead to peritonitis or abdominal compartment syndrome; laparoscopy allows clot evacuation and hemostasis.

Important note: *Objectives of Laparoscopy in the Presence of Hemoperitoneum*

1. *Evacuate Hemoperitoneum*: Decreases intra-abdominal pressure and pain; minimizes the risk of peritoneal irritation and abdominal compartment syndrome.
2. *Inspect the Organ In Situ (Spleen/Liver)*: Confirms the absence of active extravasation after embolization; detects hidden capsular tears.
3. *Rule Out Concomitant Sources of Bleeding*: Reduces the likelihood of delayed NOM failure due to undiagnosed associated injuries, such as mesenteric tears.

Bilomas, Bile Leaks, or Intra-Abdominal Abscesses

- In liver trauma, small biliary leaks can evolve into bilomas or infected collections.
- Laparoscopy can drain collections, place drains, and inspect liver parenchyma.

Splenic Sequelae Post-NOM

- Splenic infarction, pseudoaneurysm rupture, or large subcapsular hematomas with increasing size.
- In selected cases, partial laparoscopic splenectomy or even total splenectomy can be performed safely.

Persistent Unexplained Fever or Sepsis

- When CT-guided drainage fails or source is unclear, laparoscopy may assist in identifying and resolving the origin.

Laparoscopy can also be employed for peritoneal lavage to assess contamination or bleeding, guiding the decision for further intervention.

It is important to mention that there are also formal contraindications for laparoscopy, as hemodynamic instability and other absolute contraindications, like:

- Hypovolemic shock, stage II (non-responsive to fluid resuscitation), III, and IV
- Septic shock
- Severe cardiopulmonary dysfunction

- Severe head trauma
- Impossibility of performing pneumoperitoneum

Most contraindications are relative and exclusively determined based on surgeon's assessment and experience. Among them:

- Diffuse peritonitis.
- Severe chronic obstructive pulmonary disease with Hypercapnia.
- Obvious evisceration.
- Significant intra-abdominal adhesions.
- Previous abdominal surgery.
- Abdominal mass.
- Cardiorespiratory disease.
- Peritoneal tuberculosis.
- Insufficient pneumoperitoneum.
- Obesity.
- Umbilical hernia.
- Diaphragmatic hernia.

Timing of Laparoscopy

The optimal timing for laparoscopy after NOM is guided by clinical evolution:

- *Early laparoscopy (within 72 h)* is usually reserved for diagnostic dilemmas or evolving instability.
- *Delayed laparoscopy (after 5–7 days)* is more common in resolving complications such as bilomas or retained hemoperitoneum.

Delayed presentations are increasingly common, and in such cases, laparoscopy is often both diagnostic and therapeutic, reducing the need for major open surgery and promoting faster recovery [5–9].

Technical Considerations and Laparoscopic Strategies After NOM

Laparoscopy after non-operative management (NOM) of liver and splenic injuries requires a tailored approach that balances safety, diagnostic yield, and therapeutic potential. Post-traumatic patients may present anatomical distortions, adhesions, or organized hematomas, and the surgical team must be prepared for a wide range of intra-abdominal findings [9–12].

Preoperative Preparation

Patient selection and timing are crucial. Ensure that:

- Hemodynamic status is stable or responsive to fluid resuscitation.
- Imaging studies (CT scan with contrast, duplex ultrasound) have been fully interpreted. Remember: Every patient undergoing laparoscopy for trauma must have a CT angiography to allow a thorough evaluation of the abdominal cavity, especially to rule out retroperitoneal injuries.
- The indication is clearly defined (e.g., suspected bile leak, unexplained peritonitis, worsening hemoperitoneum, delayed pseudoaneurysm rupture).

Antibiotics should be administered preoperatively, especially if contamination or bile/infectious collections are suspected [3–7].

Cross-matched blood should be readily available in case of bleeding.

Operating Room Setup

- *Team*: Senior trauma surgeon with laparoscopic experience, assistant, scrub nurse familiar with advanced laparoscopy, anesthesiologist experienced with patients with potential intra-abdominal bleeding.
- *Positioning*: Supine with arms abducted. Trendelenburg or reverse Trendelenburg can be used as needed to mobilize intestines.
- *Pneumoperitoneum*: CO_2 insufflation is initiated carefully (typically via open Hasson technique at the umbilicus), particularly in patients with prior intra-abdominal injury or unknown adhesions.

Technical Aspects of Laparoscopy

Patient positioning typically involves a supine or slight reverse Trendelenburg position to optimize visualization of the upper abdomen. Trocar placement generally includes an umbilical port for the camera and additional working ports in the left and right upper quadrants tailored to the injury location [7].

Trocar Placement

Standard configuration involves:

- *Umbilical trocar (10 mm)* for the camera.
- *Left subcostal (5 mm)* and *right iliac fossa (5 mm)* trocars for instrumentation.
- Additional ports are placed under direct vision as required.

Placement can be modified based on the region of interest (Fig. 31.1):

- For *liver* exploration: subxiphoid or right upper quadrant port.
- For *spleen*: left upper quadrant and anterior axillary line access.

Exploration begins with a systematic survey of the peritoneal cavity, inspecting the liver, spleen, diaphragm, and hollow viscera. Identification of bile leaks is aided by the presence of bilious fluid or by using intraoperative cholangiography or dye tests [6–13].

- Hematomas and delayed bleeding are assessed by careful inspection and control of bleeding vessels using laparoscopic clips, sutures, or energy devices.
- Conversion to laparotomy should be considered if visualization is inadequate, there is extensive contamination, or uncontrolled bleeding is encountered.

Systematic Exploration Strategy

A methodical, quadrant-based approach helps avoid missed injuries (Fig. 31.2):

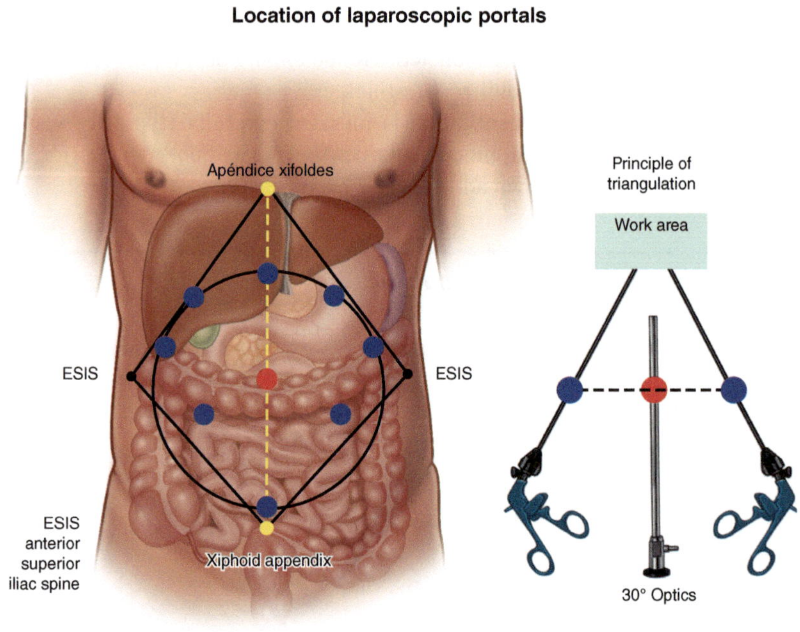

Fig. 31.1 Suggested trocar placement for laparoscopic evacuation of post-traumatic hemoperitoneum. This figure should illustrate the recommended positioning of trocars for laparoscopic evacuation following blunt or penetrating abdominal trauma. A 30° laparoscope is introduced through a supra-umbilical midline port. Working trocars are aligned in a triangular configuration directed toward the injured quadrant (liver or spleen). Anatomic landmarks—the xiphoid process and the anterior superior iliac spine (ASIS)—should be included to demonstrate spatial orientation and ensure proper spacing. Emphasis should be placed on triangulation principles, which: maximize instrument reach, minimize "sword-fighting," and maintain a stable optical apex, ensuring a broad and safe operative field [6–13]

1. *Diaphragms*: Check for occult ruptures, especially on the left side.
2. *Liver*: Assess segments for bile staining, lacerations, or active bleeding. Look for bilomas or subcapsular hematomas.
3. *Gallbladder and ducts*: In case of a bile leak, consider intraoperative cholangiography or drain placement.
4. *Spleen*: Evaluate the capsule, hilum, and parenchyma. Look for infarcts, subcapsular hematomas, or active bleeding.
5. *Intestines and mesentery*: Assess for missed perforations or hematomas.
6. *Pelvis and retroperitoneum*: Examine for pooled blood or collections, particularly after splenic or liver injury.

Specific Techniques for Common Complications

Clot Evacuation

- Gentle irrigation and suction.
- Avoid aggressive manipulation of liver or splenic parenchyma.
- Use endo-bags to remove large clots.

Control of Bleeding

- Low-pressure pneumoperitoneum (8–10 mmHg) may help reduce venous bleeding.
- Bipolar or advanced energy devices (e.g., Ligasure, Harmonic).
- Fibrin glue, hemostatic agents (Surgicel, TachoSil), or hemostatic sutures.

Bile Leak Management

- Drain placement near the leak.
- Clip or suture visible ductal leaks (caution with major bile ducts).
- Consider intraoperative cholangiography if anatomy is unclear.

Partial or Total Splenectomy

- Reserved for infarcted or bleeding spleens refractory to conservative management.
- Laparoscopic splenectomy may be completed using vascular staplers or energy devices.
- Always retrieve spleen in a bag to prevent seeding.

Drain Placement

- Always under direct vision.
- Consider double-drain technique (subhepatic + pelvic) in bilomas or infected hemoperitoneum. It is always recommended to use a closed-system silicone drain (Blake or Jackson-Pratt drains).

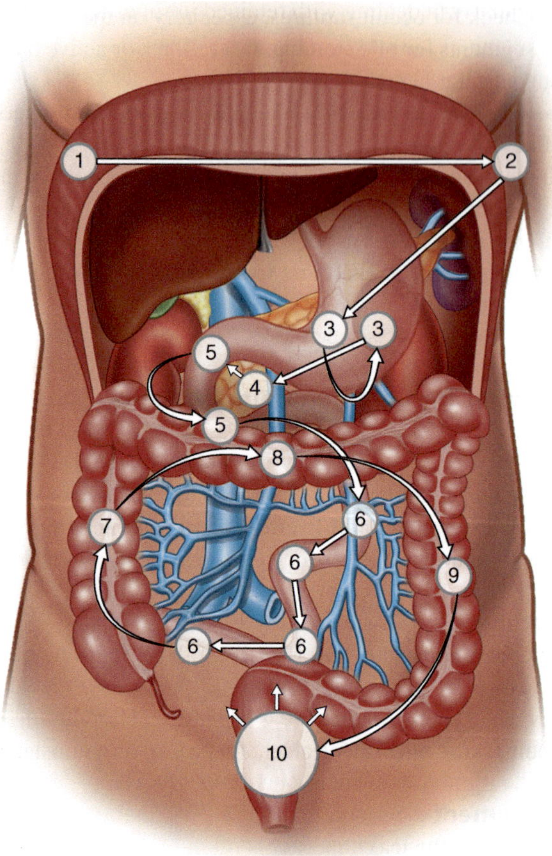

Fig. 31.2 Systematization of the laparoscopic abdominal exploration. This figure should depict an anatomically realistic human abdomen, demonstrating the recommended sequence for systematic exploration during laparoscopy to ensure safety and completeness: Right diaphragm and liver; Left diaphragm and spleen; Stomach (front and back). Pancreas (behind); Duodenum (above and below); Small bowel from the Treitz ligament to the cecal valve (forward and backward); Right colon and behind; Transverse colon and behind; Left colon and behind; Rectum and pelvis; Once the first evaluation is completed, a second exploration should be performed following the same sequence. The design should be anatomically accurate and visually clear, with directional indicators illustrating the sequence of inspection [13]

Focused Intervention, Improved Outcomes

As mentioned before, in recent decades, the paradigm shift in the management of blunt hepatic and splenic injuries has favored non-operative management (NOM) for hemodynamically stable patients. NOM has proven to be safe and effective in selected cases, significantly reducing the morbidity associated with exploratory laparotomies. However, as the scope of NOM widens, so does the recognition of its limitations—particularly in dealing with retained intraperitoneal collections such as clotted hemoperitoneum or bile leaks [11].

In this context, laparoscopy emerges not as a failure of NOM, but as an extension of its philosophy—a minimally invasive, organ-preserving strategy designed to intervene only when clinically necessary. Specifically, targeted laparoscopy performed after NOM offers substantial advantages in removing old blood, bile, or inflammatory fluid collections and modulating the systemic inflammatory response, often with minimal physiological disturbance to the patient.

Evacuation of Retained Hemoperitoneum

Following blunt injury to the liver or spleen, hemoperitoneum is a frequent CT finding that usually reabsorbs on its own. When the initial bleed is large or the injury is high-grade, however, intraperitoneal blood may persist, clot, and evolve into encapsulated or loculated collections. These retained pools can become a focus for infection, sustain the inflammatory response, and cause ongoing abdominal pain, ileus, or fever. In this scenario, laparoscopy offers a minimally invasive complement to non-operative management.

Its objectives are threefold. First, evacuating the retained hemoperitoneum lowers intra-abdominal pressure, relieves pain, and helps prevent both prolonged peritoneal irritation and abdominal compartment syndrome. Second, direct inspection of the injured organ in situ—whether spleen or liver—verifies that no active extravasation remains after embolization or observation, while allowing the surgeon to identify occult capsular tears that imaging may have missed. Third, a systematic survey of the peritoneal cavity rules out concomitant bleeding sources such as mesenteric or ligamentous injuries, thereby reducing the risk of delayed failure of non-operative management.

By suctioning old blood under direct vision and avoiding a full laparotomy, laparoscopy removes undrained collections with markedly lower morbidity, reinforcing the safety and success of conservative treatment in appropriately selected trauma patients [9, 11–13].

Management of Bile Leaks

In hepatic trauma, particularly in grade III–V injuries, disruption of intrahepatic bile ducts can result in bile peritonitis or bilomas. While many of these cases are self-limited or amenable to ERCP with biliary stenting, certain scenarios benefit from surgical intervention.

Laparoscopy provides an excellent platform for both diagnosis and treatment of bile leaks, especially when ERCP access is delayed or inconclusive. Through minimally invasive access, surgeons can drain bilomas, lavage the peritoneal cavity, and even place targeted suction drains. This reduces ongoing peritoneal irritation and enhances patient comfort while supporting faster recovery [11].

Modulation of Inflammatory Response

Beyond mechanical drainage, *l*aparoscopy plays a subtler, immunomodulatory role. Persistent peritoneal contamination by blood, bile, or necrotic tissue fuels a systemic inflammatory response syndrome (SIRS), potentially escalating into sepsis or multi-organ dysfunction. The early laparoscopic clearance of irritants helps interrupt this process by:

- Decreasing *cytokine load* within the peritoneal cavity.
- Limiting systemic absorption of pro-inflammatory mediators.
- Reducing *peritoneal macrophage activation* and neutrophil migration.
- Enhancing *immune homeostasis* and restoring gut barrier function.

As such, laparoscopy functions not only as a mechanical tool but as a biological reset, mitigating secondary inflammatory complications that would otherwise prolong ICU stay, hospital length of stay, or necessitate escalation to laparotomy. Another strength of laparoscopy in this context is its diagnostic capability. While CT imaging and ultrasound remain the cornerstone for monitoring post-NOM patients, they may fall short in distinguishing between sterile fluid collections, bile, pus, or active bleeding. Laparoscopy permits direct visualization, often guiding management toward less invasive resolution and preventing unnecessary open procedures. Importantly, the minimally invasive nature of the technique translates to less postoperative pain, faster mobilization, shorter length of stay, and lower risk of adhesion formation or incisional hernia—benefits that are particularly meaningful in the trauma population. The optimal role of laparoscopy is in patients who are clinically stable yet showing signs of NOM-related complications—persistent fever, leukocytosis, abdominal pain, or imaging suggestive of organized fluid. The timing is also critical: early laparoscopy (within 5–10 days) has shown better outcomes than late intervention, as the collections become less organized and more amenable to minimally invasive drainage. In the modern trauma algorithm, laparoscopy after NOM is not a sign of therapeutic failure—but rather a symbol of maturity in trauma care. It represents the seamless integration of precision surgery with organ preservation, physiologic respect, and inflammatory modulation. The focused use of laparoscopy for suctioning old blood or bile leverages all the strengths of minimally invasive access while offering meaningful clinical benefits. In skilled hands, it becomes a tailored, elegant extension of NOM—one that favors healing over heroics [3–8, 11–13].

Clinical Scenarios and Case Series

Example 1 A 30-year-old male with a Grade III splenic injury managed initially by NOM presented on day 5 with sudden abdominal pain and hypotension. CT showed increasing hemoperitoneum without active extravasation. Diagnostic laparoscopy revealed a bleeding subcapsular hematoma, controlled laparoscopically with hemostatic agents, avoiding laparotomy.

Example 2 A 45-year-old female with a Grade III liver laceration developed bile peritonitis on day 7 post-injury. Laparoscopy identified a bile leak from the left lobe, which was repaired laparoscopically with drainage placement, leading to recovery without open surgery.

Several recent case series demonstrate the safety and feasibility of laparoscopy in these scenarios, with reduced morbidity and hospital stay compared to traditional open surgery.

Advantages and Limitations

Advantages:

- Minimally invasive with less postoperative pain and faster recovery
- Improved diagnostic accuracy over imaging alone
- Ability to treat certain complications without laparotomy
- Reduced risk of wound infections and hernias

Limitations:

- Potential for missed injuries, especially in polytrauma or complex trauma
- Requires advanced laparoscopic skills and experience in trauma surgery
- Limited utility in unstable patients or those with extensive contamination
- Risk of delaying definitive treatment if laparoscopy is unsuccessful

Evidence from the Literature

Key studies published in journals such as *The Journal of Trauma and Acute Care Surgery*, *Annals of Surgery*, and *Surgery* have documented the expanding role of laparoscopy after failed NOM of liver and splenic injuries.

Meta-analyses comparing laparoscopy to open conversion after failed NOM suggest laparoscopy reduces hospital stay and postoperative complications without increasing missed injuries.

Recent prospective studies emphasize the importance of patient selection, surgical expertise, and institutional resources for successful implementation.

Future Directions

The role of laparoscopy is expected to grow with advances in surgical technology, including integration with robotic platforms providing enhanced dexterity and visualization.

Laparoscopy may also play an increasing role in damage control strategies, allowing staged minimally invasive interventions.

Enhanced recovery after surgery (ERAS) protocols and improved postoperative monitoring using telemetry and point-of-care ultrasound will complement laparoscopy, optimizing patient outcomes.

Conclusion

Laparoscopy is emerging as a valuable tool following failed NOM of liver and splenic injuries, offering minimally invasive diagnostic and therapeutic options. Early recognition of NOM failure, careful patient selection, and surgical expertise are paramount to success. As technology and trauma care evolve, laparoscopy will increasingly bridge the gap between conservative and open surgical management in blunt abdominal trauma.

References

1. Smith J, et al. Role of laparoscopy in blunt abdominal trauma: a review. J Trauma Acute Care Surg. 2022;92(3):450–6. https://doi.org/10.1097/TA.0000000000003540.
2. Lee C, et al. Outcomes of laparoscopy after failed nonoperative management of splenic injury. Ann Surg. 2021;273(4):654–60. https://doi.org/10.1097/SLA.0000000000003855.
3. Zago TM, Pereira BM, Calderan TR, Hirano ES, Rizoli S, Fraga GP. Blunt hepatic trauma: comparison between surgical and nonoperative treatment. Rev Col Bras Cir. 2012;39(4):307–13.
4. Broecker J, Forssten S, Forssten M, Mohseni S, Ribeiro MAF Jr. Survey of minimally invasive surgery usage for traumatic injuries among high-income and low-middle income countries. Panam J Trauma Crit Care Emerg Surg. 2025;14(2):1–5. https://doi.org/10.5005/jp-journals-10030-14803.
5. Zago TM, Pereira BM, Calderan TRA, Godinho M, Nascimento B, Fraga GP. Nonoperative management for patients with grade IV blunt hepatic trauma. World J Emerg Surg. 2012;7(Suppl 1):S8.
6. Pereira BM. Non-operative management of hepatic trauma and the interventional radiology: an update review. Indian J Surg. 2012;74(1):22–8. (volume e páginas atualizados conforme base da revista).
7. Zago TM, Pereira BM, Nascimento B, Alves MSC, Calderan TRA, Fraga GP. Trauma hepático: uma experiência de 21 anos. Rev Col Bras Cir. 2013;40(4):318–22.
8. Ribeiro Junior MAF, Tebar GK, Salgueiro JLR, Galindo GFC, Hughes JD, AlSayari A, DeSoucy ES, Mohseni S. Role and limitations of laparoscopy in abdominal trauma Med Res Arch. 2023;11(8). https://doi.org/10.18103/mra.v11i8.4333.
9. Gonzalez F, et al. Diagnostic and therapeutic laparoscopy in liver trauma: a multicenter study. Surgery. 2023;174(2):331–8. https://doi.org/10.1016/j.surg.2023.01.005.
10. Nasr A, Mello AL, de Magalhães AC, Gonçalves FL, Oliveira M, Vasconcelos PO, de Campos T, Ribeiro MA Jr. Nonoperative management of liver trauma: results of the consensus of SBAIT (Brazilian Trauma Society). Panam J Trauma Crit Care Emerg Surg. 2025;14(1):5–12. https://doi.org/10.5005/jp-journals-10030-1480.
11. Tanaka H, et al. Laparoscopic management of complications following nonoperative treatment of blunt hepatic trauma. World J Emerg Surg. 2020;15:45. https://doi.org/10.1186/s13017-020-00328-5.
12. Kumar A, et al. Meta-analysis of laparoscopy versus open surgery after failed nonoperative management of abdominal trauma. J Trauma Acute Care Surg. 2024;95(1):110–7. https://doi.org/10.1097/TA.0000000000003842.
13. Koto MZ, Matsevych OY, Aldous C. Diagnostic laparoscopy for trauma: how not to miss injuries. J Laparoendosc Adv Surg Tech A. 2018;28(5):506–13. https://doi.org/10.1089/lap.2017.0562.

Trauma Laparoscopy Complications

32

Marcus Cezillo, Robson Uwagoya, Germano Andrade Maranduba, Dirceu de Castro Rezende Júnior, and Ricardo de Deus Honorato

Introduction

Videolaparoscopy has become a powerful tool in the management of polytrauma patients, offering diagnostic and therapeutic benefits, particularly in hemodynamically stable patients with thoracoabdominal injuries. The primary indications for diagnostic laparoscopy (DL) include evaluating unnoticed injuries in stable patients with blunt or penetrating trauma and therapeutic laparoscopy (TL) for managing specific conditions identified during DV. However, the procedure's success is critically dependent on strict adherence to steps that guarantee the safety and effectiveness of the method. These include hemodynamic stability, nasogastric and bladder catheterization, cardiac monitoring, general anesthesia with endotracheal pressure control, controlled gas insufflation, trocar insertion under direct vision, smooth handling of structures, and strict safe surgery protocols used in open trauma surgeries. These aspects, associated with the presence of a qualified surgical team with trauma expertise and access to appropriate equipment and instruments, can minimize the risk of complications [1, 2].

M. Cezillo (✉)
Trauma Surgery Department, Hospital de Base do Distrito Federal (HBDF), Brasília, DF, Brazil

R. Uwagoya
FAM (Centro Universitário das Américas), Department of Medicine Departament of Pediatric Surgery at Antônio Giglio Municipal Hospital, São Paulo, Brazil

G. A. Maranduba
Hospital de Base (HBDF) Brasília / DF, Brasília, Brazil

D. de Castro Rezende Júnior
Hospital de Base do Distrito Federal (HBDF), Faculty of Medicine Unieuro DF, Brasília/DF, Brasília, Brazil

R. de Deus Honorato
Grupo de Pesquisa e Extensão em Cirurgia (GPEC), Hospital Municipal Antônio Giglio (HMAG), Osasco, Brazil

© The Author(s), under exclusive license to Springer Nature Switzerland AG 2026

M. Cezillo, B. M. Pereira (eds.), *Minimally Invasive Surgery Trauma*,
https://doi.org/10.1007/978-3-032-28971-1_32

Conversely, contraindications such as hemodynamic instability, peritoneal irritation, evisceration, or patients with high Injury Severity Scores (ISS) requiring immediate laparotomy must be carefully respected. Failure to follow these criteria or a bad indication significantly increases the risk of complications, including delayed diagnosis of life-threatening injuries, uncontrolled hemorrhage, or worsening of existing physiological derangements [1, 2].

The complications associated with laparoscopy in trauma range from intraoperative issues, such as iatrogenic injuries to organs, inadvertent insufflation site to postoperative problems, including infections and delayed recognition of missed injuries. Additionally, physiological alterations induced by pneumoperitoneum, such as hypercapnia and reduced visceral perfusion, pose unique challenges in polytrauma patients. Preventing these complications requires not only careful patient selection and adherence to criteria but also the involvement of skilled surgical teams, rigorous intraoperative monitoring, and well-established protocols [1, 2].

Although videolaparoscopy continues to expand its role in trauma care, a clear understanding of its limitations, potential risks, and the necessity of respecting its indications is essential for optimizing its application and improving clinical outcomes [1, 2].

Complications in Laparoscopy for Polytrauma Patients

Laparoscopy presents unique physiologic and technical challenges of trauma care that expose patients to a variety of complications. These complications are broadly described and manners to prevent are presented [1, 2]:

1. Equipment malfunction and failure
2. Laparoscopic access
3. Injuries related to inappropriate handling of organs
4. Missed injuries
5. Safety considerations in laparoscopic surgery

Equipment Malfunction and Failure

Although infrequent, some failures may occur during the setup and initiation of laparoscopic surgery, such as inadequate supply of insufflation gas, damaged laparoscopic light source/fiber optic conduit, faulty camera, malfunctioning instruments, or software-related issues [1, 3].

It's important to check the equipment and availability of all necessary materials prior to the surgery. If it cannot be promptly resolved, the surgeon should choose laparotomy. If the problem arises during the procedure, the surgeon must quickly decide whether to attempt to resolve the failure or convert the procedure to laparotomy. Keep in mind that, in many cases, polytrauma patients cannot hold on delays during their diagnosis and treatment, as clinical deterioration can occur rapidly over time [1].

These events can often be prevented by performing daily, controlled checks of the available resources and ensuring their functionality. Furthermore, all components used should be stored securely and protected from external factors, such as contamination and moisture, access to the equipment must be controlled and users identified every time [1].

There are a lot of different brands and types of equipment. Trauma team must know their available tools and how to deal with possible problems by the trauma team in the operating room or other personnel in the hospital. [1]

Laparoscopic Access

Pneumoperitoneum Induced by Carbon Dioxide (CO_2)

When the pneumoperitoneum increases intra-abdominal pressure, it can reduce venous return, resulting in bradycardia and hypotension, which can aggravate preoperative intravascular depletion after additional hypovolemia followed by hypoperfusion. Other complications related to gas insufflation include bradyarrhythmias due to peritoneal stretch receptor-mediated stimulation of vagal nerves during pneumoperitoneum [1, 4]

Initial establishment of pneumoperitoneum should occur at a slow rate, with the patient in a supine/flat position. If the patient becomes hypotensive or hemodynamically unstable during any part of the procedure, the pneumoperitoneum should be released and the patient returned to a neutral/flat position or even placed in the Trendelenburg position [5].

In rare cases, the laparoscopic approach may need to be aborted, depending on the operative stage of the procedure. In patients with associated chest trauma, pneumoperitoneum may worsen contralateral lung collapse [1, 4, 5].

To prevent these complications, we must limit the IAP to <12 mmHg and continuous monitoring of blood pressure, oxygen saturation, and end-tidal CO_2 [1].

Besides being considered an inert gas, the use of CO_2 can cause significant physiologic changes and decrease of the pH while the pneumoperitoneum is established, affected by the increase in carbon dioxide partial pressure ($PaCO_2$). This occurs due to a significant local peritoneal acidosis and it is independent of systemic pH and its effect promptly returns to a normal value after the desufflation. It shows that pneumoperitoneum, during trauma laparoscopy, causes temporary localized peritoneal non-systemic acidosis that is central to the mechanism of CO_2-mediated attenuation of the inflammatory response following laparoscopic surgery [4–6].

Pneumoperitoneum used during laparoscopic cholecystectomy (LC) may cause numerous changes in the cardiovascular, hormonal, and neuroendocrine systems, including activations of coagulation-fibrinolysis and endothelial activation, according to some articles, despite the paucity of publications on pH-based CO_2 and coagulopathy. The longer pneumoperitoneum stay revealed more noticeable changes in endothelial activation, decreased fibrinolysis, and enhanced coagulation. These changes may indicate an unbalanced coagulation-fibrinolysis state and raise the risk of venous thrombosis [7].

Dommez (2016) observed the effects of applying pressures of 10 mmHg or 14 mmHg on human hemodynamics and metabolism and described a notable rise in coagulation factors. Higher CO_2 pressure (14 mmHg) pneumoperitoneum has a greater detrimental influence on fibrinolysis and the coagulation cascade, but all of these changes were reversible. No pulmonary embolism was observed pulmonary emboli or clinical or ultrasonographic deep vein thrombosis (DVT) [8].

Based on this information, it's advisable to use the lower pneumoperitoneum pressure (10 mmHg) if possible, but the higher pressure (14 mmHg), if indicated, must be used, in order to offer adequate view and mobilization field for laparoscopic maneuvers. In this situation, stay always alert to the monitor and signs of respiratory distress, cardiac changes and coagulopathy derangement, indicating the moment to reduce the pressure or converting the proceeding to an open approach [7, 8].

Complication from Access

Some of the approaches used to do the first access to the abdominal cavity include the Hasson approach (under direct vision), single trocar insertion (blind insertion), or trocar insertion guided by camera. All these techniques are unique in their advantages and possible risks. Access-related complications are not so frequent, but when they do occur, they involve injuries to either the abdominal wall or intra-abdominal vessels, bowel perforation, and injury to hollow viscera like the bladder, stomach, or intestines. Such complications are not good; however, most of them are not serious enough to cause hemorrhagic shock, peritonitis, or multi-organ dysfunction syndrome, particularly when swift recognition and intervention have been possible [9, 10].

Patients who are at higher risk for such complications typically include those who are obese, those with a low body mass index, individuals with underlying conditions like hepatomegaly or splenomegaly, as well as those with coagulation disorders or patients who are on anticoagulant therapy. These risk factors can complicate the procedure, making it more challenging for the surgeon to access the abdominal cavity safely and to manage any unforeseen events that may arise during the process. Proper preoperative assessment and careful technique can significantly reduce the incidence of these complications [1, 9, 10].

One method to mitigate the risk of complications during peritoneal cavity access is by employing the technique of direct visualization. This can be achieved through two approaches. Currently, specialized cannulas, such as the Endoscopic Threaded Imaging Ports (EndoTIP), are specifically designed for this purpose. These devices obviate the need for traditional trocars and facilitate a layer-by-layer entry into the peritoneal cavity under continuous direct visualization of the anatomical structures. The application of rotational force, parallel to the skin surface, minimizes the risk of injury to critical structures, including blood vessels and viscera. Furthermore, this rotational insertion technique prevents the alignment of injuries across the muscle, fascia, and peritoneum, thereby significantly reducing the incidence of incisional hernias and soft tissue trauma, as supported by both clinical and experimental studies [11, 12].

In facilities where such specialized devices are unavailable, an alternative adaptation can be implemented using standard trocars. During the insertion of the initial trocar, the laparoscope may be positioned within the trocar itself, enabling real-time direct visualization. This approach facilitates the identification and avoidance of critical structures, thus enhancing the safety and precision of the procedure [13].

Both the use of specialized cannulas and the adaptation of conventional trocars with direct visualization represent effective strategies to minimize the occurrence of severe complications, thereby improving the overall safety profile of laparoscopic access [1].

Injuries Related to Inappropriate Handling of Organs

Inappropriate handling of organs includes injuries from inadequate instruments or excessive traction of structures and manipulation of organs. Avoiding iatrogenic injuries is essential during laparoscopy because additional and non-expected lesions can lead a controlled situation to an imminent disaster. The right laparoscopic instruments must be chosen and used in each specific situation, adapting a certain to a determined tissue. It's necessary to compare the kind of tissue (tough vs. delicate), the instrument's properties (traumatic vs. non-traumatic), and the anticipated purpose (dissection vs. retraction), all these characteristics influence the instrument selection [1, 15]·

Tools frequently used in laparoscopic procedures include tissue graspers, laparoscopic scissors, clip applicators, needle holders, staplers, and suction devices have their classification based on the surface properties of the jaw blades and the force used by the surgeon [1, 14, 15].

Organs with thin serosa like small or large intestine, esophagus (absence of serosa), biliary tree, ureter, veins, arteries, and nerves are sensitive structures that shouldn't be handled with Maryland's forceps because they are a traumatic tool neither with other traumatic instruments. For these structures non-traumatic forceps should be utilized instead. It is important to remember that, if not handled carefully, even atraumatic graspers can cause tissue damage. Even using atraumatic graspers, instruments that have handles with ratchet must not be locked or if they have a single handle, it must grab the tissue gently, using the minimum strength necessary to move the structure without sliding out the grasper jaws. Organs with thick serosa, like stomach and bladder, despite the lower risk of perforation, compared to the thin-serosa organ, can damage the serosa if a traumatic instrument is used, increasing the morbidity and risk of secondary perforation. For these organs, the atraumatic grasper is also indicated [15, 16].

Solid organs such as the liver, kidneys, pancreas, and spleen must not be grabbed. It's mobilization is better done using a gauze ball for leaning on the instrument jaw or with the jaws open it can lean under the solid organ surface or from its side and gently move, taking care to distribute the strength on the greater possible surface and respecting the limit of the pressure exerted on each point [15, 16].

Blunt dissections can be made using Maryland's forceps, with their pointing jaws or using suction cannula for moving tissue away. Another efficient way to do blunt dissection is using a gauze by grabbing (with Maryland's forceps) the gauze two-time folded or rolling the gauze on the forceps and rub it on the structure to detach tissues and isolate main structures [15, 16].

Always utilize sharp equipment under direct vision, such as diathermy hooks and laparoscopic scissors. Because it can burn or cut structures that are not in that exact frame of the image [17].

Excessive traction can lead to avulsion of mesentery, blood vessels, bile ducts, or hollow viscera. It's necessary to realize the limit of the mobilization that each structure tolerates. The running bowel must be conducted in an area as restricted as possible avoiding large mobilizations, especially at areas with fixed loops like duodeno-jejunal ligament and ileocecal valve. Eventually, adherences can create acquired fixed loops which can be handled with additional care. The colon, except the sigmoid portion, has the mobilization limited by its retroperitoneal attachment. Its mobilization is safer when grabbed by its taeniae coli, which are ribbon-like bands of thickened smooth muscle where you can grab and lift with more safety. If necessary, colon detachment by medial rotation maneuver must be performed in order to have more range of mobilization [18].

Missed Injuries

Beyond complications related to cavity manipulation and surgical access, one must consider unnoticed injuries, which often progress unfavorably, potentially leading to conditions such as sepsis and multiple organ dysfunction. During the early era of diagnostic laparoscopies, the incidence of unnoticed injuries in cases of abdominal trauma ranged from 41% to 77%. However, with advancements in laparoscopic equipment, the refinement of surgical techniques, and the improvement of surgeons' learning curves, this figure has decreased to less than 1% [19].

This minimal rate of unnoticed injuries underscores the efficacy of laparoscopy in managing hemodynamically stable patients with polytrauma. In contrast, laparotomies provoke a substantially greater metabolic and immunological response, and the average rate of non-therapeutic laparotomies remains as high as 61% [20, 21].

The most effective strategy to prevent unnoticed injuries lies in the meticulous adherence to well-defined steps, ensuring that both the indication for the procedure and its execution are satisfactory. As previously emphasized, laparoscopy is contraindicated in patients who are hemodynamically unstable or in situations where the surgical team does not possess the requisite expertise. In cases of penetrating trauma, whenever feasible, the utilization of computed tomography (CT) is highly recommended to assess potential injuries and to trace the trajectory of projectiles or blades. This imaging modality facilitates preoperative planning and improves surgical outcomes [22].

It is essential that the surgical team adheres strictly to the predefined, step-by-step protocol for diagnostic laparoscopy. This includes systematically evaluating the abdominal cavity in stages, ensuring that no anatomical structures are overlooked, as outlined in detail in Chap. 11. Such a systematic approach enhances diagnostic accuracy and minimizes the risk of missed injuries. Lastly, the surgeon must achieve complete satisfaction with the procedure and the thorough exploration of the abdominal cavity, ensuring that no additional benefit would be gained from converting to an open laparotomy [23].

As previously discussed, laparoscopy is a minimally invasive procedure with high diagnostic sensitivity and low rates of unnoticed injuries. Additionally, it is less metabolically and immunologically aggressive for the patient, leading to shorter hospital stays and reduced morbidity and mortality. The key for not having inconvenient bad surprises is to follow step-by-step procedures that give you the confidence to bail out fully satisfied with your searching method and findings related to the trauma mechanism. It is paramount that the procedure can be performed with a strict, methodical, and systematic approach to minimize the risk of complications and ensure optimal outcomes [1, 20, 22].

Safety Considerations in Laparoscopic Surgery

Trauma surgeons should consider safety aspects during the preoperative, intraoperative, and postoperative moment that avoid unexpected situations and preventable complications, contributing to the success of the proceeding [24].

Preoperative Moment

Despite the surgical urgency that involves the trauma laparoscopy, it's ideal to check the medical history for possible patient allergies and early administration of drugs during the preoperative moment. Antibiotic prophylaxis (AP) in surgery is critical to prevent surgical site infections. It is defined as the prevention of infectious complications by administering an effective antimicrobial agent before exposure to contamination during surgery. Prolonged AP (24 h) and/or antibiotic therapy should be considered in patients with hollow viscus injury (blunt or penetrating) with surgical repair, covering Gram-negative and anaerobic organisms, and its continuity depends on the source control achievement [24].

AP is not indicated routinely in blunt liver and splenic trauma treated non-operatively. In case of kidney trauma, it may need AP for patients with risk of infectious complication, such as presence of devitalized tissue, presence of urinoma, associated bowel and pancreatic injury, multiple comorbidities, and immunosuppression. AP is also indicated for patients sustaining pancreatic trauma with severe pancreatitis or concomitant bowel injury [25].

Both high and low energy forces can cause penetrating wounds, caused by stab wounds and gunshot wounds, respectively. High-energy wounds cause the most soft tissue damage, which usually leads to ischemia or necrotic tissue, which is the ideal medium for bacterial growth. AP should not be administered for longer than 24 h after an isolated intestinal injury, according to all research; however, few studies have accounted for the type of penetrating lesion [26].

All patients with penetrating hollow viscus injury should get a single preoperative dose of prophylactic antibiotics with broad-spectrum aerobic and anaerobic coverage (to be continued for no more than 24 h). No additional antibiotics are needed if there is no hollow viscus lesion or if there are isolated solid abdominal organs. The dosage of antibiotics given to patients who are admitted with hemorrhagic shock may be doubled or tripled, and this process may be repeated after each ten units of blood transfusion until no further blood loss occurs. If at all possible, avoid aminoglycosides in patients with severe injuries because to their inadequate activity. Change the prior empiric therapeutic antibiotic to another guided by the intraoperative findings, if relevant [27].

It's essential to ensure that there are no malfunctions or inadequacies in the functionality of the instrument. When an instrument's functionality is compromised, the surgeon may need to exert more force or perform broader, more forceful movements to complete dissection or clipping, which increases the stress and risk of injury [28].

Intraoperative Moment

In addition to causing musculoskeletal pain, poor ergonomic practices during surgery have an impact on the surgeon's performance and personal life. A good ergonomics depends on the height of the operating table, which should be set between 64 and 77 cm from the floor since elbow-height instruments cause the least amount of discomfort and make operations easier. When the monitor image is at or within 25 ideal degrees below the eye's horizontal plane, it provides the best vision for a laparoscopy. Based on existing research, this results in the least amount of neck strain. A "chin-up" position on the part of the surgeon is not recommended. The second monitor is crucial during operations where surgeons switch ports and postures because it relieves neck strain on assistance. Trocars are typically positioned in a triangle (triangulation) to allow for easy instrument handling and sufficient visualization during laparoscopy. The distance between the target organ and the port where the optical trocar is positioned should be 15 to 20 cm. The two remaining trocars are typically positioned 5–7 cm on either side of the optical trocars, in the same 15–20 cm arc as the reference point. This eliminates the issue of abdominal wall interference and long handles caused by ports that are positioned too close or too far from the target tissue, allowing the instruments to operate at an angle of 60° to 90°. To prevent instrument collisions, two additional auxiliary ports can be positioned laterally in the same arc if needed [29].

Occasionally, the arc formed will be positioned as one of the lateral port trocars and lack the optical characteristics of the central trocar. When a 10 mm optical trocar is inserted into the inframumbilical region during appendicectomy, this technique is frequently employed. Laterally, two more trocars are positioned beneath these. Depending on the surgical aim, this configuration can provide a better laparoscopic vision and a dramatically different hand-eye coordination, providing greater exposition and work space. The elevation angles and the manipulation have a direct relationship. The equivalent ideal elevation angle that produces the quickest execution time and the best quality performance is 60° when the manipulation angle is 60° [30].

For optimum performance and work efficiency, wide elevation angles are required for wide manipulation angles. Since this combination has the quickest execution time, the elevation angle should likewise be 30° when the patient's anatomy or build requires a 30° manipulation angle. The ideal ergonomic configuration for endoscopic surgery includes equal azimuth angles and a manipulation angle between 45° and 75°. Obesity, pregnancy, and certain abdominal conditions caused by adhesions, for instance, may necessitate a work angle larger than the optimal range; in these cases, it may be necessary to forward or forback the trocar position (taking into account the insufflated abdomen's circular shape) in order to reach the goal. The position of the work trocars should be determined following the formation of the pneumoperitoneum, the evaluation of the cavity using the camera view, the surgical target, and any potential areas to be examined [31].

Every time that the exposure of a certain structure is not adequate or one trauma surgeon's hand is being used for presenting any other structure, it's advisable to use an additional 5 mm port. The trauma surgeon's hands must be (both) free for dissecting and manipulating with free mobility to all directions, it cannot be restricted to any presentation or exposure, when it happens, maybe it's time to add an extra 5 mm port [32].

The trauma surgeon must consider a second opinion in situations that are new or when there are low options of technical repertoire to deal with a problem. In these cases, it's better to ask for a second opinion for other trauma team members (ideally an experienced member) or consider backing out and take another strategy if unsafe to proceed. Don't hand-over in the middle of the procedure, in case of total lack of options and the absence of a plan by insufficient experience in that particular situation, think about the patient's safety and consider converting to an open procedure [32].

Pneumoperitoneum may be lost during laparoscopy as a result of excessive aspiration or suction, unintentional trocar valve opening, or equipment malfunction. When that occurs, even for a few seconds, the surgeon cannot see the tip of the instrument. When that occurs, the tools must be removed right away without slowly closing the jaws. It prevents unintentional burning, perforation, and severe traction of structures [33].

Excessive fog from cauterization, condensation-induced optic blurring, and the buildup of smoke, blood, and particulate matter on the scope glass can all reduce visibility. By leaving the trocar valve partially open for gas exchange and, consequently, aspirating liquids with gauze to reduce gas suction, it can be managed. Insufflator devices that use heated and humidified gas, antifogging solutions, or even heating the optic lens with hot saline water can all help to reduce temperature and humidity differences between the cavity and the lens. Compared to anti-fog solution or chlorhexidine solution, the use of warm saline results in a much lower number of fogging occurrences, improving surgical continuity. Avoiding close contact with the entering gas by placing the insufflation hose in a trocar that is 10 to 12 mm apart from the optic trocar is another related suggestion [34].

Following port withdrawal, proper hemostasis must be maintained and all port sites should be examined for bleeding. To make sure all planned procedures have been completed, surgeons should conduct an appropriate "time out" and ultimately verify the operating count with nurses. Surgical specimens and specimen retrieval bags should be included in the operative count because it is usual for laparoscopic surgeons to leave a specimen or retrieval bag intra-abdominally for subsequent removal. Verify that all intended procedures were completed and that all materials used inside the abdomen, including specimens and bags used for laparoscopic retrieval, were included in the operating count. Avoid placing drains in ports that are 10–15 mm in diameter [35, 36].

Surgeons ought to think about sealing off all internal flaws and 15 mm port locations. However, some research has found that non-bladed laparoscopic trocars are a safe method that can view dissection through layers of the abdominal wall to make the tiniest port dissection without causing bleeding or severing muscle fibers. The surgeon can avoid closing the 10–12 mm fascial defect by splitting the muscles of the abdominal wall. Others advise closing the 10–12 mm port sites, unless the patient is extremely obese or the ports (blunt trocar) were slanted during implantation [37].

Effective communication among the members of the surgical team is vital. This includes clear communication about the patient's condition, the procedure, and any potential complications that may arise during the surgery. Team briefings and debriefings can help in identifying any issues that may impact patient safety [38, 39].

Postoperative Moment

We advise the surgeon to take a moment at the end of the procedure to think back on it. Specifically, they should consider whether all planned procedures were completed, all foreign bodies, including tonsil swabs, retrieval bags, and previously placed foreign bodies, like gastric bands and specimens, were removed, and all ports that needed to be closed were closed [40].

Venous thromboembolism (VTE) risk needs to be customized for every patient and circumstance. When polytraumatized patients have limited mobility, mechanical thromboprophylaxis (TPX) following trauma surgery may not be feasible, and pharmaceutical TPX should not be used in cases of moderate to severe bleeding [40].

Pharmacological TPX should be initiated within 48 h of the solid organ injury (SOI), with blunt SOI receiving non-operative treatment, provided there is no ongoing bleeding or other contraindications. The indication of TPX for piercing solid organs or other polytrauma involving hemorrhage management needs to be evaluated daily [41, 42].

Conclusion

Despite its numerous advantages, laparoscopy in trauma care presents distinct challenges, primarily due to the severity of injuries and the confidence to use minimally invasive approaches. Comprehensive knowledge of potential complications and the implementation of appropriate prophylactic measures and early identification are crucial to minimizing risks and improving clinical outcomes. With adequate training and meticulous patient management, laparoscopy will remain an invaluable tool in the care of polytrauma patients.

References

1. Kindel T, Latchana N, Swaroop M, Chaudhry UI, Noria SF, Choron RL, et al. Laparoscopy in trauma: an overview of complications and related topics. Int J Crit Ill Injury Sci. 2015;5(3):196. https://doi.org/10.4103/2229-5151.165004.
2. Zantut LF, Ivatury RR, Smith RS, Kawahara NT, Porter JM, Fry WR, et al. Diagnostic and therapeutic laparoscopy for penetrating abdominal trauma. J Trauma. 1997;42(5):825–31. Ovid Technologies (Wolters Kluwer Health). https://doi.org/10.1097/00005373-199705000-00012.
3. Sosa JL, et al. Laparoscopy in 121 consecutive patients with abdominal gunshot wounds. J Trauma. 1995:501–6. Ovid Technologies (Wolters Kluwer Health). https://doi.org/10.1097/00005373-199509000-00017.
4. Wenham TN, Graham D. Venous gas embolism: an unusual complication of laparoscopic cholecystectomy. J Minim Access Surg. 2009;5(2):35. https://doi.org/10.4103/0972-9941.55105.
5. Hanly EJ, Aurora AR, Fuentes JM, Shih SP, Marohn MR, De Maio A, Talamini MA. Abdominal insufflation with CO2 causes peritoneal acidosis independent of systemic pH. J Gastrointest Surg 2005;9(9):1245–51; discussion 1251–2.
6. Kwak HJ, Jo YY, Lee KC, Kim YB, Shinn HK, Kim JY. Acid–base alterations during laparoscopic abdominal surgery: a comparison with laparotomy. Br J Anaesth. 2010;105(4):442–7.
7. Yan M, Lou X, Chen Y, Yu Y, Fei X. Effect of duration of carbon dioxide pneumoperitoneum on coagulation, fibrinolysis and endothelial activation in elderly patients. Chin J Geriatr. 2011;12:365–8.
8. Donmez T, Uzman S, Yildirim D, Hut A, Avaroglu HI, Erdem DA, Cekic E, Erozgen F. Is there any effect of pneumoperitoneum pressure on coagulation and fibrinolysis during laparoscopic cholecystectomy? PeerJ. 2016;4:e2375.
9. Ahmad G, O'Flynn H, Duffy JM, Phillips K, Watson A. Laparoscopic entry techniques. Cochr Datab Syst Rev. 2012. John Wiley & Sons, Ltd. https://doi.org/10.1002/14651858.cd006583.pub3.
10. Hashizume M, Sugimachi K. Needle and trocar injury during laparoscopic surgery in Japan. Surg Endosc. 1997;11:1198–201. https://doi.org/10.1007/s004649900568.
11. Bhoyrul S, Vierra MA, Nezhat CR, Krummel TM, Way LW. Trocar injuries in laparoscopic surgery. J Am Coll Surg. 2001;192:677–83. https://doi.org/10.1016/s1072-7515(01)00913-9.
12. Campos FGCM, Roll S. Complicações do acesso abdominal e do pneumoperitônio em cirurgia laparoscópica. Causas, prevenção e tratamento. Rev bras vídeo-cir. 2003;1(1):21–8.
13. Munro MG. Laparoscopic access: complications, technologies, and techniques. Curr Opin Obstet Gynecol. 2002;14(4):365–74. https://doi.org/10.1097/00001703-200208000-00002.

14. Den Boer KT, de Jong T, Dankelman J, Gouma DJ. Problems with laparoscopic instruments: opinions of experts. J Laparoendosc Adv Surg Tech. 2001;11(3):149–55. https://doi.org/10.1089/10926420152389297.
15. Nordestgaard AG, Bodily KC, W.Osborne R, Buttorff JD. Major vascular injuries during laparoscopic procedures. Am J Surg. 1995;169(5):543–5. https://doi.org/10.1016/s0002-9610(99)80214-1.
16. Brierley G, Arshad I, Shakir F, Visvathanan D, Arambage K. Vascular injury during laparoscopic gynaecological surgery: a methodological approach for prevention and management. Obstetr Gynaecol. 2020; https://doi.org/10.1111/tog.12664.
17. Anderson PL, Lathrop RA, Webster RJ III. Robot-like dexterity without computers and motors: a review of hand-held laparoscopic instruments with wrist-like tip articulation. Expert Rev Med Devices. 2016;13:661–72.
18. Riojas KE, Anderson PL, Lathrop RA, Herrell SD, Rucker DC, Webster Iii RJ. A hand-held non-robotic surgical tool with a wrist and an elbow. IEEE Trans Biomed Eng. 2019;66:3176–84.
19. Boni L, Benevento A, Rovera F, Dionigi G, Giuseppe MD, Bertoglio C, Dionigi R. Infective complications in laparoscopic surgery. Surg Infect. 2006;7(supplement 2):s–109–11. https://doi.org/10.1089/sur.2006.7.s2-109.
20. Hajibandeh S, Hajibandeh S, Gumber AO, Wong CS. Laparoscopy versus laparotomy for the management of penetrating abdominal trauma: a systematic review and meta-analysis. Int J Surg. 2016;34:127–36. https://doi.org/10.1016/j.ijsu.2016.08.524.
21. Matsevych OY, Koto MZ, Aldous C. Trauma laparoscopy: a prospect of skills training (cohort study). Int J Surg. 2018;55:117–23. https://doi.org/10.1016/j.ijsu.2018.05.033.
22. Targarona EM, Balague C, Knook MM, Trias M. Laparoscopic surgery and surgical infection. Br J Surg. 2000;87(5):536–44. https://doi.org/10.1046/j.1365-2168.2000.01429.x.
23. Koto MZ, Matsevych OY, Aldous C. Diagnostic laparoscopy for trauma: how not to miss injuries. J Laparoendosc Adv Surg Tech. 2018;28(5):506–13. https://doi.org/10.1089/lap.2017.0562.
24. Coccolini F, Sartelli M, Sawyer R, Rasa K, Ceresoli M, Viaggi B, Catena F, Damaskos D, Cicuttin E, Cremonini C, Moore EE, Biffl WL, Coimbra R. Antibiotic prophylaxis in trauma: Global Alliance for Infection in Surgery, Surgical Infection Society Europe, World Surgical Infection Society, American Association for the Surgery of Trauma, and World Society of Emergency Surgery guidelines. J Trauma Acute Care Surg. 2024;96(4):674–82.
25. Kanlerd A, Auksornchart K, Boonyasatid P. Non-operative management for abdominal solid-organ injuries: a literature review. Chin J Traumatol. 2022;25(5):249–56.
26. Farrell MS, Agapian JV, Appelbaum RD, Filiberto DM, Gelbard R, Hoth J, Jawa R, Kirsch J, Kutcher ME, Nohra E, Pathak A, Paul J, Robinson B, Cuschieri J, Stein DM. Surgical and procedural antibiotic prophylaxis in the surgical ICU: an American Association for the Surgery of Trauma Critical Care Committee clinical consensus document. Trauma Surg Acute Care Open. 2024;9:e001305.
27. Goldberg SR, Anand RJ, Como JJ, Dechert T, Dente C, Luchette FA, Ivatury RR, Duane TM. Eastern Association for the Surgery of trauma. Prophylactic antibiotic use in penetrating abdominal trauma: an Eastern Association for the Surgery of Trauma practice management guideline. J Trauma Acute Care Surg. 2012;73(5 Suppl 4):S321–5.
28. Aaron KA, Vaughan J, Gupta R, Ali NE, Beth AH, Moore JM, Ma Y, Ahmad I, Jackler RK, Vaisbuch Y. The risk of ergonomic injury across surgical specialties. PLoS One. 2021;16(2):e0244868.
29. Supe AN, Kulkarni GV, Supe PA. Ergonomics in laparoscopic surgery. J Minim Access Surg. 2010;6(2):31–6. https://doi.org/10.4103/0972-9941.65161.
30. Hanna GB, Shimi SM, Cuschieri A. Optimal port locations for endoscopic intracorporeal knotting. Surg Endosc. 1997;11(5):397–401. https://doi.org/10.1007/s004649900385
31. World Laparoscopic Hospital. Prioritizing ergonomics in laparoscopic surgery: Balancing comfort, efficiency, and precision for optimal surgical outcomes. Available on: https://www.laparoscopyhospital.com/worldlaparoscopyhospital/index.php?pid=293&p=&cat_id=2&search=. Accessed 28 Jan 2025.

32. Yeola (Pate) ME, Gode D, Bora AK. Ergonomics in laparoscopy. Int J Recent Surg Med Sci. 2017;3(2):102–8
33. Srivastava A, Niranjan A. Secrets of safe laparoscopic surgery: Anaesthetic and surgical considerations. J Minim Access Surg. 2010;6(4):91–4.
34. Lawrentschuk N, Fleshner NE, Bolton DM. Laparoscopic lens fogging: a review of etiology and methods to maintain a clear visual field. J Endourol. 2010;24(6):905–13.
35. Song T, Lee DH. A randomized comparison of laparoscopic LEns defogging using Anti-fog solution, waRm saline, and chlorhexidine solution (CLEAR). Surg Endosc. 2020;34(2):940–5.
36. Deerenberg EB, Henriksen NA, Antoniou GA, Antoniou SA, Bramer WM, Fischer JP, Fortelny RH, Gök H, Harris HW, Hope W, Horne CM, Jensen TK, Köckerling F, Kretschmer A, López-Cano M, Malcher F, Shao JM, Slieker JC, de Smet GHJ, Stabilini C, Torkington J, Muysoms FE. Updated guideline for closure of abdominal wall incisions from the European and American Hernia Societies. Br J Surg. 2022;109(12):1239–50.
37. Liu CD, McFadden DW. Laparoscopic port sites do not require fascial closure when nonbladed trocars are used. Am Surg. 2000;66(9):853–4.
38. Morohashi H, Hakamada K, Kanno T, et al. Construction of redundant communications to enhance safety against communication interruptions during robotic remote surgery. Sci Rep. 2023;13:10831.
39. Omar I, Graham Y, Singhal R, Wilson M, Madhok B, Mahawar KK. Identification of common themes from never events data published by NHS England. World J Surg. 2021;45:697–704. https://doi.org/10.1007/s00268-020-05867-7.
40. Rappold JF, Sheppard FR, Carmichael SP II, Cuschieri J, Ley E, Rangel E, Seshadri AJ, Michetti CP. Venous thromboembolism prophylaxis in the trauma intensive care unit: an American Association for the Surgery of Trauma Critical Care Committee Clinical Consensus Document. Trauma Surg Acute Care Open. 2021;6:e000643.
41. Yorkgitis BK, Berndtson AE, Cross A, Kennedy R, Kochuba MP, Tignanelli C, Tominaga GT, Jacobs DG, Marx WH, Ashley DW, Ley EJ, Napolitano L, Costantini TW. American Association for the Surgery of Trauma/American College of Surgeons-Committee on Trauma Clinical Protocol for inpatient venous thromboembolism prophylaxis after trauma. J Trauma Acute Care Surg. 2022;92(3):597–604.
42. Madhok B, Nanayakkara K, Mahawar K. Safety considerations in laparoscopic surgery: a narrative review. World J Gastrointest Endosc. 2022;14(1):1–16.

Laparoscopic Management of Post-traumatic Ventral Hernias

33

Marcelo L. Furtado

Introduction

Ventral hernias following trauma, particularly after blunt abdominal injury or previous abdominal surgery (including damage control laparotomy), represent a complex surgical challenge. Ventral hernias are defects of the abdominal wall that can occur as a sequela of trauma. These may be the result of blunt force injury, penetrating trauma, or iatrogenic factors related to surgical interventions. In the context of trauma, they can present immediately or as delayed complications. Traditional open repair techniques, while effective, are associated with increased morbidity, longer recovery, and higher infection rates. Laparoscopic techniques offer significant advantages in appropriate candidates, including reduced postoperative pain, shorter hospital stays, and lower rates of wound complications. The advent and evolution of minimally invasive techniques, particularly laparoscopy and robotic surgery, have revolutionized the management of these hernias [1, 2].

Minimally invasive surgery, specifically laparoscopic or endoscopic techniques and Robotic surgery, is a viable option for repairing incisional hernias after abdominal trauma, offering advantages like smaller incisions and potentially faster recovery. While open surgery remains a suitable choice for complex or large defects, minimally invasive approaches are increasingly utilized, especially for smaller hernias [3, 4]

This chapter focuses on the indications, preoperative evaluation, surgical technique and outcomes of laparoscopic repair of post-traumatic ventral hernias.

M. L. Furtado (✉)
Fellow of the Brazilian College of Surgeons, General, Bariatric and Digestive Surgery, Brazilian Society of Minimally Invasive and Robotic Surgery—SOBRACIL-SP, São Paulo, Brazil

© The Author(s), under exclusive license to Springer Nature Switzerland AG 2026

M. Cezillo, B. M. Pereira (eds.), *Minimally Invasive Surgery Trauma*,
https://doi.org/10.1007/978-3-032-28971-1_33

Epidemiology and Etiology

Post-traumatic ventral hernias are relatively rare but increasingly recognized due to improved trauma care and patient survival. The mechanisms include:

- *Blunt abdominal trauma* leading to abdominal wall disruption
- *Penetrating injuries* causing fascial defects
- *Postoperative incisional hernias* following emergency laparotomies (damage control surgery)

Abdominal trauma often results in extensive muscle and fascial damage. In open trauma, laparotomy is mandatory, often requiring multi-layer surgery and closure by secondary intention. In blunt trauma, the need for surgery may be delayed or selective, with less initial damage to the abdominal wall.

Risk Factors
Surgical site infection (wound dehiscence)
Prolonged cavity opening (open abdomen/controlled damage)
Enteric fistulas
Early return to physical activity
Malnutrition and obesity
Use of synthetic meshes in a contaminated environment
Multiple laparotomies
Increased intra-abdominal pressure during recovery

Clinical Presentation

Patients may present with:

- Abdominal bulge at the site of previous trauma or incision
- Pain or discomfort, especially during physical activity
- Bowel symptoms (e.g., obstruction) in incarcerated or strangulated hernias

Imaging, particularly *CT scans with Valsalva maneuver*, is invaluable in assessing hernia size, contents, and loss of domain.

Classification of Incisional Hernias

Different grading scores have been proposed to classify ventral hernias, and classifications are important to allow better understanding in operative reports, databases, and trials. The EHS published a comprehensive classification for both primary and incisional hernias that is easy to use and understand [5]. It defines localization of the defect, if it is recurrent or not, and its size, as shown in Table 33.1.

Table 33.1 European Hernia Society classification for incisional abdominal wall hernias

EHS incisional hernia classification			
Midline		Subxiphoidal	M1
		Epigastric	M2
		Umbilical	M3
		Infraumbilical	M4
		Suprapubic	M5
Lateral		Subcostal	L1
		Flank	L2
		Iliac	L3
		Lumbar	L4
Recurrent incisional hernia?		Yes O	No O
Length: cm		Width: cm	
Width cm	W1 <4 cm O	W2 ≥4–10 cm O	W3 ≥10 cm O

Besides the EHS classification, Rosen et al. proposed a grading score based on the likelihood of SSI (Surgical Site Infection) occurrence [6]. It is based on the CDC wound classification, but proposes a three-grade score only, with grade 1 cases without any risk factor, grade 2 patients with comorbidity, and grade 3 contaminated cases.

Indications for Laparoscopic Repair

- Symptomatic hernias
- Reducible defects without extensive adhesion or contamination
- Stable patients with completed trauma recovery
- Absence of active infection or enterocutaneous fistula

Contraindications may include:

- Extensive intra-abdominal adhesions
- Active infection or contamination
- Severe cardiopulmonary comorbidities

Conservative Management

The low risk of developing complications of a ventral hernia, such as strangulation and/or intestinal obstruction, has strengthened nonoperative treatment in asymptomatic patients. Assessment of comorbidities and postoperative risks is key in this decision process. Bellows et al. observed a small cohort of patients over a period of 24 months, and there was no effect on quality of life and only one episode of incarceration during this time period [7]. A prospective cohort of 636 patients (295 with incisional hernia and 341 with umbilical/epigastric hernia) showed that active surveillance is a safe strategy in anterior abdominal wall hernias [8].

Preoperative Evaluation

- *History and Physical Examination*
- Focus on previous trauma, surgeries, comorbidities, and hernia symptoms.
- *Imaging*
- Contrast-enhanced CT to assess defect size, contents, and abdominal wall status.
- Rule out active intra-abdominal pathology.
- *Optimization*
- Smoking cessation, glycemic control, weight management.
- Nutritional assessment and optimization.

Preoperative Evaluation

In general, if a patient is a medically appropriate candidate for open hernioplasty, then he or she could be considered a candidate for the laparoscopic approach. Patients that have significant cardiac decompensation may experience physiological abnormalities during the procedure because of the insufflation and resulting decrease in venous return. Lower insufflation pressures may decrease the hemodynamic fluctuations [9]. Preoperative preparation of the patient is important because postoperative complications are predictors of recurrence [10].

Generally, almost all hernias are candidates for the LIVH. Even the smaller hernias in obese individuals could be repaired with this technique. Recurrence rates have been shown to be higher in obese patients [11, 12]. Yet the benefits of less wound complications and the ability to identify the occult defects that are missed during an open approach make LIVH a viable option for obese patients. One may opt to use the open approach in a thin patient if it is apparent that the defect is 3 cm or less [13]. Some even recommend the avoidance of hernia surgery at all if the body mass index is greater than 50 [13]. The laparoscopic method, however, is preferred in this group of patients [14].

A very large fascial defect that nearly encompasses the entire anterior abdominal wall may pose a difficult problem. A laparoscopic approach, however, may be feasible. The decision to attempt the laparoscopic method should be based upon the experience of the surgeon, the number of prior operative procedures, mesh repairs, the type of prosthetic utilized in any previous repair(s), and the location of the potential hernia sites. In those patients with very large defects, a reasonable option would be to commence the operation laparoscopically and convert to an open repair if that appears to be the best alternative. More often than not, this proves to be unnecessary. A probable exception to this sequence are those individuals that exhibit a "loss of domain" of the abdominal contents. In these patients, it is usually impossible to actually enter the abdomen behind the abdominal wall musculature because this musculature has been displaced so far laterally (Fig. 33.1). In these cases, conversion to the open method would occur earlier rather than later. More commonly, however, prudence dictates that the entire procedure should be of the open type rather than even attempting the laparoscopic approach.

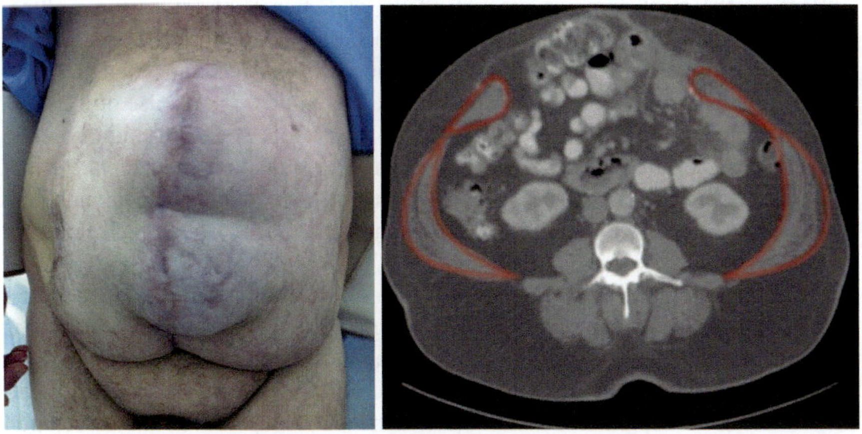

Fig. 33.1 Significant separation of the rectus abdominis in a patient with incisional hernia after laparotomy and colostomy due to abdominal trauma caused by a firearm

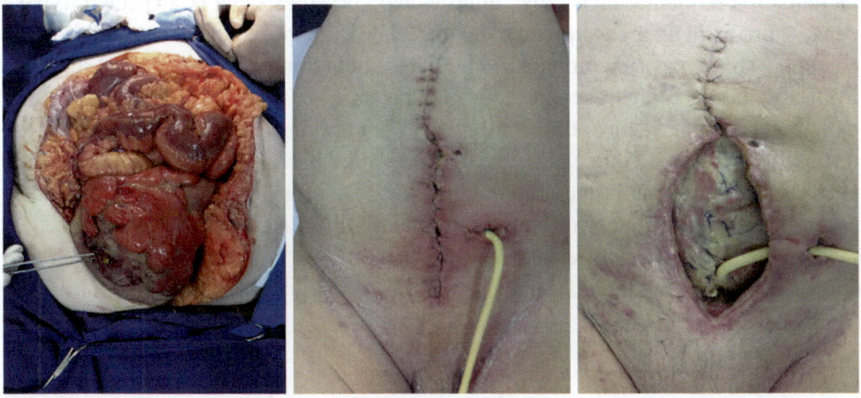

Fig. 33.2 Intra-abdominal and abdominal wall infection (surgical site) in a patient who suffered blunt abdominal trauma with perforation of the cecum and bladder

Absolute contraindications to the use of the laparoscopic method would be the presence of an acute surgical abdomen. A relative contraindication is intra-abdominal or abdominal wall (surgical site) infection from any source (Fig. 33.2). The use of a prosthetic biomaterial in the site of an overt infection may preclude the use of such a product. However, primary closure of the hernia defect with the assistance of a laparoscopic suture passer and biologic mesh [15] may have a role in such instances though an open repair may be indicated for gross contamination. There is data to support the use of mesh in contaminated fields, however [16]. Similarly, while the presence of incarcerated bowel does not prevent the performance of the procedure, strangulation of the bowel necessitates an open hernioplasty.

Because the most common incision of the abdomen is placed in the midline, most incisional hernias (approximately 90%) occur in the midline. When a surgeon begins to perform laparoscopic incisional hernioplasty, it is recommended that he or she should repair midline defects initially to gain confidence in the use of the laparoscopic technique. Once this is accomplished, the presence of a non-midline defect or multiple defects that are not adjacent to each other should not preclude the use of laparoscopy (Fig. 33.3). Appropriate positioning of the patient and accurate placement of the trocars will permit an approach to the entire abdominal cavity in most cases.

Previous intra-abdominal surgery is a major consideration in the evaluation of a patient for the laparoscopic procedure. The number and type of earlier operations will influence the choice of patient position, the method of abdominal entry, trocar placement, and the position of the monitors. This preoperative assessment will allow the surgeon to plan the operative procedure and the operative suite based upon these findings. Any previous open laparotomies will, of course, be associated with more potential for adhesion formation than procedures that were performed laparoscopically. Additionally, those patients in whom a previous incisional hernia repair included the implantation of any "unprotected" prosthesis can be expected to have dense scarring in all areas in which the material was exposed to the intra-abdominal contents. This is very uncommon today. This should not deter experienced surgeons from attempting a laparoscopic approach because as many as one-third of these patients will not have any adhesions at all. It is important to note, however, that the difficulty of the procedure can be greatly magnified because of the dissection of the tenacious scarring that is encountered involving the prosthesis and the bowel and/or omentum. The risk of enterotomy is significantly increased in such instances.

Patients in whom there is an additional need for a surgical procedure such as a cholecystectomy, fundoplication of the stomach, inguinal herniorrhaphy, or biopsy

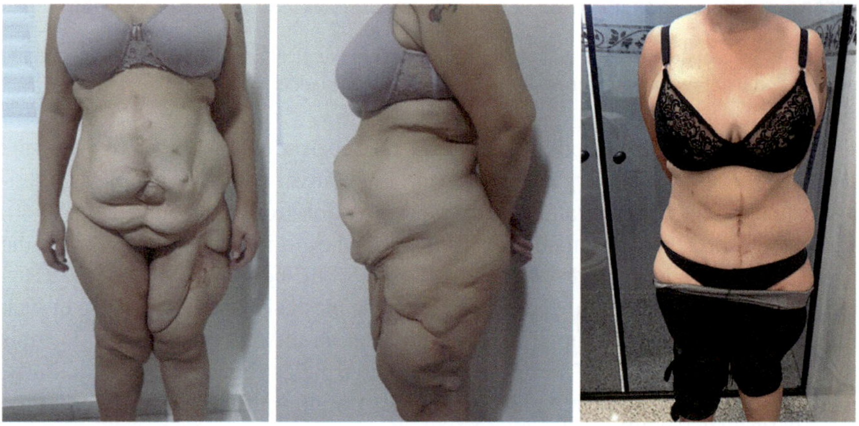

Fig. 33.3 Patient with multiple automobile trauma presenting with multiple abdominal and left flank hernias after laparotomy and nephrectomy

of an intra abdominal or retroperitoneal structure are special subsets that deserve careful consideration.

Laparoscopic incisional hernioplasty should be individualized in patients with known ascites because it may be challenging to maintain a watertight closure that averts ascitic fluid leakage postoperatively. Moreover, these patients usually have a metabolic problem (e.g., chronic renal failure or hepatic disease) that can cause poor healing and predispose them to development of a hernia at the trocar sites. The use of the 5 mm trocars, however, has made this less problematic, and these patients may also be considered on occasion. Special trocars that do not cut into the abdominal muscle but dilate the tissues to enter through the wall of the abdomen should be used in these patients. The site of entry will be smaller than the actual trocar itself after it is removed, thereby further minimizing the risk of leakage of ascitic fluid or subsequent herniation. Though the use of a prosthesis in patients with overt ascites is scarcely reported, some have achieved success with the LIVH in these patients with maximal optimization of ascites [17, 18].

LIVH patients are admitted to the day surgery unit of the hospital because they can usually be considered for discharge on the day of surgery. The number and type of comorbid conditions of the patient, the type and location of the hernia(s), the presence of incarceration, and the amount of adhesiolysis required will influence the decision of timing of discharge from the hospital. Many patients now undergo laparoscopic or robotic incisional hernia repair surgery in an ambulatory surgery center. Appropriate laboratory testing should be obtained prior to entry on the day of surgery. Patients are routinely given a preoperative dose of either a first-generation cephalosporin or a fluoroquinolone. If a patient has a history of methicillin-resistant *Staphylococcus aureus* (MRSA), vancomycin is used for preoperative prophylaxis. If there has been a prior mesh infection, it is preferable to delay surgery for 6 months, if possible, and give the antibiotic used to treat the prior mesh infection preoperatively.

Standardized preoperative workup for all hernia patients is imperative, regardless of hernia location. This begins with a detailed history, physical examination, and biochemical studies to assess the patient's baseline health. Defect number and size, prior or current wound infections, presence of an ostomy, excess skin, and contour abnormalities are part of the physical exam and critical in the selection of the proper operative approach for hernia patients.

Special effort and attention should be made to review prior medical and surgical records in order to gain a thorough understanding of patients' prior interventions and their anatomy and the presence of any mesh or fixation devices in the case of patients presenting with recurrent hernia disease. To further supplement your understanding and preparation, we recommend all patients undergo an up-to-date computed tomography study of their abdomen and pelvis for preoperative planning.

Any patient with a large panniculus, excess, thinned, or ulcerated skin may benefit from open repair with concomitant panniculectomy (Fig. 33.4). Additionally, patients with active infection should be treated with properly selected antimicrobial therapy with resolution of their infection before implantation of synthetic mesh compounds.

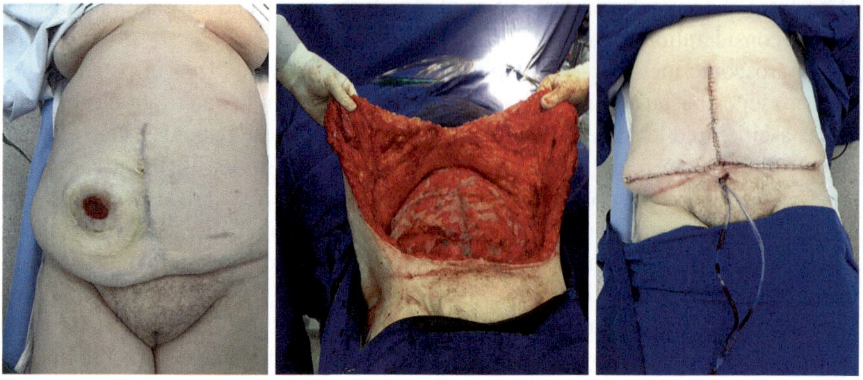

Fig. 33.4 Bowel transit reconstruction + incisional hernia repair + panniculectomy after blunt abdominal trauma with cecum explosion

Flank hernias should also be considered for defect closure and proper mesh overlap. Parastomal hernias may be repaired utilizing a modified Sugarbaker technique. Subxiphoid defects pose a significant challenge with regard to defect closure due to their proximity to the costal margin and fascial resistance to reapproximation. Finally, suprapubic hernias require a detailed understanding of the myopectineal orifice anatomy.

Regardless of hernia location, a multidisciplinary approach should be utilized to optimize patients for surgical intervention.

The preoperative condition of the patient can strongly impact the surgical outcomes in ventral repairs. Several risk factors should be analyzed and pre-optimization is a key step for best results. The modifiable risk factors should be addressed.

Obesity

Obesity is the number one patient-modifiable risk factor predictive of SSI [19]. There is no magical cutoff BMI. Some groups do not perform elective ventral repairs in patients over a BMI of 35; others are more liberal and have a BMI of 40 as a cutoff. The International Endohernia Society guidelines for the treatment of ventral hernias point out that a BMI over 30 brings increased risk of bigger defects and recurrence [3]. A strategy to lose weight should be implemented in the preoperative period for elective incisional hernias. Self-diets and exercises have very high failure rates. A medical weight loss specialist should be consulted, but good results usually happen only in very motivated patients. Bariatric surgery is an option, and a sleeve gastrectomy is the procedure of choice, once the traditional gastric bypass requires small bowel mobilization, which requires hernia content mobilization. The hernia defect and content management are very critical during the bariatric surgery. If possible, the content and defect should not be touched. If content mobilization is necessary, the defect left open can lead to small bowel obstruction. Primary closure of the defect prevents this complication, but when it is not feasible, an omental patch can be sutured to the edges of the defect to avoid new bowel incarceration. The definitive hernia repair should be done once the weight loss is stable, usually after 6 months.

Diabetic Control

Hyperglycemia adversely affects wound healing through multiple mechanisms. These include collagen glycosylation, which impairs collagen degradation and remodeling and results in reduced scar strength, as well as decreased granulation tissue formation, reduced dermal fibroblast activity, and impaired leukocyte function, including chemotaxis, oxidative burst, and phagocytosis. The level of hemoglobin A1c correlates to SSI. HA1c higher than 8 is correlated to a twofold incidence of an SSI in cardiothoracic surgery [20]. A strict preoperative control of DM and glucose/HA1c levels should be implemented.

Smoking

Tobacco is still a huge world business with a global market over US$ 700 billion, and yearly growth around 4%, with over 5 trillion cigarettes produced per year. Smoking results in abnormal wound healing, reduced neutrophil blood count, alteration in collagen metabolism, and reduced levels of vitamin C [21]. Tobacco use is a significant independent predictor of wound infection in ventral repair [22]. Abstinence partially reverses the effects and should be requested for at least 4–6 weeks prior to surgery. A nicotine blood test should be done in the week before the surgery to prove abstinence.

Prevention of Infection

MRSA (methicillin-resistant Staphylococcus aureus) decolonization with intranasal mupirocin and chlorhexidine bathing has been shown to reduce the incidence of S. aureus surgical site infections (SSIs). Universal decolonization may be performed instead of screening-based protocols, as it appears to be more cost-effective [23]. Although no randomized trial has directly compared antibiotic prophylaxis with no prophylaxis in prosthetic incisional hernia repair, most surgeons consider preoperative systemic antibiotic administration to be standard practice. Furthermore, the addition of a second antibiotic dose has been associated with a significant reduction in wound infections, even in clean surgical procedures without contamination [24]. In patients with additional risk factors, such as diabetes, obesity, or a previous surgical site infection, antibiotic prophylaxis should be strongly considered.

Nutrition

The preoperative nutritional status is very important for any major operation, and the ventral repairs should not be different. Preoperative albumin is the single best predictor of overall procedure risk [25]. Besides adequate nutrition, arginine supplementation seems to decrease overall infection rates and hospital stay in elective surgery and can be given for 5–7 days before the surgery [26].

Loss of Domain

The definition of loss of domain has been very subjective, and no reliable criterion has been published. In huge and obvious cases, it is not difficult to make the diagnosis, but in some smaller cases, it may not be that easy. The volume calculation of the hernial sac and the abdominal cavity by CT scan can give a ratio between these two variables that, when it reaches over 25%, gives the diagnosis of loss of domain as described by Tanaka et al. [27] (Fig. 33.5).

Pneumoperitoneum as an Aid in Surgical Treatment of Giant Hernias

Management of giant incisional hernia is often compromised by obesity, intrahernial adhesions, and contraction in the volume of the abdominal cavity—the hernial contents have lost their "right of domain." The use of pneumoperitoneum before

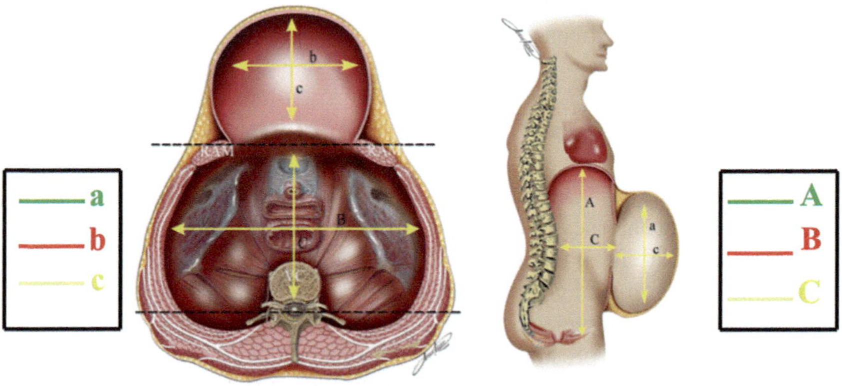

Volume saco herniário(VSH) ≈ a x b x c x 0,52
Volume cavidade abdominal (VCA) ≈ A x B x C x 0,52

Relação de Volumes (RV)=VSH/VCA

Fig. 33.5 Tanaka et al. [27]

attempting definitive repair of giant hernias was originally suggested by Moreno in 1940 [28]. The advantages of the technique are:

- Stretching of the abdominal wall, creating a larger cavity into which the hernial contents can be replaced.
- Reduction of edema in the mesentery, omentum, and viscera in the hernial sac, creating less mass to be reduced.
- Stretching of the hernial sac leading to elongation of adhesions, making dissection and reduction easier [29].
- Increased tone of the diaphragm, allowing preoperative respiratory and circulatory adaptation to the elevation of the diaphragm [30].

The technique has evolved during the last decades, and recently a simpler technique using a double-lumen intra-abdominal catheter inserted through a Veress needle in the left hypochondrium has been popularized [31]. Daily insufflations of ambient air are utilized over a period or an average of 9.3 days. A total of between 1000 and 4000 cc of air is insufflated, depending on patient comfort. The maximum intra-abdominal pressure reached should be no greater than 15 mm of mercury (measured by sphygmomanometer). Successful hernia repair is subsequently possible in most patients.

In practice, the patient is ready for operation at about 2 weeks after induction of the pneumoperitoneum, the end point being judged by the tension of the abdominal wall, which should feel as tight as a drum, especially in the flanks. The patient should be operated on at this stage—if possible, most of the dissection should be performed with the hernial sac unpunctured and distended. When this dissection has been completed, puncture of the sac allows easy reduction of contents, and the slack parietes will facilitate repair. Air is only slowly absorbed from the peritoneal cavity, and often after the first 2 or 3 days, absorption is so reduced as to become inconsequential.

Contraindications to pneumoperitoneum include abdominal wall sepsis, prior cardiorespiratory decompensation, and suspected strangulation of hernial contents. Complications, which are very rare, include visceral puncture, hematoma, and the risk of an embolism into a solid organ if the liver or spleen is needled prior to insufflation. Mediastinal and retroperitoneal surgical emphysemas are rare complications. Prophylactic anticoagulation for DVT and respiratory physiotherapy are key to avoid complications and should be routine.

Botulinum Toxin Injection

Ibarra et al. had shown that botulinum toxin injections are a potential preoperative means to counteract abdominal wall tension, reduce hernia size, and facilitate fascial closure during the definitive procedure [32]. A recent meta-analysis showed a significant hernia width reduction (almost 6 cm) and an increase in lateral abdominal wall muscle lengthening (more than 3 cm), showing a potential use especially in complex ventral hernia management [33]. These excellent results were corroborated by other systematic reviews demonstrating excellent results with the use of botulinum toxin in abdominal wall defects [34].

Surgical Technique

The optimal management of ventral abdominal wall hernias has undergone significant transformation over the last several decades.

The first laparoscopic ventral and incisional hernia repairs (LVIHR) were performed by LeBlanc and Booth in 1993 [36]. They introduced a safe, feasible, and reproducible minimally invasive approach that later became referred to as intraperitoneal onlay mesh placement (IPOM) repair (Fig. 33.6). The procedure consists of reducing the hernia contents and patching the abdominal wall defect with an overlapping nonabsorbable synthetic mesh, which is tacked to the abdominal wall. In LeBlanc's original technique, the tacks were metallic. Their experience in the first 100 patients led to reinforcement of the tacked mesh with additional penetrating transfascial mesh-fixing sutures, which decreased their hernia recurrence rate from 9 to 4% in the next 100 patients [37]. This repair has withstood the test of time for over two decades with low recurrence rates and wound morbidities. However, debate continues among surgeons regarding the benefits of defect closure versus a bridged repair [35].

In recent years, the fascial closure technique with IPOM reinforcement in LVIHR, referred to as IPOM-Plus (Fig. 33.7), has progressively gained support and appeared in the guidelines for the laparoscopic treatment of ventral and incisional abdominal wall hernias published by the International Endohernia Society (IEHS) in 2014 [3]. In addition, the Society of American Gastrointestinal and Endoscopic Surgeons (SAGES) newest guidelines endorse closure of fascial defect when possible [38]. Despite this change, modern ventral hernia repair techniques remain founded on the principles and techniques used by Rives and Stoppa [39].

Their concept of placing synthetic mesh in the retrorectus position revolutionized the field of hernia surgery (Fig. 33.8). Furthermore, the component separation

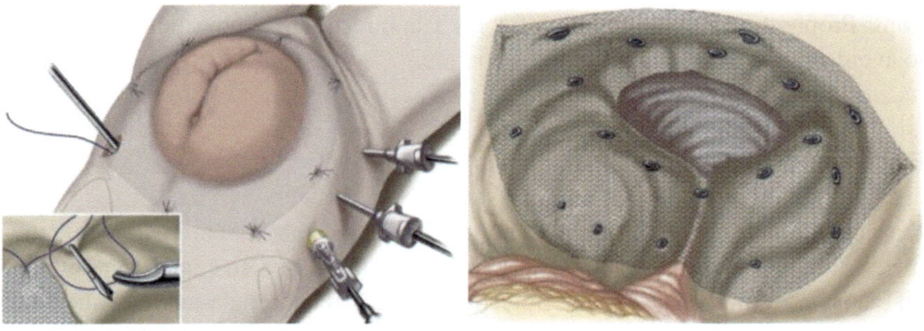

Fig. 33.6 IPOM technique: LeBlanc and Booth [36].

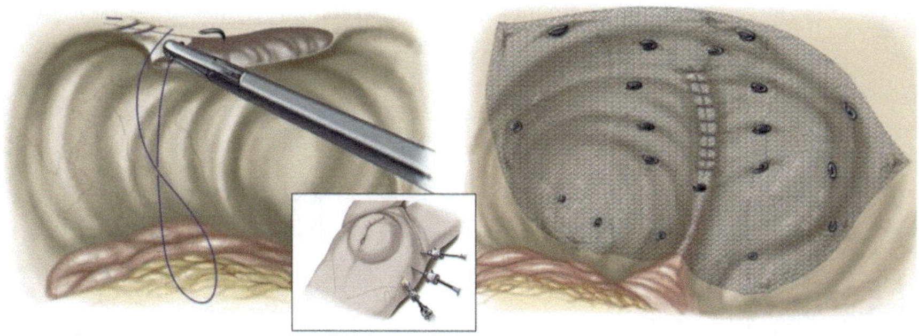

Fig. 33.7 IPOM PLUS technique: Bittner et al. [3]

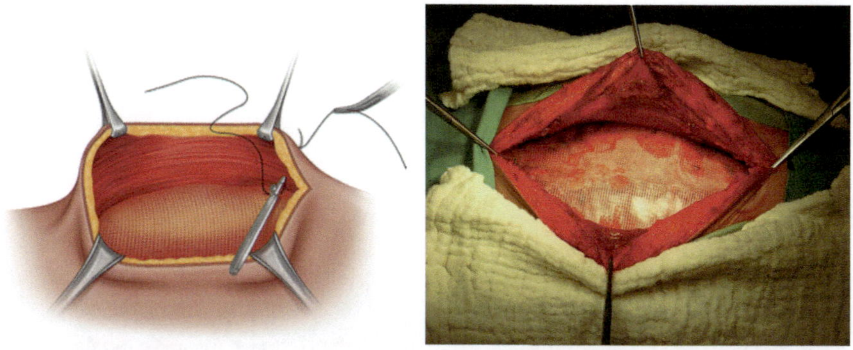

Fig. 33.8 Rives J, et al. Treatment of large eventrations, Rives-Stoppa technique: Published with kind permission of © Yuri Novitsky 2017. All Rights Reserved

techniques (CST) were introduced by Ramirez [40] in 1990, which provided an additional tool for closure of large, complex ventral hernias (Fig. 33.9). Adding to these techniques recently, Novitsky introduced the transversus abdominis release (TAR) as a retromuscular repair, essentially extending the Rives-Stoppa dissection laterally via a posterior component separation [41]. This created a large retromuscular myofascial release and a well-vascularized compartment which is protected from the abdominal viscera. This space allows significant overlap of the defect with synthetic mesh for reinforcement of the repair (Fig. 33.10).

As the field of hernia surgery continues to evolve via technological advancements and increasing use of evidence-based decisions, so will the techniques and platforms that cutting-edge surgeons use today. Since the introduction of robotic surgery, this approach has gained popularity. Surgeons have adapted this approach in a wide array of specialties ranging from cardiac and thoracic surgery to gynecology and urology. The robotic platform was first used to perform a retrorectus Rives-Stoppa hernia repair by Abdalla [42]. Since then, it has become apparent that many of the open techniques can now be performed with robotic assistance while utilizing a minimally invasive approach. This makes robotic ventral hernia repair a great

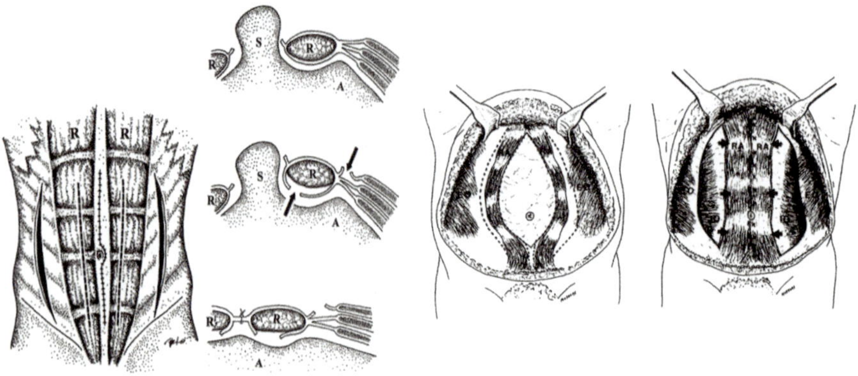

Fig. 33.9 Ramirez et al. [40]

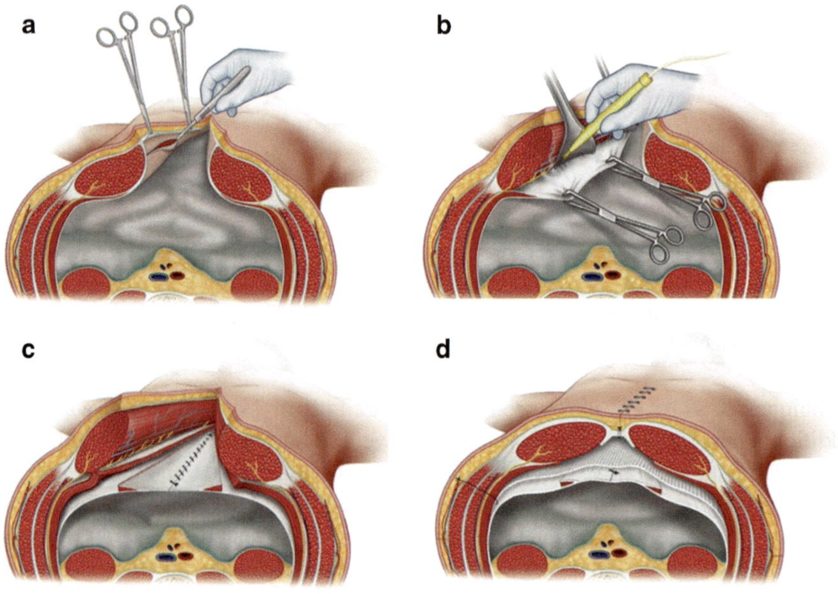

Fig. 33.10 TAR technique: Novitsky et al. [41]

combination of conventional open surgery but with the benefits of minimal access to the abdominal cavity. This statement gained strength after the description of a new method of placing the mesh in the retromuscular space through the lateral access of the rectus abdominis sheath by Novinsky when describing the e-TEP and Re-TEP techniques [41], now widespread throughout the world thanks to the advancement of the robotic platform, especially the Da Vinci Xi™ system where bilateral access is facilitated by the rotation of the axis of the robotic arms.

While there is a paucity of convincing evidence to support the use of robotics in ventral hernia repair, we believe there are several advantages the robot can provide which are not possible through an open or laparoscopic approach. Robotic assistance makes it possible to perform conventional open hernia repair through minimal incisions that would otherwise be very difficult with standard laparoscopy. This affords several advantages including being able to restore abdominal wall anatomy through a minimally invasive approach, limiting the wound burden to the patient, creating a well-vascularized space in which to place mesh with significant overlap of the defect, improving ergonomics and visualization, and avoiding the placement of intraperitoneal mesh. Disadvantages include cost, time, and training staff specifically for robotic surgery. What little evidence does exist seems to favor robotic ventral hernia repair when compared to open with regard to decreased length of stay and lower incidence of wound infections [43, 44].

Laparoscopic Considerations

Creation of a Pneumoperitoneum

Since incisional hernias most commonly result from a previous laparotomy, the surgeon is often faced with the task of opening a re-operative abdomen. The primary objective of this step is to establish pneumoperitoneum and obtain visualization without damaging the viscera. We prefer the conservative approach of an open cutdown. The abdominal layers are incised sequentially with careful identification of the abdominal wall structures. It is prudent to enter the abdomen away from the site of the previous incision. Even when exercising proper caution, bowel injury may be unavoidable.

Another approach to a re-operative abdomen is the Veress needle approach. The Veress needle is a small, spring-loaded needle, which is inserted away from the site of the prior operation, usually in Palmer's point in the left upper quadrant, two-finger breadths under the costal margin in the midclavicular line. Optical trocars offer an opportunity for entry under laparoscopic visualization and have become quite popular in these operations.

Conversion to Open

Conversion of a laparoscopic procedure to open should not be considered a complication but may be a safety measure to obtain better exposure when laparoscopy is deemed inadequate or unsafe by the surgeon. It has been said that conversion is dependent largely on the skill and comfort level of the surgeon to proceed with laparoscopic lysis of adhesions, control of hemorrhage, organ repair, or definitive exposure. As such, conversion rates vary greatly in the literature depending on the study setting, patient selection, and procedure choice. Conversion rate data is important for research purposes and patient counseling in terms of postoperative expectations of laparoscopic versus open procedures and the relative odds of each. In their review of literature, Carlson et al. identified 180 (3.3%) conversions in 5411 operations. The reason for conversion to an open repair was reported in 157 cases, extensive adhesions (48%) and intraoperative complications (29%) being the most common. Whether conversion to an open procedure impacts hernia repair outcomes is impossible to estimate because the predominant factor is likely to be the reason for conversion itself; cases converted from laparoscopic to open, perhaps, should be analyzed separately and not included in the open or laparoscopic category in the surgical outcome research.

Outcomes

Numerous studies have demonstrated that laparoscopic repair of ventral hernias, including those post-trauma, is associated with:

- Lower rates of surgical site infection
- Faster recovery and return to function
- Comparable or reduced recurrence rates vs open repair

Recurrence is more common in high-risk patients (e.g., smokers, obese, large defects) and those with inadequate mesh fixation.

Risk Factors for Recurrence

An important step in minimizing the risk of recurrence is identification of risk factors that may predict recurrence or complications in a particular patient [45, 46]. The defect size, mesh size, operative time, and complications all correlate with each other and together reflect the complexity of a repair but do not appear to increase the risk of recurrence in some series [47–49]. Despite mixed evidence, most surgeons agree that significant risk factors for recurrence include surgical site infections (discussed separately), previous recurrence history, and a complex interplay of mechanical factors such as obesity, hernia size, fixation methods, and mesh material.

In their retrospective review of 146 cases, Bencini et al. found significantly higher recurrence in patients with prior recurrences (67 vs. 16%) and smokers (58 vs. 23%), but the latter was not an independent predictor in their model [50]. In their analysis of 9 recurrences out of 505 laparoscopic repairs, Wassenaar et al. found that 8 of 9 patients had a first-time incisional hernia with no differences in age, sex, ASA score, OR time, mesh size, and hospital stay compared to the rest; seven of nine recurrences had no other postoperative complications. Approximately half of the recurrences had transfascial suture fixation; the others had tacks only [51].

Mesh selection, positioning, and fixation play a significant role in recurrence after laparoscopic hernia repair. The most popular and time-tested technique for intraperitoneal underlay synthetic mesh placement is transfascial suture fixation followed by tacks around the mesh perimeter [52, 53]. Variations of this technique as well as selection of mesh, sutures, and tacks are abundantly described in the literature. Berger and colleagues used sutures to position the mesh but secured it solely with tacks, resulting in a 2.7% (4/147) recurrence at a mean follow-up of 15 months [51]. Several groups reported using no fixation sutures but a "double crown" (two circumferential rows) of tacks [54] resulting in a 4.4% (12/270) recurrence rate at 44 months mean follow-up [55] and 3.5% (7/200) with 22.5 months follow-up. Bageacu et al. reported 15% (19/121) recurrence over a mean follow-up of 49 months and attributed the high recurrence rate to inadequate mesh fixation with metallic tacks alone [56]. In fact, the pull-off strength of suture fixation of the mesh to the abdominal wall is higher compared to the tacks [57]. In open repair, proper technique, including fascial closure, the choice of whether to use mesh, and mesh positioning, also affects recurrence rate. As discussed above, mesh repair significantly reduces the risk of recurrence in ventral and incisional hernias as compared to suture repair [58].

Special Considerations

Hernias After Damage Control Laparotomy

- Often involve large defects and loss of domain.
- May require staged abdominal wall reconstruction.
- Preoperative progressive pneumoperitoneum or Botox may be considered.

Traumatic Flank Hernias

- Rare, often require tailored port placement.
- May need hybrid open-laparoscopic approaches.

Future Directions

- Robotic-assisted approaches are emerging with enhanced dexterity for complex cases.
- Biologic and biosynthetic meshes under evaluation for contaminated fields.
- Long-term outcome studies needed in trauma-specific populations.

Conclusion

Minimally invasive surgery (Laparoscopic and Robotic) repair of post-traumatic ventral hernias is a safe, effective, and increasingly preferred technique in appropriately selected patients and in the hands of surgeons experienced in the treatment of abdominal wall hernias. A meticulous surgical approach, proper patient selection, and thorough preoperative planning are essential to achieving optimal outcomes.

References

1. LeBlanc KA. Laparoscopic incisional and ventral hernia repair: complications—how to avoid and handle. Hernia. 2004;8:323.
2. Novitsky YW, et al. Outcomes of laparoscopic ventral hernia repair in trauma patients. Surg Endosc. 2010;25:1452–7.
3. Bittner R, Bingener Casey J, Dietz U, International Endohernia Society (IEHS), et al. Guidelines for laparoscopic treatment of ventral and incisional abdominal wall hernias (International Endohernia Society [IEHS])-part 1. Surg Endosc. 2014;28:2–29.
4. LeBlanc KA, Kingsnorth A, Sanders DL. Management of Abdominal Wall. Springer Nature Book; 2018.
5. Muysoms FE, Miserez M, Berrevoet F, et al. Classification of primary and incisional abdominal wall hernias. Hernia. 2009;13:407–14.
6. Kanters AE, Krpata DM, Blatnik JA, Novitsky YM, Rosen MJ. Modified hernia grading scale to stratify surgical site occurrence after open ventral hernia repairs. J Am Coll Surg. 2012;15(6):787–93.
7. Bellows CF, Robinson C, Fitzgibbons RJ, Webber LS, Berger DH. Watchful waiting for ventral hernias: a longitudinal study. Am Surg. 2014;80(3):245–52.
8. Kokotovic D, Sjølander H, Gögenur I, Helgstrand F. Watchful waiting as a treatment strategy for patients with a ventral hernia appears to be safe. Hernia. 2016;20(2):281–7.
9. O'Malley C, Cunningham A. Physiologic changes during laparoscopy. Anesthesiol Clin North Am. 2001;19(1):1–19.
10. Mercoli H, Tzedakis S, D'Urso A, Nedelcu M, Memeo R, Meyer N, Vix M, Perretta S, Mutter D. Postoperative complications as an independent risk factor for recurrence after laparoscopic ventral hernia repair: a prospective study of 417 patients with long-term follow-up. Surg Endosc. 2017;31(3):1469–77.
11. Hesselink VJ, Luijendijk RW, de Wilt JH, et al. An evaluation of risk factors in incisional hernia recurrence. Surg Gynecol Obstet. 1993;176(3):228–34.
12. Sauerland S, Korenkov M, Kleinen T, et al. Obesity is a risk factor for recurrence after incisional hernia repair. Hernia. 2004;8:42–6.
13. Liang MK, Holihan JL, Itani K, Alawadi ZM, Gonzalez JR, Askenasy EP, Ballecer C, Chong HS, Goldblatt MI, Greenberg JA, Harvin JA, Keith JN, Martindale RG, Orenstein S, Richmond B, Roth JS, Szotek P, Towfigh S, Tsuda S, Vaziri K, Berger DH. Ventral hernia management: expert consensus guided by systematic review. Ann Surg. 2017;265(1):80–9.
14. Novitsky YW, Cobb WS, Kercher KW, Matthews BD, Sing RF, Heniford BT. Laparoscopic ventral hernia repair in obese patients: a new standard of care. Arch Surg. 2006;141(1):57–61.
15. Franklin M, Gonzalez J, Glass J, et al. Laparoscopic ventral and incisional hernia repair: an 11 year experience. Hernia. 2004;8:23–7.
16. Carbonell AM, Criss CN, Cobb WS, Novitsky YW, Rosen MJ. Outcomes of synthetic mesh in contaminated ventral hernia repairs. J Am Coll Surg. 2013;217(6):991–8.
17. Sarit C, Eliezer A, Mizrahi S. Minimally invasive repair of recurrent strangulated umbilical hernia in cirrhotic patient with refractory ascites. Liver Transpl. 2003;9:621–2.
18. Mekeel K, Mulligan D, Reddy KS, Moss A, Harold K. Laparoscopic incisional hernia repair after liver transplantation. Liver Transpl. 2007;13(11):1576–81.
19. Krpata DM, Blatnik JA, Novitsky YW, Rosen MJ. Evaluation of high-risk, comorbid patients undergoing open ventral hernia repair with synthetic mesh. Surgery. 2013;153(1):120–5.

20. Latham R, Lancaster AD, Covington JF, Pirolo JS, Thomas CS Jr. The association of diabetes and glucose control with surgical-site infections among cardiothoracic surgery patients. Infect Control Hosp Epidemiol. 2001;22(10):607–12.
21. Lorensen LT, Toft BG, Rygaard J, Ladelund S, Paddon M, James T, Taylor R, Gottrup F. Effect of smoking, smoking cessation, and nicotine patch on wound dimension, vitamin C, and systemic markers of collagen metabolism. Surgery. 2010;148(5):982–90.
22. Finan KR, Vick CC, Kiefe CI, Neumayer L, Hawn MT. Predictors of wound infection in ventral hernia repair. Am J Surg. 2005;190(5):676–81.
23. Huang SS, Septimus E, Kleinman K, et al. Targeted versus universal decolonization to prevent ICU infection. N Engl J Med. 2013;368:2255–65.
24. Rios A, Rodriguez JM, Munitz V, Alcaraz P, Perez FD, Parrilla P. Antibiotic prophylaxis in incisional hernia repair using a prosthesis. Hernia. 2001;5:148–52.
25. Khuri SF, Daley J, Henderson W, et al. Risk adjustment of the post- operative mortality rate for the comparative assessment of the quality of surgical care: results of the National Veterans Affairs surgical risk study. J Am Coll Surg. 1997;185(4):315–27.
26. Drover JW, Dhaliwal R, Weitzel L, Wischmeyer PE, Ochoa JB, Heyland DK. Perioperative use of arginine-supplemented diets: a systematic review of the evidence. J Am Coll Surg. 2011;212(3):385–99.
27. Tanaka EY, Yoo JH, Rodrigues AJ Jr, Utiyama EM, Birolini D, Rasslan S. A computerized tomography scan method for calculating the hernia sac and abdominal cavity volume in complex large incisional hernia with loss of domain. Hernia. 2010;14(1):63–9.
28. Moreno IG. Chronic eventuation and large hernias. Surgery. 1947;22:945–53.
29. Hamer DB, Duthie HL. Pneumoperitoneum in the management of abdominal incisional hernia. Br J Surg. 1972;59:372–5.
30. Forrest J. Repair of massive inguinal hernia with pneumo-peritoneum and without mesh replacement. Arch Surg. 1979;114:1087–8.
31. Mayagoitia JC, Suarez D, Arenas JC, Diazdeleon V. Preoperative progressive pneumoperitoneum in patients with abdominal-wall hernias. Hernia. 2006;10:213–7.
32. Barra-Hurtado TR, Nuño-Guzmán CM, Miranda-Díaz AG, Troyo-Sanromán R, Navarro-Ibarra R, Bravo-Cuéllar L. Effect of botulinum toxin type A in lateral abdominal wall muscles thickness and length of patients with midline incisional hernia secondary to open abdomen management. Hernia. 2014;18(5):647–52.
33. Weissler JM, Lanni MA, Tecce MG, Carney MJ, Shubinets V, Fischer JP. Chemical component separation: a systematic review and meta-analysis of botulinum toxin for management of ventral hernia. Plast Surg Hand Surg. 2017:1–9.
34. Alam NN, Narang SK, Pathak S, Daniels IR, Smart NJ. Methods of abdominal wall expansion for repair of incisional hernias: a systematic review. Hernia. 2016;20(2):191–9.
35. Tandon A, Pathak S, Lyons NJ, et al. Meta-analysis of closure of the fascial defect during laparoscopic incisional and ventral hernia repair. Br J Surg. 2016;103:1598–607
36. LeBlanc KA, Booth WV. Laparoscopic repair of incisional abdominal hernias using expanded polytetrafluoroethylene: preliminary findings. Surg Laparosc Endosc. 1993;3:39–41.
37. LeBlanc KA, Whitaker JM, Bellanger DE, et al. Laparoscopic incisional and ventral hernioplasty: lessons learned from 200 patients. Hernia. 2003;7(3):118–24.
38. Earle D, Roth JS, Saber A, SAGES Guidelines Committee, et al. SAGES guidelines for laparoscopic ventral hernia repair. Surg Endosc. 2016;30(8):3163–83.
39. Rives J, et al. Treatment of large eventrations (apropos of 133 cases). Minerva Chir. 1977;32(11):749–56.
40. Ramirez OM, Ruas E, Dellon AL. "Components separation" method for closure of abdominal-wall defects: an anatomic and clinical study. Plast Reconstr Surg. 1990;86(3):519–26.
41. Novitsky YW, et al. Transversus abdominis muscle release: a novel approach to posterior component separation during complex abdominal wall reconstruction. Am J Surg. 2012;204(5):709–16.
42. Abdalla RZ, et al. Modified robot assisted Rives/Stoppa videosurgery for midline ventral hernia repair. Arq Bras Cir Dig. 2012;25(2):129–32.

43. Warren JA, Cobb W, Ewing J, Carbonell AM. Prospective observational cohort study of robotic vs open Rives-Stoppa retrorectus incisional hernia repair. Hernia. 2015;19:S177–86.
44. Warren JA, et al. Standard laparoscopic versus robotic retromuscular ventral hernia repair. Surg Endosc. 2016;31(1):1–9.
45. Burger JW, Luijendijk RW, Hop WC, Halm JA, Verdaasdonk EG, Jeekel J. Long-term follow-up of a randomized controlled trial of suture versus mesh repair of incisional hernia. Ann Surg. 2004;240:578–83. discussion 83–5
46. Koehler RH, Voeller G. Recurrences in laparoscopic incisional hernia repairs: a personal series and review of the literature. JSLS. 1999;3:293–304.
47. Wassenaar EB, Schoenmaeckers EJ, Raymakers JT, Rakic S. Recurrences after laparoscopic repair of ventral and incisional hernia: lessons learned from 505 repairs. Surg Endosc. 2009;23:825–32.
48. Perrone JM, Soper NJ, Eagon JC, et al. Perioperative outcomes and complications of laparoscopic ventral hernia repair. Surgery. 2005;138:708–15. discussion 15–6.
49. Parker HH, Nottingham JM, Bynoe RP, Yost MJ. Laparoscopic repair of large incisional hernias. Am Surg. 2002;68:530–3. discussion 3–4.
50. Bencini L, Sanchez LJ, Bernini M, et al. Predictors of recurrence after laparoscopic ventral hernia repair. Surg Laparosc Endosc Percutan Tech. 2009;19:128–32.
51. Wassenaar E, Schoenmaeckers E, Raymakers J, van der Palen J, Rakic S. Mesh-fixation method and pain and quality of life after laparoscopic ventral or incisional hernia repair: a randomized trial of three fixation techniques. Surg Endosc. 2010;24:1296–302.
52. Heniford BT, Park A, Ramshaw BJ, Voeller G. Laparoscopic repair of ventral hernias: nine years' experience with 850 consecutive hernias. Ann Surg. 2003;238:391–9. discussion 9–400.
53. Asencio F, Aguilo J, Peiro S, et al. Open randomized clinical trial of laparoscopic versus open incisional hernia repair. Surg Endosc. 2009;23:1441–8.
54. Eriksen JR, Poornoroozy P, Jorgensen LN, Jacobsen B, Friis-Andersen HU, Rosenberg J. Pain, quality of life and recovery after laparoscopic ventral hernia repair. Hernia. 2009;13:13–21.
55. Carbajo MA, Martp del Olmo JC, Blanco JI, et al. Laparoscopic approach to incisional hernia. Surg Endosc. 2003;17:118–22.
56. Bageacu S, Blanc P, Breton C, et al. Laparoscopic repair of incisional hernia: a retrospective study of 159 patients. Surg Endosc. 2002;16:345–8.
57. van't Riet M, de Vos van Steenwijk PJ, Kleinrensink GJ, Steyerberg EW, Bonjer HJ. Tensile strength of mesh fixation methods in laparoscopic incisional hernia repair. Surg Endosc. 2002;16:1713–6.
58. den Hartog D, Dur AH, Tuinebreijer WE, Kreis RW. Open surgical procedures for incisional hernias. In: Cochrane Database Syst Rev, vol. 3; 2008. p. CD006438.

Robotic Surgery and Trauma: Future Perspectives

34

Bruno Monteiro Pereira, Andrea Pakula, Rafael L. Curado, and Marcus Cezillo

Introduction

Robot-assisted surgery (RAS) is gradually being adopted and incorporated into the routine surgical practice of multiple specialties, including general surgery, urology, gynecology, spine and orthopedics, neurosurgery and even cardiac surgery. Its applications are expanding rapidly as more institutions are equipped with a robotic platform, and this model of surgery gains more acceptance in the global surgical community.

In 1985, the first use of the RAS is described in literature for a brain biopsy procedure, when the robotic arm provided more precise and stable guidance when compared to the human arm's natural movements. Ten years later, a project from the Stanford Research Institute, financed by DARPA—the Defense Advanced Research Projects Agency, which for 60 years has held to the mission of making pivotal investments in breakthrough technologies for national security—initially focusing on remote surgical intervention for those wounded in war. This gave rise to Intuitive Surgical, which eventually developed the da Vinci surgical systems. This company has the largest number of platforms currently distributed around the world and is the developer of much of the technology available now for this type of surgical technique.

B. M. Pereira (✉)
University of Vassouras, Surgical Group® President, Campinas Brazil. World Society of the Abdominal Compartment Past-President, Campinas, Brazil

A. Pakula
Adventist Health, Simi Valley, CA, USA

R. L. Curado
Grupo Surgical, Campinas, Brazil

M. Cezillo
Trauma Surgery Department, Hospital de Base do Distrito Federal (HBDF), Brasília, DF, Brazil

© The Author(s), under exclusive license to Springer Nature Switzerland AG 2026

M. Cezillo, B. M. Pereira (eds.), *Minimally Invasive Surgery Trauma*,
https://doi.org/10.1007/978-3-032-28971-1_34

Up to now, there are three types of RAS platforms in use: active, semi-active and master-slave systems. Active systems essentially function autonomously (remaining under the control of the operating surgeon) and perform pre-programmed tasks. Semi-active systems allow a surgeon-driven element to complement the pre-programmed element of the active robot systems, while master-slave systems are completely dependent on the surgeon's activity. The da Vinci Surgical System was designed as a master-slave robotic platform; it obtained FDA approval for general laparoscopic procedures in 2000 and later became the first operative surgical robot in the World. Since then, RAS has registered increasing growth year after year for multiple surgical procedures, as have commercial competitors and the technologies used in this field [1, 2].

Through the application of 3D visualization, 4 to 8 K definition, optimal ergonomic positioning, and precise instrument manipulation, this documented expanded interest of surgical community has also been observed in acute surgical critical care, including trauma. However, RAS is not yet widely used for emergency general surgery due to multiple reasons, but it is becoming more prevalent and is being associated with better results, reduced conversion to open surgery, and decreased length of stay, which undoubtedly guarantees the stimulus for new research and improvement of technique and docking in the field of emergency surgery [3].

As emergency surgery and trauma surgery go hand in hand as a specialty in most health services around the world, new training programs involving robotic surgery and acute care surgery appear, corroborating a trend with no return [4–6]. Although there is much more evidence out there regarding non-trauma acute care cases, RAS for trauma is feasible as this is another modality for minimally invasive surgery (MIS). Robotic surgery represents an evolution of the laparoscopy; therefore offers all the advantages of an MIS approach already established for trauma.

Why Use RAS in Trauma

RAS was created to overcome the difficulties and ameliorate the disadvantages of conventional laparoscopy, offering a three-dimensional stereoscopic vision, a 10× magnification, much greater precision with tremor control, range of motion, surgeon camera control, and an ergonomically efficient position for the surgeon. Additionally, robotic surgery appears to have a shorter learning curve than laparoscopy for certain procedures. A robotic approach may allow overcoming some technical difficulties encountered in trauma laparoscopy that would often lead to conversion to open surgery, and this will ultimately lead to lower morbidity rates and reduced hospital stays, making the application of robotics in emergencies, such as trauma, highly interesting (Table 34.1).

Viewing exposure can be improved with RAS due to greater illumination, magnification (which, along with motion scaling, can improve vision and accuracy), better viewing angles, and immersive vision. Optimal surgical lighting provides sufficient ambient light with the ability to focus on the surgeon's operative field even at difficult angles such as the pelvis, without shadow, glare, and artifact

Table 34.1 Main comparison points between laparoscopy and robotic-assisted surgery

	Laparoscopy	RAS
View	Monocular 2D	Binocular 3D
Camera Control	Assistant	Surgeon
Peripheral vision	No	Yes
Depth perceptions	–	+
Ergonomics	No	Yes
Movements amplitude	Limited	Wider
Tremor filtering	–	+

production. The modern robotic console can provide a better stereopsis experience for surgeons compared to traditional 3D images created by shuttering or polarizing imaging. The da Vinci robotic system uses two separate optical trains with two independent three-chip cameras and display systems to present slightly different images to each eye, mimicking binocular vision. The optical system minimizes geometric distortion across the entire field of view, enabling stereo fusion of images even close to the edges [7].

Moreover, RAS brings back camera control to the surgeon on a stable platform, resulting in a more stable view of the operative field with better centering, horizon, and depth adjustment, zoom control, and instrument visualization, promoting altogether an extraordinary surgical field experience [8].

The fact that robotic ergonomics is superior to laparoscopy, the literature has already proven [9]. With the robotic system, the use of clutch control that allows greater movement of the robotic arms from the smaller limits of the surgeon's console makes surgical movements smoother and more delicate. There is less muscular effort when compared to laparoscopy, less effort with the hands, with less tremors and much greater precision and accuracy in the activity of the surgeon's hands, as well as a greater range of rotation of the robotic forceps and arms due to their advanced joints [9].

Since the expiration of patents held by Intuitive Surgical, novel robotic surgical systems have been created and are now gradually becoming available for use. The Versius, Hugo, and Senhance robotic systems provide an open console system that requires the use of 3D polarizing glasses. The open console design may or may not allow for better verbal and non-verbal communication between surgical team members. Ergonomic viewing considerations for the closed da Vinci system would be different for the open console systems but were not directly compared. Viewing advantages of the open console system include improved camera control and less reliance on visual cues for haptic feedback. However, with the recent release of the newest daVinci 5 surgical system, there is a large focus on improved ergonomics as well as force feedback technology, which allows the surgeon to complement learned visual cues with the feeling of forces being applied to tissues. The Senhance surgical system offers the additional advantage of controlling the camera by eye movements through an infrared eye tracking system. Versius and Senhance robotic systems offer haptic feedback from the handles. The visualization disadvantages of the open console system are related to the need to use polarized glasses, as in three-dimensional laparoscopic surgery, and include decreased brightness of the operative field, need for horizontal gauze, less stereopsis, and more visual fatigue [10]. In one way or another, after Intuitive's patent expires, many other robotic systems for surgery are being launched by many different countries such as India, China, and Japan.

Another important WHY that stimulates the use of RAS in acute care surgery and trauma is the near-infrared fluorescence (NIRF). NIRF imaging is a promising tool that is being explored as a method to improve visualization of perfusion during various types of surgery. Fluorescence is the property of certain molecules called fluorochromes (indocyanine green, for instance), capable of emitting fluorescent radiation when excited by a laser beam or exposed to near-infrared light at specific wavelengths. Thus, fluorescence can be detected using specific scopes and cameras.

With the continuous use of NIRF, this technique is now widely used in general surgery, mainly to evaluate esophageal, gastric, hepatic, splanchnic or colorectal perfusion, with the aim of verifying adequate organic blood perfusion as well as newly created anastomoses and ultimately reducing the incidence of anastomotic leaks. The immunofluorescent technology (Fig. 34.1) is also becoming standard during cholecystectomy for the identification of critical biliary structures during both elective and emergency cases. For emergency cases, it is reasonable to realize that all these resources exist to help, as is the case in elective surgical scenarios.

After all technical aspects were mentioned, as an MIS model, RAS will obviously keep the advantages of lower metabolic response to surgical trauma, higher diagnostic accuracy and fewer negative laparotomies, less postoperative pain, lower rate of adhesions, incisional hernias, surgical site infection, and faster recovery.

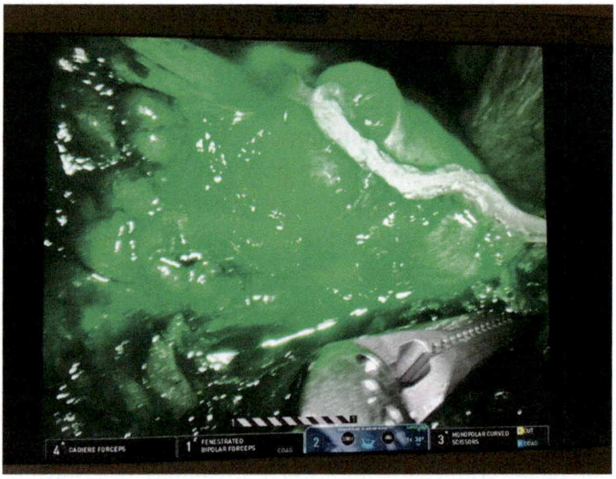

Fig. 34.1 Use of indocyanine green. (Courtesy of Prof. Bruno M Pereira, MD, MSc, PhD)

When Use RAS in Trauma

First, to use RAS in trauma the whole team must be trained in robotics. This includes not only surgeons but also nurses, scrub techs, and anesthesiologists.

Secondly, it is essential to remember that all RAS begins with a laparoscopy. Just before docking, a mandatory step is to observe the inside of the abdomen, for instance, with the endoscope and take any measures that may be necessary, such as releasing abdominal adhesions in this example or adjust optimal organ positioning such as transverse colon. That said, it is reasonable to understand that many laparoscopic indications can also be applied to robotics, but not all. Once the robot is attached, moving the surgical table is prohibitive (a clear disadvantage of the RAS, favoring laparoscopy); however, surgeons can start the procedure with laparoscopy and once the need to use the robot to assist the surgery is identified, the gadget is there and only docking will be necessary.

It is important to remember that trauma-injured patients must be stable to be eligible for a minimally invasive procedure such as laparoscopy or robotics. Hemodynamic instability is an absolute contraindication as are severe traumatic brain injuries and the inability to withstand pneumoperitoneum. However, with the improved visualization and maintenance of camera stability, cases can be performed at much lower insufflation pressures, which aid in the completion of these procedures in patients with or at risk of hemodynamic instability [11].

Table 34.2 summarizes some possible indications for RAS in trauma. Other indications may also apply.

Table 34.2 Possible indications for RAS in trauma

Absolute Indication	Hemodynamic stability
Relative Indications	Lower tracheal and bronchial injuries
	Esophageal injuries
	Diaphragmatic complex injury (penetrating or blunt)
	Stable hepatic or splenic injury with surgical indication
	High-grade pancreatic injuries
	Retroperitoneal injuries
	Hepatic, Splenic or Pancreatic Complications after NOM
	Grade IV renal injuries
	Ureteral injuries
	Intraperitoneal complex bladder rupture
	High-grade rectal injuries
	Complex pelvic trauma with low rectal injuries
	Peritonitis or peritoneal-free air
	Free fluid with no parenchymal injury

Timing of a robotic procedure in trauma patients is an important issue to take into consideration. The timing of a laparoscopy, for example, can be immediate or delayed, as we have done several times to repair a missed injury or improve NOM with laparoscopic blood aspiration and diversion of hepatic or pancreatic fistulas. While the laparoscopic procedure may be necessary upon admission for diagnostic purposes, robotic surgery will certainly not be applicable for this intent. On the other hand, RAS will possibly have an open scope for participation in second-look non-operative treatment or resolution of complex injuries that are also difficult to access, such as mediastinal, retroperitoneal, hepatic, pancreatic, complex bladder, and rectal injuries, overcoming technical difficulties that in laparoscopy could exist.

To date, there is little data on the use of RAS in trauma; however, evidence on emergency surgery is becoming increasingly available and strong new evidence in this segment will certainly emerge soon [12].

How

Robot-assisted surgery (RAS) in acute care surgery fundamentally depends on structured training and effective multidisciplinary teamwork. Acute care surgery academic programs have expanded substantially worldwide, with some centers reporting nearly a 100% increase in activity within a single year [5]. Acute care surgeons perform more than 850,000 procedures annually in the United States alone, highlighting the growing demand for advanced surgical approaches in this field. As increasing numbers of acute care and trauma surgeons become trained in RAS, the global adoption of robotic procedures in emergency settings is expected to rise naturally [4].

The implementation of a successful robotic surgery program requires coordinated administrative planning and close collaboration among multidisciplinary teams to ensure seamless integration into daily clinical practice. Continuous 24/7 support from industry technology specialists may further facilitate the safe and efficient progression of robotic procedures. Importantly, emergency and trauma cases should not interfere with elective surgical schedules. This limitation may restrict the use of RAS in institutions equipped with only a single robotic platform.

Although laparoscopic surgery already faces important limitations in trauma care, RAS introduces additional challenges. In both minimally invasive approaches, hemodynamically unstable patients remain a relative contraindication, depending on the experience and comfort level of the operating surgeon. Nevertheless, both laparoscopy and robotics may be used diagnostically in selected trauma patients. If the patient tolerates insufflation and the injury is amenable to minimally invasive repair, either approach may be considered.

Currently, robotic surgery is most applicable in carefully selected complex scenarios and in the management of surgical complications. Extremely urgent cases that cannot tolerate delays associated with robotic platform availability are generally not suitable candidates for RAS. Therefore, careful operating room organization is essential, and some institutions have successfully incorporated up to two robotic emergency procedures per day into their workflow [5].

Despite being in an early stage of development within emergency and trauma surgery, the use of RAS represents a clear and growing trend. The position paper published by the World Society of Emergency Surgery states that robotic surgery in emergency settings can be considered safe and feasible when performed by appropriately trained surgical teams [13–15]. Preliminary unpublished data also suggest that robotic-assisted surgery may significantly reduce conversion rates to open procedures in several emergency general surgery scenarios [13].

Several barriers may limit the adoption of robotic surgery among trauma surgeons. These surgeons often have fewer elective surgical cases, reduced exposure to advanced minimally invasive procedures, limited experience with complex laparoscopy, and lower robotic surgical volumes. For these reasons, we strongly support the integration of elective general surgery or digestive tract surgery into trauma surgeons' practice to facilitate the development and maintenance of advanced minimally invasive surgical skills [15].

After establishing an acute care robotic surgery program with appropriate training and workflow organization, the next step is optimizing the robotic operating room structure and processes. In our institution, the da Vinci Surgical System is used for RAS. The system is composed of three main components: the vision cart, the patient cart, and the surgeon console, as illustrated in Fig. 34.2.

As mentioned above, minimal personnel trained in robotic surgery are obviously required, including the surgeon and his assistants, anesthesia staff, nurses, scrub nurses, and OR technicians. A dedicated operating room with plenty of space is recommended to accommodate the robotic system and to allow free movement of OR personnel. In addition, it will grant the robot to be fitted from different angles depending on the type of surgery and must be organized in such a way that the surgeon has a clear view of the patient from the console.

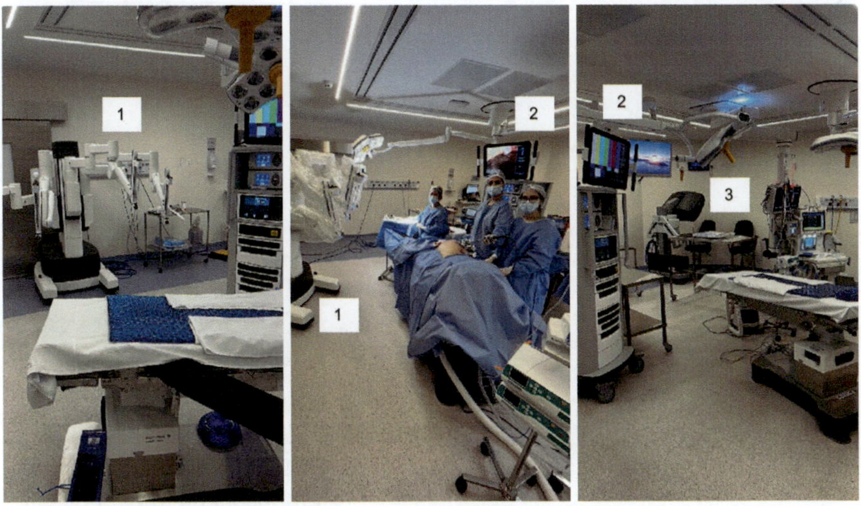

Fig. 34.2 (1) Patient-side Cart (da Vinci X system, Intuitive Surgical Inc.), (2) Vision Cart, (3) Surgeon Console. (Courtesy of Prof. Bruno M Pereira, MD, MSc, PhD)

The next question is how to dock the robot for trauma cases. Well, at first a question that seems difficult turns out to be not. Considering that in most cases the proposed robotic treatment has already been defined, docking is at the discretion of the treatment focus. This does not, of course, prevent multiple dockings from taking place in the same procedure, as already occurs in some elective cases. For cases of abdominal trauma, an in-line or arc-shaped trocar position after docking toward the pelvis or upper abdomen, depending on where to operate, may be the best option. Thoracic, pulmonary, bronchial, mediastinal, and esophageal injuries may require lateralization of the patient (left or right lateral recumbent) or prone position (Fig. 34.3). In the latter cases, it is mandatory to analyze each case to assess whether the patient can support these varied positions after trauma. Care must be taken when performing RAS to protect the patient from contact with the hard parts of the robot with a specific cushion, as exposed in Fig. 34.4.

After all these, surgeons should keep the RAS standard of using monopolar and bipolar energies in the right and left hands respectively, and advanced energies or staplers when necessary.

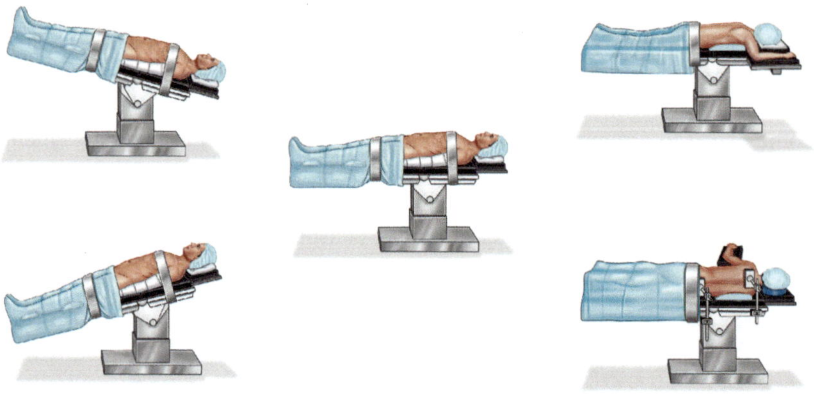

Fig. 34.3 Common OR Bed positions in Trauma RAS [16]

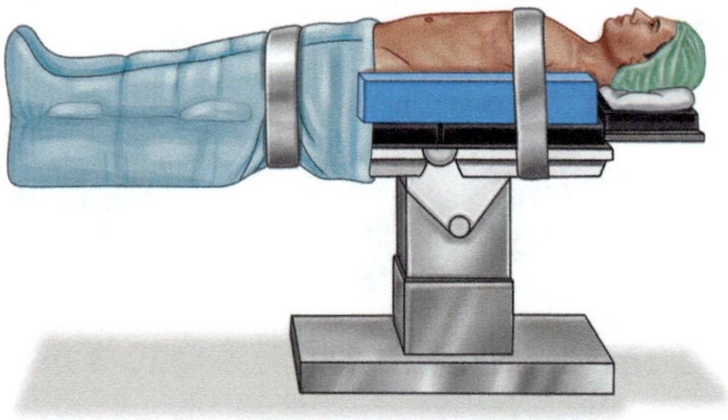

Fig. 34.4 Patient protection from contact with the hard parts of the robot with a specific cushion [16]

Final Commentaries

Although there are already records and even guidelines describing the use of RAS in acute care surgery [15–17], no literature specifically on trauma was found until the conclusion of this chapter. However, the tendency for this to happen seems natural. In cases of Acute Care Surgery, the RAS is already well established, including with highly complex cases, and as more trained teams become available, the easier it will be to use the RAS method in trauma. There are many advantages of robotic surgery in trauma:

1. Improved visualization and improved ergonomics compared to laparoscopy and open surgery.
2. Improved dexterity compared to conventional laparoscopy, which may facilitate some techniques.
3. Facilitated standardization of surgical steps, as performed during elective surgeries.
4. Near-infrared fluorescence imaging.

Currently, for non-trauma cases RAS has performed very well. Reinisch et al. retrospectively evaluated 30 studies with a total of 703 patients submitted to non-trauma acute care surgeries, followed by 9 studies including incarcerated hernias (199 patients). The feasibility of robotic operations has been demonstrated for all indications. No robotics-specific issues or extensive complication rates were reported [18]. Several urgent operations in general surgery can be performed robotically without increased risk, and it looks like trauma will shortly be the same. Robotics can be integrated into your Acute Care Surgery and Trauma practice but requires initial dedication to training and then continued use at the beginning of the learning curve. Cholecystectomy is often the initial case of acute care surgery entry into robotics and can be used to enhance your initial knowledge of basic skills until you level up for trauma complex surgeries [18, 19].

References

1. Kwoh YS, Hou J, Jonckheere EA, Hayati S. A robot with improved absolute positioning accuracy for CT guided stereotactic brain surgery. IEEE Trans Biomed Eng. 1988;35:153–60.
2. Bianchi G, Martínez-Pérez A, de 'Angelis N. Chapter 30: Robotics. In: Textbook of emergency general surgery. Springer; 2023. p. 457–69.
3. Lunardi N, Abou-Zamzam A, Florecki KL, et al. Robotic technology in emergency general surgery cases in the era of minimally invasive surgery. JAMA Surg. 2024;159(5):493–9.
4. Torres CM, Florecki K, Haghshenas J, Manukyan M, Kent A, Lawrence C, Sakran JV. The evolution and development of a robotic acute care surgery program. J Trauma Acute Care Surg. 2023;95(4):e26–30.
5. Gage D, Neilson T, Pino MG, Eiferman D, Knight-Davis J. Establishment of a 24/7 robotic acute care surgery program at a large academic medical center. Surg Endosc. 2024;38(8):4663–9.

6. Haghshenas J, Florecki K, Torres CM, Manukyan M, Kent A, Lawrence C, Sakran JV. Incorporation of a robotic surgery training curriculum in acute care surgical fellowship. J Trauma Acute Care Surg. 2023;95(2):e11–4.
7. Wong SW, Crowe P. Visualisation ergonomics and robotic surgery. J Robot Surg. 2023;17(5):1873–8.
8. Kim JS, Piozzi GN, Kwak JM, Kim J, Kim T, Choo J, Yang G, Lee TH, Baek SJ, Kim J, Kim SH. Quality of laparoscopic camera navigation in robot-assisted versus conventional laparoscopic surgery for rectal cancer: an analysis of surgical videos through a video processing computer software. Int J Med Robot. 2022;18(4):e2393.
9. Wee IJY, Kuo LJ, Ngu JC. A systematic review of the true benefit of robotic surgery: ergonomics. Int J Med Robot. 2020;16(4):e2113.
10. Koukourikis P, Rha KH. Robotic surgical systems in urology: what is currently available? Investig Clin Urol. 2021;62(1):14–22.
11. Andrews BC, Dietrich CS III, Stanley Z, Ali S. Robotic-assisted laparoscopic surgery: lower insufflation pressures reduced the risk of hemodynamic instability. J Minim Invasive Gynecol. 2021;28, 11
12. Ceresoli M, Pisano M, Abu-Zidan F, Allievi N, Gurusamy K, Biffl WL, et al. Minimally invasive surgery in emergency surgery: a WSES survey. World J Emerg Surg. 2022;17(1):18.
13. Custom Hospital Analytics Database (CHA database) 2017–2023.
14. Pakula AM. The application of robotics for the acute care surgeon. SAGES: a view through the scope—past, present, & future. 2019.
15. de'Angelis N, Khan J, Marchegiani F, Bianchi G, Aisoni F, Alberti D, Ansaloni L, Biffl W, Chiara O, Ceccarelli G, Coccolini F, Cicuttin E, D'Hondt M, Di Saverio S, Diana M, De Simone B, Espin-Basany E, Fichtner-Feigl S, Kashuk J, Kouwenhoven E, Leppaniemi A, Beghdadi N, Memeo R, Milone M, Moore E, Peitzmann A, Pessaux P, Pikoulis M, Pisano M, Ris F, Sartelli M, Spinoglio G, Sugrue M, Tan E, Gavriilidis P, Weber D, Kluger Y, Catena F. Robotic surgery in emergency setting: 2021 WSES position paper. World J Emerg Surg. 2022;17(1):4.
16. Lee-Ong A, Buenafe AA. Operating room setup and patient positioning in MIS. In: Lomanto D, Chen WTL, Fuentes MB, editors. Mastering endo-laparoscopic and thoracoscopic surgery. Singapore: Springer; 2023.
17. Milone M, Anoldo P, de'Angelis N, Coccolini F, Khan J, Kluger Y, Sartelli M, Ansaloni L, Morelli L, Zanini N, Vallicelli C, Vigutto G, Moore EE, Biffl W, Catena F, ROEM Collaborative Group. The role of RObotic surgery in EMergency setting (ROEM): protocol for a multicentre, observational, prospective international study on the use of robotic platform in emergency surgery. World J Emerg Surg. 2024;19(1):20.
18. Reinisch A, Liese J, Padberg W, Ulrich F. Robotic operations in urgent general surgery: a systematic review. J Robot Surg. 2023;17(2):275–90.
19. Wu J, Martin MJ, Kirkpatrick V, Cassaro S, Pérez Rodríguez F. The great debate: robotic vs traditional surgical approach in the acute care setting. Am SurgTM. 2024;90(10):2357–61.

Correction to: Minimally Invasive Approaches in Cardiac Injuries

Patrizio Petrone, José A. Pezati Tenani,
Bruno Monteiro Pereira, John McNelis,
and Corrado P. Marini

Correction to:
Chapter 14 in: M. Cezillo, B. M. Pereira (eds.),
Minimally Invasive Surgery Trauma,
https://doi.org/10.1007/978-3-032-28971-1_14

The affiliation of the author John McNelis was inadvertently published wrongly in Chap. 14 and has now been updated in both the chapter and the List of Contributors:

Department of Surgery, Albert Einstein College of Medicine, Jacobi Medical Center, Bronx, NY, USA

The updated version of this chapter can be found at
https://doi.org/10.1007/978-3-032-28971-1_14

© The Author(s), under exclusive license to Springer Nature Switzerland AG 2026

M. Cezillo, B. M. Pereira (eds.), *Minimally Invasive Surgery Trauma*,
https://doi.org/10.1007/978-3-032-28971-1_35

Index

© The Editor(s) (if applicable) and The Author(s), under exclusive license to Springer Nature Switzerland AG 2026

M. Cezillo, B. M. Pereira (eds.), *Minimally Invasive Surgery Trauma*,
https://doi.org/10.1007/978-3-032-28971-1

GPSR Compliance

The European Union's (EU) General Product Safety Regulation (GPSR) is a set of rules that requires consumer products to be safe and our obligations to ensure this.

If you have any concerns about our products, you can contact us on ProductSafety@springernature.com

In case Publisher is established outside the EU, the EU authorized representative is:

Springer Nature Customer Service Center GmbH
Europaplatz 3
69115 Heidelberg, Germany

Batch number: 10726133

Printed by Printforce, the Netherlands